# Bioresorbable Scaffolds

## From Basic Concept to Clinical Applications

# Bioresorbable Scaffolds

## From Basic Concept to Clinical Applications

Edited by

Yoshinobu Onuma

Patrick W.J.C. Serruys

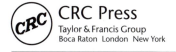

**CRC Press**
Taylor & Francis Group
Boca Raton  London  New York

CRC Press is an imprint of the
Taylor & Francis Group, an **informa** business

CRC Press
Taylor & Francis Group
6000 Broken Sound Parkway NW, Suite 300
Boca Raton, FL 33487-2742

© 2017 by Taylor & Francis Group, LLC
CRC Press is an imprint of Taylor & Francis Group, an Informa business

No claim to original U.S. Government works

Printed and bound in India by Replika Press Pvt. Ltd.

Printed on acid-free paper

International Standard Book Number-13: 978-1-4987-7974-6 (Pack - Hardback and eBook)

This book contains information obtained from authentic and highly regarded sources. While all reasonable efforts have been made to publish reliable data and information, neither the author[s] nor the publisher can accept any legal responsibility or liability for any errors or omissions that may be made. The publishers wish to make clear that any views or opinions expressed in this book by individual editors, authors or contributors are personal to them and do not necessarily reflect the views/opinions of the publishers. The information or guidance contained in this book is intended for use by medical, scientific or health-care professionals and is provided strictly as a supplement to the medical or other professional's own judgement, their knowledge of the patient's medical history, relevant manufacturer's instructions and the appropriate best practice guidelines. Because of the rapid advances in medical science, any information or advice on dosages, procedures or diagnoses should be independently verified. The reader is strongly urged to consult the relevant national drug formulary and the drug companies' and device or material manufacturers' printed instructions, and their websites, before administering or utilizing any of the drugs, devices or materials mentioned in this book. This book does not indicate whether a particular treatment is appropriate or suitable for a particular individual. Ultimately it is the sole responsibility of the medical professional to make his or her own professional judgements, so as to advise and treat patients appropriately. The authors and publishers have also attempted to trace the copyright holders of all material reproduced in this publication and apologize to copyright holders if permission to publish in this form has not been obtained. If any copyright material has not been acknowledged please write and let us know so we may rectify in any future reprint.

**Visit the Taylor & Francis Web site at**
**http://www.taylorandfrancis.com**

**and the CRC Press Web site at**
**http://www.crcpress.com**

# Contents

# Contributors

**Alexandre Abizaid**
Department of Interventional Cardiology
Instituto Dante Pazzanese de Cardiologia
São Paulo, Brazil

**Manuel de Sousa Almeida**
Department of Cardiology
Hospital Santa Cruz
Carnaxide, Portugal

**Rasha Al-Lamee**
International Centre for Circulatory Health
Imperial College London
United Kingdom

**Daniele Andreini**
Centro Cardiologico Monzino
IRCCS
University of Milan
and
Department of Clinical Sciences and Community Health
Cardiovascular Section
University of Milan
Milan, Italy

**Liew Houng Bang**
Clinical Research Centre (CRC)
Department of Cardiology
Queen Elizabeth Hospital 2
Kota Kinabalu, Malaysia

**Peter Barlis**
Melbourne Medical School
Faculty of Medicine
Dentistry and Health Sciences
The University of Melbourne
Melbourne, Australia

**Antonio L. Bartorelli**
Centro Cardiologico Monzino
IRCCS
University of Milan
and
Department of Clinical Sciences and Community Health
Cardiovascular Section
University of Milan
Milan, Italy

**Peter Behrens**
Institute for Biomedical Engineering
University Medicine Rostock
Rostock, Germany

**Susann Beier**
Mercy Angiography
Auckland, New Zealand

**Sanjeev Bhatt**
Meril Life Sciences Pvt. Ltd.
Vapi, Gujarat, India

**Christos V. Bourantas**
Barts Heart Centre
Barts Health NHS Trust
and
Institute of Cardiovascular Sciences University College London
London, United Kingdom

**A.J. Van Boven**
Department of Cardiology
Medical Center Leeuwarden
Leeuwarden, the Netherlands

**Adam J. Brown**
Department of Interventional Cardiology
Papworth Hospital
Cambridge, United Kingdom

**Gianluca Campo**
Cardiovascular Institute
Azienda Ospedaliero-Universitaria S. Anna
Cona, Ferrara, Italy

**Carlos M. Campos**
Department of Interventional Cardiology
Heart Institute (InCor)
University of São Paulo Medical School
and
Department of Interventional Cardiology
Hospital Israelita Albert Einstein
São Paulo, Brazil

**Davide Capodanno**
CardioThoracic-Vascular Department
Ferrarotto Hospital, Azienda Ospedaliero-Universitaria
(AOU)
Policlinico-Vittorio Emanuele
Catania, Italy

**Piera Capranzano**
Department of Cardiology
Ferrarotto Hospital
University of Catania
Catania, Italy

**Didier Carrié**
Department of Cardiology
Hopital de Rangueil
Toulouse, France

**Angel Ramón Cequier Fillat**
Director Heart Disease Clinic
Bellvigte University Hospital
Barcelona, Spain

**Daniel Chamié**
Cardiovascular Research Center
São Paulo, Brazil

**Bernard Chevalier**
Institut Jacques Cartier
Massy, France

**Alaide Chieffo**
Interventional Cardiology Unit
San Raffaele Scientific Institute
Milan, Italy

**Roisin Colleran**
Deutsches Herzzentrum München
Munich, Germany

**Carlos Collet**
Department of Cardiology
Academic Medical Center
University of Amsterdam
Amsterdam, the Netherlands

**Antonio Colombo**
Interventional Cardiology Unit
San Raffaele Scientific Institute
and
Interventional Cardiology Unit
EMO-GVM Centro Cuore Columbus
Milan, Italy

**J. Ribamar Costa Jr.**
Department of Interventional Cardiology
Instituto Dante Pazzanese de Cardiologia
São Paulo, Brazil

**Ricardo Costa**
Cardiovascular Research Center
São Paulo, Brazil

**Tom Crake**
Department of Cardiology
Barts Heart Centre
and
Department of Cardiovascular Sciences
University College London
London, United Kingdom

**Hubertus Degen**
Medical Clinic I
Städtische Kliniken Neuss
Lukaskrankenhaus GmbH
Neuss, Germany

**Joseph M. Deitzel**
Center for Composite Materials
University of Delaware
Newark, Delaware

**Jouke Dijkstra**
LKEB–Division of Image Processing
Department of Radiology
Leiden University Medical Center
Leiden, the Netherlands

**Nienke Simone van Ditzhuijzen**
Thorax Centre
Erasmus University Medical Centre
Rotterdam, the Netherlands

**Marcello Dominici**
Interventional Cardiology Unit
S. Maria University Hospital
Terni, Italy

**Dariusz Dudek**
Jagiellonian University
Department of Cardiology and Cardio Vascular
Interventions
University Hospital
Krakow, Poland

**Stephen G. Ellis**
Department of Cardiovascular Medicine
The Cleveland Clinic
Cleveland, Ohio

**Matthias Epple**
Inorganic Chemistry and Center for Nanointegration
Duisburg-Essen (CeNIDE)
University of Duisburg-Essen
Essen, Germany

**Raimund Erbel**
Cardiology Department
West German Heart Center Essen
Essen, Germany

**Simona Espejo**
Department of Radiology
Hospital Universitario Reina Sofía
Córdoba, Spain

**Bert Everaert**
Thoraxcenter
Erasmus University Medical Centre
Rotterdam, the Netherlands

**Babu Ezhumalai**
Fortis Escorts Heart Institute
New Delhi, India

**Jiang Ming Fam**
Department of Interventional Cardiology
Thoraxcenter
Erasmus University Medical Center
Rotterdam, the Netherlands
and
National Heart Centre Singapore
Singapore

**Cordula M. Felix**
Thoraxcenter
Erasmus University Medical Center
Rotterdam, the Netherlands

**Filippo Figini**
Interventional Cardiology Unit
San Raffaele Scientific Institute
and
Interventional Cardiology Unit
EMO-GVM Centro Cuore Columbus
Milan, Italy

**Aloke V. Finn**
CVPath Institute Inc.
Gaithersburg, Maryland

**Nicolas Foin**
National Heart Centre Singapore
and
Duke-NUS Medical School Singapore
Singapore

**Anna Franzone**
Department of Cardiology
Bern University Hospital
Bern, Switzerland

**Runlin Gao**
Department of Cardiology
Fu Wai Hospital
National Center for Cardiovascular Diseases
Chinese Academy of Medical Sciences
Beijing, China

**Hector M. Garcia-Garcia**
Department of Interventional Cardiology
Thoraxcenter
Erasmus University Medical Center
and
Cardialysis
Rotterdam, the Netherlands

**Junbo Ge**
Department of Cardiology
Zhongshan Hospital
Fudan University
Shanghai, China

**Robert-Jan M. van Geuns**
Department of Interventional Cardiology
Thoraxcenter
Erasmus University Medical Center
Rotterdam, the Netherlands

**Giuseppe Giacchi**
Cardiology Department
Thorax Institute
Hospital Clínic
University of Barcelona
Barcelona, Spain

**Daniele Giacoppo**
Deutsches Herzzentrum München
Munich, Germany

**Josep Gomez-Lara**
Interventional Cardiology Department
Hospital Universitari de Bellvitge
Catalunya, Spain

**Tommaso Gori**
Department of Cardiology
University Hospital Mainz
and
DZHK Standort Rhein-Main
Mainz, Germany

**Juan F. Granada**
CRF-Skirball Center for Innovation
Columbia University Medical Center
New York

**Maik J. Grundeken**
AMC Heart Center
Academic Medical Center
University of Amsterdam
Amsterdam, the Netherlands

**Yaling Han**
Department of Cardiology
The General Hospital of Shenyang Military Region
Shenyang, China

**Tatsuhiko Hata**
Department of Cardiology
Shiga Medical Center for Adults
Shiga, Japan

**Michael Haude**
Medical Clinic I
Städtische Kliniken Neuss
Lukaskrankenhaus GmbH
Neuss, Germany

**Steffen Helqvist**
Rigshospitalet
University of Copenhagen
Copenhagen, Denmark

**Stephen P. Hoole**
Department of Interventional Cardiology
Papworth Hospital
Cambridge, United Kingdom

**Shigeru Ikeguchi**
Department of Cardiology
Shiga Medical Center for Adults
Shiga, Japan

**Andrés Iñiguez**
Interventional Cardiology Unit
Cardiology Department
Hospital Alvaro Cunqueiro
University Hospital of Vigo
Vigo, Spain

**Yasutaka Inuzuka**
Department of Cardiology
Shiga Medical Center for Adults
Shiga, Japan

**Javaid Iqbal**
South Yorkshire Cardiothoracic Centre
Sheffield, United Kingdom

**Yuki Ishibashi**
Division of Cardiology
Department of Internal Medicine
St. Marianna University School of Medicine
Kawasaki, Japan

**Richard J. Jabbour**
San Raffaele Scientific Institute
and
EMO-GVM Centro Cuore Columbus
Milan, Italy
and
Imperial College London
United Kingdom

**Nigel Jepson**
Eastern Heart Clinic
Prince of Wales Hospital
Randwick, New South Wales, Australia

**Michael Joner**
CVPath Institute Inc.
Gaithersburg, Maryland

**Antonios Karanasos**
Department of Interventional Cardiology
Thoraxcenter
Erasmus University Medical Center
Rotterdam, the Netherlands

**Adnan Kastrati**
Deutsches Herzzentrum München
and
DZHK (German Centre for Cardiovascular Research)
Partner Site Munich Heart Alliance
Munich, Germany

**Yuki Katagiri**
Academisch Medisch Centrum
Amsterdam, the Netherlands

**Hiroyoshi Kawamoto**
Interventional Cardiology Unit
San Raffaele Scientific Institute
and
Interventional Cardiology Unit
EMO-GVM Centro Cuore Columbus
Milan, Italy

**Dean J. Kereiakes**
The Christ Hospital Heart and Vascular Center
and The Carl and Edyth Lindner Center for Research
and Education at The Christ Hospital
Cincinnati, Ohio

**Takeshi Kimura**
Department of Cardiovascular Medicine
Kyoto University Hospital
Kyoto, Japan

**Frank D. Kolodgie**
CVPath Institute Inc.
Gaithersburg, Maryland

**Jacques Koolen**
Cardiologie
Catharina Ziekenhuis
Eindhoven, the Netherlands

**Tobias Koppara**
CVPath Institute Inc.
Gaithersburg, Maryland

**Kunihiko Kosuga**
Department of Cardiology
Shiga Medical Center for Adults
Shiga, Japan

**R.P. Kraak**
AMC Heartcenter
Academic Medical Center
University of Amsterdam
Amsterdam, the Netherlands

**Eisho Kyo**
Kusatsu Heart Center
Shiga, Japan

**Antoine Lafont**
Laboratory of hemodynamic (LADHYX)
Ecole Polytechnique
Saclay, France
and
Department of Cardiology
Hôpital Européen Georges Pompidou
University Paris Descartes
Paris, France

**Byron J. Lambert**
Abbott Vascular
Santa Clara, California

**Azeem Latib**
Interventional Cardiology Unit
San Raffaele Scientific Institute
and
Interventional Cardiology Unit
EMO-GVM Centro Cuore Columbus
Milan, Italy

**Laura E. Leigh Perkins**
Abbott Vascular
Santa Clara, California

**Wenjiao Lin**
Research and Development Center
Lifetech Scientific (Shenzhen) Co Ltd
Shenzhen, China

**Daniel Lootz**
Biotronik AG
Buelach, Switzerland

**Dieter Mairhörmann**
ROFIN-BAASEL Lasertech GmbH
Starnberg, Germany

**Charis Mamilou**
Department of Cardiology
University Hospital Mainz
and
DZHK Standort Rhein-Main
Mainz, Germany

**Carlo Di Mario**
Biomedical Research Unit
Royal Bromton NHS Trust and Imperial College London
United Kingdom

**Alessio Mattesini**
Department of Heart and Vessels
AOUC Careggi
Florence, Italy

**Dougal McClean**
Christchurch Hospital
Christchurch, New Zealand

**Pau Medrano-Gracia**
Department of Anatomy with Medical Imaging
University of Auckland
Auckland, New Zealand

**Lynn Morrison**
Elixir Medical Corporation
Sunnyvale, California

**Takashi Muramatsu**
Fujita Health University Hospital
Kutsukake, Toyoake, Japan

**Shimpei Nakatani**
Thoraxcenter
Erasmus University Medical Center
Rotterdam, the Netherlands

**Jaryl Ng**
National Heart Centre Singapore
Singapore

**Koen Nieman**
Cardialysis BV
and
Erasmus Univeristy Medical Center
Rotterdam, the Netherlands

**Soji Nishio**
Kusatsu Heart Center
and
Department of Cardiology
Shiga Medical Center for Adults
Shiga, Japan

**Masaharu Okada**
Department of Cardiology
Shiga Medical Center for Adults
Shiga, Japan

**Yoshinobu Onuma**
Thoraxcenter
Erasmus University Medical Center
and
Cardialysis
Rotterdam, the Netherlands

**John A. Ormiston**
Mercy Angiography
and
Cardiology Department
Auckland City Hospital
and
University of Auckland
Auckland, New Zealand

**Erica Pacheco**
CVPath Institute Inc.
Gaithersburg, Maryland

**Manuel Pan**
Section Head Hemodynamics
Hospital Universitario Reina Sofía
Córdoba, Spain

**Raffaele Piccolo**
Department of Cardiology
Bern University Hospital
Bern, Switzerland

**Jan Piek**
Academic Medical Center
University of Amsterdam
Amsterdam, the Netherlands

**Haiping Qi**
Research and Development Center
Lifetech Scientific (Shenzhen) Co Ltd
Shenzhen, China

**Hong Qiu**
Department of Cardiology
Fu Wai Hospital
National Center for Cardiovascular Diseases
Chinese Academy of Medical Sciences
Beijing, China

**Nagarajan Ramesh**
Elixir Medical Corporation
Sunnyvale, California

**Richard J. Rapoza**
Abbott Vascular
Santa Clara, California

**Evelyn Regar**
Department of Interventional Cardiology
Thoraxcenter
Erasmus University Medical Center
Rotterdam, the Netherlands

**Sebastian Reith**
Institute for Physical Chemistry
Georg-August University of Göttingen
Göttingen, Germany

**Neil Ruparelia**
Interventional Cardiology Unit
San Raffaele Scientific Institute
and
Interventional Cardiology Unit
EMO-GVM Centro Cuore Columbus
Milan, Italy
and
Department of Cardiology
Imperial College
London, United Kingdom

**Manel Sabaté**
Cardiovascular Institute
University Hospital Clinic
Institut d'Investigacions Biome`diques August Pi i Sunyer
(IDIBAPS)
University of Barcelona
Barcelona, Spain

**Teguh Santoso**
Department of Cardiology
Medistra Hospital
Jakarta, Indonesia

**Janarthanan Sathananthan**
Auckland City Hospital
Auckland, New Zealand

**John J. Scanlon**
Hartlon, LLC
Wilmington, Delaware

**Wolfram Schmidt**
Institute for Biomedical Engineering
University Medicine Rostock
Rostock, Germany

**Klaus-Peter Schmitz**
Institute for Implant Technology and Biomaterials
IIB e.V. Associated Institute of the University of Rostock
Rostock-Warnemünde, Germany

**Junya Seki**
Department of Cardiology
Shiga Medical Center for Adults
Shiga, Japan

**Antonio Serra**
Cardiology Department
Hospital de la Santa Creu i Sant Pau
Barcelona, Spain

**Patrick W.J.C. Serruys**
Emeritus Thorax Center
Thoraxcenter
Erasmus University Medical Center
Rotterdam, the Netherlands
and
International Centre for Cardiovascular Circulatory Health
Imperial College
London, United Kingdom

**Ashok Seth**
Fortis Escorts Heart Institute
New Delhi, India

**Li Shen**
Department of Cardiology
Zhongshan Hospital
Fudan University
Shanghai, China

**Pieter Smits**
Cardiology Department
Maasstad Ziekenhuis
Rotterdam, the Netherlands

**Yohei Sotomi**
Department of Cardiology
Academic Medical Center
University of Amsterdam
Amsterdam, the Netherlands

**Gregg W. Stone**
Division of Cardiology
New York Presbyterian Hospital
Columbia University Medical Center
and
The Cardiovascular Research Foundation
New York

**Solomon Su**
Manli Cardiology Ltd
Singapore

**Ayyaz Sultan**
Royal Albert Edward Infirmary
Wigan, United Kingdom

**Ajay Suri**
Department of Cardiology
Barts Heart Centre
London, United Kingdom

**Pannipa Suwannasom**
Department of Cardiology
Academic Medical Center
University of Amsterdam
Amsterdam, the Netherlands
and
Northern Region Heart Center
Faculty of Medicine
Chiang Mai University
Chiang Mai, Thailand

**Shinsaku Takeda**
Department of Cardiology
Shiga Medical Center for Adults
Shiga, Japan

**Yuzo Takeuchi**
Department of Cardiology
Shiga Medical Center for Adults
Shiga, Japan

**Corrado Tamburino**
Department of Cardiology
Ferrarotto Hospital
University of Catania
Catania, Italy

**Akihito Tanaka**
San Raffaele Scientific Institute
and
EMO-GVM Centro Cuore Columbus
Milan, Italy

**Erhan Tenekecioglu**
Thoraxcentre
Rotterdam, the Netherlands

**Vikas Thondapu**
Department of Cardiology
Melbourne Medical School
Faculty of Medicine
Dentistry and Health Sciences
and
Department of Mechanical Engineering
University of Melbourne
Melbourne, Australia

**Ryo Torii**
Department of Mechanical Engineering
University College London
United Kingdom

**Sho Torii**
CVPath Institute Inc.
Gaithersburg, Maryland

**Sara Toyloy**
Elixir Medical Corporation
Sunnyvale, California

**Takafumi Tsuji**
Kusatsu Heart Center
Shiga, Japan

**Jors van der Sijde**
Department of Interventional Cardiology
Thoraxcenter
Erasmus University Medical Center
Rotterdam, the Netherlands

**Pratik Vasani**
Meril Life Sciences Pvt. Ltd.
Vapi, Gujarat, India

**Stefan Verheye**
Interventional Cardiology
Antwerp Cardiovascular Center
ZNA Middelheim
Antwerp, Belgium

**Michel Vert**
Institute for Biomolecules Max Mousseron
CNRS Unité Mixte de Recherche (UMR) 5247
University of Montpellier-CNRS, CRBA
Faculty of Pharmacy
Montpellier, France

**Renu Virmani**
CVPath Institute Inc.
Gaithersburg, Maryland

**Ron Waksman**
Division of Cardiology
MedStar Washington Hospital Center
Georgetown University
Washington, DC, USA

**Bruce Webber**
Cardiology
Mercy Angiography
Auckland, New Zealand

**Mark W.I. Webster**
Mercy Angiography
and
Cardiology Department
Auckland City Hospital
and
University of Auckland
Auckland, New Zealand

**Nick E.J. West**
Department of Interventional Cardiology
Papworth Hospital
Cambridge, United Kingdom

**Stephan Windecker**
Department of Cardiology
Bern University Hospital
Bern, Switzerland

**Eric Wittchow**
CVPath Institute Inc.
Gaithersburg, Maryland

**Roland Wölzein**
ROFIN-BAASEL Lasertech GmbH
Starnberg, Germany

**Philip Wong**
National Heart Centre Singapore
Singapore

**Chao Wu**
Department of Cardiology
Fu Wai Hospital
National Center for Cardiovascular Diseases
Chinese Academy of Medical Sciences
Beijing, China

**Joanna J. Wykrzykowska**
AMC Heartcenter
Academic Medical Center
University of Amsterdam
Amsterdam, the Netherlands

**Ying Xia**
Research and Development Center
Lifetech Scientific (Shenzhen) Co Ltd
Shenzhen, China

**Kazuyuki Yahagi**
CVPath Institute Inc.
Gaithersburg, Maryland

**Bu-Chun Zhang**
Department of Interventional Cardiology
Thoraxcenter
Erasmus University Medical Center
Rotterdam, the Netherlands

**Deyuan Zhang**
Research and Development Center
Lifetech Scientific (Shenzhen) Co Ltd
Shenzhen, China

**Gui Zhang**
Research and Development Center
Lifetech Scientific (Shenzhen) Co Ltd
Shenzhen, China

**Yao-Jun Zhang**
Department of Cardiology
Nanjing First Hospital
Nanjing Medical University
Nanjing, China

# PART 1

# Introduction

# Early development of bioresorbable scaffold

PATRICK W.J.C. SERRUYS AS INTERVIEWED BY CARLOS COLLET AND YOSHINOBU ONUMA

In September 1986, I had the privilege to implant the first endoluminal prosthesis (wall stent), as we called the stent at that time, in our first patient in Rotterdam just a few months after the pioneering cases of Jacques Puel in Toulouse and Ulrich Sigwart in Lausanne. In 1986, there was not yet an official Ethics Committee established at the Thoraxcenter, and it was only with the blessing of the chairman of cardiology and the permission of Paul Hugenholtz and with the support of the chief of surgery Egbert Bos that I was allowed to implant the first stent. Following the implantation, I performed an angioscopy, as it was available in Europe at that time. I was shocked by the vision of the shiny metal embedded in this delicate structure that is a human coronary artery. I felt guilty to have introduced in that very delicate biological structure such a rough device as a self-expanding stent. Honestly, I left the cath-lab with a tremendous feeling of guiltiness, having the impression that I had carried out something irreversible that would leave this human coronary artery caged forever. As ominously predicted by our chief surgeon... by the third case, I experienced my first stent thrombosis despite extensive platelet antiaggregation and anticoagulation with aspirin, heparin, warfarin, persantine and reomacrodex. On the same, day I started to reflect on the fact whether it could be possible to scaffold a vessel without using a permanent metallic implant to keep the vessel largely patent.

Scaffold was the word used by Ulrich Sigwart to describe the stenting process since at that time the word "stent" was not even mentioned in any dictionary of the English language. I told my colleagues that it would be possible to achieve the same kind of results with a device that would disappear with time. Immediately, my colleague Wim van der Giessen mentioned that a structure made of a polymer such as poly-lactide could do the trick, having heard that Richard Stack at Duke University was working on a biodegradable stent. I met Richard Stack at the American Heart Association 1988 and for more than one hour we shared our interest in developing a new field of bioresorbable stenting and later on it became evident that it would be a very complex and difficult endeavour, since nobody else including manufacturers and major device companies like Schneider, Boston Scientific, or Cordis showed interest in the development of biodegradable technologies. They had enough issues on their hands with the bare metallic stents.

Back in the Netherlands, Wim van der Giessen and myself kept working on the concept of developing a stent with a biostable polymer with the major Dutch corporation AkzoNobel. The results of this scaffold implantation in the coronaries of the pig model were very satisfactory and were published in the *Journal of Interventional Cardiology* in 1992 [1]. I will never forget the visit of the chief of cardiology Paul Hugenholtz, to the headquarters of AkzoNobel Company, who specialised in polymers to encapsulate the telephonic and electrical cable under the Atlantic Ocean for telecommunication between Europe and the United States. When I mentioned to the CEO of the company that a stent had on average a length of 14 mm and a diameter of 3 mm, the discussion came quickly to an end and clearly the microscopic need of polymers to manufacture a stent did not excite him excessively and did not steer his imagination or his vision as a captain of the industry.

In 1995, I went to the Mayo and Cleveland Clinics. We created a working group to test a family of bioresorbable polymers and biostable polymers, all attached on the external surface of a Wictor stent. I guess that the model was inappropriate, creating an eccentric and asymmetric configuration of the implant that induced major mechanical injury and inflammatory reactions. It was with anxiety that we all met at the American Heart Association in 1996, each academic group having experienced terrible animal results and we concluded that it was not the way to go. In the year 2000, Dr. Igaki and Dr. Tamai came to Rotterdam and in a meeting at the Hilton Hotel showed me a self-expanding thermolabile biodegradable scaffold, the so-called Igaki-Tamai stent. I will never forget the demonstration in the bathroom of their hotel, filing a glass with hot water from the tap and then dropping the stent into the glass and then expanding. Convinced by this experience and seeing for the first time a clinical product, we convinced the ethics committee to conduct a short series of 10 clinical implantations.

As the matter of fact, we carried out the implantation with Dr. Tamai during his stay in Rotterdam, and unfortunately by the seventh case the device got somewhat dislodged from the balloon and subsequently was pulled out with the balloon semi-inflated, which was a good reason to stop working with this device. The reader has to understand that we had to inflate the balloon with hot contrast medium at 60°C to obtain thermolabile self-expansion which was another reason to terminate the clinical trial. Dr. Tamai had the courage to complete a series of 55 patients and 10 years later we published together, after his death, the results of the 10 years' follow-up of these patients in *Circulation Journal* [2].

July 1999 was for me the discovery of stents with a permanent coating eluting called Rapamycin at the headquarters of Cordis Johnson and Johnson. Our first experience was in Rotterdam and in Sao Paulo with the Cypher® Stent. And of course, the Cypher stent for a few years overshadowed any development in the field of biodegradable scaffolds. It is Hans Bonier, one of my ex-trainees, who drew my attention to the idea of a German Professor of Cardiology, Heublein, who had developed the concept of a metallic bioresorbable stent using magnesium. I found the idea fascinating, but obviously, Biotronic being a German company, the technology went to Raymund Erbel and Michael Haude in order to be investigated. I followed the development and gave my advice to them on several occasions. So when Abbott made known that they were ready with their first bioresorbable scaffold, the so-called ABSORB Cohort A, the first iteration of an everolimus bioresorbable scaffold, I was fully committed to investigate that product the best I could. John Ormiston had the privilege to perform the first historical implantation. At the Thoraxcenter, we implanted 16 of the first 30 scaffolds. And from the very beginning, I used the combination of optical coherence tomography, virtual histology, grayscale intravascular ultrasound, angiography, and multislice CT scan to assess the results (Figure 1.1.1). Later on, it appeared that this combination

of invasive and noninvasive imaging was essential and critical in the understanding of the bioresorbable concept. Yoshi Onuma joined me at that time and became instrumental in collecting and analyzing the 6-month and 2-year results of the Cohort A. We came to the conclusion that the integrity of the device was subsiding too quickly and could not counteract fully the constrictive reaction of the vessel wall following the barotrauma of the implantation. A second iteration was designed since the late loss with the first device was 0.44 mm, a loss judged by myself unacceptable, taking into account that even a stent like the Taxus® stent had a loss of 0.39 mm [3,4]. The second generation, the so-called ABSORB Cohort B, was a real success in the sense that we lowered the late loss to 0.23 mm with long-term results that were mimicking the results of Cohort A [5]. From Cohort A, although the results at 6 months were not acceptable, we learned that the later follow-up with positive remodeling and late lumen enlargement had tremendous potential and should be duplicated by this second iteration device, providing a better late loss could be obtained. This was going to be achieved with Cohort B1 and B2.

As usual, I have been extremely optimistic about new technology and made some overenthusiastic statement about the future, but I keep mentioning that a coronary artery should not be caged by a metallic corset, but a vessel should be transiently scaffolded and then the phenomenon of restenosis being by definition a transient phenomenon, the scaffold should disappear and provide us with a healing process close to the natural healing process of the vessel. I am convinced of the solid foundation of this concept, and the future will have to prove to me that I am wrong before I lose my interest in the bioresorbable scaffold. I am convinced that within the end of the decade of investigation of this device, metal in the coronary artery will sound like something incongruous, and clearly other developments in the field of biomolecular technology (i.e., nanotherapy) will maybe surpass and redefine the bioresorbable technology as old-fashioned; I keep saying that if the future is unrealistic it will remain the future, which is a good thing, if the future is realistic it will soon become the past. I hope that biodegradable will have a life between these two extremes.

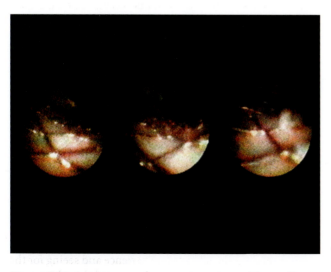

Figure 1.1.1 Angioscopy of a coronary artery with a wall stent implanted showing prolapse of tissue trough the struts.

## REFERENCES

1. van der Giessen WJ, Slager CJ, van Beusekom HM, van Ingen Schenau DS, Huijts RA, Schuurbiers JC et al. Development of a polymer endovascular prosthesis and its implantation in porcine arteries. *J Interv Cardiol.* 1992;5(3):175–85.
2. Nishio S, Kosuga K, Igaki K, Okada M, Kyo E, Tsuji T et al. Long-Term (>10 years) clinical outcomes of first-in-human biodegradable poly-l-lactic acid coronary stents: Igaki-Tamai stents. *Circulation.* 2012;125(19):2343–53.
3. Ormiston JA, Serruys PW, Regar E, Dudek D, Thuesen L, Webster MW et al. A bioabsorbable everolimus-eluting coronary stent system for

patients with single de-novo coronary artery lesions (ABSORB): A prospective open-label trial. *Lancet.* 2008;371(9616):899–907.

4. Stone GW, Ellis SG, Cox DA, Hermiller J, O'Shaughnessy C, Mann JT et al. A polymer-based, paclitaxel-eluting stent in patients with coronary artery disease. *N Engl J Med.* 2004;350(3):221–31.

5. Ormiston JA, Serruys PW, Onuma Y, van Geuns RJ, de Bruyne B, Dudek D et al. First serial assessment at 6 months and 2 years of the second generation of absorb everolimus-eluting bioresorbable vascular scaffold: A multi-imaging modality study. *Circ Cardiovasc Interv.* 2012;5(5):620–32.

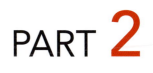

# PART 2

# Principles of bioresorption, vascular application

# Degradable, biodegradable, and bioresorbable polymers for time-limited therapy

MICHEL VERT

## INTRODUCTORY TERMINOLOGY*

For thousands of years, **biopolymers** (i.e., natural polymeric compounds like proteins, polysaccharides, etc.) have been used as **materials** (substances exploited by humans for practical applications) or as sources of materials after chemical modification by humans, including for therapy [1]. In the nineteenth century appeared the first **artificial** (non-natural synthesized by humans) organic compounds useable as materials like Bakelite® but the exact chemical structure of the matter was still unidentified. It was in 1922 that H. Staudinger recognized plastics as made of long molecules (**macromolecules**) composed by the repetition of small organic entities chemically linked and not associated as it was believed before, the so-called **repeating or monomer units**. He received the Nobel Prize for this in 1953 [2]. Once people realized that combining small organic molecules bearing two or more chemical sites susceptible to react was the condition to attach these molecules together repetitively, the door was largely opened to invent new macromolecules associated to make macroscopic materials (often referred to as **plastics or resins** improperly) that are now named **polymers**. According to the International Union for Pure and Applied Chemistry (IUPAC), the term "polymer" reflects a material composed of "macromolecules" although it is often used improperly as an alternative to macromolecule [3].

Polymers, known as poly(methyl methacrylate), silicones, polyethylene, polyamides, polyurethanes, and so on, were invented and developed industrially to replace advantageously materials of natural origin [4]. Artificial polymers have revolutionized and invaded almost all human activities. However, people realized soon that using long-lasting materials for time-limited applications is nonsense

and generates residues and wastes postexploitation. Nature solved the problem long ago via complex biological machineries involving enzymes and cellular entities to eliminate the organic matters produced naturally and to achieve the turnover typical of living organisms. The first stage of this turnover based on the activities of cells, organs, and organisms is specifically named **biodegradation** in opposition to **degradation** that is more general and is reserved for chemical breakdown of macromolecules. To be precise and rigorous, the term **degradable** is generally complemented by the phenomenon that causes the degradation. Biodegradation is a contraction of **biotic** (related to biological activities) **degradation** whereas **photodegradation, thermodegradation, hydrolytic degradation, chemical degradation, enzymatic degradation, physical degradation**, and so on, result from the actions of electromagnetic phenomena, heath, water, chemical reagent, enzymes, physical stresses, and so on, respectively. In the case of solid state devices, biodegradation occurs generally at the surface because cells are located there and active enzymes are large molecules that cannot penetrate inside. The process is named **bioerosion**. Surface degradation referred to as **erosion** can be observed under abiotic conditions when the aggressive phenomenon is limited to the surface.

This is the case of hydrolytic degradation when the rate of degradation is faster than the rate of water penetration, a feature that can be confused with bioerosion. Physical degradation is a generic term for **fragmentation, disintegration,** or **dismantling** of a polymer or a polymeric device without systematic breakdown of constituting macromolecules. If biopolymers are intrinsically biodegradable, their material properties lack reproducibility and are difficult to control. These two features constitute severe drawbacks for engineers and engineering.

The search for artificial polymeric materials that may disappear once their time-limited material mission is

* Note: Terms in bold in the text reflect the terminology recommended by IUPAC for "Biorelated Polymers" [5].

completed started in the early 1960s for therapeutic purposes. The first so-called **"bioabsorbable"** therapeutic device of this kind was a suture made of hydrolytically degradable poly(glycolic acid) (PGA) artificial aliphatic polyester composed of glycolyl units derived from the glycolic acid metabolite. This suture appeared on the US market in the late 1960s [6,7].

The term "bioabsorbable" is presently considered inappropriate because absorption reflects disappearance and not necessarily breakdown of macromolecules into shorter macromolecular segments. The human body is a close space for macromolecules that cannot cross skin and mucosa. This is an important feature that nature set up because a huge number of soluble biopolymers like proteins and polynucleotides contribute to biological processes. Being macromolecular, artificial polymeric compounds and devices are also entrapped and remain therein for the rest of the patient's life. This is an advantage for permanent prostheses but not for time-limited applications based on polymers. To be eliminated through natural pathways (lungs and kidneys) macromolecules must first be degraded to shorter soluble molecules that can then be **biomineralized** (turned to carbon dioxide and water) or excreted via glomerula filtration. The term **bioresorption** was introduced to indicate that degradation goes up to elimination of the foreign residues. Sometimes, PGA, and its superior analogue poly(lactic acid) (PLA), a generic abbreviation that actually reflects a large family of macromolecules, are referred to as "biopolymers." This is again inappropriate because the human body has no cell machinery or associated enzyme to make and cleave the PGA or PLA inter-unit ester links. Therefore, PGA and PLA and their copolymers PLAGA are **hydrolytically degradable** only. PLA is known as degradable by some bacterial enzymes like proteinase K, but this enzyme is not present in the human body. Under these conditions, biodegradable is not applicable and a polymer degraded by an enzyme *in vitro* (under **abiotic** conditions) must be identified as **enzymatically degradable**. Using biodegradable is misleading and confusing when *in vivo* behaviors are considered. PGA, like PLAs, is only hydrolytically degradable *in vivo*, a feature that permits long functional time prior to weakening. In comparison, cell-mediated enzyme-dependent processes are generally very fast and difficult to control.

## POLYMERS REPUTED DEGRADABLE

Literature is very rich in polymers said to be degradable and/or biodegradable in the environment, *in vitro* and less frequently *in vivo*. In the human body, biodegradation is of little interest because the cleavage of macromolecules and pathogens is rather fast like in the case of collagen, hyaluronic acid, bacteria, and viruses as well. In the case of artificial polymers, degradation can result from an attack by the radicals present in biochemistry or from chemical processes like hydrolysis and/or oxidation. There is no implanted polymer or polymeric device that is absolutely stable. Sooner or later, the initial properties are affected either physically or chemically or both. Therefore, one has to distinguish the desired and useful degradation from the undergone one that is detrimental. The degradation of interest is the beneficial one. The loss of integrity should occur preferably when the temporary biomaterial function is completed but when the tissue healing process is still in progress to take advantage of the limited period of tissue healing. These are the reasons why the number of degradable polymers that are exploited in medicine and pharmacology is rather small (Table 2.1.1) [8].

Basically any degradable or biodegradable polymer has a potential to be exploited in time-limited therapeutic systems like those listed in Table 2.1.2 where approximate functional durations are indicated. In translational research, degradation is not sufficient and many other requisites are to be taken into account since clinical and commercial developments are final targets. Table 2.1.3 lists these requisites from a general viewpoint; however, each criterion has to be confronted to the specificity of an application, a stage that results in drastic selection and excludes many candidates, especially those whose chemical nature does not provide exploitable means to adapt properties to requirements.

Some of these applications require macromolecules soluble in aqueous media, especially body fluids; some others must self-assemble in these fluids like micelles and aggregates. This is the domain of amphiphilic macromolecules. Last but not least, applications that require mechanical properties are relevant to thermoplastic polymers. The main phenomenon that commands the behavior of this class of materials and thus of polymeric biomaterials is the **glass transition temperature**, Tg. In practice, solid state properties of a prosthetic device depend very much on the position of Tg with respect to the temperature of exploitation of this device. Above Tg, a thermoplastic polymer is in the rubbery state and can be deformed more or less rapidly when submitted to mechanical stresses. Below Tg, the same solid polymer is rigid and resistant to stresses but it is brittle, i.e., it breaks at low degree of deformation. Tg is normally well defined for a given polymer. However, many factors can affect this transition, especially the presence or the uptake of plasticizing small molecules (**plasticizers**) that shifts it toward lower temperatures. Other compounds (**fillers** like carbon fibers, mineral radio-opacifiant, some drug particles, etc.) can be present that do not affect Tg because they are not compatible with the polymer. The body temperature being imposed, the Tg of a polymer must be below or above 37°C depending on whether one wants deformation or rigidity. When macromolecules are composed of monomer units repeated regularly, they can assemble in regular arrays and crystallize more or less partially, a physical **semi-crystalline** state characterized by a **melting temperature** (actually a melting zone because macromolecules do not have the same length, a feature referred to as **polydispersity**) and a **degree of crystallinity**.

**Table 2.1.1** Major artificial and biopolymer-derived degradable polymers in relation to *in vivo* applications or potential applications

| Polymer | Chemical formula | Remarks |
|---|---|---|
| Poly(glycolic acid) | | Exploited to make fibers and sutures |
| Poly(L-lactic acid) | | Exploited to make pins, staples, bone surgery devices and stents |
| Lactic acid stereocopolymers | | Exploited to make bone surgery devices and stents (crystalline ones) and drug delivery devices and stent coatings (amorphous ones) |
| Poly(lactic acid-co-glycolic acid) | | Exploited to make drug delivery devices, coatings: proposed to make porous scaffolds in tissue engineering and stents |
| Polycaprolactone | | Fast biodegradation by outdoor microorganisms, exploited for long-term drug delivery |
| Poly(β-alkanoates)s | | Bacterial polymers biodegradable by outdoor microorganisms, very slowly hydrodegradable *in vivo* |
| Poly(para-dioxanone) | | Exploited as rather long-lasting bioresorbable sutures. Proposed to make stents |
| Poly(trimethylene carbonate) | | Slow degradation. Exploited as copolymers for sutures |
| Poly(tyrosine carbonate)s | | Hydrodegradable. Proposed to make stents and drug delivery |
| Poly(salicylate anhydride ester)s | | Exploited for stents in mixtures. Proposed for drug delivery |
| Polyorthoesters | | Exploited for drug delivery |
| Polyanhydrides | | Hydrodegradable, exploited for drug delivery |
| Polyphosphazenes | | Hydrodegradable. Proposed for many biomedical applications |
| Collagen and gelatine, chitosans, glycosamino glycans, alginates, silk | Extracted from more or less chemically modified natural compounds or tissues | Proposed for various applications, frequently as gels; risks of immune reactions because of the presence of protein residues |

Table 2.1.2 Examples of time-limited devices that can take advantage of suitable degradable materials and approximate required lifetimes prior to degradation

| Domain | Time-limited device | Tissue | Lifetime |
|---|---|---|---|
| Surgery | Suture, staple | Skin | 15 days |
| | Bone plates, screws, nails | Bones | 2–6 months |
| | Bone defect fillers | Bones | 1–4 months |
| Dentistry | Membrane for GTR[a] | Gengiva and bone | 1–2 months |
| Pharmacology (drug delivery) | Implants and hydrogels | Soft | 15 days–2 years |
| | Microparticles | Any except blood | 15 days–6 months |
| | Nanoparticles, micelles and tiny aggregates | Blood | |
| | DNA complexes | Cells (post blood) | 1 day |
| Cardiology | Stent | Blood vessels | 2–3 months |
| Tissue engineering | Porous matrices | Soft and hard | Tissue–dependent |

a Guided tissue regeneration.

Table 2.1.3 General properties that condition the potential of materials involved in time-limited therapeutic devices

| Biocompatibility[a] | Biofunctionality | |
|---|---|---|
| | Material-related properties | Exploitation-related properties |
| Acceptable acute toxicity | Chemical | Easy to use |
| No long term toxicity | Physical | Sterilization-resistant |
| No immunogenicicity | Physico-chemical | Stability on storage |
| No mutagenicity | Thermal | Programmed degradation |
| No thrombogenicity | Mechanical | Bioresorption |
| | | Conform to regulations |

a Parent material and degradation-by products.

# MAJOR DEGRADABLE POLYMERS AND POTENTIAL OR EFFECTIVE APPLICATIONS (TABLE 2.1.1)

## Poly(glycolic acid) (PGA)

Poly(glycolic acid) macromolecules are linear and composed of repeated glycolyl units. The regular linear structure and the absence of side-chains are in favor of chain packing, crystallinity, and tensile strength, three properties typical of good fiber-forming polymers. PGA has a high melting temperature (~220°C) a rather high crystallinity (~50%), high tensile strength, and Tg = ~34°C, slightly below body temperature. Furthermore, the density of ester bonds and the presence of only one $CH_2$ group between them are in favor of hydrophily. PGA is hydrolytically degradable and bioresorbable with the glycolic acid metabolite as ultimate degradation by-product. All these characteristics led to exploitation as threads, sutures, and meshes, despite a trend to be inflammatory [9]. During the rather fast degradation and probably because of the release of glycolic acid and soluble oligomers and the formation of highly crystalline residues, PGA sutures are sources of irritation but the disagreement is acceptable. PGA is not recommended to make large devices like bone plates and screws because of dramatic local inflammation [10].

## Poly(L-lactic acid) (PLLA)

Poly(L-lactic acid) macromolecules, generally referred to as PLLA in the literature, are also linear with high stereoregularity. In contrast to PGA chains that are achiral, the chains of PLLA are composed of chiral units with the same L (S) configuration each bearing a methyl pendent group. If the density in ester bonds is similar to that of PGA, the presence of the methyl groups along the main chain generates steric hindrance and hydrophobicity. These features are the sources of lower melting temperature (~175°C), lower crystallinity (30%), higher Tg (~60°C), and lower hydrophily than PGA. As a result, poly(L-lactic acid) absorbs less water and thus its hydrolytic degradation is much slower than that of PGA. Degradation rate is difficult to indicate because it depends on many more or less interrelated factors. Therefore, there is not one PLLA but a number of polymers having the same basic chemical structure but different behaviors depending on the synthesis route. A PLLA can be spun to fibers; however, these fibers are highly crystalline and their degradation can require up to several years depending on purity and morphology. These dependencies are at the origin of the controversial data and findings frequently found in literature. This polymer is not appropriate to make bioresorbable sutures, basically. PLLA is less inflammatory than PGA. Inflammation is observed right after implantation, like for any material. After a period of low reaction, a secondary inflammation can be observed associated with the beginning of the release of soluble degradation by-products. However, this release is very slow and causes acceptable mild foreign body reactions only. A third period of inflammation can occur very late when tiny crystalline residues, if any, are left. This may be the actual cause of the late dramatic reaction observed with bone plates made of very high molecular mass and highly crystalline as polymerized PLLA reported many years ago [11]. Since then, PLLA polymers have found applications in bone surgery as bone plates, screws, and so on, and in interventional cardiology as degradable stents.

## Poly(D-lactic acid) (PDLA)

Basically, poly(D-lactic acid) generally referred to as PDLA in the literature, the mirror image of PLLA, has the same chemical and physico-chemical and material characteristics, including hydrolytic degradation ones. It is degradable and bioresorbable. However, the derived polymer has not been exploited thus far primarily because the D-lactic acid precursor is less accessible than the L-isomer.

## Poly(lactic acid) stereocopolymers

Poly(lactic acid) stereocopolymers and the previous homopolymers have the same basic chemical structure but the linear chains that form the macromolecules are composed of L- and D-lactyl units in various proportions. The pendent methyl groups localized on both sides of the chains occupied a larger volume than in homopolymers, a feature that results in a looser packing of macromolecules in the solid phase. This particularity affects thermal and hydrolytic degradation characteristics that are then dependent on the composition. Relatively minor attention was paid to lactic acid-stereocopolymers in the literature compared with PLLA. L- and D-rich stereocopolymers are semicrystalline with melting temperatures decreasing with the increase in the other isomer up to a certain composition (~8%) beyond which solids stereocopolymers are amorphous. Tg varies also but only slightly (55°C–60°C). To distinguish stereocopolymers from homopolymers, a specific mode of abbreviation was introduced based on PLAx where x stands for the percentage in L-units [12]. The increase of irregularities due to the presence of more or less D-units in the chains acts in favor of water uptake and thus the lifetime decreases from PLA100 (PLLA) to PLA50 also referred to as PDLLA, the stereocopolymer derived from the racemic mixture of L- and D-lactides. Semi-crystalline L-rich stereocopolymers like PLA98 or PLA96 are suitable to make devices for bone surgery whereas amorphous ones are more adapted to

make micro- and nanoparticles for sustained drug delivery. Among them, PDLLA appears frequently in literature. Again, it is rather difficult to assign a specific degradation rate because of the number of interrelated factors that condition it [13]. Made of metabolites, PLA50 and higher stereocopolymers are hydrolytically degradable and bioresorbable.

## Poly(lactic acid-co-glycolic acid) and other LA and GA-based copolymers

Lactic and glycolic acid-based copolymers and stereocopolymers form a large family of degradable compounds with different properties and behaviors. In the literature, abbreviations like PLGA and PLAGA are frequent. However, they fail to reflect the fine composition of linear macromolecules in which irregularities due to chirality are complemented by those due to the presence of GA units. A more informative abbreviation, namely PLAxGAy where x and y stand for percentage in L-lactyl and glycolyl units, was introduced [12]. This general abbreviation mode is applicable to homopolymers, copolymers, and stereocopolymers since x can vary from 100 to 0 and y from 0 to 100, i.e., from PLA100 to PGA. Only polymers with low or high x or y values are semicrystalline (except for block copolymers). All the others are amorphous. PLA8GA92, which has lower crystallinity than PLA100, is slightly less inflammatory than PGA and has been exploited to make sutures (Vicryl®) and many other devices [7]. Among other PLAGA copolymers, PLA50GA50 and PLA25GA50 are used more mainly to make micro- and nanoparticles and coatings for sustained drug delivery.

Many other biocompatible degradable copolymers derived from lactides and/or glycolide and other monomers are present in the literature and have been proposed to make various therapeutic devices that have a potential for applications as degradable material. Some have reached the level of clinical application and commercialization like Maxon® sutures made of PGA-co-TMC (trimethylene carbonate). Some others like PLA-PEO-PLA (PEO = poly[ethylene oxide]) have a potential for effective applications as drug delivery systems or as scaffolds in tissue engineering [14].

## Poly(ε-caprolactone)

Macromolecules of poly(ε-caprolactone) (PCL) are of the aliphatic polyester-type like PGA and PLA. However, the ester bonds are separated by five $CH_2$ groups instead of one. This structure leads to high crystallinity but rather low melting temperature (~50°C), low Tg (~–60°C), and rather high hydrophobicity. Therefore, stressed PCL polymers are prone to deform at body temperature. PCL is frequently considered biodegradable. This is true in the environment because bacteria and fungi degrade PCL very rapidly, i.e., in a couple of days. In contrast, PCL is not biodegradable *in vivo*. It is hydrolytically degradable only and the rate of hydrolysis is very slow so that PCL can last for a long time in the human body, despite the fact that lipases are able to degrade PCL *in vitro*. Under these conditions, PCL is enzymatically degradable and not biodegradable. Because of its resistance to degradation *in vivo* and its lipophily, PCL is exploited to make long-term drug delivery of hydrophobic drugs, especially for contraception (Capronor®). Different copolymers containing PCL segments have been proposed for therapeutic applications. Some like PGACL are exploited as soft sutures (Monocryl®).

## Poly(β-hydroxy alkanoate)s (PHAs) and poly(β-hydroxy butyrate) (PHB)

These polymers are also of the aliphatic polyester-type. Their chains are composed of similar backbone with two carbon atoms between ester bonds. The difference between the members of the family comes from the nature of the substituent located in beta position with respect to the carbonyl group in repeating units that are thus chiral. The first member of the family, namely, poly([R]-β-hydroxy butyrate) (PHB) is produced by microorganisms, mainly bacteria, and like any biopolymer, it is biodegraded by bacteria and enzymatically degraded by bacteria depolymerase *in vitro*. PHB melts at 177°C but its Tg is 9°C. It is a stiff and relatively brittle polymer. When bacteria are fed by suitable chemicals, they can make copolymers with longer and different side-chains in lower yields. The repeating units of all bacterial PHAs have the same *R* absolute configuration and are thus semicrystalline with high crystallinity. Like PCL these polyesters are hydrophobic. Like for PCL, there is some confusion in the literature of therapeutic biomaterials. PHB and sometimes PHAs are often said to be biodegradable. Actually PHAs are not biodegradable in the human body because the specific depolymerases are not part of the available pool of enzymes. Implanted PHB and PHA-based devices are hydrolytically degradable and they can last for a long time [15]. Despite these shortcomings, PHB and PHAs are frequently proposed for many biomedical uses in the literature, including making a stent that showed large recoil [16,17]. Thus far, there has been no effective development for the biomedical applications listed in Table 2.1.2 that require rather short lifetimes.

## Poly(para-dioxanone) (PDO)

This polyester derives from 1,4-dioxane-2-one, a cyclic monomer that leads to repeating units linked by ester bonds with an oxygen atom and three methylene groups between them. The presence of an oxygen atom makes the spatial structure of macromolecules different with respect to the previous polymers. PDO is semicrystalline with a rather low melting temperature (~110°C). It is rather resistant to hydrolytic degradation and is exploited to make sutures (PDS), occasionally with antibacterial drug, that retain their strength for approximately 3 months prior to resorption via kidney filtration and maybe metabolization [18].

## Poly(trimethylene carbonate) (PTMC)

The repeating units of this polymer and those of the previous poly(para-dioxanone) have the same gross composition but the atoms are located differently. This polymer is not aliphatic polyester, the units being connected by carbonate functions. *In vitro*, PTMC degraded about 20 times less rapidly than PCL and degraded more rapidly *in vivo* than *in vitro*, a difference that was assumed due to biodegradation [19]. Only PTMC with molecular mass above 100,000 g/mol shows exploitable mechanical properties. Copolymers with glycolic acid are exploited to make sutures (Maxon). Cross-linking by γ-irradiation can lead to systems with better mechanical properties.

## Poly(tyrosine carbonate)s

This is a particular class of hydrolytically degradable and bioresorbable macromolecules with repeating units composed of an esterified amino acid, namely tyrosine, linked to a deaminated analog of tyrosine and linked by water-sensitive carbonate functions. The properties can be modified by changing the R substituent [20]. These polymers degrade rather slowly. The poly(tyrosyl carbonate) with R = ethyl processed as pins exhibited a good contact with bony tissue and was proposed for applications in bone reconstruction. Presently, a bioresorbable stent is under evaluation (REVA Co.) that is based on a polymer of this type composed of a poly(tyrosine carbonate) that includes iodine atoms attached to some tyrosine moieties to provide radio opacity [21].

## Poly(salicylate anhydride ester)s

This rather recent family of polymers exploits the hydrolytic cleavage of anhydride and ester functions that are present in repeating units [22]. The anhydride functions are easily cleaved and full degradation after 90 days was observed *in vitro* when R = $(CH_2)_8$. Degradation releases salicylate, a well-known anti-inflammatory compound. Polymers of this family are involved in some sustained drug delivery systems and also to make a bioresorbable stent [23].

## Polyorthoesters

The structure of macromolecules of this type gives access to hydrolytically degradable polymers with different properties. These polymers are hydrophobic. The rate of water penetration is slow with respect to the rate of degradation. Therefore, degradation occurs at the surface according to a process named **erosion**. The first commercial drug delivery system was based on a matrix of this type developed for ophthalmic applications (ALZA Co.). Tg is rather low so that polyorthoesters are past-like, an interesting property for formulation with drugs. Erosion and low Tg are favorable features to deliver drug progressively. Lately, erosion is combined with bulk degradation [24].

## Polyanhydrides

Poly(anhydride)s are the most hydrolytically unstable polymers. This is again a class of hydrophobic compounds. Degradation occurs generally by erosion and the degradation rate decreases when aromatic groups are present in the chains. The family is large and includes compounds with different properties. Most of the members are semicrystalline with a rather high degree of crystallinity (~60%). Major applications are in the field of drug delivery because of the erosion process [25].

## Polyphosphazenes

Polyphosphazenes are hydrolytically degradable polymers with no common structural characteristics with the previous copolymers. The backbone is composed of alternating phosphorus and nitrogen atoms and properties depend on the substituents R. A great number of polyphosphazenes have been synthesized. They are very hydrophobic, except when side chains contain hydrophilic ionisable groups. Polyphosphazenes have been proposed for many applications but to the most of our knowledge, none has reached the level of exploitation [26].

## Collagens and gelatine

Collagens are fibrous proteins of natural origin present in all mammals. There are different collagens whose properties depend on the tissue they come from. Collagens used in therapy are not genuine. In most cases, they are denaturized to tropocollagen and resulting chains are occasionally cross-linked. Despite these physical and chemical modifications, the resulting compounds remain biodegradable with short lifetimes unless the degree of modification is too high. To avoid immunogenicity, biodegradable collagenic compounds have to be purified to eliminate residues of other proteins. Many therapeutic systems (films, membranes, meshes, etc.) are marketed as wound dressings and tissue cultures. They also received applications in drug delivery. The main shortcoming is the lack of reproducibility of properties, including *in vivo* degradation. Solutions of collagen in water can be obtained after destructuration and deorientation of macromolecules. Collagen solutions are referred to as gelatines [27].

## Chitosans

This family of polymers derives from an abundant natural polysaccharide, namely chitin, a poly(N-acetyl glucosamine) that forms the shells of shellfish. This rigid biopolymer is chemically modified by deacetylation to yield a family of copolymers bearing primary amine functions. The properties of these copolymers depend on the degree of deacetylation, especially biocompatibility, degree of crystallization, and solubility in aqueous media. Therefore, there is not one chitosan but many of them. Chitosans are involved in many effective or potential applications. Most commercial applications use chitosans with less than 20% of residual N-acetyl glucosamine units. Because of the presence of many amine groups, the properties of chitosans depend also on the pH of aqueous media. Chitosans are enzymatically degradable by lysozyme *in vitro* and *in vivo* as well

although degradability depends very much on the residual acetylation. Enzymatic degradation and biodegradation depend on crystallinity and are minimal for a low degree of N-acetylation, in agreement with the fact that lysozyme degrades the poly(N-acetyl glucosamine) segments. Therefore, the degradation of chitosans may leave amino deacetylated units or segments as basic residues that can interact with negative entities present in body tissues (cell membranes) and fluids (negative proteins). Chitosans (and too often chitosan in singular without any structural information) have been proposed as having potential interest for many biomedical applications (drug delivery, scaffolds for tissue engineering, wound dressings, etc.) but exploitations are primarily in other domains [28].

## Glycosamino glycans

This class of polymers is also derived from biopolymers that are generally impaired by extraction processes, even if they keep biological activities. The family is composed of many different polymeric compounds characterized by disaccharidic repeating units composed of N-acetyl galactosamine or N-acetyl glucosamine and a uronic acid (glucuronate or iduronate). In therapy, the main exploited members are hyaluronic acid and heparin. Both names should be in the plural because their properties depend very much on the tissues they are extracted from and the process used. Both compounds are enzymatically degradable and biodegradable by hyaluronidase and heparinase, respectively. Most of their applications are in pharmacology although hyaluronate gels can be cross-linked to increase lifetime. However, the chemical cross-linking can affect the biodegradability [8]. These highly functionalized polymers are not suitable for making solid state devices or coatings.

## Alginates

The members of this large family are extracted from algae and like other polymeric compounds extracted from living tissues, the original structures can be altered during extraction and lead to different compositions. Alginate chains are characterized by units composed of α-L-glucuronic acid and β-D-mannuronic acid of different sizes and proportions. The main material property of alginates is their ability to form hydrogels either by chemical cross-linking or by complexation cross-linking by calcium ions, the latter depending on the proportion of glucuronate units. Alginates are stable in neutral aqueous media. They do not have the reputation of being biodegradable *in vivo*. One of the main proposed applications is the encapsulation of Langerhans islets in alginate gel to treat diabetes [8–29]. Alginates are not suitable to make solid state devices or coatings.

## Silks

Silks are fibrous proteins composed of glycine, serine, and alanine. Their molecular structures are rather complex and depend on their origin. The outstanding strength of silk fibers comes from the presence of a number of crystalline domains separated by disordered ones. In practice, silk fibroin is purified from sericin. As most of polymeric compounds derived from biopolymers, silks can be processed to gels, films, sponges, and also chemically modified. Silk proteins degrade via the action of proteases, like any protein. The degradation by-products of silk are peptides and amino acids. The rate of silk fibroin degradation depends on structure, morphology, and mechanical and biological conditions at the location of implantation. The degradation of silk-based polymeric compounds by enzymes is well documented *in vitro* where degradation is rather fast. Much less information is available for *in vivo* degradation where fibroin-based materials seem to fragment with variable fragmentation times. Many applications are proposed [30].

## HOW TO CHOOSE A DEGRADABLE POLYMER FOR EFFECTIVE DEVELOPMENT

As previously shown with selected examples, there are many polymeric compounds that can degrade *in vivo*, regardless of the mechanism. If studying degradation is of interest for the progress of science and to better know the fundamental behaviors of degradable polymers, this is by far not enough for translational research. Effective clinical application and commercial development requires consideration paid to many other more important criteria, i.e., specific criteria imposed to a time-limited application. Degradation is a plus that must be tuned to cell machineries whereas bioresorption is necessary to exhaust the body from any residual foreign compounds or molecules. Table 2.1.3 lists the main criteria to be taken into account that can be grouped under the biocompatibility and biofunctionality headings.

Accordingly, development of a time-limited therapeutic device or macromolecule-based systems is always a matter of difficult-to-find compromises resulting from collaborations between many specialists of complementary disciplines.

## CONCLUSION

Among the most common degradable or biodegradable polymers presented before, only a few are suitable to make solid state devices for time-limited biomedical applications. Aliphatic polyesters are predominant because intrachain ester links can be cleaved by hydrolysis, a chain cleaving process more easily controlled by engineers than biodegradation. Some of the aliphatic polyesters like PHAs and PCL are biodegradable in the environment, enzymatically degradable *in vitro*, and only slowly hydrolytically degradable *in vivo* because of rather high hydrophobicity and high degrees of crystallinity. Although they have been extensively studied in the literature, they are not well adapted to make solid state devices. Among aliphatic polyesters, polymers, copolymers, and stereocopolymers derived from lactic and/or glycolic acids are then the most studied and are the more versatile by far. They offer large possibilities to adjust mechanical properties and degradability. Basically, semicrystalline members of the family are more suitable to make devices that require mechanical properties and stability *in vivo*. Amorphous ones that have larger free volume available are better suited for sustained drug delivery. Lifetimes can be adjusted by stereocopolymerization and by copolymerization as well, especially with glycolide [31–33]. Many members of the family are currently exploited clinically and commercially in surgery, cardiology, pharmacology, and dentistry as temporary therapeutic devices and to help *in situ* tissue reconstruction provided the degradation rate is adjusted to occur during the remodeling phase of the tissue healing machinery. These multiple applications result from their biocompatibility and from the outstanding possibilities of tuning material and degradation properties through macromolecule chemical and configurational structures, molecular mass, chemical modification of chain ends, chain orientation, crystallinity, and formulation, these factors acting on the level and the rate of water uptake. It is important to note that lactic acid-based polyesters have mechanical characteristics of the same order of magnitude provided they are in dry and glassy state (i.e., below the glass transition temperature [$T_g$]). Once in contact with an aqueous medium, the absorbed water affects more or less the mechanical and degradation characteristics because of the increase in local hydrophilicity, the adsorbed water acting as a plasticizer.

## REFERENCES

1. Ratner BD, A history of biomaterials, in *Biomaterials Science: An Introduction to Materials in Medicine*, Ratner BD, Hoffman AS, Schoen FJ, Lemons JE, Eds., Academic Press, San Diego, CA, 2012, p. xli.
2. Morris PJ, *Polymer Pioneers: A Popular History of the Science and Technology of Large Molecules*, Beckman Center for the History of Chemistry, Philadelphia, PA, 2005.
3. Jenkins AD, Kratochvil P, Stepto RFT, Suter UW, Glossary of basic terms in polymer science (IUPAC recommendations 1996). *PAC*. 1996; 68:2287–2311.
4. http://www.bpf.co.uk/Plastipedia/Polymers/Default.aspx
5. Vert M, Doi Y, Hellwich K-H, Hess M, Hodge P, Kubisa P, Rinaudo M, Schue F, Terminology for biorelated polymers and applications (IUPAC Recommendations 2012). *PAC*. 2012; 84:377–408.
6. Frazza EJ and Schmitt EE, A new absorbable suture. *J Biomed Mater Res Part A*. 1971; 2:43–58.
7. Shalaby SW, Absorbable and degradable polymers, in *Advanced in Polymeric Biomaterials Series*, Shalaby SW and Burg KJL, Eds., CRC Press, Boca Raton, FL, 2003.

8. Piskin E, Biodegradable polymers in medicine, in *Biodegradable Polymers: Principles and Applications*, Scott G, Ed., Kluwer Academic Publishers, Dordrecht, the Netherlands, 2002, p. 321.

9 Burg KLG, Shalaby SW, Atkins GG, Polymer biocompatibility and toxicity, in *Absorbable and Degradable Polymers*, Shalaby SW and Burg KJL, Eds., CRC Press, Boca Raton, FL, 2004, pp. 143–156.

10. Personal unpublished data.

11. Bersgma EJ, Rozema FRM, Bos RR, De Bruijn WC, Foreign body reactions to resorbable poly (L-Lactide) bone plates and screws used for the fixation of unstable zygomatic fractures. *J Oral Maxillofac Surg.* 1993; 51:666–670.

12. Vert M, Chabot F, Leray J, Christel P, Bioresorbable polyesters for bone surgery. *Makromol Chem.* 1981; Suppl. 5:30–41.

13. Li S and Vert M, Biodegradation of aliphatic polyesters, in *Biodegradable Polymers, Principles and Applications,* Scott G and Gilead D, Eds., Chapman & Hall, London, 2002, pp. 43–87.

14. Bathia SR and Tew GN, PLA-PEO-PLA hydrogels: Chemical structure; Self-assembly and Mechanical properties, in *Biodegradable Polymers and Materials: Principle and Practice*, 2nd ed., Khemani K and Scholz C, Eds., ACS Symposium Series 1114, 2012, pp. 313–324.

15. Marois Y, Zhang Z, Vert M, Deng X, Lenz RW, Guidoin R, Mechanism and rate of degradation of polyhydroxyoctanate films in aqueous media: A long term in vitro study. *J Biomed Mater Res.* 2000; 49:216–224.

16. Williams SF and Martin DP, Applications of PHAs in medicine and pharmacy, in *Biopolymers for Medical and Pharmaceutical Applications*, Steinbüchel A and Marchessault RH, Eds., Wiley-VCH Verlag, Weinhein, Germany, 2005, pp. 89–126.

17. Unverdorben M, Schywalsky M, Labahn D, Hartwig S, Laenger F, Lootz D, Behrend D et al., Polyhydroxybutyrate (PHB) biodegradable stent-experience in the rabbit. *Am J Cardio.* 1998; 82:5S–5S, Special Issue: SI.

18. Ray JA, Doddi N, Regula D, Williams JA, Melveger A, Polydioxanone (PDS), a novel monofilament synthetic absorbable suture. *Surg Gynecol Obstet.* 1981; 153:497–507.

19. Zhu KJ, Hendren RW, Jensen K, Pitt CG, Synthesis, properties and biodegradation of poly(trimethylene carbonate). *Macromolecules.* 1991; 24:1736–1740.

20. Johnson PA, Luk A, Demtchouk A, Pate H, Sung HJ, Treiser MD, Gordonov S et al., Interplay of anionic charge, poly(ethylene glycol), and iodinated tyrosine incorporation within tyrosine-derived polycarbonates: Effects on vascular smooth muscle cell adhesion, proliferation, and motility. *J Biomed Mater Res Part A.* 2010; 93A:505–514.

21. Baluca EG, N-Substituted monomers and polymers, patent no. US 20080112999, Appl. Oct. 2007.

22. Erdmann L and Uhrich KE, Synthesis and degradation characteristics of salicylic acid-derived poly(anhydride-esters). *Biomaterials.* 2000; 21:1941–1946.

23. Jabara R, Chronos N, Robinson K, Novel fully bio-absorbable salicylate-based sirolimus-eluting stent. *EuroIntervention.* 2009; 5 Suppl. F:F58–F64.

24. Heller J and Gurny R, Polyorthoesters, in *Encyclopedia of Controlled Drug Delivery* Vol. II, Mathiowitz E, Ed., John Wiley, New York, 1999, pp. 60–71.

25. Gopferic A, Biodegradable polymers: Polyanhydrides, in *Encyclopedia of Controlled Drug Delivery* Vol. I, Mathiowitz E, Ed., John Wiley, New York, 1999, pp. 60–71.

26. De Jaeger R and Gleria M, Polyorganophosphazenes and related compounds: Synthesis, properties and applications. *Prog Polym Sci.* 1998; 23:179–276.

27. Brodsky B, Werkmeister JA, Ramshaw JA, Collagen and gelatins, in *Biopolymers for Medical and Pharmaceutical Applications* Vol. 2, Steinbüchel A and Marchessault RH, Eds., Wiley-VCH Verlag, Weinhein, Germany, 2005, pp. 791–826.

28. Peter MG, Chitin and chitosan from animal resources, in *Biopolymers for Medical and Pharmaceutical Applications* Vol. 1, Steinbüchel A and Marchessault RH, Eds., Wiley-VCH Verlag, Weinhein, Germany, 2005, pp. 419–512.

29. Draget KI, Smidsrod O, Skjäk-Braek G, Alginates from algae, in *Biopolymers for Medical and Pharmaceutical Applications* Vol. 1, Steinbüchel A and Marchessault RH, Eds., Wiley-VCH Verlag, Weinhein, Germany, 2005, pp. 235–298.

30. Kundu B, Kurland NE, Bano S, Patra C, Engel FB, Yadavalli VK, Kundu SC, Silk proteins for biomedical applications: Bioengineering perspectives. *Prog Polym Sci.* 2014; 39:251–267.

31. Tsuji H, Polylactides, in *Biopolymers for Medical and Pharmaceutical Applications* Vol. 1, Steinbüchel A and Marchessault RH, Eds., Wiley-VCH Verlag, Weinhein, Germany, 2005, pp. 183–232.

32. Vert M, Polyglycolide and copolyesters with glycolide, in *Biopolymers for Medical and Pharmaceutical Applications* Vol. 1, Steinbüchel A and Marchessault RH, Eds., Wiley-VCH Verlag, Weinhein, Germany, 2005, pp. 159–182.

33. Inkinen S, Hakkarainen M, Albertsson A-C, Södergard A, From lactic acid to poly(lactic acid) (PLA): Characterization and analysis of PLA and its precursors. *Biomacromolecules.* 2011; 12:523–532.

# Lactic acid-based polymers in depth

MICHEL VERT AND ANTOINE LAFONT

Among the various polymers and polymeric compounds known as degradable that are involved in the search for suitable time-limited therapeutic applications [1], lactic acid-based polymers are the most frequently appearing in scientific and patent literatures. The potential of these polymers is primarily due to chirality that provides exceptional possibilities to reach the compromises imposed by the multiple criteria that have to be respected if clinical use is the goal.

The use of the abbreviation PLA frequently found in literature is inappropriate because there is not one lactic acid-based polymer but many of them which can be referred to as PLAs [2]. Like any polymer, PLAs' properties depend on molecular mass, molecular mass distribution, and processing history. However, they also depend on many other factors.

## ORIGINS OF THE MULTITUDE OF PLAS

### The synthesis route

Like polyesters in general, lactic acid-based polymers can be synthesized by polycondensation, i.e., by formation of ester links between the alcohol and the carboxylic acid function present in the lactic acid molecule. In general, this route does not lead to high molecular mass macromolecules and thus corresponding polymers are rather weak, though that high molecular mass lactic acid-based polycondensates have been reported in the literature [3]. The use of PLAs obtained by the polycondensation route has not been prospected for biomedical applications yet.

The route to make high molecular mass PLAs with exploitable mechanical properties is referred to as ring opening polymerization (ROP) of cyclic dimers of lactic acid named lactides as shown below. PLAs of this type are actually polydimers since two lactyl units are added to a growing chain as shown below:

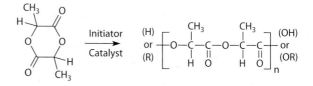

Whereas PLA-type macromolecules made by polycondensation are terminated by an OH function at one chain end and a COOH one at the other end, those made by ROP have one of the chain ends that bears a residue of the initiator or of the catalyst, at least basically. A great number of compounds can initiate the ROP of lactides [4]. However tin octoate and zinc lactate are predominant in the literature of biomedical applications. In the case of tin octoate, hydrophobic residues of the initiator or of the catalyst are present at one end or as pollutants and resulting polyesters are rather hydrophobic [5]. In contrast, zinc lactate and zinc metal lead to lactyl end units similar to those of polycondensates. This particularity leads to PLAs that are more hydrophilic. Hydrophilicity also depends on the presence of unreacted monomer and of additives and impurities [6,7]. Nature is an outstanding chemist in the sense that she is able to synthesize biopolymers repeatedly that have the same molecular mass (isomolecular), the same structure, and the same bioactivity. Thus far, polymer chemists are not able to make isomolecular artificial polymers. Polymers are always made of macromolecules of different length and thus different molecular mass whose values depend on the techniques used to determine them. Some techniques count the macromolecules, others weigh them. Counting leads to a number average molecular mass (Mn) whereas weighting leads to a mass average molecular mass (Mw). The ratio Mw/Mn is called polydispersity, a factor that reflects the broadness of molecular mass heterogeneity. Most polymer properties depend asymptotically on the molecular mass of the forming macromolecules to become independent in the high molecular mass range. In general, to correctly identify a polymer, polydispersity must be provided at the top of molecular mass, composition and presence of residual monomer and other present small molecules. Molecular mass and polydispersity command the number of chain ends. The influence of chain ends is generally ignored in literature because high molecular mass polymers are generally considered as to which contributions of chain ends are very small with respect to the rest of the macromolecules. Accordingly the effects of chain ends on most of the properties are negligible, except on hydrolytic degradation as we will see later on. Syntheses and major properties of PLA polymers have been recently reviewed extensively [8].

## The chirality

There are not one but two lactic acids that have the same chemical reactivity but opposite rotatory effects on a plane polarized light. These molecules are mirror images and thus are similar in terms of chemistry: this is what is called chirality. In the case of polycondensation, a feed composed of the sole L- or D-enantiomer leads to homopoly(L-lactic acid) and homopoly(D-lactic acid), respectively. Historically, L and D were used to distinguish the configurations (localization of subtituents of the central carbon atom in the space) of the two lactic acid isomers relative to a standard chiral simple molecule, namely the glyceraldehyde enantiomer that rotates the plane polarized light clockwise that was given a D-configuration. The use of L- and D-relative configurations is an old, confusing, and often incorrect method of specifying configurations which was devised in the early years of the twentieth century by Emil Fischer, a German organic chemist who worked extensively with carbohydrates [9]. Later on, chemists selected the use of S and R referred to as absolute configurations according to the Cahn, Ingold, and Prelog convention [10]. Despite its unsuitability, the use of D and L in the case of old chemicals remains traditional with correspondences S = L and R = D for L and D in the particular case of lactic acid enantiomers. When two enantiomers are combined, their chirality leads to various chiral lactide diastereoisomers, namely L-lactide derived from two L-lactic acid molecules, D-lactide derived from two D-lactic acids, and meso-lactide derived from one L- and one D-lactic acid molecule. There is also a racemic mixture of L- and D-lactides known as racemic lactide.

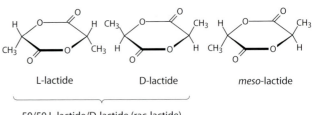

L-lactide        D-lactide        meso-lactide

50/50 L-lactide/D-lactide (rac-lactide)

Basically the ring opening polymerization of a feed composed of L- or D-lactides leads to poly(L-lactide) and poly(D-lactide), respectively, that are similar to homopoly(L-lactic acid) and homopoly(D-lactic acid) when chain ends are OH and COOH. In the case of racemic lactide, meso-lactide and unbalanced mixtures of racemic lactide in favor of one of the diastereoisomers, the pair addition leads to macromolecules with different configurational structures. Macromolecules derived from racemic lactides are enriched in pairs of similar configurations (isotacticity) whereas those derived from meso-lactide are enriched in pairs of opposite configurations (syndiotacticity). Mixtures of poly(L-lactide) and poly(D-lactide) can form a polymeric racemate referred to as stereocomplex. Table 2.2.1 shows the schematic representation of the various unit distributions depending on the monomer feed together with abbreviations. This table clearly emphasizes that abbreviations frequently found in literature like PLLA and PDLLA are acceptable for poly(L-lactide) and the stereocopolymer derived from the 50/50 mixture of L- and D-lactides improperly known as racemic polylactide, but they do not reflect the differences between unit distributions in macromolecules derived from the meso-lactide or involved in the stereocomplex that are also composed of 50% L- and 50% D-lactyl units. This is the reason why a more indicative mode of abbreviating was proposed many years ago which is based on the indication of the percentage X of L-units in lactic acid-based PLA macromolecules [11]. PLLA becomes PLA100, PDLA becomes PLA0. Stereocopolymers are thus PLAX and indices $i$, $s$ for preferentially isotactic and preferentially syndiotactic, respectively, can be added when necessary to distinguish similar gross compositions with different unit distributions. The index $c$ can be used to indicate the presence of stereocomplexed segments. Chain configurations can be distinguished at the level of the ester

Table 2.2.1 Feed-dependent unit distributions and abbreviations of lactic acid-based polymers obtained by ring opening polymerization

| Monomer feed | Abbreviation(s) | Distribution of chiral units |
| --- | --- | --- |
| L-lactide | PLA100 (PLLA) | -LLLLLLLLLLLLLLLLLLLLLL- |
| D-lactide | PLA0 (PDLA) | -DDDDDDDDDDDDDDDDDDDD- |
| 50/50 L/D lactides | PLA50i (PDLLA)[a] | -LLDDLLDDLLLLDDDDLLDD- |
| meso-lactide | PLA50s (PDLLA)[a] | -LDDLDLLDLDDLDLDLLDLD- |

[a]  These two polymers have the same gross composition in L- and D-lactyl units but different unit distribution along the chains and thus different macroscopic properties, including degradation. The use of the PDLLA abbreviation does not reflect the difference and thus is confusing.

carbon atom resonances observed in $^{13}$C NMR spectra at approximately 150–160 ppm [12].

Many PLA stereocopolymers with other chiral unit distributions and chain ends can be obtained depending on the polymerization mechanism. The interest of these PLAs is primarily academic. More important is the fact that unit distributions that depend on the monomer feed and on the mechanism of polymerization can be dramatically modified when PLA sterocopolymers are processed above 120°C because of transesterifaction reactions that cause unit interchanges.

This detailed analysis of the most important particularities related to chirality clearly shows that the PLA family provides outstanding possibilities to tune structural and material properties, possibilities adopted remarkably by nature for biopolymers.

## The morphology

Combined with the general effects of molecular mass, molecular mass polydispersity, and chirality-related configurational structures, morphology is a factor that conditions PLAs' properties. PLA-type polymers and stereocopolymers are primarily linear polymers that are more or less stereoregular as indicated previously. To exemplify the complexity of chain structure-morphology dependence, let us consider some lactic acid-based stereocopolymers with similar gross composition, namely 50/50 L/D. Such stereocopolymers can be made from racemic lactide and from *meso*-lactide, by stereoselective polymerization of racemic lactide, and also by stereocomplexation of poly(L) and poly(D) homopolymers. Basically, the first two are amorphous; the third one will be likely semicrystalline depending on the length of the stereoblocks, whereas the last one is highly crystalline with a high melting temperature (~240°C). Crystallinity is generally observed for macromolecules rich in L-units (or D-units). In the case of PLAX stereocopolymers, crystallinity increases from X = 92 to X = 100. However, the morphology of semicrystalline PLAs depends on quenching and annealing and thus on processing conditions, as for any crystalline polymer.

For thermoplastic polymers like PLAs, the glass transition temperature (Tg) that reflects the reversible passage between glassy (rigid) and rubbery (deformable) solid states must be as high as possible if rigidity and shape preservation are required. Tg is related to the amorphous phase and its value for lactide-based homopolymers and stereocopolyesters in the solid state is in the range of 55°C–60°C, depending on chirality, on how data are collected, and on how the polymer is processed (annealed or quenched). Significant decreases are observed when the polymers are in contact with water which is a plasticizer, i.e., a small molecule that decreases Tg. Tg conditions phenomena like relaxation and creeping, two critical phenomena for applications that require shape retention under mechanical stresses as it is the case for a degradable scaffold that is in a particular liquid environment at 37°C and must stay rigid under these conditions. The crystalline zones present in a matrix made of semicrystalline PLAs contribute to rigidity when a sample is submitted to fast cyclic deformations like those caused by heartbeats. However, fast deformation below Tg when the polymer is rigid can be the source of cracking and breaking. This is the reason why the deployment of a PLA-based stent must be conducted slowly.

## The hydrolytic degradation

The hydrolysis of a polyester chain depends on the local concentration in water and also on the presence of catalysts such as bases or acids. The cleavage of ester bonds generates more and more acidic and alcoholic chain ends. As a result, the matrix is more and more hydrophilic and the rate of ester cleavage increases according to a phenomenon named "autocatalysis." Typically, once a device made of a lactic acid-based polymer is in contact with an aqueous medium, water penetrates more or less rapidly and the hydrolytic cleavage of ester bonds starts. The local acidity increases in the bulk and hydrolysis speeds up. For a time, the partially degraded macromolecules remain insoluble in the outer medium and thus stay entrapped in the matrix. There is no mass loss. However, as soon as partially degraded macromolecules become soluble, diffusion starts from the surface to the outer aqueous phase.

In the case of PLAs, solubility in the outer aqueous medium, especially body fluids, appears when oligomeric degradation by-products become small enough. The device loses weight and a gradient of acidity is formed in the bulk because soluble fragments entrapped well inside continue to generate acidity and cause a faster degradation inside. Sometimes, a residual outer membrane appears with a void inside [13].

To summarize, the whole process depends on several factors: (1) the amount of absorbed water molecules initially absorbed that depends on the hydrophobicity of the matrix (the rate of water absorption being rather rapid with respect to the rate of ester cleavage); (2) the rate of ester cleavage that depends on the structure of macromolecules; (3) the rate of diffusion of macromolecular degradation products through the hydrated matrix provided a gradient of concentration is established by the products soluble in the outer medium, and (4) the solubility of these degradation products in the receiving medium, a factor that depends on the affinity of degradation b-products for the medium. Any phenomenon that can affect one or several of these main factors will affect degradation characteristics too. A number of such factors have been identified. Let us mention molecular mass, polydispersity, presence of acid or base or impurities, outer medium, chirality, and so on, including chain ends. Hydrolysis occurs preferentially in amorphous domains and thus crystallinity increases. Degradation-resistant crystalline residues can even appear during the degradation of an initially amorphous matrix [13,14]. Shape and size of an object are also important. The smaller the size, the slower the degradation rate is [15]. The degradation characteristics and thus the lifetime of a device are defined provided the polymer is pure and in the absence of other influencing factors. Let us mention hydrophobic chain ends or additives and drugs or other compounds such as residual monomer, solvent, or catalyst as possible modifying factors [13].

Basically, a highly pure PLLA (PLA100) polymer made of high molecular mass macromolecules with low polydispersity is highly crystalline and thus resists degradation for many years, especially if the size is small [11]. However, the factors mentioned previously can affect these intrinsic properties. This is one of the reasons to have so many discrepancies regarding the material characteristics and lifetimes one can find in the literature associated to the abbreviation PLA in the absence of more precise identification.

This rapid survey of structural and degradation particularities justifies the outstanding potential of the PLA family to provide thermoplastic degradable materials going from rapidly degraded wax to very rigid long-lasting solids.

## WHICH PLAS ARE BASICALLY SUITABLE TO MAKE A DEGRADABLE AND BIORESORBABLE STENT?

To make a biomedical device exploitable for a particular application, it is essential to consider the list of specific requirements, including biological ones [16,17]. Such a list is composed of two classes of criteria referred to as biocompatibility and biofunctionality, the latter including material-related properties and exploitation-related properties.

Insofar as biocompatibility criteria are concerned, polymers are rather inert unless macromolecules or surfaces include ionic or interactive functional groups to interact and trigger the defenses against foreign bodies [18,19]. Problematic biological responses can appear when macromolecules are soluble, especially polyelectrolytes (charged macromolecules) than can interact with blood charged elements and body fluids proteins and perturb cell membranes. Other sources of perturbing compounds are degradation when macromolecule fragments are small enough to become soluble, and small molecules or ions present as additives or pollutants when they diffuse up to body fluids. From a general viewpoint, polymers with no chemical function or group susceptible of reacting with biological entities like PLAs are biocompatible. This statement is supported by many applications and tests in humans [20–23]. Basically, similar comments are valuable for immunogenicity unless immunogenic residues or pollutants issued from biopolymers are released. In the case of artificial polymers, regardless whether they are degradable or biostable, there has been no report of mutagenic actions unless a mutagenic pollutant or drug is present and released. Absence of thrombosis is a more severe criterion because blood coagulation can be triggered by charged surfaces and macromolecules via the coagulation cascade or by the complement activation after deposition of opsonins. It is then an adverse reaction.

Insofar as material-related properties are concerned, proportion and distribution of chiral units have minor influence on mechanical characteristics at body temperature that is rather far below their Tg. It is not the case when a lactic acid-based polymeric matrix is in contact with an aqueous medium or with a body fluid. The latter is more like a mixture of an organic solvent with water than water. In pure and salted aqueous medium, the absorbed water plays a plasticizing role that increases with degradation. On the other hand, some lipophilic elements present in body fluids can be absorbed and cause Tg decreasing. In parallel, these elements can increase the hydrophobic character of the matrix and act against water uptake as it is the case when hydrophobic drugs are dispersed therein as solid solution. Resistance to heat is important when a PLA-type matrix is processed at high temperature (above ~180°C). Heat can change the unit distribution via transesterification reactions, increase the hydrophilicity because of chain cleavage, and decrease because of average molecular masses. Generation of lactide is also possible if catalyst residues are present than can help thermic backbiting (degradation inverse of polymerization). *In vivo*, physico-chemical properties (temperature, pH, ionic strength, presence of proteins and other chemicals) of local fluids (blood, lymph, vitreous, bile, extracellular liquids, etc.) are imposed. Furthermore, tissue healing is based on a series of events, namely inflammation that promotes activation of local tissue reconstruction machinery (cells and growth factors) and leads to consolidation followed by remodeling and finally restoration of normal and functional tissue as much as possible [18]. The duration of the whole process depends on the tissue. More time to heal is necessary for a bone fracture than for a soft tissue injury.

As for exploitation-related properties, PLA-type polymers, especially amorphous ones, can absorb water slowly from a humid atmosphere which can cause slow hydrolytic degradation that results in undesired aging. Rearrangements of more or less oriented chain conformation, a phenomenon referred to as chain relaxation, can occur very slowly below Tg to affect dimensions and stability on storage. Sterilization is also a source of problems because there is a risk of fast deformation (above Tg) and thermal degradation if heat is used. In the case of radiation-based sterilization, severe decreases of molecular mass are observed and cross-linking has been suggested. Sterilization by cold plasma seems to be the best characteristic-respecting process with very small molecular weight decreases although some surface functionalization may change protein adsorption.

Many companies are trying to take advantage of the versatility of lactic acid-based polymers to make degradable stents. To be suitable as a source of bioresorbable scaffold, a member of the PLA family has to provide solutions to corresponding specific requirements that are listed in Table 2.2.2 with main issues.

Several companies have reached the First-in-Man trial level with bioresorbable scaffolds made of lactic acid-based polymers. Different strategies are under way. Some are based on PLLA with lactic acid-based polymer or copolymer coating used to deliver an antiproliferative drug locally

Table 2.2.2 Requirements and issues specific faced by a PLA candidate to bioresorbable stenting

| Requirements | Issues |
|---|---|
| Suitable polymer | Hydrolytically degradable |
| Biocompatibility | With arterial tissues and blood |
| Design | Strut thinness |
| Processing | Moulding vs. extrusion + laser cutting |
| Sterilization | Respect of molecules, shape and size |
| Crimping on a balloon | No relaxation |
| Crimping stability | High Tg or sheath |
| Circulation up to the heart | Flexibility |
| Deployment | Shape memory or ballooning |
| Absence of recoil (size stability) | High Tg or locking |
| Radial strength | Suitable material and design |
| Scaffolding duration | Match the restoration cell machinery |
| Bioresorbability | Mineralization to $H_2O$ and $CO_2$ or kidney filtration |
| Stability on storage | Packaging under dry atmosphere |
| Cost | Social security limits |

(Abbott's BVS [23]; Elixir medical's DeSolve BRS [24]); or without (Tamai's stent [25]). ART selected a strategy based on the PLA98 stereocopolymer without coating [26]. Blends of copolymers with coating + drug are also under investigation (Huuan Biotechnology's Xinsorb BRS [27]). Abbott's BVS 150 μm received CE mark approval in 2011, Elixir Medical's Desolve BRS 150 and 100 μm in 2013 and 2014, respectively, and ART's pure BRS in 2016. The mechanical and physical properties and the safety from strut fracture of side branch and post-dilatation strategies were compared drug eluting 150 μm BVS and 100 μm BRS scaffolds were compared. Both stents recoiled after deployment, the DESolve enlarged between 10 mins and 1 hour returning to the immediate postdeployment diameter ("self-correction"). In 3.0 mm stents/scaffolds, the main branch postdilatation safe threshold without fracture for ABSORB was 3.8 mm at 20 atm and 5.0 mm for DESolve. For side branch dilatation with a 3.0 mm noncompliant balloon, the threshold before the ABSORB fractured was 10 atm whereas the DESolve did not fracture at 22 atm. The safe threshold for mini-kissing balloon postdilatation in 3.0 mm scaffolds/stents with 3.0 mm noncompliant balloons was 5 atm for the ABSORB whereas the DESolve did not fracture up to 20 atm [28].

Only Abbott's second generation BVS is now at the commercial level with struts composed of PLLA (PLA100) [29] coated by a thin layer of PDLLA (PLA50) loaded with Everolimus as antiproliferative drug. The company found solutions to most of the requirements listed in Table 2.2.2. However, the approximately 2-year scaffolding time is considered too long and over-expending is still problematic.

The possibility to take advantage of configuration-dependent degradation of PLA50, PLA75, and PLA92 stereocopolymers to vary the scaffolding functional period was previously demonstrated in the rabbit model [30]. More recently, it was shown that an experimental drug-free stent based on PLA98 was able to dismantle after approximately 3 months in the pig animal model [31]. For arterial tissue, the required scaffolding time is assumed to be 3 months.

## THE RESPONSE OF ARTERIAL REMODELLING TECHNOLOGIES (ART)

As soon as 1992, researchers at the origin of ART decided to take advantage of lactic acid stereocopolymers in attempt to fulfil the requirements specific to the development of a drug-free bioresorbable stent up to the clinical level [30–32]. A long-term interdisciplinary program led to the ARTDIVA First-in-Man trial started in July 2013 with promising results recently reported [33].

Briefly, the scaffolding provided by the ART bioresorbable stent was intended to be transitory and provide radial force, avoid acute recoil, and release the cage effect as soon as 3 months. As previously recalled, mechanical properties of semicrystalline lactic acid-based aliphatic polyesters at body temperature are rather independent of the composition provided that the polymer is not plasticized by too much absorbed water and/or by the presence of residual small molecules or degradation by-products, and/or by a too broad molecular mass dispersity. In the case of the ART stent, the material requirements, the trend of polymers to relax (recoil in the case of a stent), and early dismantling at 3 months were obtained by selecting a 98% L/2% D lactic acid stereocopolymer (PLA98) associated with an optimized protocol that includes particular polymer synthesis, design, moulding + laser cutting, crimping, and macromolecule-respecting sterilization stages. The observed faster degradation with respect to PLLA results from the presence of chain structural defects due to the few D-lactyl units inserted between PLLA segments that generate sites of preferential chain cleavage by local hydrolysis with decrease of molecular mass and thus increase of end groups and inner acidity. Some concerns are sometimes raised about more or less dramatic effects due to acidity on the basis of some dramatic effects reported many years ago [34]. Actually, body fluids are efficient buffers and the release of degradation by-products is very slow, except in the case of rapidly degrading polyesters. In animals as well as in humans acute recoil was comparable to that of a metallic stent (Vision, Abbott) [26]. Moreover, one of the requests of a polymeric scaffold is the ability to be over-expanded like a standard metallic stent permits. The ART scaffold can be over-expanded by 25%, i.e., deployed from 3 to 4 mm without any fissures or fractures with a 30-day control showing a persistent deployment without recoil. This performance can be explained by the greater proportion of amorphous domains in PLA98 than in PLLA, thus giving some reserve to further overstretch with respect to oriented annealed crystalline domains.

Two major simultaneous studies showed that the artery after balloon angioplasty was healed at 3 months in humans [35,36]. Therefore, at this time, the "cage" effect of the scaffold can be progressively suppressed to give back flexibility to the remodelling artery. Early dismantling and late recoil observed in preclinical studies are two of the original features of the ART scaffold. It has already been shown that early dismantling did not result in late loss but in late gain starting at 6 months in a porcine coronary artery [26].

The degradability, the bioresorbability, and the biocompatibility of PLA-type polymers are now proved by many applications in humans, including for the PLA98 stereo-copolymer [37]. Although the hydrolytic degradation of lactic acid-based polymers depends on many factors that can speed up or slow down the degradation rate of PLLA taken as reference, the PLA 98 scaffold is expected to degrade completely between 18 and 24 months leaving no foreign residues thus reducing the need for extended dual antiplatelet therapy [31]. Altogether, the choice of the polymer and suitable processing and conditioning provided a device with early mechanical properties comparable to those of a standard metallic device with the advantage of degradation and bioresorption periods adapted to take advantage of the healing and the remodeling properties of a coronarian artery.

## CONCLUSION

Lactic acid enantiomers appear as outstanding precursors to make hydrolytically degradable macromolecular polymer with different composition, chirality, unit distribution, morphology, and hydrolytic degradation characteristics. Combining all these factors appears as a means to approach a suitable compromise to meet the requirements of bioresorbable stenting in coronarian interventional cardiology on the basis of a drug-free strategy. This does not preclude extension to drug elution in combination with proper coating. Longer-term investigation is still necessary.

## REFERENCES

1. Piskin E, Biodegradable polymers in medicine, in *Biodegradable Polymers: Principles and Applications*, 2nd ed., Scott G, Ed., Kluwer Academic Publishers, Dordrecht, the Netherlands, (2002), pp. 321–378.
2. Vert M, Lactic acid-based polymers, in *Handbook of Biodegradable Polymers*, Bastioli C, Ed., SmithersRapra, UK, (2015), Chapter 9.
3. Kimura Y, Molecular, structural, and material design of bio-based polymers, *Polym.* (2009) 41, 797–807.
4. Kleine J and Kleine H, Unber hochmolekulare, insbesondere optische aktive polyester des milch-säure, ein beitrag zur stereochemie makromoilekularer verbindungen. *Makromol Chem.* (1959) 30, 23–38.
5. Schwach G, Coudane J, Engel R, Vert M, More about the initiation mechanic of lactide polymerization in the presence of stannous octoate. *J Polym Sci Polym Chem.* (1997) 35, 431–440.
6. Schwach G, Coudane J, Engel R, Vert M, Ring-opening polymerization of DL-lactide in the presence of zinc-metal and zinc lactate. *Polym Int.* (1998) 46, 177–182.
7. Schwach G, Coudane J, Engel R, Vert M, Zn lactate as initiator of DL-lactide ring opening polymerization and comparison with Sn octoate. *Polym Bull.* (1996) 37, 771–776.
8. Inkinen S, Hakkarainen M, Albertsson A-C, Södergård A, From lactic acid to poly(lactic acid) (PLA): Characterization and analysis of PLA and its precursors. *Biomacromolecules.* (2011) 12, 523–532.
9. Slocum DW, Surgarman D, Tucker SP, The two faces of L and D nomenclature. *J Chem Educ.* (1971) 48, 597.
10. Cahn RS, Ingold CK, Prelog V, The specification of asymmetric configuration in organic chemistry. *Experimentia.* (1956) 12, 81–94.
11. Vert M, Chabot F, Leray J, Christel P, Bioresorbable polyesters for bone surgery. *Makromol Chem.* (1981) Suppl. 5, 30–41.
12. Chabot F, Vert M, Chapelle S, Granger P, Configurational structures of lactic acid stereocopolymers as determined by $^{13}C$-$^1H$-NMR. *Polymer.* (1983) 24, 53–59.
13. Li S and Vert M, Biodegradation of aliphatic polyesters, in *Biodegradable Polymers, Principles and Applications*, 2nd ed., Scott G, Ed., Kluwer Academic Publishers, Dordrecht, the Netherlands, (2002) pp. 71–132.
14. Vert M, Bioresorbable synthetic polymers and their operation field, in *Biomaterials in Surgery*, Walenkamp G, Ed., Georg Thieme Verlag, Stuttgart, (1998), pp. 97–101.
15. Grizzi I, Garreau H, Li S, Vert M, Biodegradation of devices based on poly(DL-lactic acid): Size dependence. *Biomaterials.* (1995) 16, 305–311.
16. Vert M, Not any new functional polymer can be for medicine: What about artificial biopolymers? *Macromol Biosci.* (2011) 11, 1653–1661.
17. Vert M, Degradable polymers in medicine: Updating strategies and terminology. *Int J Artif Organs.* (2011) 34, 76–83.
18. Anderson JM, Rodriguez A, Chang DT, Foreign body reaction to biomaterials. *Semin Immunol.* (2008) 20, 86–100.
19. Babensee JE, Anderson JM, McIntire LV, Mikos AG, Host response to tissue engineered devices. *Adv Drug Deliv Rev.* (1998) 33, 111–139.
20. Vert M, After soft tissues, bone, drug delivery and packaging, PLA aims at blood. *Eur Polym J.* (2015) 68, 516–525.
21. Barber FA and Dockery WD, Long-term absorption of poly-L-lactic acid interference screws. *Arthroscopy.* (2006) 22, 820–826.

22. Tsuji H, Polylactides, in *Biopolymers: Biology, Chemistry, Biotechnology, Applications, Polyesters* III. Doi Y and Steinbüchel A, Eds., Verlag GmbH, Weinhiem, Germany: Wiley-VCH, (2002) pp. 129–178.

23. Ormiston JA, Serruys PW, Regar E, Dudek D, Thuesen L, Webster MWI, Onuma Y et al., A bioabsorbable everolimus-eluting coronary stent system for patients with single de-novo coronary artery lesions (ABSORB): A prospective open-label trial. *Lancet.* (2008) 371, 899–907.

24. Verheye S, First-in-man results with a myolimus-eluting bioresorbable PLLA-based vascular scaffold. *TCT.* 2012.

25. Nishio S, Long-term (>10 years) clinical outcomes of first-in-man biodegradable poly-l-lactic acid coronary stents. *EuroIntervention.* (2010) 6, H44.

26. Durand E, Sharkawi T, Leclerc G, Raveleau M, van der Leest M, Vert M, Lafont A, Head-to-head comparison of a drug-free early programmed dismantling polylactic acid bioresorbable scaffold and a metallic stent in the porcine coronary artery six-month angiography and optical coherence tomographic follow-up study. *Circ Cardiovasc Interv.* (2014) 7, 70–79.

27. Shen L, Wang Q, Wu Y, Xie J, Ge J, Short-term effects of sirolimus elutingfully bioabsorbable polymeric coronary stents in a porcine model. *TCT.* 2011.

28. Ormiston JA, Webber B, Ubod B, Darremont O, Webster MW, An independent bench comparison of two bioresorbable drug-eluting coronary scaffolds (Absorb and DESolve) with a durable metallic drug-eluting stent (ML8/Xpeditio). *EuroIntervention.* (2015) 11, 60–67.

29. Onuma Y, Dudek D, Thuesen L, Webster M, Nieman K, Garcia-Garcia HM, Ormiston JA et al., Five-year clinical and functional multislice computed tomography angiographic results after coronary implantation of the fully resorbable polymeric everolimus-eluting scaffold in patients with de novo coronary artery disease. *JACC Cardiovasc Interv.* (2013) 6, 999–1009.

30. Lafont A, Li S, Garreau H, Cornhill F, Vert M, PLA stereocopolymers as sources of biresorbable stents: Preliminary investigation in rabbit. *J Biomed Mater Res B Appl Biomater.* (2006) 77B, 349–356.

31. Nakano M, Pacheco E, Acampado E, Otsuka F, Sakakura K, Kolodgie F, Lafont A et al., Optical coherence tomography evaluation of a PLA bioresorbable stent in a swine coronary artery model. *J Am Coll Cardiol.* (2013) 61, E1648, Supplement: S.

32. Lafont A, Le "STENT" biorésorbable comme moyen de prévention de la resténose: Exploration à l'aide d'un modèle artériel chez le lapin. *Thèse de Doctorat de l'Université de Montpellier,* December 17, 1996.

33. Fajadet J, Carrie D, Durand E, Barragan P, Coste P, Sharkawi T, Vert M et al., ARTDIVA: A first in man evaluation of a bare Poly((D+L)-lactic acid) coronary bioresorbable scaffold. *The Lancet.* submitted, 2015.

34. Bersgma EJ, Rozema FRM, Bos RR, De Bruijn WC, Foreign body reactions to resorbable poly (L-Lactide) bone plates and screws used for the fixation of unstable zygomatic fractures. *J Oral Maxil Surg.* (1993) 51, 666–70.

35. Nobuyoshi M, Kimura T, Nosaka H, Mioka S, Ueno K, Yokoi H, Hamasaki N et al., Restenosis after successful percutaneous transluminal coronary angioplasty: Serial angiographic follow-up of 229 patients. *J Am Coll Cardiol.* (1988) 12, 616–623.

36. Serruys PW, Luijten HE, Beatt KJ, Geuskens R, de Feyter PJ, van den Brand M, Reiber JH et al., Incidence of restenosis after successful coronary angioplasty: A time-related phenomenon. A quantitative angiographic study in 342 consecutive patients at 1, 2, 3, and 4 months. *Circulation.* (1988) 77, 361–371.

37. Vert M, After soft tissues, bone, drug delivery and packaging, PLA aims at blood. *Eur Polym J.* (2015) 68, 516–525.

# Scaffold processing

JOHN J. SCANLON, JOSEPH M. DEITZEL, DIETER MAIRHÖRMANN,
AND ROLAND WÖLZEIN

Mature manufacturing processes developed for the production of plastic parts and metal stents have been successfully adapted to produce bioresorbable scaffolds. The processing conditions of a bioresorbable polymer significantly impact the mechanical properties of the scaffold and must be carefully controlled during fabrication. Composite materials that can be converted into scaffolds using similar processes are being investigated to broaden the applicability of bioresorbable scaffolds.

## POLYMERS

A scaffold is produced from a tube that is converted into a scaffold by removing portions of the tube's wall thickness with a laser that leaves behind a series of sinusoidal-shaped, interconnected rings. The crests and valleys of the adjacent rings are offset, so that the scaffold can be crimped onto a balloon catheter and delivered through the vascular lumen in a smaller profile. The resultant strut pattern is designed to allow the scaffold to be longitudinally flexible during delivery and radially stiff during the treatment time.

To understand the process of manufacturing a bioresorbable scaffold, a fundamental understanding of polymers is necessary. The workhorse polymer used to produce a bioresorbable vascular scaffold is poly(L-lactide). Poly(L-lactide) was chosen because its mechanical properties are sufficient to support a vascular lumen after percutaneous coronary intervention (PCI) and it degrades into biocompatible absorbable byproducts after the treatment time. Poly(L-lactide) can be characterized as a stiff material that provides functionality similar to durable metals.

Poly(L-lactide) is a thermoplastic homopolymer produced by polymerization of a monomer comprised of L-lactide. Polymerization is the process of converting the L-lactide monomer molecules into a polymer. A polymer is a large molecule, or macromolecule, comprised of many repeating interconnected monomer subunits. Lactide is derived from lactic acid (2-hydroxypropanoic acid), which is formed by bacterial fermentation of dextrose.

Poly(L-lactide) is produced by ring-opening polymerization using hydroxyls as initiators. The polymerized poly(L-lactide) is typically produced in the form of pellets that are converted into other shapes by extrusion, molding, or spinning processes.

The poly(L-lactide) pellets are converted into new shapes by either melting or dissolving the polymer in an organic solvent so that it is transformed into a liquid phase that is formable. Poly(L-lactide) is semi-crystalline, which means it is comprised of amorphous and crystalline regions. In the crystalline region, the molecules are tightly packed and exhibit long-range positional order in three dimensions. In the amorphous region, the molecules are entangled with only short-range order. When the polymer is melted or dissolved, the molecules comprising the polymer become mobilized and can slide past each other, which allows the polymer to be reconfigured into a new shape. As the polymer cools or the solvent evaporates, the molecules become frozen in their newly molded shape.

During processing the molecules orient in the direction of flow. If solidification occurs before the molecules are fully relaxed to their state of equilibrium, molecular orientation is locked into the formed part. The orientation introduces anisotropic, nonuniform shrinkage and mechanical properties in the directions parallel and perpendicular to the direction of flow.

The crystallinity of poly(L-lactide) is primarily dependent on its thermal history. When the polymer is held at a crystallization temperature, polymer crystals begin to form and grow until they impinge on one another. These crystals can adopt a number of characteristic morphologies dependent on the processing conditions. These include chain folded lamella (solution grown), extend chain (high pressure or high shear), and spherulites (melt processing). The spherulitic morphology is most commonly seen in melt processed materials. As depicted in Figure 2.3.1, stacks of lamellar crystals grow in time from individual nuclei and radiate outward in three dimensions forming spheres called spherulites [1]. As illustrated, in semi-crystalline polymers

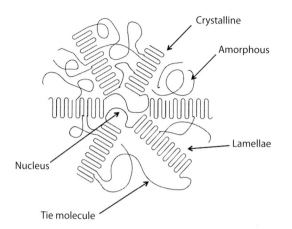

Figure 2.3.1 Spherulite [1].

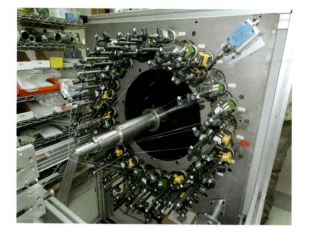

Figure 2.3.2 Microbraiding machine. (Photograph provided by HARTLON LLC [USA].)

fractions of the polymer remain uncrystallized and the amorphous polymer becomes trapped between the growing crystals. It is common for long chain molecules to meander in and out of the lamellae, which are plate-like crystals. The meandering molecules are referred to as tie-molecules.

The crystallinity of the polymer can be modified during the cooling of the melted polymer or by heating an amorphous polymer to the crystallization temperature until crystals form. Poly(L-lactide) spherulitic morphology is generally observed at temperatures above the glass transition temperature but below about 145°C. At higher temperatures, a smaller amount of spherulites are formed due to a decrease in nucleation density. This leads to larger spherulites. It is believed that the optimum crystallization temperature for poly(L-lactide) is in the range of 100°C–130°C [2]. It has also been observed that cooling poly(L-lactide) from a melt produces larger spherulites than heating an amorphous polymer to the crystallization temperature. It is believed that smaller spherulites produce stronger scaffolds.

The crystalline regions are rigid and the amorphous regions are flexible. Semicrystalline polymers can be tough with the ability to bend without breaking. Polymer scaffolds are strengthened by molecular orientation. After extruding or molding the tube used to produce a scaffold, the tube's wall thickness is stretched to increase its diameter and length [3]. The tube is stretched at conditions above the glass transition temperature of the polymer. Above the glass transition temperature, the polymer molecules are mobile so that their position can be rearranged during the orientation process. The biaxial orientation is generally performed by first increasing the length of the tube to prevent the ring connectors from cracking during delivery followed by increasing the diameter of the tube to increase radial strength during the treatment time. The orientation process moves the crystalline and amorphous regions so that they are aligned in the direction of deformation and frozen in this position when the polymer is cooled below the glass transition temperature. The glass transition temperature of poly(L-lactide) is about 60°C–65°C, which is well above the body temperature of 37°C so that the scaffold is dimensionally stable in its deployed size under physiological conditions.

Polymer orientation increases the strength of a polymer but decreases its ductility [4]. The reduced ductility limits the amount a polymer scaffold can be expanded in diameter during deployment. To achieve the same level of ductility as a durable metal stent, the scaffold would be expandable in diameter during deployment by 40%–50% [5]. To increase the ductility of the scaffold wall thickness, producing the scaffold of a composite including fiber instead of an extruded or molded wall thickness is being investigated. Fibers having high tensile strength are formed into a scaffold wall thickness by microbraiding, as shown in Figure 2.3.2, and electrospinning processes.

Poly(L-lactide) is resorbed by first undergoing scission of the tie-molecules in the amorphous region. The crystalline regions are less prone to absorb water than the amorphous regions so they are resorbed later [6]. The scission of the tie-molecules results in a reduction in scaffold strength. To obtain dimensional and mechanical stability during storage and the treatment time, it is important to achieve the optimum balance of amorphous and crystalline regions in the semicrystalline polymer during the production of the scaffold. Since the last heating and cooling cycle determines crystallinity of the scaffold, the sequence of manufacturing operations wherein the polymer experiences temperatures above the glass transition temperature is carefully managed.

## EXTRUSION

Extrusion is used to produce simple parts of a single profile like a rod or tube. Scaffolds are produced from rigid, extruded tubes. Extrusion is a manufacturing process in which a melted polymer is forced to flow through a die orifice to produce a long continuous product whose cross-sectional shape is determined by the shape of the orifice. Polymer pellets stored in a hopper are gravity fed into the rear of the barrel of the extruder. Inside the barrel a rotating screw conveys the polymer pellets forward, heating the pellets until they transform into a pressurized, viscous liquid that is forced at a constant flow rate through the annular orifice of the die. A circular orifice having a mandrel centered in the opening forms the tubular shape as the melt flows through the die. The mandrel is held in position by supports that bridge the gap between the outer surface of the mandrel and the inner surface of the die. The melt flows around the supports when passing through the orifice to reunite in a monolithic tube wall. The mandrel commonly includes an air channel through which air is blown to maintain the hollow form of the extrudate during hardening. After exiting the die, the extrudate is cooled as it is pulled through a sealed water bath, which is maintained under a vacuum to keep the newly formed tube from collapsing until the polymer is at a temperature below its glass transition temperature [7]. The outer surface of the extruded tube is smooth to avoid abrasion of the anatomical lumen during diastole and systole.

Since poly(L-lactide) is sensitive to hydrolytic, thermal, and mechanical degradation during processing, special steps are taken to preserve the degree of polymerization. One precaution is to dry the polymer to low moisture content prior to processing. Another preservation step is to process the polymer at temperatures slightly above the melting temperature to lower the melt viscosity to reduce shear stress during extrusion. Finally, the air blown through the mandrel filling the hollow space in the tube can be replaced with an inert gas like nitrogen to minimize oxidation–degradation of the polymer.

## MOLDING

Injection molding is used to make complex and intricate parts formed of polymer. The polymer is melted and forced to flow under high pressure into a mold cavity where it solidifies. On cooling, the molded part is removed from the cavity. A part is typically produced in 10–30 seconds, but sometimes a cycle time of one or more minutes is required. The mold may contain multiple cavities to improve productivity. A mold requires a large capital investment, so injection molding is generally limited to parts produced in large quantities. The injection molding process is comprised of two components. The injection unit operates like an extruder by melting and delivering polymer to the mold. Like an extruder, pellets of polymer are gravity fed from a hopper into the barrel where a screw rotates to transfer the pellets through a melting zone toward the mold. The screw of the injection unit is different than an extruder in that it moves right and left laterally to meter and inject polymer into the mold. The clamping unit opens and closes the mold during each injection cycle. The clamping unit holds two mold halves in proper alignment and keeps the mold closed with sufficient clamping force to resist the injection force. When multiple parts are molded a hot runner mold is used to convey melted polymer from the injection nozzle to two or more cavities. A mold includes water channels within the wall thickness of the mold to cool the melt to a solid [7]. Molds must be designed to account for part shrinkage as the polymer molecules crystalize and reach a new state of equilibrium during solidification.

Blow molding is a molding process in which hot air pressure is used to inflate softened plastic in a mold cavity. Blow molding is useful for making one-piece hollow plastic parts like bottles. A blow molded part is formed by first forming a starting tube called a parison through extrusion or injection molding and then inflating the parison to the desired shape. Extrusion blow molding consists of extruding the parison, pinching the parison at the top and sealing the bottom around a metal blow pin as the two mold halves come together, inflating the tube to take the shape of the mold cavity, and opening the mold to remove the solidified part. Injection blow molding consists of injection molding a parison around the metal blow pin, opening the injection mold and transferring the parison to a blow mold, inflating the parison to conform to the cavity of the blow mold, and opening the blow mold to remove the solidified part. Stretch blow molding consists of first injection molding a parison, elongating the parison by pushing the blow pin against the bottom of the parison, inflating the parison to conform to the cavity of the blow mold, and opening the blow mold to remove the solidified part [7].

## SPINNING AND MICROBRAIDING

A fiber is a long, thin strand whose length is many times its cross-sectional thickness. Incorporating fibers into the wall thickness of a scaffold is an experimental concept for increasing the strength of a scaffold. Subjecting the fibers to hot or cold drawing to align the crystal structure along the direction of the lengthwise axis strengthens fibers. Drawn fibers are typically elongated by 2–10 times their originating length. Stretching the fiber between two spools where the winding spool is rotating faster than the unwinding spool performs drawing.

Spinning produces bioresorbable fibers. The term spinning is a holdover from methods used to draw and twist natural fibers into yarn or thread [8]. For bioresorbable fibers, spinning means extruding a polymer melt or solution through a spinneret and then drawing the extrudate. A spinneret is a die with multiple orifices. There are four variations of spinning: (1) melt spinning, (2) dry spinning, (3) wet spinning, and (4) electrospinning.

Melt spinning consists of the steps of squeezing a melted polymer through a circular orifice in a spinneret, drawing the extrudate from a thicker to a thinner cross-sectional thickness and a shorter to longer length, and cooling the polymer so that it resolidifies. Wet spinning consists of the steps of producing a polymer solution by dissolving the polymer in a volatile solvent, extruding the polymer solution through a circular orifice in a spinneret, drawing the extrudate from a thicker to a thinner cross-sectional thickness and a shorter to longer length, and solidifying the polymer by evaporating the solvent. Dry spinning consists of the steps of producing a polymer solution by dissolving the polymer in a nonvolatile solvent, extruding the polymer solution through a circular orifice in a spinneret, drawing the extrudate from a thicker to a thinner cross-sectional thickness and a shorter to longer length, and solidifying the polymer by immersing the fiber in a nonsolvent that coagulates or precipitates the polymer into fibers.

Electrospinning is a process by which submicron diameter fibers, as shown in Figure 2.3.3, are produced through use of an electrostatically driven jet of polymer solution or melt [9]. A standard lab scale approach fundamentally consists of the steps of: (1) delivering the polymer liquid to the tip of a spinneret at a fairly slow rate (~mL/h) resulting in the formation of a pendent droplet and (2) application of an electric potential (5–30 kV) between the spinneret tip and grounded collector. In the presence of the applied electric field, the shape of the pendent drop deforms into that of a cone first described in detail by Taylor [9]. When the electric field strength at the tip of this cone exceeds a critical value, a jet of polymer is ejected and proceeds toward the nearest grounded target. The charged, continuous jet of liquid polymer streams from the cone toward the collecting surface, initially in a straight line, but transitions into a sinusoidal whipping action before reaching the collector. The amplitude of this lateral instability is influenced by number of solution/melt variables such as dielectric constant, surface tension, and viscosity [10]. In the case where a polymer melt is being spun, solidification occurs through cooling. When fibers are electrospun from a polymer solution, the solvent evaporates leaving a solid filament on the collection plate.

A wide variety of modifications to the basic spinning setup described here exist [11]. To increase productivity, commercially available electrospinning machines have been developed that replace the nozzle with a cylindrical-shaped electrode that rotates through a bath of liquefied polymer. In this case, the applied electric field distorts the surface of the liquid layer on the drum inducing the formation of large numbers of jets simultaneously, which can be collected on a grounded target of choice (drum, mandrel, conveyor belt, etc.).

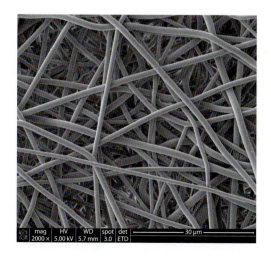

**Figure 2.3.3** Electrospun bioresorbable nanofibers. (Photograph provided by NANOFIBER SOLUTIONS [USA].)

Nanofibers are of interest because theoretically over 150 discrete fibers can be layered into the wall thickness of a strut. The small diameter of these filaments provides a specific surface area that can be as much as two orders of magnitude higher than conventional polymer fibers, providing greater interaction between the reinforcing fibers and the polymer matrix. Furthermore, electrospun membranes can be produced with uniaxially oriented filaments through a number of ways, including collection on a high speed drum, use of electrostatic lens to control deposition [9,10,12], or through use of solvents with low dielectric constants to minimize the lateral bending instability described earlier. Such unidirectional fabrics enable optimization of fiber orientation in a composite. Based on the details of the electrospinning setup, these fibers can be aligned in the wall thickness perpendicular to the scaffold lengthwise axis, obliquely, or in a nonwoven configuration to achieve the desired mechanical properties, such as strength, stiffness, and coefficient of thermal expansion (CTE). These fabrics can be incorporated into composites using standard processing techniques such as hand lay-up, resin infusion, and pultrusion among others. The nanoscale morphology of these fibers is also of interest in producing a scaffold because smaller poly(L-lactide) fibers degrade by hydrolysis slower than larger samples do [13].

Producing a fiber from a solution has several advantages over melt spinning. One advantage is that ultra high molecular weight polymers (Mw $>10^6$ g/mol) can be converted into dilute solutions suitable for spinning into high strength fibers. Starting with an ultra high molecular weight polymer can offset the partial reduction of molecular weight obtained during scaffold sterilization. Polymers can lose as much as 78% of their viscosity-average molecular weight after gamma sterilization [14]. Moreover, ultra high molecular weight polymers tend to have a ductile failure rather than the brittle failure mode found in low molecular weight polymers [15]. The low viscosity solution processing performed at room temperature also preserves molecular weight because the polymer experiences less degradation related to thermal, hydrolytic, and shear stresses [16]. Polymers can lose as much as 66% of their viscosity-average molecular weight after extrusion and drawing [14]. Finally, the dilute solutions tend to separate and detangle molecular chains so that they can be more easily extended in length and oriented to increase the tensile strength and elastic modulus during drawing of the fiber along its lengthwise axis [16]. Fiber produced from solution spun, hot drawn poly(L-lactide) has been produced having an increase in tensile strength from 40 MPa to 2.3 GPa [16]. Therefore, under the right conditions poly(L-lactide) fiber can be produced having tensile strength that is competitive with metal alloys used in durable stents. For example, cobalt-chromium L605 has a tensile strength of >1000 MPa and platinum-chromium has a tensile strength of 834 MPa [17].

There is a greater potential to improve the mechanical properties of a polymer in the form of a fiber than in the form of a tube because larger draw ratios are possible in the form of a fiber. The tensile strength of a melt spun, hot drawn poly(L-lactide) fiber is increased from about 40 MPa to 530 MPa when having a draw down ratio of about 10 and increased to about 200 MPa when having a draw down ratio of about 4 [18]. Likewise, the Young's modulus of elasticity of a melt spun, hot drawn poly(L-lactide) fiber is increased from about 3.5 GPa to about 9.0 GPa when having a draw down ratio of about 9 and increased to about 5.5 GPa when having a draw down ratio of about 4 [19]. Tubes suitable for use in the production of a scaffold have physical limitations that prevent an expansion ratio above 4. For example, a 3 mm inner diameter tube having an expansion ratio of 4 would have a parison having an inner diameter of 0.75 mm prior to expansion. Because fibers can be processed without physical constraints, there is more opportunity to increase the mechanical properties of a fiber.

Spun fibers typically have a thickness in the range of 5 to 50 microns. The fibers are formed into tubes by braiding. For easier handling, the thinner fibers are braided in bundles of 5 to 10 fibers. Interlacing about 10 to 20 fibers obliquely aligned in the tube's wall thickness forms a 3–5 mm diameter tube. Some of the fibers run from the upper left to lower right and the other fibers run from the upper right to lower left when the tube is viewed from its side. Electrospun nanofibers have a thickness in the range of about 200 nm to about 1 micron. Nanofibers are configured in the shape of a tube by directly depositing the nanofiber or by wrapping sheets of nanofiber around a cylindrical-shaped mandrel and interconnecting the sheets with seams.

Reproducing the exceptional mechanical properties of melt-spun, hot drawn or solution-spun, hot drawn poly(L-lactide) fiber in electrospun poly(L-lactide) nanofiber is challenging. In many cases, existing data show that the mechanical properties of electrospun nanofiber are inferior to the bulk polymer [20]. The reasons for this are most likely related to insufficient molecular orientation due to the absence of post-drawing processes, residual solvent in the polymer, and fiber porosity [20]. Positive mechanical property improvements have been demonstrated by alignment of nanofiber in mats followed by annealing [20].

Although nonisotropic fibers have relatively high tensile strength, they have the drawback of low compressive strength and are extremely flexible due to their high aspect ratio. This means that tubes comprised solely of fiber without a matrix exhibit excellent resistance to forces applied during expansion by a balloon catheter but they have insufficient crush resistance to provide support during the treatment time. The fibrous tubes are stiffened to increase crush resistance by increasing the crystallinity of the fibers, filling the void space between the fibers with a bioresorbable matrix material, and/or by interconnecting the nanofiber at crossover points. Increasing the crystallinity by annealing of unconstrained fibers at temperatures over the glass transition temperature of the polymer may reduce the molecular orientation imparted on the fiber during previous drawing operations [21].

## STRUT PATTERN CUTTING

A scaffold is created from a polymer tube by laser micromachining a strut pattern in the tube's wall thickness. Laser cutting of metal implants like stents using a thermal process has been in use since the early 1990s and commonly used for cutting stainless steel, cobalt-chromium, and platinum-chromium stents. Since bioresorbable polymers have a melting temperature in the range of 170°C–230°C, thermal laser cutting damages the material. Recently, in response to the material change, the industry has developed a cold laser cutting process suitable for cutting bioresorbable scaffolds.

The laser cuts a strut pattern in the tube by focusing a laser beam on the tube during cutting, as shown in Figure 2.3.4. The laser beam delivery and the motion system, which moves the tube under the laser beam, are mounted on a high precision granite base to isolate the cutting process from ambient vibrations that could impact cutting accuracy. High precision multidirectional axes move the tube under the laser during machining. Lasers do not touch the tube during machining. The laser following computer generated instructions machines a strut pattern in the tube by focusing a laser beam on the tube. The design of the scaffold is modeled using computer aided design/computer aided manufacturing (CAD/CAM) software. Separate software adds laser specific details like cut sequence, pierce holes, destroy cuts, and finally converts the information into cutting instructions which are uploaded into the laser machinery in preparation for converting the tube into a scaffold comprised of a series of sinusoidal-shaped rings separated by connectors.

To avoid changes in the mechanical properties of polymer tubes during cutting, scaffolds are produced using a cold laser cutting process that imparts no thermal damage to the polymer. Excessive generation of heat during cutting can reduce the molecular weight and change the crystallinity of the polymer. To minimize heat generation, ultra-short pulse lasers are employed. Ultra-short pulse lasers have pulses in the range of 300–800 femtoseconds and

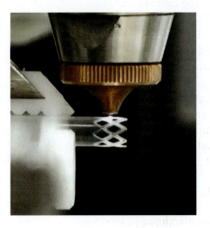

Figure 2.3.4 Laser machining bioresorbable scaffold. (Photograph provided by ROFIN-BAASEL LASERTECH GmbH [Germany].)

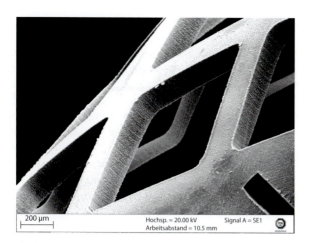

**Figure 2.3.5** Precision cut by ultra-short pulse, femtosecond laser. (Photograph provided by ROFIN-BAASEL LASERTECH GmbH [Germany].)

wavelengths ranging from about 500–1100 nm. As a general rule, lasers can cut features about 10–15 wavelengths in size. Therefore, a laser has the capability of easily cutting a precise strut pattern in a tube having strut width less than 100 microns.

Femtosecond laser ablation is a multi-photon absorption process. The laser converts the polymer from a solid into a gas during ablation. As the laser machines the tube, the polymer in the cutting area is vaporized in the form of a plasma plume producing no debris other than the small sections that are cut out between the rings and connectors. As shown in Figure 2.3.5, the laser beam creates a smooth cut in the wall thickness without producing micro-cracks that could potentially propagate through the wall thickness as the scaffold expands and contracts during systole and diastole pulsatile pressures for over 18 million cycles during the treatment time.

Since the width of the scaffold struts is typically less than 160 microns, the tubes must have low dimensional variation. In general, to successfully cut a strut pattern the tubes should be as round as possible having the highest concentricity. Wall thickness variations should not be less than 20 microns. If the tubes are elliptical in shape or not sufficiently straight, the strut width will have unacceptable variations and this will finally influence the mechanical properties of the scaffold.

Industrially proven ultra-short pulsed lasers with pulse durations of several hundred femtoseconds are readily available. Recently, hybrid-MOPA-configuration lasers combining fiber and rod laser technology are available and have been commercially introduced providing the right average power levels, repetition rates, and robustness to cope with industrial cutting speeds in a 24/7 production environment.

## CONCLUSION

Mature manufacturing processes used to produce metal stents and other products have been successfully adapted to produce bioresorbable scaffolds comprised of polymers. The first generation, commercial bioresorbable scaffolds have relatively thick struts and the clinical application is limited to relatively simple lesions [22,23]. Further refinement of manufacturing processes to preserve the degree of polymerization during scaffold formation and sterilization may lead to more a versatile bioresorbable scaffold. Experimentation with composite scaffolds employing fibers as reinforcements and/or bioresorbable fillers as stiffeners may also contribute to development of more versatile bioresorbable scaffolds in the future.

## GLOSSARY

**Amorphous:** A polymer where the molecules are oriented randomly and are intertwined, much like cooked spaghetti.

**Annealing:** A process of heating and cooling a plastic part slowly to relieve the stress introduced into the part during manufacturing processes (e.g., extruding, molding).

**Blow molding:** A manufacturing process for producing hollow parts.

**Braiding:** A manufacturing process comprising interweaving three or more strands of fiber.

**Composite:** A combination of two or more distinct materials, each of which retains its own distinctive properties, to create a new material with properties that cannot be achieved by any of the components acting alone.

**Crystalline:** A portion of a polymer where the molecules are arranged closely and in a discernible order.

**Degree of polymerization:** The number of monomeric units in a molecule of a polymer.

**Drawing:** A manufacturing process that uses tensile forces to stretch a polymer to impart orientation on the polymer.

**Ductility:** A measure of a material's ability to undergo appreciable plastic deformation before fracture; it is usually expressed as percent elongation in a tensile test.

**Elasticity:** The property of complete and immediate recovery of a material from an imposed displacement on release of the load.

**Extrusion:** A manufacturing process for producing parts of a fixed cross-sectional profile, where polymer is pushed through a die of the desired cross-section to form a continuous object.

**Glass transition temperature:** The reversible transition in amorphous materials (or in amorphous regions within semicrystalline materials) from a hard and relatively brittle "glassy" state into a molten or rubber-like state, as the temperature is increased.

**Hydrolysis:** Chemical decomposition of a material in which the compound is split into other compounds by reacting with water.

**Injection molding:** A manufacturing process for producing discrete parts by injecting polymer into a mold.

**Matrix:** A continuous material that connects one or more reinforcements in a composite material; generally the reinforcement is much stronger and stiffer than the matrix.

**Molecular orientation:** A process of aligning molecular chains in a specific direction, which results in higher strength in the direction of orientation and lower strength perpendicular to the direction of orientation.

**Molecular weight:** The mass of a molecule, which is calculated as the sum of the mass of each constituent atom multiplied by the number of atoms of that element in the molecular formula.

**Monomer:** A chemical compound that can undergo polymerization.

**Morphology:** The arrangement of molecules in a polymer on a large scale.

**Polymer:** A chemical compound that is made of small molecules that are arranged in a simple repeating structure to form a larger molecule.

**Polymerization:** A chemical reaction in which two or more molecules combine to form larger molecules that contain repeating structural units.

**Screw:** A device that feeds polymer in the form of pellets, granules, flakes, or powders from a hopper into the barrel of the extruder; the material is gradually melted by the mechanical energy generated by the turning screw and by heaters arranged along the barrel.

**Semicrystalline:** A polymer including amorphous and crystalline portions.

**Spinning:** A manufacturing process for creating polymer fibers that employs a specialized form of extrusion that uses a spinneret to form multiple continuous filaments.

**Tensile strength:** The resistance of a material to breaking under tension.

**Thermoplastic:** A material capable of softening when heated and of hardening again when cooled.

**Young's modulus of elasticity or elastic modulus:** A measure of an elastic material's stiffness.

# REFERENCES

1. Dietzel J, Kleinmeyer D, Harris D, Tan N, The effect of processing variables on the morphology of electrospun nanofibers and textiles. *Polymer.* 2001, 42, 8163: 261–272.
2. Sun Z, Deitzel J, Knopf J, Chen X, Gillespie J, The effect of solvent dielectric properties on the collection of oriented electrospun fibers. *J Appl Appl Polym Sci.* 2012, 125, 2585–2594.
3. Yao J, Bastiaanesen C, Peijs T, High strength and high modulus electrospun nanofibers. *Fibers.* 2014, 2, 158–187.
4. Penning J, Dijkstra H, Pennings A, Preparation and properties of absorbable fibres from L-lactide copolymers. *Polymer.* 1993, 34, 5: 4, Figure 3.
5. Zang X, *Fundamentals of Fiber Science, Part III, Fiber Properties,* Chapter 15, Mechanical properties of fiber, Lancaster, PA: DEStech Publications, 2014: 288–289.
6. Henton D, Gruber P, Lunt J, Randal R, Polylactic Acid Technology, In *Natural Fibers, Biopolymers, and Biocomposites,* Taylor & Francis, 2005: 558.
7. Nuutinen JP, Cleric C, Reinikainen R, Törmälä P, Mechanical properties and in vitro degradation of bioresorbable self-expanding braided stents. *J Biomater: Sci Polym Edn.* 2003, 14, 3: 263.
8. Venkatraman S, Poh TL, Vinalia T, Mak KH, Boey F, Collapse pressure of biodegradable stents. *Biomaterials.* 2003, 24, 12: 2107.
9. Agrawal CM, Haas KF, Leopold DA, Clark HG, Evaluation of poly (L-lactic acid) as a material for intravascular polymeric stents. *Biomaterials.* 1992, 13, 3: 177–178.
10. Penning J, Dijkstra H, Pennings A, Preparation and properties of absorbable fibres from L-lactide copolymers. *Polymer.* 1993, 34, 5: 4, Figure 1.
11. Kereiakes D, What's important in a stent? Flexibility and conformity in the synergy stent and Absorb BVS. *Cath Lab Digest.* 2013, 1, 3: 1.
12. Dzavik V, Colombo A, The absorb bioresorbable vascular scaffold in coronary bifurcations, insights from bench testing. *JACC Cardiovasc Interv.* 2014, 7, 1, ISSN 1936-8798: 82.
13. Foin N, Sen S, Di Mario, Davies JE, Stent maximal expansion capacity with current DES platforms: A critical factor for stent selection during treatment of left-main bifurcations? *EuroIntervention.* 2013, 8, Supplement N: 1.
14. Foin N, Lee R, Torii R, Guiterrez-Chico J, Matteshini A, Nijjer S, Sen S, Petraco R, Davies J, Di Mario C, Joner M, Virmani R, Wong, Impact of stent strut design in metallic stents and biodegradable scaffolds. *Int J Cardiol.* 2014: 6, Table 6.
15. Park S, Park K, Yoon H, Son J, Min T, Kim G, Apparatus for preparing electrospun nanofibers: Designing an electrospinning process for nanofiber fabrication. *Polym Int.* 2007, 56, 11: 1361–1366.
16. Deitzel J, Kleinmeyer J, Hirvonen J, Tan N, The effect of processing variables on the morphology of electrospun nanofibers and textiles. *Polymer.* 2001, 42: 261–272.
17. University of South Carolina Upstate, Polymer Chemistry, www.uscupstate.edu/academics /arts_sciences.
18. Kariduraganavar M, Arjumand K, Ravindra K, Polymer synthesis and processing, natural and synthetic biomedical polymers. *Nat Synth Biomed Polym.* 2014, Chapter 1: 25–26.
19. Gueriguian V, Gale D, Huang Bin, Fabricating a stent from a blow molded tube, U.S. Patent No. 7,829,008, filed May 30, 2007: 1–5.
20. Groover M, *Fundamentals of Modern Manufacturing: Materials, Processes, and Systems,* 4th Edition, Chapter 13: Shaping Processes for Plastics, Section 13.14, Fiber and Filament Production (Spinning), Hoboken, NJ: John Wiley & Sons, Inc., 2010, ISBN 978-0470-467008: 284.

# Basics of magnesium biodegradation

MICHAEL HAUDE, DANIEL LOOTZ, HUBERTUS DEGEN, AND MATTHIAS EPPLE

## INTRODUCTION

Magnesium was identified in the eighteenth century and its first samples produced on an industrial scale were used for pyrotechnical applications and flashlights of the upcoming photographic industry [1,2]. Owing to its low specific weight (30% lighter than aluminium) and the relatively high strength and stiffness, magnesium has become the third most commonly used structural metal after iron and aluminium, with the main application in the automotive, aerospace, and lightweight electronics industry. As a non-noble metal, magnesium is reactive and has poor corrosion resistance, especially in aqueous solutions containing chloride ions [3].

The ability of magnesium to corrode in a saline environment, such as body fluids, has attracted interest in bioabsorbable magnesium implants that can temporarily assist in wound healing after cardiovascular, musculoskeletal, or general surgery [1]. The explorations started approximately in 1878, when Edward C. Huse ligated bleeding blood vessels with magnesium wires [1]. In the next decades, several designs of magnesium tubes, plates, sheets, screws, fixtures, and woven wires were tested as sutures, osteosynthetic devices, and intestine, vessel, or nerve connectors [1,4]. Although they exhibited favorable biocompatibility and full bioabsorption, magnesium implants have not reached commercial application, mainly due to the inability to control the fast degradation rate [1]. The interest in this biomaterial subsided in the 1980s and was rekindled in the 1990s when new magnesium alloys were developed for improved corrosion and mechanical properties.

The first generation of magnesium alloy-based scaffolds for cardiovascular interventions, manufactured by BIOTRONIK AG (Bülach, Switzerland), underwent clinical investigation between 2003 and 2006 [5,6]. The scaffold design was thereafter optimized in several ways [7–9]. The key modification was the addition of the BIOlute coating composed of the bioresorbable poly-L-lactic acid (PLLA) polymer matrix loaded with the antiproliferative drug sirolimus [7,9]. This chapter provides the fundamental information on the resorption of magnesium.

## MAGNESIUM FROM A MATERIAL SCIENTIFIC PERSPECTIVE

### Basic information

Magnesium is an essential nutrient for humans, animals, and plants. Magnesium salts, which make up to 17% of sea salt, are released to the atmosphere as sea spray. The general population is exposed to magnesium compounds via inhalation of ambient air, ingestion of food and drinking water, and dermal contact with compounds and consumer products containing magnesium compounds.

Magnesium is essential for many biological processes in the human body. For example, at the molecular level, magnesium is required as a cofactor for a large number of enzymes and has a key function in regulating the concentration of $Ca^{2+}$ and other molecular signaling pathways.

Increased serum magnesium levels resulting from excessive intake of magnesium are reduced via excretion of magnesium through the kidney. There is no indication that a moderate intake of magnesium supplements is problematic.

However, an insufficient intake of magnesium can be a health issue since it increases the risk for a large number of diseases. One example is coronary artery disease. Low magnesium levels increase the incidence and mortality of this disease by promoting inflammatory processes in the artery wall and thrombogenesis. Increased magnesium level is thought to have the opposite effect and suppress inflammation [10].

Magnesium is essential for human health and is involved in most if not all processes in the human body [11]. The biological role of magnesium involves supporting function of more than 600 enzymes, binds to DNA and ATP, and is regulating signaling processes as an antagonist to $Ca^{2+}$. The signaling process is relevant for understanding how magnesium acts as a vasodilator and may also be involved in mediating the anti-inflammatory function [12].

The endothelium is located at the interface between the blood and the vessel wall and an important function is to provide a nonchromogenic environment and to influence inflammatory reactions. Defective functioning of the endothelium is a key process in the pathogenesis of atherosclerosis and thrombosis [13].

Many studies in animal models and humans have shown that magnesium suppresses inflammatory processes [14,15] in the endothelium. As a result, magnesium reduces the risk of coronary artery disease [16–18].

Magnesium acts as a vasodilator [19] and this may explain why certain magnesium levels reduce blood pressure [20] and potentially reduce the risk of myocardial infarction in humans. The mechanism of magnesium in vasodilatation is probably linked to its inhibitory effects on $Ca^{2+}$ signaling, a cascade that regulates vasodilatation in vascular smooth muscle cells.

In addition to the fact that magnesium is involved in preventing inflammation, the vasodilator function provides an additional explanation why sufficient magnesium is important for reducing the mortality of coronary artery disease.

## Metallic magnesium structure

With the atomic number 12 and the density of 1.74 g/cm³, magnesium is the lightest of all structural metals and has good casting capabilities, making it attractive for handling during manufacture or use. Magnesium mostly serves as an alloying agent. Two key features of solid magnesium dominate the physical metallurgy of its alloys: (1) the hexagonal crystal lattice structure (Figure 2.4.1) and (2) the atomic diameter (0.320 nm) facilitating solid solubility of magnesium with a plethora of solute elements that have a similar (±15%) atomic diameter. Due to the hexagonal crystal structure, magnesium alloys are much more workable at elevated temperatures, whereas room temperature allows only mild deformations around generous radii.

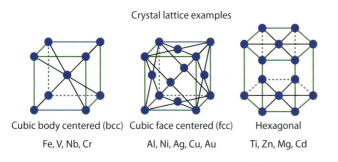

Crystal lattice examples

Cubic body centered (bcc)    Cubic face centered (fcc)    Hexagonal
Fe, V, Nb, Cr                Al, Ni, Ag, Cu, Au           Ti, Zn, Mg, Cd

Figure 2.4.1 Schematic representation of crystal structure of metallic elements.

## Magnesium alloys

Alloying elements, such as aluminum, calcium, manganese, rare earth elements, yttrium, zinc, and zirconium, are added to pure magnesium to adjust the mechanical properties (e.g., strength, hardness) and physical characteristics (e.g., degradation rate) of magnesium-based implants [21]. The designation system of magnesium alloys is following the nomenclature of the American Society for Testing and Materials (ASTM) and uses a letter-figure combination indicating the two major alloying components and their (rounded) relative contribution to the material weight. Compared with pure magnesium, the magnesium alloy used for the BIOTRONIK scaffold offers higher creep (deformation) resistance and high-temperature stability, in combination with excellent mechanical properties, a 12-month degradation process, and light weight [21–24].

The detailed metallurgical and metal physical reasons for the use of various components in magnesium alloys have been described in the literature [25,26]. An increasing amount of an alloying element added to the bulk material usually increases proportionally the specific physical or mechanical effect of this element [4,26]. There are many possibilities for alloy composition and processing, resulting in various microstructure-property relationships and in great differences in the strength, ductility, creep resistance, and resorption time of the alloy [4,21]. A wide range of mechanical properties can be obtained by varying the working environment the scaffold is made in [26].

Magnesium alloys contain impurities, such as iron, copper, or nickel. The amounts of trace elements depend on the alloy's composition, the technology for production, and the progress in alloy development [21]. For biomedical applications, impurities have to be strictly controlled and kept minimal. Numerous standardization documents issued by the ASTM (e.g., B90/B90M, B107/B107M) and the International Standards Organisation (ISO) (e.g., 3116) cover the structure, composition, mechanical testing, and corrosion testing of magnesium-based material.

## Corrosion of magnesium-based materials

Corrosion means the degradation of metals by chemical surface reactions with aggressive components of the environment. Only noble metals are immune to corrosion under normal conditions. For other metals and their alloys, the chemical reaction with oxygen is spontaneous and exergonic, i.e., it involves a net gain in free enthalpy of the metal/environment system [27]. Corrosion mechanisms of magnesium and its alloys have been thoroughly investigated for a variety of applications, including aerospace, automotive, transportation, and medical implant technology [3,24].

In nature, magnesium occurs only in combination with other elements. The free element can be produced artificially and is highly reactive. Once produced, magnesium is coated with a thin layer of oxide, which partly inhibits its reactivity. In humid conditions, magnesium oxide transforms into magnesium hydroxide ($Mg(OH)_2$). In aqueous electrolytes, corrosion of magnesium alloys is dominated by anodic magnesium dissolution and cathodic water reduction, according to [21]:

$$Mg(s) \rightarrow Mg^{2+}(aq) + 2e^- \quad \text{(anodic reaction)}$$

$$2\,H_2O(aq) + 2e^- \rightarrow 2\,OH^-(aq) + H_2(g) \quad \text{(cathodic reaction)}$$

$$Mg^{2+}(aq) + 2\,OH^-(aq) \rightarrow Mg(OH)_2(s) \quad \text{(production formation)}$$

Magnesium hydroxide serves as a corrosion protective layer in water, but when the chloride concentration rises, magnesium hydroxide starts to convert into highly soluble magnesium chloride, promoting pitting corrosion. Magnesium and its alloys are highly susceptible to microgalvanic corrosion because impurities like iron, copper, and nickel are known to form efficient cathodic centers for galvanic corrosion, increasing the corrosion rate to more than 50 times that of pure magnesium [3,21–23,28]. The accompanying hydrogen evolution can form gas cavities which are of potential concern for orthopedic implants in tissues with a low diffusion coefficient of hydrogen [1,21,28]. Although necessary to modify physical properties of the implants, most alloying elements are, like impurities, susceptible to microgalvanic corrosion [24,28].

Corrosion pits during exposure of the magnesium alloy to saline solution are believed to be related to the galvanic coupling between the magnesium matrix and rare earth containing intermetallic compounds or secondary or impurity phases [3,21–23]. Not only the distribution and elemental composition of the grain structure, but also the surface conditioning of the implant material by mechanical, chemical, electrochemical (e.g., polymeric coating), physical (e.g., ion implantation and deposition), and thermal-oxidation methods is of significant importance for the resorption behavior of the BIOTRONIK scaffold and worth of optimization [3,4,22,24,29–31].

In addition to the materials characteristics, the reaction depends on environmental conditions [3,21,28]. To simulate the *in vivo* environment, the material can be immersed in physiological solutions such as simulated body fluids, Hank's buffered solution, artificial blood plasma, and other electrolyte media [3,23]. Other influential factors are

- The buffering system (e.g., HEPES) used to regulate the pH value of the physiological solution [4,23].
- The presence of inorganic ions. For example, chloride ions accelerate the reaction by breaking down the protective oxide/hydroxide layer, while phosphate ions retard it by the precipitation of insoluble phosphate salts [4].

- The presence of proteins and other organic molecules that can slow down the whole process by building a protective layer around magnesium [4,21,22,32].
- Temperature, as it can influence the absorption of proteins onto the material surface and some other mechanisms of the biological response [21,22].
- The mechanical stress, since material exposed to different kinds of mechanical loads, including tension, compression, and fluid sheer stress, may change 10 times faster than unstressed material [21].
- The flow of electrolyte that can slow down or accelerate corrosion by influencing the deposition of corrosion products, by taking away locally generated $OH^-$ ions, by modifying local pH value, and by bringing the oxygen onto the metal surface [21,22].

*In vitro* tests are simple and helpful for material screening, quality control, and studying degradation mechanisms [4,22,23]. However, magnesium degradation is faster *in vitro* than *in vivo* by several orders of magnitude, and *in vitro* test findings are not directly transferable to human patients [32]. This is explained by the presence of proteins, blood flow, ions, and a specific pH. Also, the contact of the implanted device with the tissue and with blood cells can influence the corrosion rate by providing a passive protective layer for the implant and by altering local metabolic processes [22].

Because of the different *in vitro* methodologies, the magnesium corrosion rate can vary greatly between tests and should always be carefully verified by *in vivo* studies [21] such as mass loss measurement, scanning electron microscopy (SEM) analysis, and energy dispersive x-ray (EDX) analysis performed on a retrieved sample from a sacrificed animal [4,33].

## THE DEGRADATION PROCESS *IN VIVO*

The use of resorbable magnesium alloys as medical implant materials requires extended knowledge of their degradation in biological environments in order to ensure biocompatibility, the mechanical integrity, and the disintegration of implants. Many publications are available on the physiological resorption of magnesium implants (i.e., *in vitro* degradation), yet only a few focus on the characterization of explanted materials [3,24,28,34–37].

### Magnesium metabolism

The human body contains 22–26 g of magnesium, making it the eleventh most abundant element in the Earth's crust by mass and the fourth most abundant cation (metallic element) in the human body [38]. The majority of magnesium (99%) is found inside cells. Most intracellular magnesium is located in bones (60% of the total volume), skeletal muscles (20%), and in other soft tissues (19%). Thirty percent of the magnesium found in bones is exchangeable and functions as a reservoir to stabilize the serum concentration [39]. The remaining 1% of magnesium that is located extracellularly is encountered in blood serum. The magnesium concentration in blood plasma is 0.7–1.1 mmol/L. The recommended daily dietary allowance in adults is 270–400 mg magnesium [40]. Magnesium is absorbed mainly in the small intestine as well as in the colon in small portions.

It is interesting to note that calcium and magnesium have antagonist roles. Indeed, the excess of calcium may partially inhibit the absorption of magnesium.

Magnesium is excreted into the digestive tract by the bile, pancreatic, and intestinal juices. There is an apparent obligatory urinary loss of magnesium, which is about 12 mg/day. The urine is the major route of excretion under normal conditions. In the blood plasma, about 65% is in ionic form while the remainder is bound to protein. Excretion also occurs in the sweat and milk [19].

During the resorption of a magnesium implant, high concentrations of magnesium can be achieved in the local microenvironment. This raises no concern because magnesium grants cardiovascular protection and is beneficial for the cells of the vascular wall, as discussed in section "Basic information" [41].

## Results from animal studies

This section summarizes the current understanding of the BIOTRONIK magnesium scaffold resorption, based on detailed analyses of samples from various studies in the porcine coronary artery model [33].

In brief, it was found that the degradation process takes place in two steps. The first step is the anodic reaction of the magnesium alloy in water, resulting in magnesium hydroxide. The second step is the conversion of magnesium hydroxide to a calcium phosphate phase via a magnesium (hydrogen) phosphate phase. Overall, by means of anions and cations exchange the reaction slowly converts the metallic alloy to a final phase consisting mainly of amorphous calcium phosphate with high water content.

The degradation process starts from the surface of the scaffold backbone. The physiological electrolytes have access to the metallic surface by diffusion through the polymeric coating. In aqueous environment, magnesium is converted into magnesium hydroxide according to:

$$Mg + 2\,H_2O \rightarrow Mg(OH)_2(s) + H_2(g)$$

Because of the low reaction rate, the hydrogen release ($H_2$) does not reach harmful concentrations; the small amount of released hydrogen is easily dissolved in the blood stream. The covering layer of magnesium hydroxide grows slowly by the proceeding degradation of the scaffold backbone.

The contact of blood and neointimal cells with the scaffold allows a slow in-diffusion of phosphate, calcium, sodium, potassium, and other ions and their precipitation in the reaction area. Hydrogen phosphate ions and calcium ions react with the magnesium oxide to form a calcium phosphate:

$$Mg(OH)_2(s) + HPO_4^{2-}(aq) + Ca^{2+}(aq) + H_2O(l)$$
$$\rightarrow Ca_x(PO_4)_y \cdot n\,H_2O(s) + H_3O^+(aq) + Mg^{2+}(aq)$$

The above reaction equation is not stochiometrically balanced, but indicates the main participating compounds because biologically precipitated calcium phosphate always contains hydrogen phosphate, carbonate, and other substituting ions like sodium, potassium, or magnesium out of the extracellular matrix.

Bowen et al. [34] have found a magnesium-substituted calcium phosphate after the *in vivo* implantation of magnesium stents into rat arteries. However, the exact identification of the calcium phosphate phase remains challenging because of its complex composition, its amorphousness, and its heterogeneity. Despite this, the given equation gives a good approximation for the experimental results.

The corrosion process may also occur via the intermediate formation of a calcium-free magnesium phosphate/magnesium hydrogen phosphate phase [42]. In this case, solid phases like $Mg_3(PO_4)_2$ and $MgHPO_4 \cdot 3\,H_2O$ may form which later convert to a less soluble calcium phosphate as indicated above. Note that magnesium which is present in the calcium phosphate phase is known to inhibit the crystallization of calcium phosphate (Figure 2.4.2) [43]; therefore, it is not surprising that the solid phase does not form crystals of calcium phosphate and remains largely amorphous, even after long-term implantation.

The formed magnesium-containing calcium phosphate is in equilibrium with its dissolution products (i.e., the corresponding ions) which may eventually lead to its dissolution in the blood stream. Depending on the perfusion conditions and the local pH, the dissolution will continue until the original scaffold material gets absorbed by the body (Figure 2.4.3) [44]. The fact that the whole degradation/conversion occurs without swelling of the implant indicates that most magnesium is rapidly diffusing from the implantation side in the early and intermediate stages of degradation. Otherwise, the degraded implant would have a strongly increased volume when converting from Mg to $Mg(OH)_2$, $Mg_3(PO_4)$, and finally to $Ca_x(PO_4)_y \cdot n\,H_2O$. This can be easily derived from a comparison of the molar volumes of these solid phases, without even taking into account the additional presence of water in the degrading implant.

Due to the relatively high concentrations of phosphate and calcium ions in body fluids, the conversion process is slow. Only a minor part of the original strut areas is converted to magnesium oxide/hydroxide after 90 days, and the complete conversion of the implanted material to an amorphous calcium phosphate with high water content requires up to 360 days. Figure 2.4.2 illustrates the degradation progress using different colors for chemical elements.

All chemical reactions occur in a complex biological environment with high water content, including ions

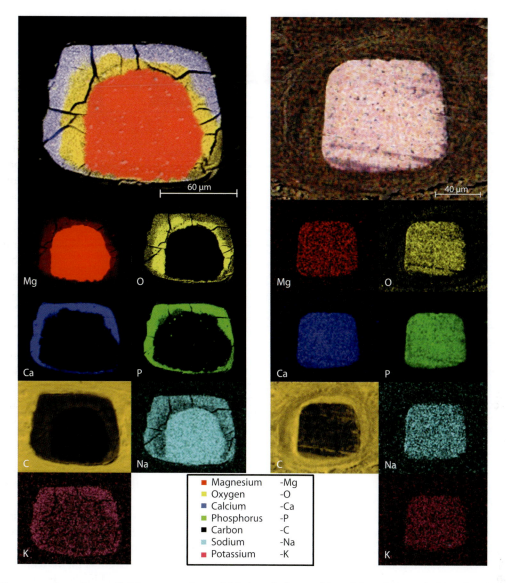

**Figure 2.4.2** Cross-section of a scaffold strut explanted 90 days (left panels) and 360 days (right panels) after a magnesium (Mg) alloy scaffold implantation in a porcine coronary artery. The degradation process and the distribution of chemical elements were visualized by energy dispersive x-ray spectroscopy combined with scanning electron microscopy. At 90 days, the *in vivo* degradation process is still ongoing and two layer zones are seen around the residual Mg alloy core. The first layer (adjacent to the core) consists mainly of an Mg hydroxide phase. The second (outer) layer contains a magnesium (hydrogen) phosphate and in later stages, an amorphous calcium phosphate. After 360 days, the elution of magnesium from the metallic backbone is largely completed in the majority of examined struts, and the former strut area is mostly filled amorphous calcium phosphate with high water content.

and biomolecules, and precise stoichiometric descriptions of the precipitated compounds can therefore not be given. In addition to the chemical processes mentioned in Figure 2.4.3 deemed to be essential for magnesium bioresorption, other reactions may occur in parallel (caused by other ions).

The thickness of the reaction layer is often not uniform because of the local character of the reaction and the comparatively uneven access of physiological fluids through the polymeric coating of the metallic surface. No debris or particles were found to be detached from the degrading struts. The original shape of the strut cross-sections was preserved,

with no obvious enlargement or swelling of the degradation products. It is important to note that the presence of amorphous calcium phosphate doesn't seem to trigger vascular calcification.

## Magnesium scaffold improvements

Based on the insights from animal studies [33,45,46] and clinical trials [6,8], the initial magnesium scaffold (AMS-1) for human coronary arteries was redesigned iteratively to achieve slower biodegradation, better scaffolding properties, and a reduction of the neointimal growth [7,47]. The

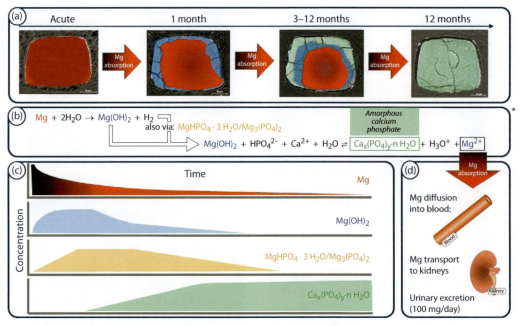

* Simplified chemical process equations

**Figure 2.4.3** Schematic presentation of the biodegradation of a coronary scaffold made of a magnesium (Mg) alloy: cross-section of the scaffold strut (panel **a**), simplified chemical equations summarizing the 12-month degradation process (panel **b**), the concentration of Mg and the key chemical compounds over time (panel **c**), and the path of Mg bioresorption (panel **d**). Mg and water corrode to Mg hydroxide, which reacts with phosphate to solid Mg (hydrogen) phosphate. Subsequently, calcium ions convert this magnesium (hydrogen) phosphate phase into an amorphous calcium phosphate.

latest generation, DREAMS 2G (known as Magmaris) [9], is made of a refined, slower-degradable magnesium alloy, and has a modified electro-polished strut cross-sectional profile ($150 \times 150$ µm$^2$) to slow down fracture and resorption [7]. The 6-crown 2-link geometrical design is used to increase radial force and bending flexibility. The scaffold is coated with the BIOlute system composed of a 7 µm thick bioresorbable PLLA polymer matrix [48,49] loaded with the potent antiproliferative drug sirolimus (1.4 µg/mm$^2$) [50]. The BIOlute system with the identical dose density and release rate of sirolimus was previously used in the commercially available Orsiro drug-eluting stent (BIOTRONIK AG) and showed excellent clinical performance [51].

## ADVANTAGES, DISADVANTAGES, AND STATUS OF MAGNESIUM-BASED IMPLANTS

Magnesium scaffolds offer good radial strength, low acute recoil, high compliance to the vessel geometry [47] and can therefore be implanted via a single-step inflation. Moreover electropolishing of magnesium scaffolds produces soft, rounded edges for good trackability, deliverability [9], and flow dynamics. On the other hand, there still is room to improve the resorption process as well as the overall strut thickness of the scaffold [47,52].

Biodegradable coronary scaffolds increasingly deliver what they promise: by offering controlled scaffolding time, the benefits of an uncaged artery and potentially by preventing late unfavorable effects such as stent thrombosis, they appear to be the obvious next step in PCI treatment [9,47].

Indisputably, the most advanced clinical applications of magnesium implants are biodegradable coronary scaffolds. Magnesium alloys have also been investigated as bone implants [3,4,21], chips for vertebral fusion in spinal surgery of sheep [53], and load bearing (open-porous) biomaterials for tissue engineering [21,54]. Although cardiovascular commercial implants containing magnesium and its alloys are still not available, the advantages and obvious benefits from biodegradable metallic implants are still the inspiration and hope of many researchers and clinicians [1,55]. Moreover, the favorable clinical performance of the Magmaris scaffold in the BIOSOLVE-II study [9] resulted in the submission for CE mark approval.

## CONCLUSION

In this chapter we provide fundamental information on the corrosion of magnesium, mostly from the perspective relevant for coronary scaffolds, currently the most advanced clinical application of magnesium implants. After implantation, magnesium is converted into magnesium hydroxide, which reacts with phosphate ions into magnesium phosphate, and, with calcium ions, into amorphous calcium phosphate with high water content. As a result, magnesium ions diffuse from the matrix and are excreted in urine. Only a minor portion of the scaffold strut areas is degraded to magnesium hydroxide after 90 days. After 360 days, the elution of magnesium from the metallic backbone is largely completed, and the strut areas are replaced by amorphous calcium phosphate with high water content. The scaffold resorption may allow uncaging of the treated coronary artery segment and restoration of the vessel wall physiology and vasomotion.

## ACKNOWLEDGMENTS

We would like to thank Dr. Dejan Danilovic and Ludovica Visciola for the assistance in manuscript preparation and Dr. Heinz Müller and Philipp Ruppelt for the assistance by characterizing the magnesium degradation.

## REFERENCES

1. Witte F. The history of biodegradable magnesium implants: A review. *Acta Biomater.* 2010;6(5): 1680–92.
2. Weeks ME. Discovery of the elements. *J Chem Educ.* 1956, 523.
3. Atrens A, Liu M, Abidin NIZ. Corrosion mechanism applicable to biodegradable magnesium implants. *Mater Sci Eng B.* 2011;176(20):1609–36.
4. Zheng YF, Gu XN, Witte F. Biodegradable metals. *Mater Sci Eng R.* 2014;77:1–34.
5. Bosiers M, Deloose K, Verbist J, Peeters P. First clinical application of absorbable metal stents in the treatment of critical limb ischemia: 12-month results. *Vasc Dis Manag.* 2005;2(4):86–91.
6. Erbel R, Di Mario C, Bartunek J, Bonnier J, de Bruyne B, Eberli FR, Erne P et al. Temporary scaffolding of coronary arteries with bioabsorbable magnesium stents: A prospective, non-randomised multicentre trial. *Lancet.* 2007;369(9576):1869–75.
7. Campos CM, Muramatsu T, Iqbal J, Zhang YJ, Onuma Y, Garcia-Garcia HM, Haude M et al. Bioresorbable drug-eluting magnesium-alloy scaffold for treatment of coronary artery disease. *Int J Mol Sci.* 2013;14(12):24492–500.
8. Haude M, Erbel R, Erne P, Verheye S, Degen H, Bose D, Vermeersch P et al. Safety and performance of the drug-eluting absorbable metal scaffold (DREAMS) in patients with de-novo coronary lesions: 12 month results of the prospective, multicentre, first-in-man BIOSOLVE-I trial. *Lancet.* 2013;381(9869):836–44.
9. Haude M, Ince H, Abizaid A, Toelg R, Lemos PA, von BC, Christiansen EH et al. Safety and performance of the second-generation drug-eluting absorbable metal scaffold in patients with de-novo coronary artery lesions (BIOSOLVE-II): 6 month results of a prospective, multicentre, non-randomised, first-in-man trial. *Lancet.* 2015.
10. Maier JA. Endothelial cells and magnesium: Implications in atherosclerosis. *Clin Sci.* 2012;122(9):397–407.
11. de Baaij JH, Hoenderop JG, Bindels RJ. Magnesium in man: Implications for health and disease. *Physiol Rev.* 2015;95(1):1–46.
12. Lin CY, Tsai PS, Hung YC, Huang CJ. L-type calcium channels are involved in mediating the anti-inflammatory effects of magnesium sulphate. *Br J Anaesth.* 2010;104(1):44–51.
13. Cines DB, Pollak ES, Buck CA, Loscalzo J, Zimmerman GA, McEver RP, Pober JS et al. Endothelial cells in physiology and in the pathophysiology of vascular disorders. *Blood.* 1998;91(10):3527–61.
14. Zartner P, Buettner M, Singer H, Sigler M. First biodegradable metal stent in a child with congenital heart disease: Evaluation of macro and histopathology. *Catheter Cardiovasc Interv.* 2007;69(3):443–6.
15. Kum CH, Cho Y, Young YK, Choi J, Park K, Seo SH, Park YS, Ahnb DJ, Han DK. Biodegradable poly (l-lactide) composites by oligolactide-grafted magnesium hydroxide for mechanical reinforcement and reduced inflammation. *J Mater Chem B.* 2013;1(21):2764–72.
16. Abbott RD, Ando F, Masaki KH, Tung KH, Rodriguez BL, Petrovitch H, Yano K, Curb JD. Dietary magnesium intake and the future risk of coronary heart disease (the Honolulu Heart Program). *Am J Cardiol.* 2003;92(6):665–9.
17. He K, Liu K, Daviglus ML, Morris SJ, Loria CM, Van Horn L, Jacobs DR, Jr. et al. Magnesium intake and incidence of metabolic syndrome among young adults. *Circulation.* 2006;113(13):1675–82.
18. Zhang W, Iso H, Ohira T, Date C, Tamakoshi A. Associations of dietary magnesium intake with mortality from cardiovascular disease: The JACC study. *Atherosclerosis.* 2012;221(2):587–95.
19. Klaasen CD. *Casarett and Doull's Toxicology. The Basic Science of Poisons.* 6th ed. New York: McGraw-Hill Professional; 2001, p. 843.
20. Sontia B, Touyz RM. Role of magnesium in hypertension. *Arch Biochem Biophys.* 2007;458(1):33–9.
21. Witte F, Hort N, Vogt C, Cohen S, Kainer KU, Willumeit R, Feyerabend F. Degradable biomaterials based on magnesium corrosion. *Curr Opin Solid Mater Sci.* 2008;12:63–72.
22. Kalb H. Mikroskopisches Korrosionsmodell für Magnesiumlegierungen und Grenzen der elektrochemischen Rauschanalyse (PhD Thesis in German). Erlangen-Nürnberg, Germany: Der Naturwissenschaftlichen Fakultät der Friedrich-Alexander-Universität; 2012.
23. Schrenk S. Abbauverhalten degradierbarer Magnesiumlegierungen in körperähnlichen Elektrolyten (PhD Thesis in German). Erlangen-Nürnberg, Germany: Der Naturwissenschaftlichen Fakultät der Friedrich-Alexander-Universität; 2011.

24. Kalb H, Rzany A, Hensel B. Impact of microgalvanic corrosion on the degradation morphology of WE43 and pure magnesium under exposure to simulated body fluid. *Corros Sci.* 2012;57:122–30.

25. Friedrich HE, Mordike BL. *Magnesium Technology.* Berlin, Germany: Springer-Verlag; 2006.

26. Avedesian M, Baker H. *ASM Specialty Handbook: Magnesium and Magnesium Alloys.* Materials Park, OH: ASM International; 1999.

27. Kaesche H. *Corrosion of Metals. Physicochemical Principles and Current Problems.* Berlin, Germany: Springer-Verlag; 2003.

28. Persaud-Sharma D, McGoron A. Biodegradable magnesium alloys: A review of material development and applications. *J Biomim Biomater Tissue Eng.* 2012;12:25–39.

29. Hanzi AC, Gunde P, Schinhammer M, Uggowitzer PJ. On the biodegradation performance of an Mg-Y-RE alloy with various surface conditions in simulated body fluid. *Acta Biomater.* 2009;5(1):162–71.

30. Zheng Y, Lia Y, Chen J, Zou Z. Surface characteristics and corrosion resistance of biodegradable magnesium alloy ZK60 modified by Fe ion implantation and deposition. *Progr Nat Sci Mater Int.* 2014;24:547–53.

31. Coy AE, Viejo F, Skeldon P, Thompson GE. Susceptibility of rare-earth magnesium alloys to microgalvanic corrosion. *Corros Sci.* 2010;52:3896–906.

32. Charyeva O, Feyerabend F, Willumeit R, Szakacs G, Agha NA, Hort N, Gensch F et al. In vitro resorption of magnesium materials and its effect on surface and surrounding environment. *MOJ Toxicol.* 2015;1(1):00004.

33. Wittchow E, Adden N, Riedmuller J, Savard C, Waksman R, Braune M. Bioresorbable drug-eluting magnesium-alloy scaffold: Design and feasibility in a porcine coronary model. *EuroIntervention.* 2013;8(12):1441–50.

34. Bowen PK, Drelich J, Goldman J. Magnesium in the murine artery: Probing the products of corrosion. *Acta Biomater.* 2014;10(3):1475–83.

35. Harrison R, Maradze D, Lyons S, Zheng Y, Liu Y. Corrosion of magnesium and magnesium–calcium alloy in biologically-simulatedenvironment. *Progr Nat Sci Mater Int.* 24 (2014): 539–546.

36. Kalb H, Rzany A, Hensel B. Impact of microgalvanic corrosion on the degradation morphology of WE43 and pure magnesium under exposure to simulated body fluid. *Corros Sci.* 57 (2012) 122–130.

37. Wang H, Shi Z. In vitro biodegradation behavior of magnesium and magnesium alloy. *J Biomed Mater Res B Appl Biomater.* (Aug. 2011);98B(2):203–9.

38. Swaminathan R. Magnesium metabolism and its disorders. *Clin Biochem Rev.* 2003;24(2):47–66.

39. Swaminathan R. Magnesium metabolism and its disorders. *Clin Biochem Rev.* 2003;24(2):47–66.

40. Baghurst K. *Nutrient Reference Values for Australia and New Zealand.* Australia: National Health and Medical Research Council; 2005.

41. Castiglioni S, Maier JAM. Magnesium alloys for vascular stents: The biological bases. *BioNanoMaterials.* 2015;16(1):23–9.

42. Verbeck RMH, De Bruyne PAM, Driessens, FCM, Verbeek, F. Solubility of magnesium hydrogen phosphate trihydrate and ion-pair formation in the system magnesium hydroxide-phosphoric acid-water at 25 degree C. *Inorg Chem.* 1984;23(13):1922–26.

43. Salimi MH, Heughebaert JC, Nancollas GH. Crystal growth of calcium phosphates in the presence of magnesium ions. *Langmuir.* 1985;1:119–122.

44. Seitz JM, Eifler R, Bach FW, Maier HJ. Magnesium degradation products: Effects on tissue and human metabolism. *J Biomed Mater Res A.* 2014;102(10):3744–53.

45. Heublein B, Rohde R, Kaese V, Niemeyer M, Hartung W, Haverich A. Biocorrosion of magnesium alloys: A new principle in cardiovascular implant technology? *Heart.* 2003;89(6):651–6.

46. Waksman R, Pakala R, Kuchulakanti PK, Baffour R, Hellinga D, Seabron R, Tio FO et al. Safety and efficacy of bioabsorbable magnesium alloy stents in porcine coronary arteries. *Catheter Cardiovasc Interv.* 2006;68(4):607–17.

47. Iqbal J, Onuma Y, Ormiston J, Abizaid A, Waksman R, Serruys P. Bioresorbable scaffolds: Rationale, current status, challenges, and future. *Eur Heart J.* 2014;35(12): 765–76.

48. Domb AJ, Kost J, Wiseman D. *Handbook of Biodegradable Polymers.* Boca Raton, FL: CRC Press; 1997, pp. 10–14.

49. Middleton JC, Tipton AJ. Synthetic biodegradable polymers as orthopedic devices. *Biomaterials.* 2000;21(23):2335–46.

50. Colmenarez H, Fernandez C, Escaned J. Impact of technological developments in drug-eluting stents on patient-focused outcomes: A pooled direct and indirect comparison of randomised trials comparing first- and second-generation drug-eluting stents. *EuroIntervention.* 2014;10(8):942–52.

51. Windecker S, Haude M, Neumann FJ, Stangl K, Witzenbichler B, Slagboom T, Sabate M et al. Comparison of a novel biodegradable polymer sirolimus-eluting stent with a durable polymer everolimus-eluting stent: Results of the randomized BIOFLOW-II trial. *Circ Cardiovasc Interv.* 2015;8(2):e001441.

52. Lu P, Cao L, Liu Y, Xu X, Wu X. Evaluation of magnesium ions release, biocorrosion, and hemocompatibility of MAO/PLLA-modified magnesium alloy WE42. *J Biomed Mater Res B Appl Biomater*. 2011;96(1):101–9.

53. Kaya RA, Cavusoglu H, Tanik C, Kaya AA, Duygulu O, Mutlu Z, Zengin E et al. The effects of magnesium particles in posterolateral spinal fusion: An experimental in vivo study in a sheep model. *J Neurosurg Spine*. 2007;6(2):141–9.

54. Witte F, Ulrich H, Palm C, Willbold E. Biodegradable magnesium scaffolds: Part II: Peri-implant bone remodeling. *J Biomed Mater Res A*. 2007;81(3): 757–65.

55. Heublein B, Rohde R, Kaese V et al. Biocorrosion of magnesium alloys: A new principle in cardiovascular implant technology? *Heart*. 2003;89:651–656.

# Basics of biodegradation of iron scaffold

DEYUAN ZHANG AND RUNLIN GAO

## PHYSICOCHEMICAL PROPERTIES OF IRON AND ITS CORROSION PRODUCTS

The physicochemical properties of iron and its possible corrosion products in different solutions are listed in Table 2.5.1. The possible corrosion products of iron in water or NaCl solution include corresponding hydroxides and oxides and their intermediate products [1–5]. The corrosion products also include some phosphates of iron in phosphate solution [6]. Only $Fe_3O_4$ is magnetic in all corrosion products. The volume of solid substances will increase gradually during the corrosion process of iron. Based on their density data in Table 2.5.1, the volume will increases to 1.5 times when Fe changes to $Fe_2O_3$, and 2.35 times when Fe changes to $Fe(OH)_3$. Actually, it is possible that the volume increases to 3–8 times due to the fact that the corrosion products are loose.

## THE APPROACH TO MONITORING BIOCORROSION AND BIORESORPTION OF IRON-BASED SCAFFOLD *IN VIVO*

The feasibility of microcomputed tomography (micro-CT), intravascular ultrasound (IVUS), optical coherence tomography (OCT), multi-slice computed tomography (MSCT), and magnetic resonance imaging (MRI) in monitoring biocorrosion and bioresorption of iron-based scaffolds was explored in the rabbit model. The sirolimus-eluting iron-based bioresorbable coronary scaffolds (IBS™) were implanted in the abdominal aorta of adult New Zealand rabbits. At 3 days, 6 months, and 13 months after implantation, the rabbits were checked with MSCT, MRI, IVUS, and OCT in sequence, and then the scaffolded vessel segments were explanted for Micro-CT 3D reconstruction.

### Micro-CT

The 2D images of the explanted IBS scaffolds after 3 days, 6 months, and 13 months implantation in the rabbit abdominal aorta have been obtained using micro-computed tomography (Micro-CT, Skyscan1172, Bruker, Belgium) to inspect the biocorrosion extent of the nitrided iron scaffolds. Micro-CT of type Skyscan 1172 has very high resolution (0.5 µm). The micro-CT images in Figure 2.5.1 clearly show that the nitrided iron scaffold degrades partially 6 months after implantation and almost completely corrodes except for several obviously attenuated struts 13 months after implantation. It could also be seen that the corrosion products of the nitrided iron scaffold scatter in the tissue around the struts, taking on a nebulous appearance. The reconstructed 3D scaffold profile from 2D images provides us with substantial important information. It reveals the real *in situ* scaffold shape and biocorrosion extent, helps us to determine if there is scaffold bending, kink, or fracture, and even locates the accurate fracture positions. Micro-CT could be used as a visualized and quantitative method to monitor the biocorrosion and bioresorption of the iron-based materials, however, mostly for small animal experiment and *ex vivo* investigation. Micro-CT has also been demonstrated to be capable of quantitative characterizing the degradation of implants in many other applications [7].

### OCT

OCT is an invasive modality for diagnosis of vascular diseases with high resolution [8]. OCT images of the IBS scaffolds after 3 days, 6 months, and 13 months implantation in the rabbit abdominal aorta were acquired with a commercially available Fourier-Domain OCT system (C7 XR, LightLab Imaging, St. Jude Medical, Westford, Massachusetts). OCT imaging in Figure 2.5.2 shows a nice open lumen with a high image resolution of 10–15 µm. Individual scaffold struts along the intima could be easily identified, which are represented as highly reflective structures with typical dorsal shadowing after 3 days implantation. After 6 months implantation, OCT imaging indicates that there is impressive 100% strut coverage with a thin and uniform neointimal layer and no strut malapposition or scaffold thrombus is found. A few struts remain visible in accordance with the micro-CT result,

Table 2.5.1 Physicochemical properties [9] of iron and its possible corrosion products

| Chemical name | Chemical formula | Color | Magnetism | Density (g/cm³) | Whether exists in solution | | |
|---|---|---|---|---|---|---|---|
| | | | | | Water | NaCl solution | Phosphate solution |
| Iron | Fe | Silvery-white/gray | Y | 7.87 | – | – | – |
| Ferrous hydroxide | Fe(OH)$_2$ | White-green | N | 3.4 | √ | √ | √ |
| Iron hydroxide | Fe(OH)$_3$ | Yellow | N | 3.12 | √ | √ | √ |
| Green rust (fougerite) | / | Blue-green | N | / | √ | √ | √ |
| Goethite | α-FeOOH | Red-brown | N | 4.26 | √ | √ | √ |
| Akaganeite | β-FeOOH | Orange-yellow | N | 3.51 | | √ | |
| Lepidocrocite | γ-FeOOH | Orange-brown | N | 3.96 | √ | √ | √ |
| Magnetite | Fe$_3$O$_4$ | Black/brown | Y | 5.17 | √ | √ | √ |
| Hematite | α-Fe$_2$O$_3$ | Red-brown | N | 5.25 | √ | √ | √ |
| Ferrous phosphate | Fe$_3$(PO$_4$)$_2$·8H$_2$O | Gray-blue/blue white | N | 2.58 | | | √ |
| Iron phosphate | FePO$_4$·2H$_2$O | White/gray-white | N | 2.87 | | | √ |
| Ferrous ion | Fe$^{2+}$ | / | / | / | √ | √ | √ |
| Iron ion | Fe$^{3+}$ | / | / | / | √ | √ | √ |
| / | FeOH$^+$ | / | / | / | √ | √ | √ |
| / | FeCl$^+$ | / | / | / | | √ | |
| / | FeCl$^{2+}$ | / | / | / | | √ | |

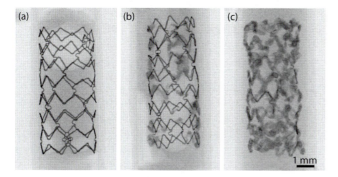

Figure 2.5.1 The 2D images of the IBS scaffolds after (a) 3 days, (b) 6 months, and (c) 13 months implantation in the rabbit abdominal aorta using microcomputed tomography (Micro-CT). (From Lin WJ, Zhang DY, Zhang G, Sun HT, Qi HP, Chen LP, Liu ZQ, Gao RL, Zheng W. *Mater Des* 2016; 91:72–79.)

which reveals that the scaffold corrodes partially 6 months after implantation. After 13 months implantation, nearly all the scaffold struts are no longer identified; however, the highlight ring surrounding the lumen in the neointima with typical dorsal shadowing is noted. This may be because the struts have completely changed into corrosion products scattering in the tissue, as demonstrated by Micro-CT. The corrosion products of the nitrided iron scaffold are found to be highly reflective. It is speculated that the highlight ring with the dorsal shadowing could disappear only after the corrosion products are cleared away from the vessel tissue. From the preliminary study, OCT seems to be an ideal technique for monitoring the biocorrosion and bioresorption of the iron based scaffold *in vivo*.

## IVUS

IVUS also has its application in monitoring degradation of the biodegradable scaffold [11]. The application of IVUS to act as an invasive method monitoring the corrosion and bioresorption process of iron-based scaffold (IBS) implanted in New Zealand rabbit abdominal aorta has been explored. The ultrasonic images of this scaffold are assumed to have a strong relationship toward its biocorrosion and bioresorption process. The IVUS (iLab, Boston Scientific) data shown in Figure 2.5.3 indicates visual changes of the ultrasonic images of the nitrided iron scaffolds, with much lower detail resolution compared with OCT. In IVUS image of 3 days post-implantation, the struts of the IBS scaffold appear as clearly visible and quantifiable hyperechogenic spots without, unlike calcified lesions, causing any acoustic shadowing. Echogenicity analyses of scaffolded segments in 6 months post-implantation show a significant increase of hyperechogenicity than in 3 days, which may be caused by the scaffold biocorrosion. At 13 months after implantation, the scaffolded segments still show a continuous further increase of hyperechogenicity due to the accumulation of the solid corrosion products. It could be expected that the nitrided iron scaffold would show a continuous decrease of its echogenicity over time with the bioresorption of the solid corrosion products. The exact relationship between these ultrasonic changes and the biocorrosion and bioresorbption process of the nitrided iron scaffold is still under investigation.

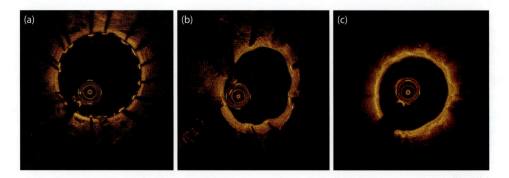

Figure 2.5.2 Optical coherence tomography (OCT) images of the IBS scaffolds after **(a)** 3 days, **(b)** 6 months, and **(c)** 13 months implantation in the rabbit abdominal aorta. (From Lin WJ, Zhang DY, Zhang G, Sun HT, Qi HP, Chen LP, Liu ZQ, Gao RL, Zheng W. *Mater Des* 2016; 91:72–79.)

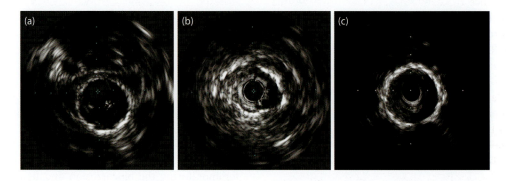

Figure 2.5.3 Intravascular ultrasound (IVUS) images of the IBS scaffolds after **(a)** 3 days, **(b)** 6 months, and **(c)** 13 months implantation in the rabbit abdominal aorta.

## MSCT

Among the advanced cardiac imaging modalities, MSCT has emerged as a reliable noninvasive method for the assessment of coronary anatomy, coronary artery disease, and cardiac function [12]. The rabbits underwent the noninvasive MSCT (Discovery CT750 HD, GE) at 3 days, 6 months, and 13 months after implantation of the IBS scaffolds, respectively. In the MSCT lateral observations, the scaffolded aorta could be identified as the highlight spot as indicated by the arrow in Figure 2.5.4, which shows no significant change with the ongoing biocorrosion of the nitrided iron scaffold. It is apparent that the limited resolution of MSCT in combination with the blooming artifacts of the dense metallic struts is the main reason for not being able to distinguish the states in corrosion process of the nitrided iron scaffold. Accordingly, MSCT is not suitable for monitoring the biocorrosion of iron-based materials, though noninvasive. However, the highlight spot would disappear with the full bioresorption of the solid corrosion products, which indicates that it is possible to adopt MSCT as an effective qualitative way to monitor the bioresorption of iron-based materials.

## MRI

Magnetic resonance imaging (MRI) is also a noninvasive technique, which could be used for diagnosis of cardiovascular diseases. Cardiovascular MRI is performed with high magnetic field, radio frequency waves, and

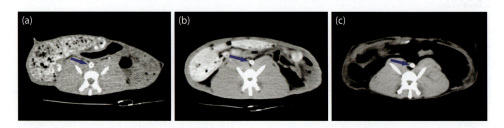

Figure 2.5.4 Multi-slice computed tomography (MSCT) examination of the IBS scaffolds after **(a)** 3 days, **(b)** 6 months, and **(c)** 13 months implantation in the rabbit abdominal aorta.

powerful computers, and typically without a need for administration of a contrast agent in most cases. There is no risk of kidney damage due to contrast and no radiation involved. Figure 2.5.5 shows the representative MR images (MAGNETOM Avanto 1.5T, Siemens, Germany) of IBS scaffolds implanted in the rabbit abdominal aorta for 3 days, 6 months, and 13 months, respectively. Each rabbit was implanted with three nitrided iron scaffolds (3.0 × 8 mm). All animals survived without any adverse cardiovascular events after MRI test, indicating the iron-based material is MRI safe, though not MRI compatible. It could be found that the MR imaging artifacts of the nitrided iron scaffolds diminish apparently with the ongoing corrosion (Figure 2.5.5). This is because the iron-based alloy becomes corrosion products with weaker magnetism in the biocorrosion process. Once the corrosion products were cleared away completely by the body, the artifacts would disappear completely accordingly.

Therefore, MRI is a suitable noninvasive method to semiquantitatively evaluate the biocorrosion and bioresorption process of iron-based materials by comparing the contrast and size of artifact in a certain imaging section. Since the iron-based materials are ferromagnetic materials which are sensitive to the gradient echo sequences, it is recommended that the fast spin echo sequences should be used for MR imaging of iron-based materials. In addition, special care should be taken for *in vivo* investigation since the iron-based materials are only MRI safe but not compatible due to the ferromagnetism. It is recommended that the clinical MRI examination be conducted after full endothelialization of the implanted iron-based alloy scaffolds, e.g., 6 months after implantation.

In summary, the effectiveness and application scopes of Micro-CT, OCT, IVUS, MSCT, and MRI for the biocorrosion and bioresorption of iron-based materials are listed in Table 2.5.2. Micro-CT is an effective method for visually and quantitatively monitoring the biocorrosion and bioresorption of iron-based materials, however, mostly for small animal experiment and *ex vivo* investigation. IVUS could be used as an invasive method *in vivo*, especially in clinical cases to determine the biocorrosion and bioresorption extent of the iron-based materials qualitatively. OCT with higher resolution than that of IVUS also demonstrates the capability to investigate qualitatively the biocorrosion and bioresorption of iron-based materials *in vivo*, especially in clinical cases. MSCT could not be used for monitoring the biocorrosion of iron-based materials due to its low-resolution; however, MSCT as a noninvasive method could be used to qualitatively judge the full bioresorption of iron-based materials. Making use of MR image artifact is a suitable noninvasive method to follow up semiquantitatively both *in vivo* and *ex vivo* cases; however, special care should be taken for clinical MRI investigation since the iron-based materials are not MRI compatible but only safe for MRI examination due to their ferromagnetism. The MRI investigation is recommended for clinical noninvasive monitoring the biocorrosion and bioresorption of iron-based materials after 6 months' implantation.

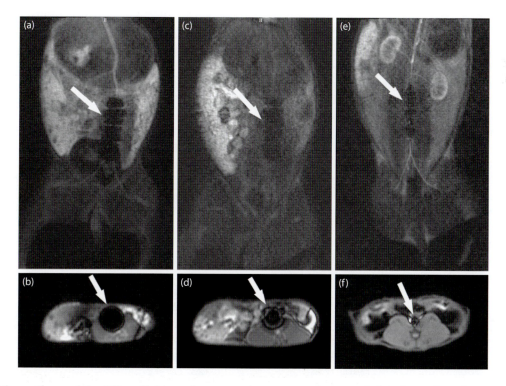

Figure 2.5.5 The artifacts of the IBS scaffolds under magnetic resonance imaging (MRI) after **(a,b)** 3 days, **(c,d)** 6 months, and **(e,f)** 13 months implantation in the rabbit abdominal aorta, axial and lateral, respectively. (From Lin WJ, Zhang DY, Zhang G, Sun HT, Qi HP, Chen LP, Liu ZQ, Gao RL, Zheng W. *Mater Des* 2016; 91:72–79.)

Table 2.5.2 Effectiveness and application scopes of Micro-CT, IVUS, OCT, MSCT, and MRI for the biocorrosion and bioresorption of iron-based scaffolds

| Method | Biocorrosion of iron | Bioresorption of rust | Application scope |
|---|---|---|---|
| Micro-CT | Quantitative | Quantitative | Small animal, *ex vivo* |
| IVUS | Qualitative | Qualitative | Clinical, animal, *ex vivo* |
| OCT | Qualitative | Qualitative | Clinical, animal, *ex vivo* |
| MSCT | NA | Qualitative | Clinical, animal, *ex vivo* |
| MRI | Semiquantitative | Semiquantitative | Clinical, animal, *ex vivo* |

## ADVANTAGES AND DISADVANTAGES

The potential advantages of iron-based materials are summarized as: (1) high strength and sufficient plasticity of iron-based materials could ensure the scaffold high mechanical performances comparable to those of the best permanent stents made of cobalt-based alloy and Pt-Cr alloy. Moreover, high strength and sufficient plasticity of iron-based materials could ensure the scaffold to have a similar design to the workhorse permanent stents, with the same over-dilation and side-branch dilation capability, specification coverage, and procedural manipulation without any compromise. These merits make the iron-based scaffold the only potential bioresorbable scaffold to cover all indications and specifications of the current permanent stents, when compared with the bioresorbable polymer-based and magnesium-based scaffolds. (2) In comparison with the polymer scaffold, corrosion speed of the iron-based scaffold can be adjusted easily by many ways to obtain the best corrosion timeframe, for example, effective scaffolding for 4 months, uncaging at 6 months and total loss of structural integrity at 1 year or so. (3) Trace alloying of carbon or nitrogen or both could significantly elevate the mechanical strength of pure iron. Consequently, biocompatibility of the iron-based materials would not deteriorate like that of the magnesium-based alloy with many toxic metallic elements alloyed, such as rare earth elements and manganese.

The disadvantages of iron-based materials are as follows according to their severity: (1) Despite the fact that the solid corrosion products of iron-based materials scattered in tissue could remain *in situ* without causing any biosafety problem, a long time is needed for them to be cleared away. (2) Iron-based materials are just MRI safe with strong image artifact before most of the iron is cleared away. (3) Production and storage of scaffolds made of iron-based materials are much more complicated and need strict control.

## REFERENCES

1. Talbot DEJ and Talbot JDR. *Corrosion Science and Technology*. Boca Raton, FL: CRC Press, 1998.
2. Revie RW and Uhlig HH. *Corrosion and Corrosion Control: An Introduction to Corrosion Science and Engineering*, 4th ed. Hoboken, NJ: John Wiley & Sons, Inc., 2008.
3. Simpson LJ and Melendres CA. Temperature dependence of the surface enhanced Raman spectroelectrochemistry of iron in aqueous solutions. *Electrochim Acta*. 1996; 41: 1727–1730.
4. Gan Y, Li Y, Lin H. Experimental study on the local corrosion of low alloy steels in 3.5% NaCl. *Corros Sci*. 2001; 43: 397–411.
5. Gismelseed A, Elzain M, Yousif A, al Rawas A, Al-Omari IA, Widatallah H, Rais A. Identification of corrosion products due to seawater and fresh water. *Hyperfine Interact*. 2004; 156–157: 487–492.
6. Sahoo G, Fujieda S, Shinoda K, Suzuki S. Influence of phosphate species on green rust I transformation and local structure and morphology of $\gamma$-FeOOH. *Corros Sci*. 2011; 53: 2446–2452.
7. Fischerauer SF, Kraus T, Wu X, Tanql S Sorantin E, Hanzi AC Loffler JF, Uqqowitzer PJ, Weinberg AM. In vivo degradation performance of micro-arc-oxidized magnesium implants: A micro-CT study in rats. *Acta Biomater*. 2013; 9: 5411–5420.
8. Lee SY and Hong MK. Stent evaluation with optical tomography. *Yonsei Med J*. 2013; 54: 1075–1083.
9. Lide DR. *CRC Handbook of Chemistry and Physics*, Boca Raton, FL: CRC Press, 2004.
10. Lin WJ, Zhang DY, Zhang G, Sun HT, Qi HP, Chen LP, Liu ZQ, Gao RL, Zheng W. Design and characterization of a novel biocorrodible iron-based drug-eluting coronary scaffold. *Mater Des*. 2016; 91: 72–79.
11. Waksman R et al. Early- and long-term intravascular ultrasound and angiographic findings after bioabsorbable magnesium stent implantation in human coronary arteries. *JACC Cardiovasc Interv*. 2009; 2: 312–320.
12. Onuma Y and Serruys PW. Bioresorbable scaffold: The advent of a new era in percutaneous coronary and peripheral revascularization. *Circulation*. 2011; 123: 779–797.

# PART 3

# From bench test to preclinical assessment

# Unlocking scaffold mechanical properties

JOHN J. SCANLON, YOSHINOBU ONUMA, PATRICK W.J.C. SERRUYS, AND JOSEPH M. DEITZEL

## INTRODUCTION

The current coronary bioresorbable scaffolds (BRSs) are composed of either an aliphatic polymer or bioresorbable metal alloy. Numerous different polymers are available, each with different chemical compositions, mechanical properties, and subsequent bioresorption times. The purpose of this chapter is to facilitate the understanding of mechanical features of the materials used for bioresorbable scaffolds.

The key mechanical traits for candidate material in coronary indications include: (1) good conformability during delivery, (2) thin struts that enable a low profile that minimizes injury during delivery, enables access to small passageways, and facilitates complete re-endothelialization after deployment, (3) large break strains to impart the ability to withstand deformations from the crimped to expanded states, (4) low yield strains to reduce the amount of recoil and over-inflation necessary to achieve a target deployment, (5) high radial strength to minimize recoil during vascular remodeling, and (6) radiopacity for visualization during delivery and deployment [1–3].

Although originally taken for granted, it is also important for a scaffold to be deformable so that it can be crimped onto a balloon catheter with a good retention and have its strut geometry easily modified *in vivo* to obtain good apposition to the interior vessel wall in the scaffolded area. Since a bioresorbable scaffold does not have stable mechanical properties like a durable material, there is also a need to maintain mechanical properties during at least 3–4 months after implantation of the device, since the restenosis would be caused by constrictive remodeling [4–8] and to a lesser extent by elastic recoil [9] or the neointimal hyperplastic healing response [10–12]. To inhibit the neointimal hyperplasia, the local delivery of the anti-proliferative drug is desirable. Finally, a bioresorbable scaffold has the new requirement that it must decompose into nontoxic byproducts.

The leading bioresorbable scaffolds are primarily comprised of poly (L-lactide) (PLLA) or magnesium alloy (WE43-type)

[13,14]. If a bioresorbable scaffold is ultimately expected to have the same range of applicability as a durable metal stent, the gap in mechanical properties must be reduced. Presently, scaffold materials have three primary limitations that prevent the use of a bioresorbable scaffold in the full PCI population:

- Insufficient ductility which impacts scaffold retention on balloon catheter and limits the range of scaffold expansion during deployment
- Low tensile strength and stiffness which require thick struts to prevent recoil during vessel remodeling [2,3,7,8]
- Instability of mechanical properties during vessel remodeling

## MATERIAL PROPERTIES

Stress–strain curves are an extremely important graphical measure of a material's mechanical properties. Perhaps the most important test of a material's mechanical response is the tensile test, in which one end of a specimen is clamped in a frame and the other is subjected to a controlled displacement, signified as $\delta$. The engineering measures of stress and strain, signified as $\sigma$ and $\varepsilon$, respectively, are determined from the measured load and displacement. A transducer connected in series with the specimen provides an electronic reading of the load corresponding to the displacement [15]. The stress is the applied load divided by the original cross-sectional area of the test specimen and the strain is the displacement divided by the original specimen length. Experimental procedures for performing stress–strain testing are provided by standards-setting organizations, notably the American Society for Testing and Materials (ASTM) and International Organization for Standardization (ISO).

The stress plotted against the strain produces an engineering stress–strain curve. Figure 3.1.1 displays an engineering stress–strain curve for a ductile material such as a metal alloy, showing strains from zero up to specimen fracture, where the red "X" signifies the fracture. A material is configured into a dog bone shaped specimen as shown in Figure 3.1.2 prior to testing and mechanically elongated by applying the load to the specimen. Generally, the specimen is elongated so that it necks down and ultimately fractures at the highest applied strain. In the lower portion of the stress–strain curve where the specimen is under low strain, materials typically used in the fabrication of a scaffold obey Hooke's law so that the stress is proportional to the strain where the constant of proportionality is the elastic modulus, which quantifies material stiffness. As the strain is increased, the material yields, which means that the stress is no longer linearly proportional to the strain. This nonlinearity is usually associated with stress-induced "plastic" flow in the specimen. Here the material is undergoing a reorganization of its internal molecular structure, in which

the atoms are being moved to new equilibrium positions. These microstructural rearrangements associated with plastic flow are usually not reversed when the specimen is unloaded [15].

As the strain increases, a neck typically forms in the specimen while it is under tension. The neck is an area where the cross-sectional area of the specimen becomes smaller than the remaining portion. Until the neck forms, the deformation is essentially uniform throughout the specimen. In metals once the neck forms all subsequent deformation takes place in the neck. As a result, under increasing strain the cross-sectional area of the neck becomes smaller and smaller until the specimen fractures.

As shown in Figure 3.1.3, an engineering stress-strain curve of a semicrystalline polymer has a slightly different appearance than a curve produced of metal material. In polymers, after yielding occurs, the stress–strain curve plateaus as the molecules begin to orient in the direction of strain. At the portion of the curve where higher strains occur, there is a dramatic upturn in load that corresponds to strain hardening. At this point, the molecules stop moving which enables them to carry higher loads until fracture. Therefore, once the neck forms in a polymeric material the neck stretches to a natural, sustainable cross-sectional thickness and at that point the neck discontinues reducing in size. Once the neck stops stretching, the material adjacent to the neck starts to be drawn down to the smaller cross-sectional thickness. Polymer specimens generally fracture when the drawing process produces a strengthened portion in the drawn down area whose breaking load is greater than needed to induce necking in the undrawn material outside of the neck. Since polymers are viscoelastic, the natural draw down ratio varies depending on the rate at which the load is applied and the temperature of the specimen. Drawing processes are sometimes used to increase the mechanical properties of scaffolds comprised of polymers.

The yield strength is the stress at which a material begins to deform plastically. At strains below the yield point, the

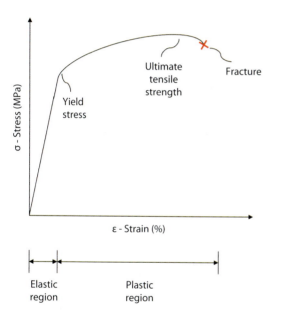

Figure 3.1.1 Exemplary engineering stress–strain curve of a ductile material.

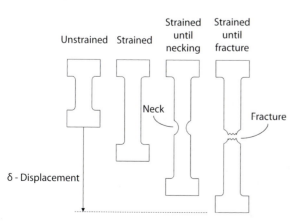

Figure 3.1.2 Material configured into a specimen for tensile testing.

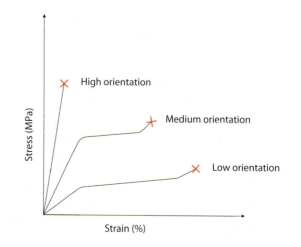

Figure 3.1.3 Result of polymer orientation on the stress-strain curves.

material will deform elastically and return to its original shape when unloaded. Once the strain passes the yield point at least some portion of the deformation will be permanent and irreversible. As shown in Figure 3.1.1, a material used in the construction of a bioresorbable scaffold has an elastic region defined by the portion of the stress–strain curve starting at the onset of loading and ending about when the material yields. The portion of the stress–strain curve starting at about the onset of yielding and ending when the material fractures defines the plastic region.

In metals, defects exist in the crystalline structure of the material. When straining a metal after it yields, new defects are created and existing defects relocate which impede plastic flow and results in strengthening of the material. In contrast, once a polymer yields the molecular chains comprising the polymer orient in the direction of strain, which increases the strength of the material in the direction of strain. The process of strengthening a material by plastic deformation is referred to in material science as strain hardening and in manufacturing as work hardening or cold working. Increasing the strength of a material by strain hardening has the consequence of lost material ductility.

The tensile strength of a material is defined by its yield stress and ultimate tensile strength. The yield stress is found at about the point where the material transitions from the elastic region to the plastic region. The ultimate tensile strength is found at the point of maximum stress. During strain hardening, the tensile strength of the specimen increases in the plastic region as evidenced by the additional stress required to increase strain. Although materials are often described by their ultimate tensile strength, engineers prefer not to employ materials past the yield stress of a material. Beyond the yield stress, strain hardened materials lose ductility and can more easily fracture. Moreover, specimens typically start necking down when strained past the ultimate tensile strength resulting in a substantially reduced cross-sectional area, which can more rapidly advance to material fracture.

Examination of the tensile properties of bioresorbable and durable materials discloses the engineering challenge of producing a bioresorbable scaffold. As shown in Table 3.1.1 and Figure 3.1.4, it is evident that there is a large difference between the strength of bioresorbable materials

and durable materials like cobalt-chromium (CoCr) or platinum-chromium (PtCr) alloys presently used in durable metallic stents having thin strut configurations. There is also a substantial difference in mechanical properties between the precursor stainless steel (SS type 316L) used to fabricate durable metallic stents having thicker strut configurations.

Both bioresorbable materials can be tuned by formulation and during manufacturing processes to improve the mechanical properties. For PLLA, the mechanical properties are improved by molecular orientation [16]. Molecular orientation is imparted on the polymer during material processing by hot drawing and crystallization of the material during formation of the tube. As depicted in Figure 3.1.3, molecular orientation increases the tensile strength substantially but has the drawback of reducing polymer ductility [17]. Although molecular orientation increases the elastic modulus, the increase is far short of what is needed to equal durable metallic materials. A material having a high elastic modulus has a steeper curve in the elastic region of the stress-strain curve. This means that a PLLA scaffold of the same volume and geometry has less stiffness than a durable metallic stent during the treatment time.

The mechanical properties of magnesium alloys are improved by inclusion of other chemical elements in the alloy formulation. Initial magnesium devices were based

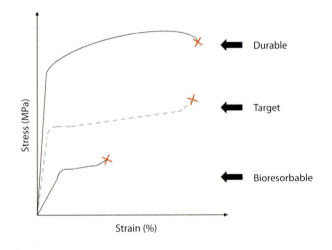

Figure 3.1.4 Approximate stress–strain curves.

Table 3.1.1 Mechanical strength of bioresorbable and durable materials

| Material | | Elastic modulus (GPa) | Ultimate tensile strength (MPa) | Elongation (%) |
|---|---|---|---|---|
| PLLA [8] | Bioresorbable | 3.1–3.7 | 60–70 | 2–6 |
| PLLA (oriented) | | <7 [9,16] | <300 [9,16] | <6 [10] |
| Mg-alloy (WE43) [7] | | 44 | 220 | 7 |
| Modified Mg-alloy [6] | | 45 | 280 | 23 |
| CoCr L605 [2] | Durable | 243 | >1000 | >50 |
| SS type 316L [2] | | 193 | 670 | 48 |
| PtCr [2] | | 203 | 834 | 45 |

on a WE43-type alloy [18,19]. Magnesium alloys are named according to ASTM specification 275. WE43 designates that the primary alloying elements are W (Yttrium) and E (other rare earth elements) with the remainder comprising magnesium and other impurities that may impact mechanical properties or corrosion resistance. Once again referring back to Table 3.1.1, the mechanical properties of WE43-type alloys show good tensile strength but relatively low ductility and elastic modulus when compared to durable metallic materials. Promotional materials show that a modified magnesium alloy exists having improved ductility but the specific alloying elements are not provided. Patent references teach that the ductility of a WE43-type alloy is improved by the addition of rare earth elements Gd, Dy, and Er [18]. Regardless of the approach, the promotional literature depicts the expansion of a 3 mm diameter magnesium alloy scaffold to 4.5 mm in diameter with low probability of strut fracture, which suggests that the modified magnesium alloy having an elongation of 23% may be adequate in a bioresorbable scaffold. As in the processing of PLLA, the mechanical properties of Mg alloys are also improved by heat-treating, aging, and deformation processes [17]. It remains unclear, however, if a material having an elastic modulus of 45 GPa is capable of producing a scaffold of the best-in-class thin strut configuration having a thickness at or below 0.100 mm.

To obtain familiar stent handling characteristics, the region of the curve between the yield stress and the ultimate tensile strength is the most interesting. Thinking of bending a paper clip as shown in Figure 3.1.5 helps you imagine the characteristics of a strut in this region of the stress-strain curve. A paper clip is formed of a ductile metal that under a load is bent into a desired shape. It is in this region of the curve that a durable metallic stent is clamped onto a balloon catheter with a clamping force so that the stent has good retention during delivery. It is also the region of the curve in which a durable metallic stent is expanded in size one or more times during deployment in pursuit of the optimum size so that good apposition is obtained with the interior vessel wall. Just like a paper clip, a strut formed of a ductile material can be bent into different shapes until the preferred shape is obtained. Finally, in PCI treatments involving stent placement at bifurcations, a ductile strut can be bent to permanently move the strut out of the way of the opening of the branched vessel. Materials having low ductility or where

the scaffold geometry is modified in the elastic region of the stress strain curve do not offer these familiar handling characteristics. Materials where the geometry of the scaffold is modified in the elastic region have a tendency to spring back to their original shape and materials with low ductility can fracture under low deformation. Although a paper clip is made of a ductile material, it can also fracture if the wire forming the clip is bent back and forth multiple times. Fracturing occurs because each time the wire is bent, the material strain hardens which means the mechanical properties are changed so that the material loses its ability to resist strain, which can result in fracture.

To have a robust scaffold that is suitable for use in a broad variety of applications, the material should be capable of being elongated by about 50% or more without fracturing [20]. A material with good range of ductility provides ample room to manipulate the size of the scaffold in situations wherein lumen size may have been misjudged due to poor visibility during delivery. Deforming the struts in the necking-down portion of the curve is undesirable because sections of the struts will become thin and most likely provide inconsistent support during the treatment time.

Approximately 20% of PCI patients receive treatment of bifurcated lesions [5]. Although the majority of patients undergoing bifurcation stenting can be treated with a single stent deployed in the main vessel, a portion also require stenting of the side branch [5]. In some cases, bifurcation stenting requires opening of the space between the struts to prevent membrane formation that can potentially restrict flow between branches. Analysis of 6 workhorse durable metallic stents revealed that the maximum expansion of 3 mm diameter stents ranged from 4.6 to 4.7 mm (53%–56%) using postdilatation with a 5.0 mm NC balloon at 14 atm [20]. Opening the struts requires plastic deformation of the material comprising the struts, which means the material must have sufficient ductility to avoid fracture or excessive thinning of the struts if necking occurs.

After deployment, the stiffness and tensile strength of the material provide support and prevent recoil. The elastic modulus as determined by the slope of the stress-strain curve in the elastic region indicates the stiffness of the scaffold. As shown in Figure 3.1.4, the slope of the stress-strain curve in the elastic region of the durable metallic material is much greater than the slope of the bioresorbable material. To make bioresorbable scaffolds suitable for use in narrow vessels, it is desirable to reduce the thickness of the struts. Thinner struts and more conformable designs also produce less injury and improve integration with the vessel wall [1]. The reduction of strut thickness is also important for increasing luminal flow capacity when overlapping struts are unavoidable. It is, however, difficult to reduce strut thickness when the bioresorbable materials have less than 25% of the elastic modulus of the predecessor durable metallic materials.

During the treatment time the scaffold is deployed in the elastic region of the stress-strain curve. Within the elastic region of the stress–strain curve, the scaffold supports the

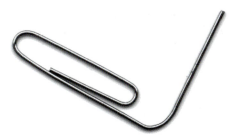

Figure 3.1.5  Bent paper clip.

vascular vessel withstanding the pulsatile flow during systole and diastole. Since the scaffold operates in the elastic region, it maintains its open, tubular configuration. If the loading would exceed the yield stress, the scaffold could collapse and stop supporting the vessel. Although bioresorbable materials have an ultimate tensile strength greater than 60 MPa for one loading cycle and pulsatile pressures typically do not exceed 0.02 MPa, engineers must consider that bioresorbable scaffold must provide support for about 14 million cycles when specifying strut thickness. Experience with reducing the strut thickness from about 0.113 mm to 0.091 mm when changing from 316 L stainless steel to a CoCr alloy required increasing the yield strength from about 275 MPa to about 413 MPa. Since the design life of a bioresorbable scaffold is about 6 months and a durable metallic stent is 10+ years or 400+ million cycles, it is reasonable that materials comprising bioresorbable scaffolds not require the same amount of increase in tensile strength as durable metallic stents. Endurance testing where specimens are loaded and unloaded for multiple cycles over time provides indications of the number of cycles to failure. Figure 3.1.6 illustrates regions of high stress in one embodiment of a scaffold during expansive loading [21].

## MECHANICAL PROPERTY STABILITY

### PLLA

The aforementioned mechanical properties are representative of the raw material properties prior to conversion into a scaffold. Because of the degradable nature of the raw materials, steps must be taken to preserve mechanical properties

during processing of the scaffold as well as during deployment and loading [22,23].

PLLA is a rigid thermoplastic homopolymer formed by polymerization of monomer comprised of L-lactide. Polymerization is the process of converting the L-lactide monomer molecules into a polymer. A polymer is a large molecule, or macromolecule, comprised of many repeating interconnected monomer subunits. Molecular weight (Mw) indicates the length of the PLLA molecule. Low molecular weight polymers generally exhibit dramatic increases in tensile strength as molecular weight increases. However at high molecular weights, the tensile strength only increases slightly with increasing molecular weight [17]. For PLLA, the tensile strength and modulus of elasticity do not change much with increasing molecular weight for polymers in the range of 330,000 to 2,198,000 g/mol [17]. The failure mode of polymers within this range, however, transitions from brittle to ductile with increasing molecular weight [24]. Therefore, higher molecular weight PLLA is viewed as a more suitable candidate for scaffold material, especially polymers having a molecular weight over 838,000 g/mol [24]. To obtain the optimum molecular weight polymer for use in a bioresorbable scaffold, the impact of thermal processing during tube formation and scaffold sterilization, which can reduce polymer molecular weight, must be taken into consideration when selecting raw materials [22].

PLLA is a semicrystalline polymer, which means that it is comprised of crystalline and amorphous regions. In amorphous regions, the molecules are oriented randomly and are intertwined like a bowl of spaghetti. In crystalline regions, the molecules are packed together in an ordered arrangement.

Semicrystalline polymers are viscous liquids at temperatures above their melting point. As a molten crystalizable

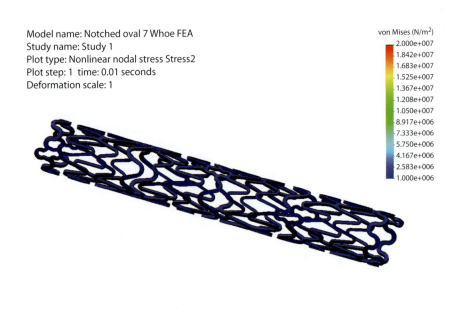

Model name: Notched oval 7 Whoe FEA
Study name: Study 1
Plot type: Nonlinear nodal stress Stress2
Plot step: 1 time: 0.01 seconds
Deformation scale: 1

von Mises (N/m²)

2.000e+007
1.842e+007
1.683e+007
1.525e+007
1.367e+007
1.208e+007
1.050e+007
8.917e+006
7.333e+006
5.750e+006
4.167e+006
2.583e+006
1.000e+006

**Figure 3.1.6** Illustration of strain on scaffold during crimping and implanting. (From Scaffold Strain Animation.)

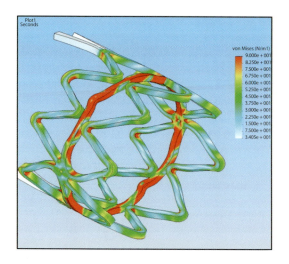

Figure 3.1.7 Crystallization of molten polymer. (Reprinted from *EuroIntervention* 5, Cottone RJ, Thatcher GL, Parker SP, Harks L, Kujawa DA, Rowland SM, Costa M, Schwartz RS and Onuma Y, OrbusNeich fully absorbable coronary stent platform incorporating dual partitioned coatings, F65–71, Copyright 2009, with permission from Europa Digital & Publishing.)

polymer cools, crystals grow from individual nuclei and radiate out like the spokes of a bicycle wheel forming spherulites as illustrated in Figure 3.1.7 [25]. In semicrystalline polymers, fractions of the polymer remain uncrystalized (or amorphous) when cooled to room temperature and the amorphous polymer becomes trapped between the crystals. These amorphous chains meander in and out of the ordered crystalline portions. Semicrystalline polymers combine the strength of crystalline polymers with the flexibility of amorphous. Semicrystalline polymer can be tough with the ability to bend without breaking.

The molecular weight of PLLA is consumed during thermal processing, sterilization, and *in vivo* application. This phenomenon is demonstrated by production and analysis of fibers comprised of PLLA. A reference shows that converting PLLA into fiber having a diameter of 0.31 mm and a starting molecular weight of 647,600 g/mol is reduced to 218,000 g/mol after thermal extrusion and drawing processes. After gamma sterilization, the molecular weight of the same material is reduced further to 48,400 g/mol [22].

Simulating anatomical conditions, fibers conditioned in a phosphate buffer solution maintained at pH of 7.4 and 37°C lost 50% of their elastic modulus and ultimate tensile strength after 23 and 8 weeks, respectively [22]. At 36 weeks the fibers lost their structural integrity and the molecular weight decreased to 9200 g/mol [22]. The reference provides additional support that it is important to preserve molecular weight by utilizing good manufacturing procedures and to produce a scaffold from high molecular weight polymer so that the molecular weight of the scaffold can be maintained above the critical ductile–brittle transition during the support phase of treatment.

Gamma irradiation sterilization is based on an exposure to gamma rays of the isotopes cobalt 60 or caesium 137. The isotopes are contained in a rack inside a concrete chamber

and a conveyor moves the scaffolds around the radiation source. The dose delivered depends on the adjusted speed of the conveyor and the amount and density of the devices in the load. The target of commercial suppliers of gamma irradiation is to guarantee the minimum dose of 25 kGy. As a drawback, gamma irradiation causes chain scission of the polymer molecules, which results in a reduction in polymer molecular weight. Sterilization, therefore, has a tendency to decrease the strength and increase the crystallinity of the polymer [26].

A PLLA scaffold starts absorbing water under physiological conditions upon deployment [23]. After water absorption, the polymer experiences a stiffness decrease. Degradation of strength begins with the start of hydrolysis in the amorphous regions [27]. The degradation is primarily due to hydrolysis of the ester linkages, which occur more or less randomly along the backbone of the polymer. PLLA exhibits a gradual reduction in molecular weight over time without an appreciable mass loss for most of the time. In larger wall thicknesses, the inside degrades faster than the outside because of the buildup of compounds containing carboxylic end groups that cause an autocatalytic reaction through acid-catalyzed chain end scission. Since hydrolysis starts by cleaving the amorphous regions of the polymer, using higher crystalline PLLA slows degradation of the mechanical properties of the scaffold after deployment [23]. PLLA hydrolyzes more slowly under neutral pH and more quickly under acidic and alkaline conditions.

## Magnesium alloy

Magnesium reacts with water and is broken down into magnesium hydroxide and hydrogen in less than 6 months [4,22,24]. Magnesium hydroxide is formed on the outside surfaces of the scaffold that produces a passivation layer that slows the corrosion process [23]. Within 9 months the residual magnesium degradative byproducts are reduced to calcium phosphate (aka hydroxyapatite) [4].

A problem with some Mg alloys is their high corrosion rate at physiological conditions, which can make their biodegradability faster than the treatment time. Another drawback of Mg alloys is the evolution of hydrogen. This gas can be accumulated in pockets next to the implant or can form in subcutaneous gas bubbles [23]. However, if the gas is generated slowly enough it can be transported away from the treatment area. To circumvent these issues alloying elements are added to Mg to slow the corrosion rate of the struts.

Since the chemical elements Fe, Ni, Co, and Cu have been found to be corrosion-causing constituents, they are excluded in an alloy having improved corrosion resistance [12]. These elements accelerate corrosion because of the large difference in electro–potential between these elements and magnesium. In corrosive environments these elements produce microgalvanic cells, which lead to corrosion [12]. Small amounts of Zn and Mn may improve a WE43-type alloy's corrosion resistance [12].

One more way to improve corrosion resistance of WE43-type alloys is to purify the alloy by including a

Table 3.1.2 Composition of material (wt.%)

| | PLLA | Mg alloy (WE43) [2] | CoCr (L605) [5] | SS (316L) [4] | PtCr [8] |
|---|---|---|---|---|---|
| Cr | | | 20 | 16 to <18 | 18 |
| Fe | | | 3 | Remainder | Remainder |
| C | | | 0.33 | 0.3 | |
| P | | | 0.04 | 0.045 | |
| S | | | 0.03 | 0.03 | |
| Si | | | 0.4 | 0.75 | |
| N | | | | 0.1 | |
| Co | | | Remainder | | |
| Pt | | | | | 33 |
| Ni | | | 10 | 10 to <14 | 9 |
| Mo | | | | 2 to <3 | 2.6 |
| Mn | | | 2.5 | 2 | <0.05 |
| Mg | | Remainder | | | |
| Ti | | | | | |
| Mg | | | | | |
| W | | | | 15 | |
| Other rare earth | | 2.4.4.4 | | | |
| Y | | 3.7–4.3 | | | |
| Zr | | 0.4 min. | | | |
| L-Lactide | 100 | | | | |

combination of Zr and Al [12]. The addition of Zr and Al combine with Fe and Ni to form an insoluble compound. This compound is precipitated in the melting crucible and settles prior to casting. Thus the addition of Al and Zr to the alloy can improve corrosion resistance by purifying the alloy by eliminating Fe and Ni impurities. To achieve this effect, at least 0.05 wt.% Zr and less than 0.3 wt.% Al must be present in the final alloy [12]. As shown in Table 3.1.2 in the highlighted cells, bioresorbable scaffolds introduce new chemical elements not previously used in durable metallic stents. The disposition of the degradative by-products of alloy impurities that slow corrosion and/or improved ductility are being investigated.

## FUTURE MATERIALS

The benefits of a bioresorbable scaffold motivate finding solutions to the shortcomings of contemporary scaffolds that limit application. The evolution of durable metallic stents provides an excellent understanding of the optimum strut pattern geometry, and for this reason, improving scaffold mechanical properties by taking this route is limited. From today's perspective, the likely pathway for developing bioresorbable scaffolds that have the full range of applicability of durable metal stents is to close the gap in material performance. It is fairly clear that the mechanical properties of a bioresorbable scaffold during the treatment time must be closer to those of a durable metallic stent as suggested by the target stress–strain curve illustrated in Figure 3.1.4 and that compensation for lower strength materials by almost doubling the strut thickness versus CoCr and PtCr stents is not the optimum solution.

Since both leading bioresorbable polymer and metallic materials have lower starting strength than their counterpart durable materials, opportunity exists for controlling the onset and rate of degradation during the treatment time to fully utilize the capability of these materials. Good advances have heretofore been achieved by manipulating material morphology by increasing polymer crystallinity, reducing alloy grain size, and reformulating alloy constituent materials. The landscape, however, does look rich in opportunity by additional research into barrier coatings that modify onset of degradative processes like hydrolysis and corrosion. Longer retention of the starting mechanical properties may be one key to unlocking significant strut size reduction in degradable scaffolds.

It also appears that opportunity exists to preserve the molecular weight of polymers during fabrication of scaffolds. Various sources highlight that polymer molecular weight is reduced during thermal processing and sterilization. Alternative manufacturing processes that enable use of higher starting molecular weight materials and retaining more degree of polymerization may hold a second key to unlocking greater mechanical property performance.

Like the success achieved by metallurgists at the US Department of Energy's National Energy Technology Laboratory (NETL), Pittsburgh, Pennsylvania, during the development of the platinum-chromium alloy (PtCr), opportunity exists to increase the mechanical properties of scaffolds through development of improved bio-corrodible alloys that have nontoxic constituents and degradative byproducts.

These alloys may be used singularly in the construction of struts or as inclusions in polymer form composites that include bio-corrodible metal fibers or spherical beads. There are a multitude of examples of boosting the mechanical properties of polymers, especially the yield strength and elastic modulus, by incorporating reinforcing materials and this approach may be yet one more key to unlocking mechanical properties in bioresorbable scaffolds.

To increase the adoption rate of bioresorbable scaffolds, there is also opportunity to manipulate the mechanical properties so that bioresorbable scaffolds have familiar handling characteristics and use the same procedures as those used for the delivery and deployment of durable metallic stents. Using existing procedures minimizes investments in training and tooling associated with technology changes. Consistent procedures also reduce the risk of human error.

The investment in resources to develop bioresorbable scaffolds suitable for use in complex lesions offers the benefit of unconstrained, treated arteries. The benefit of restoring the artery to a more natural state after resorption allows the artery to auto-regulate so that it can expand during strenuous activity when greater blood flow is required. Moreover, the artery can adaptively remodel over time to compensate for new atherosclerosis [1]. These benefits can be realized in broader applications by increasing the tensile strength, ductility, and elastic modulus of bioresorbable materials.

## REFERENCES

1. Foin N, Lee RD, Torii R, Guitierrez-Chico JL, Mattesini A, Nijjer S, Sen S et al. Impact of stent strut design in metallic stents and biodegradable scaffolds. *Int J Cardiol.* 2014;177:800–8.
2. Onuma Y and Serruys PW. Bioresorbable scaffold: The advent of a new era in percutaneous coronary and peripheral revascularization? *Circulation.* 2011;123:779–97.
3. AL-Mangour B, Mongrain R and Yue S. Coronary stents fracture: An engineering approach. *Mater Sci Appl: MSA.* 2013;04.
4. Kimura T, Kaburagi S, Tamura T, Yokoi H, Nakagawa Y, Hamasaki N, Nosaka H et al. Remodeling of human coronary arteries undergoing coronary angioplasty or atherectomy. *Circulation.* 1997;96:475–83.
5. Hoffmann R, Mintz GS, Dussaillant GR, Popma JJ, Pichard AD, Satler LF, Kent KM et al. Patterns and mechanisms of in-stent restenosis. A serial intravascular ultrasound study. *Circulation.* 1996;94:1247–54.
6. Mintz GS, Popma JJ, Pichard AD, Kent KM, Satler LF, Wong C, Hong MK et al. Arterial remodeling after coronary angioplasty: A serial intravascular ultrasound study. *Circulation.* 1996;94:35–43.
7. Di Mario C, Gil R, Camenzind E, Ozaki Y, von Birgelen C, Umans V, de Jaegere P et al. Quantitative assessment with intracoronary ultrasound of the mechanisms of restenosis after percutaneous transluminal coronary angioplasty and directional coronary atherectomy. *Am J Cardiol.* 1995;75:772–7.
8. Luo H, Nishioka T, Eigler NL, Forrester JS, Fishbein MC, Berglund H and Siegel RJ. Coronary artery restenosis after balloon angioplasty in humans is associated with circumferential coronary constriction. *Arterioscler Thromb Vasc Biol.* 1996;16:1393–8.
9. Rodriguez AE, Santaera O, Larribau M, Fernandez M, Sarmiento R, Perez B, Newell JB et al. Coronary stenting decreases restenosis in lesions with early loss in luminal diameter 24 hours after successful PTCA. *Circulation.* 1995;91:1397–402.
10. Clowes AW, Reidy MA and Clowes MM. Kinetics of cellular proliferation after arterial injury. I. Smooth muscle growth in the absence of endothelium. *Lab Invest.* 1983;49:327–33.
11. Nobuyoshi M, Kimura T, Ohishi H, Horiuchi H, Nosaka H, Hamasaki N, Yokoi H et al. Restenosis after percutaneous transluminal coronary angioplasty: Pathologic observations in 20 patients. *J Am Coll Cardiol.* 1991;17:433–9.
12. Garratt KN, Edwards WD, Kaufmann UP, Vlietstra RE and Holmes DR, Jr. Differential histopathology of primary atherosclerotic and restenotic lesions in coronary arteries and saphenous vein bypass grafts: Analysis of tissue obtained from 73 patients by directional atherectomy. *J Am Coll Cardiol.* 1991;17:442–8.
13. Erbel R, Di Mario C, Bartunek J, Bonnier J, de Bruyne B, Eberli FR, Erne P et al. Temporary scaffolding of coronary arteries with bioabsorbable magnesium stents: A prospective, non-randomised multicentre trial. *Lancet.* 2007;369:1869–75.
14. Haude M, Erbel R, Erne P, Verheye S, Degen H, Bose D, Vermeersch P et al. Safety and performance of the drug-eluting absorbable metal scaffold (DREAMS) in patients with de-novo coronary lesions: 12 month results of the prospective, multicentre, first-in-man BIOSOLVE-I trial. *Lancet.* 2013;381:836–44.
15. Roylance D. *Stress Strain Curves,* Massachusetts Institute of Technology, Cambridge, MA.
16. Penning JP, Dijkstra H and Pennings AJ. Preparation and properties of absorbable fibres from L-lactide co-polymers. *Polymer.* 1993:942.
17. Zhang X. *Fundamentals of Fiber Science.* DEStech Publications, Inc.; 2014.
18. Lyon P, Syed I, Boden J and Savage K. Magnesium alloys containing rare earths. U.S. Patent Application Publication No. US 2011/0229365 A1. 2011; 1–9.
19. Permana KD, Shuib AS and Ariwahjoedi B. A review of magnesium alloys for use in biodegradable cardiovascular stents. *World Appl Sci J.* 2014;30:375–81.
20. Foin N, Sen S, Allegria E, Petraco R, Nijjer S, Francis DP, Di Mario C et al. Maximal expansion capacity with current DES platforms: A critical factor

for stent selection in the treatment of left main bifurcations? *EuroIntervention. Journal of EuroPCR in Collaboration with the Working Group on Interventional Cardiology of the European Society of Cardiology.* 2013;8:1315–25.

21. Scaffold Strain Animation.

22. Nuutinen JP, Clerc C, Reinikainen R and Tormala P. Mechanical properties and in vitro degradation of bioabsorbable self-expanding braided stents. *J Biomater Sci-Polym Ed.* 2003;14:255–66.

23. Vieira AC, Vieira JC, Guedes RM and Marques AT. Degradation and viscoelastic properties of PLA-PCL, PGA-PCL, PDO and PGA fibres. *Mater Sci Forum.* 2010;636–637:825–32.

24. Venkatramana S, Poha TL, Vinaliaa T, Makb KH and Boeya F. Collapse pressures of biodegradable stents. *Biomaterials.* 2003;24:2105–11.

25. Cottone RJ, Thatcher GL, Parker SP, Harks L, Kujawa DA, Rowland SM, Costa M, Schwartz RS and Onuma Y. OrbusNeich fully absorbable coronary stent platform incorporating dual partitioned coatings. *EuroIntervention.* 2009;5(Suppl F):F65–71.

26. Annala T and Kellomäki M. Sterilization of bio-degradable polymers. *Degradable Polymers for Skeletal Implants*: Nova Science Publishers; 2009.

27. Cam D, Hyon S-h and Ikada Y. Degradation of high molecular weight poly(l-lactide) in alkaline medium. *Biomaterials.* 1994;16:833–43.

# Bench testing for polymeric bioresorbable scaffolds

JOHN A. ORMISTON, BRUCE WEBBER, JANARTHANAN SATHANANTHAN,
PAU MEDRANO-GRACIA, SUSANN BEIER, AND MARK W.I. WEBSTER

## INTRODUCTION

Polymeric resorbable drug-eluting scaffolds that treat coronary arterial lesions and subsequently resorb promoting normal vessel vasomotion have potential advantages over durable metallic stents [1,2]. However, polymers behave differently from the metallic alloys commonly used for stent construction. Poly-L-lactic acid (PLLA) has less ultimate tensile strength and percentage elongation compared with metallic alloys such as cobalt chromium. Hence, polymeric struts fracture more readily [3,4]. Polymeric struts are thicker and wider and have greater vessel wall coverage compared with metallic stents in order to provide sufficient radial strength, to limit recoil, and to resist fracture [5]. One consequence of thicker, wider struts is a larger delivery system crossing profile which can cause device delivery challenges.

Bench testing provides an understanding of the mechanical properties of different scaffolds and aids the interventionalist in device selection. It provides insights on how devices work, their strengths and weaknesses, and can test efficacy of design iterations and procedural changes. It can shed light on a clinical problem, aid device development, and validate potential solutions. Bench studies may validate computational modeling and aid teaching interventional techniques. Testing should be independent as some manufacturers may select tests that show their product favorably. However, manufacturers can provide detailed geometric information such as strut dimensions, polymer thickness, vessel wall coverage, and potential size of the cell between struts for side-branch access.

## HOW TO TEST POLYMERIC SCAFFOLDS

The U.S. Food and Drug Administration stipulates in its extensive guidance for industry that nonclinical (bench) testing should support the safety and effectiveness of intracoronary stents and their delivery systems (dsmica@fda.hhs.gov). The International Organization for Standardization (ISO) publication, ISO 25539-2, details minimum requirements for endovascular devices and methods of test that will enable their evaluation. For testing of polymeric scaffolds on the bench, the ASTM F2079-09 recommends immersion in a water bath that has heating and recirculation instruments to maintain the bath at $37 \pm 2°C$ because polymer behavior is greatly affected by temperature. A scaffold may need to be removed briefly from the bath for measurements.

### Bifurcation phantoms

The future of bifurcation models lies with anatomic accuracy, obedience to the scaling laws, and construction from materials with an appropriate Young's modulus. They should allow imaging of deployed stents. While the above is fundamentally important for the future, important bifurcation information to date has been derived from phantoms that do not obey these principles. The geometry of a coronary bifurcation obeys a set of geometric rules known as scaling laws. The relationship between diameters of mother and daughter vessels proposed by Murray has recently been challenged for coronary arteries (Table 3.2.1) [6,7]. Finet proposed a simpler (linear) model based on fractal arguments that hold only for Y-type but not T-type bifurcations (Table 3.2.1) [8].

### Diameters and angles for different bifurcations

An atlas of normal coronary bifurcation anatomy derived from 300 CT coronary angiograms without stenosis or calcification has been constructed. The atlas describes the distributions of diameters and angles (Figure 3.2.1) for the major coronary bifurcations [9]. From this atlas, average

Table 3.2.1 Coronary bifurcation geometric rules

| Model | Geometric relation |
|-------|--------------------|
| Murray [6] | $D_m^3 = D_l^3 + D_s^3$ |
| Huo-Kassab [7] | $D_m^{7/3} = D_l^{7/3} + D_s^{7/3}$ |
| Finet [25] | $D_m = 0.678(D_l + D_s)$ |

*Note:* $D_m$ = diameter of the mother vessel, $D_l$ and $D_s$ are diameters of daughter vessels (l = large, s = small branch).

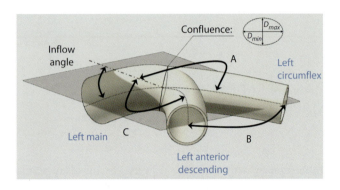

Figure 3.2.1 Left main bifurcation anatomy from an atlas of normal coronary anatomy derived from 300 normal CT coronary angiograms. A bifurcation plane (shown in gray) is automatically computed and used to calculate different angles and diameters.

population models can be 3D printed providing anatomically accurate bifurcation phantoms.

The angle between the left main coronary artery and the left circumflex is called angle A, between the left anterior descending and circumflex is angle B, between the left main and left anterior descending is angle C (Figure 3.2.1). In addition there is an inflow angle between the left main coronary and the plane of the daughter vessels. Diameters of individual vessels can be measured and mean data derived [9].

## Materials used for model construction

Ideally coronary artery phantoms should be constructed from a material with an appropriate Young's modulus matching the mechanical properties of the coronary artery. Young's modulus is a mechanical property of solid materials measuring the force per unit area needed to stretch (or compress) a material sample. The higher the Young's modulus the more rigid is the material. Historically different phantom materials have been used, and most have limitations. Troughs in Perspex plates [10] have important limitations, lacking both anatomical bifurcation accuracy and having a nontubular structure. Perspex has a very high Young's Modulus (is hard) in comparison with the human coronary arteries. These phantoms are good for light photography because there is no material between the stent and camera [10].

Glass tubes used as phantom arteries are limited by being difficult to construct with anatomical accuracy, rigidity of the wall, and distortion of light images because glass refracts light [11].

We use tubing from aliphatic polyether-based thermoplastic polyurethanes (tecoflex) when we measure radial strength and sometimes for longitudinal distortion assessment [12,13]. This tubing is difficult to make into anatomically correct bifurcations. Because translucency is limited, photographic quality is limited but it is suitable for microCT imaging.

Casts made from silicone can be anatomically accurate but need to be modified to allow quality light photography. They can be tubular and can have a suitable Young's modulus. They are suitable for microCT imaging [14].

Phantoms can be made by 3D printing using a wide range on materials with different physical properties. Excellent anatomical accuracy is possible. Conventional photography is challenging. These materials are suitable for microCT, although radioopacity may be similar to that of polymeric scaffolds limiting the differentiation of phantom wall from scaffold.

## Imaging and bench testing

The deployment of stents or scaffolds in a bifurcation phantom in a water bath and subsequent steps (e.g., proximal optimization, side-branch wire access, additional stenting) can be viewed live and recorded fluoroscopically [5,14]. The stent or scaffold can be temporarily removed from the water bath so a particular step can be photographed or a microCT image aquired. Photography through a microscope is very useful to record images of stents or scaffolds during a wide range of maneuvers. Multiple images are feasible and cost-effective. In the past we have imaged stent deployments through a borescope (pediatric endoscope) but this technique has been largely made redundant by microCT [15]. While microCT is limited by cost and imaging time required, it does allow unparalleled scaffold examination and images can be readily postprocessed with computer algorithms allowing slicing and advanced viewing such as fly-through [16]. The image reconstruction using gaming software distorts images and precludes accurate measurements. Intravascular ultrasound and optical coherence tomography are useful imaging tools for stents and scaffolds. For examining polymeric stent or scaffold coatings, we use environmental scanning electron microscopy which has very high resolution.

## DEVICE DESIGN

Device design can be readily demonstrated by photography or microCT imaging. The design of most contemporary polymeric scaffolds is sinusoidal hoops with peaks and troughs linked by three straight connectors [5]. Because most polymers are highly radiolucent, most scaffolds have radio-opaque markers at each end to enable identification radiologically. An exception is the REVA (Reva Medical Inc, San Diego, CA) design, which is radio-opaque due to polymer iodination.

## Strut dimensions, potential cell size obtained from manufacturers are summarized

Measurements were provided by the manufacturers (Table 3.2.2). The polymeric struts are thicker in a radial direction than those of the metallic drug-eluting stent, Xpedition. Their struts are also wider with a consequence that percentage of vessel wall covered by struts (27%–30%) is twice that for metallic DESs (13%) [5].

## Radial strength

We measure radial strength by deploying a stent or scaffold (usually 3.0 mm diameter device) in a tecoflex tube and then measuring cross-sectional luminal area change with increasing external pressure applied in a water bath. We derive pressure to reduce area by 10%, 25%, and that to cause stent/scaffold collapse and use the results to compare stents and scaffolds.

## Recoil

Because recoil measurements for different polymers may show time dependency (ASTM F2079-09), we compared diameter measurements of two bioresorbable scaffolds (ABSORB and DESolve) with the durable metallic MultiLink 8 stent (Abbott Vascular) over 1 hour following deployment. The polymeric scaffolds were deployed in a water bath at 37°C. The external diameters of the ABSORB and DESolve scaffolds at deployment were greater than that of the ML8 stent because of their thicker struts (Figure 3.2.2). By 1 minute after deployment, all three devices had recoiled by approximately 0.1 mm. Between 1 minute and 10 minutes there was minimal change in diameter. Between 10 minutes and 1 hour, the ABSORB scaffolds and ML8 stents showed little change but the DESolve scaffold increased in diameter to baseline dimensions ("self correction"), so that its diameter was larger than that of ML8 stent and ABSORB scaffold (Figure 3.2.2) [5]. This unique feature may correct

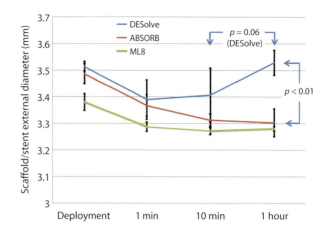

**Figure 3.2.2** Construction material influences recoil over time. Bench measurements of immediate diameter recoil for a metallic stent compared with ABSORB and DESolve BRSs at 1 hour. All were 3.0 mm devices deployed at nominal pressure. The polymeric scaffolds were deployed in a water bath at 37°C and the permanent metallic stents were deployed in air. Recoil at 1 hour for the current ABSORB scaffold was greater than for most durable metallic stents [19]. The DESolve scaffold at 1 hour was very similar to its diameter at baseline as it showed enlargement between 10 minutes and 1 hour. (From Ormiston JA, Webber B, Ben Ubod B, Darremont O and Webster MWI. *EuroIntervention* 2015; 11:60–67.)

strut malapposition and is being exploited in the design of the "Amity" scaffold (Elixir Medical) where there is at least 0.5 mm of self correction above nominal diameter which may correct scaffold malapposition after resolution of thrombus and spasm following treatment of acute myocardial infarction or chronic total occlusion. Clearly it is important to state the time after deployment that recoil measurements are made because for different polymeric scaffolds the results at 1 minute may be very different from those at, for instance, 1 hour (Figure 3.2.2).

## Lessons from the bench testing

Bench testing has provided valuable insights into real world issues with scaffold deliverability and optimization. Importantly bench testing allows potential solutions to be developed and their efficacy to be assessed.

**Table 3.2.2** Comparison of the durable Xpedition stent with ABSORB and DESolve scaffolds (3.0 mm diameter devices)

| | ML8/Xpedition | ABSORB | DESolve |
|---|---|---|---|
| Strut thickness including coating thickness, μm | 89 | 157 | 150 |
| Strut width, μm | | | |
|     Hoop | 89–112 | 191 | 165 |
|     Connector | | 140 | 100 |
| % vessel coverage by stent scaffold/stent | 13 | 27 | 30 |
| Potential cell diameter, mm | 4.2 | 3.0 | 3.2 |

## Crossing profile and delivery challenges

The crossing profile of an ABSORB scaffold (1.42 ± 0.01 mm) measured from calibrated photographs using a microscopen is larger than the crossing profile of the metallic DESs (Xpedition, 1.14 ± 0.01 mm) and may create delivery challenges. Bench testing can clarify what equipment and strategies are feasible to improve delivery (Figure 3.2.3).

## Flexibility

Flexibility of scaffolds can be measured mounted on the delivery system or after deployment in a Tecoflex tube using a 3-point bend test [17]. The expanded ABSORB polymeric scaffold is more flexible than a contemporary metallic stent [18].

## Postdilatation safety

Scaffold postdilatation may damage scaffolds by fracturing struts which may have important adverse clinical events [4]. Dilatation through the side of a scaffold causes distortion and may cause strut fracture [14,19]. We carried

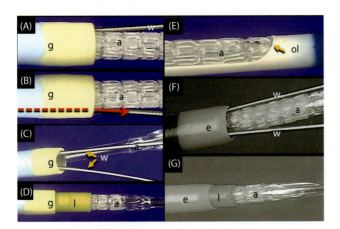

Figure 3.2.3 Strategies to facillitate ABSORB delivery. A "buddy" wire can facilitate delivery. In **A**, an ABSORB scaffold (a) and a 0.014 inch guide wire (w) are accommodated in a 6F guide catheter (g). Panel **B** shows that a guide wire can be advanced through a guide containing an ABSORB without preloading. Panel **C** shows that if the ABSORB scaffold is advanced beyond the guide into the artery, then two guide wires and the ABSORB shaft can be accommodated in the guide. Panel **D** shows that a Guideliner (Vascular Solutions Inc, Minneapolis, MN) can aid scaffold delivery if a 2.5 or 3.0 mm ABSORB is preloaded into the Guideliner (l). If the scaffold is not preloaded, its passage may be obstructed by the ostium of the Guideliner (panel **E**, l). A 7.5 F sheathless Eaucath (Asahi Intecc, Japan) (e in panels **F** and **G**) which has the same lumen as a 7F guide catheter with an outer diameter less than a 6F sheath can accommodate a 3.5 mm ABSORB and two guide wires (**F**) of a 7F guideliner and a 3.5 mm ABSORB hence is very useful for the radial approach.

out bench experiments to determine safe postdilatation strategies, safe side-branch dilatation, and safe, effective strategies to correct distortion of ABSORB and DESolve scaffolds [14,19]. To determine safe postdilatation balloon sizes, 3.0 mm diameter scaffolds were deployed unconstrained in the water bath at 37°C and then postdilated with increasing NC balloon diameters and pressures up to 20 atm pressure or until strut fracture. Stents were deployed unconstrained in air. The percentage of scaffolds with fracture was plotted against balloon diameter (Figure 3.2.4). The ML8 stent did not fracture with main branch postdilatation with balloon diameters up to 5.5 mm at 20 atm pressure. The DESolve did not fracture at diameters of 5.0 mm or less and the ABSORB did not fracture at diameters of 3.8 mm or less [19].

## Side-branch dilatation

Dilatation through the side of a scaffold causes distortion (Figure 3.2.5) similar to that caused by dilatation through the side of metallic stent [14,20]. We showed that dilatation through the side of a 3.0 mm ABSORB scaffold with a 2.0 mm balloon did not cause strut fracture. When we found that a 2.5 mm side-dilatation caused fracture in 13% of dilatations and a 3.0 balloon in 22% of inflations at 14 atm, we sought to clarify what constituted safe side-branch dilatation.

We dilated through the sides of 3.0 mm scaffolds (Figure 3.2.6) with 3.0 mm noncompliant balloons at increasing balloon pressure for individual ML8 stents, ABSORB, and DESolve scaffolds [5]. There were no fractures observed in DESolve scaffolds or ML8 stents even with side branch dilatation at 22 atm. With the ABSORB scaffold there were no fractures at 10 atm pressure or less so we concluded that for a 3.0 mm ABSORB scaffold, side-branch dilatation with a

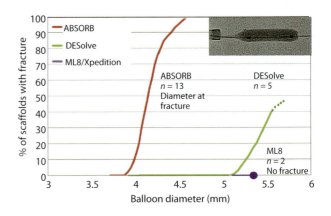

Figure 3.2.4 Percentage of scaffolds with strut fracture and balloon diameter. The ML8 did not fracture. DESolve did not fracture at diameters of 5.0 mm or less and the ABSORB did not fracture at diameters of 3.8 mm or less at 20 atm [19]. (From Ormiston JA, Webber B, Ben Ubod B, Darremont O and Webster MWI. *EuroIntervention* 2015; 11:60–67.)

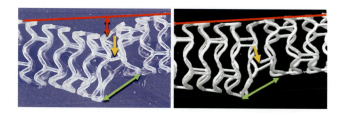

Figure 3.2.5  3.0 mm ABSORB after 3.0 mm side-branch dilatation at 16 atm (left panel) and after kissing balloon postdilatation with two 3.0 mm noncompliant balloons at 4 atm. In the left panel there is distortion with malapposition of struts opposite the side-branch (red double arrow), and narrowing of the scaffold just distal to the side-branch. The side-branch ostium has been cleared of overlying struts (green double arrow). In addition, there is a connector fracture (yellow arrow). After kissing balloon postdilatation, the malapposition and scaffold narrowing are corrected with maintenance of side-branch ostial scaffold clearance.

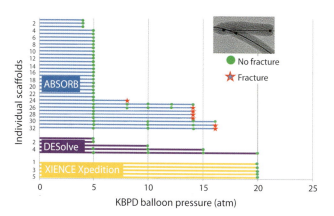

Figure 3.2.7  Mini-kissing balloon postdilatation in a 3.0 mm scaffold with two 3.0 mm noncompliant balloons with pressure for ABSORB and DESolve scaffolds. The insert in the top right corner shows balloons inflated using the mini-KBPD strategy where the proximal main branch is exposed to the diameter of only one balloon and the bifurcation to the diameters of both balloons. A green point represents a scaffold inspection with no strut fracture. The red star represents inspection with strut fracture(s) observed. There were no strut fractures in the ML8 stent or DESolve scaffold even at 20 atm pressure with mini-KBPD. With the ABSORB there were no fractures at 5 atm or less, so this is a safe threshold for mini-KBPD in a 3.0 mm ABSORB scaffold with two 3.0 mm noncompliant balloons [19]. (From Ormiston JA, Webber B, Ben Ubod B, Darremont O and Webster MWI. *EuroIntervention* 2015; 11:60–67.)

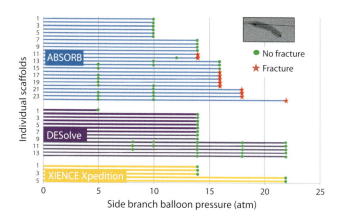

Figure 3.2.6  Side branch dilatation of a 3.0 mm scaffold with increasing 3.0 mm noncompliant balloon pressure for individual ML8 stents and ABSORB and DESolve scaffolds. The green points represent a scaffold inspection that revealed no strut fracture. The red star represents inspection with strut fracture(s) observed. There were no fractures observed in DESolve scaffolds or ML8 stents even with side branch dilatation at 22 atm. With the ABSORB scaffold there were no fractures at ≤10 atm pressure, the safe threshold [19]. (From Ormiston JA, Webber B, Ben Ubod B, Darremont O and Webster MWI. *EuroIntervention* 2015; 11:60–67.)

3.0 mm noncompliant balloon at 10 atm was safe and that all pressures were safe for the DESolve and ML8 (Figure 3.2.6).

## Correction of scaffold distortion caused by side-branch dilatation

Some of the strategies that have been tried with the hope of maintaining the side-branch ostium and correcting distortion caused by side-branch dilatation include kissing balloon postdilatation, mini-kissing balloon postdilatation [5], "hugging balloons" [5], main branch postdilatation, and final "POT" [21]. When we carried out mini-kissing balloon postdilatation with two 3.0 mm noncompliant balloons at increasing pressure, there were no strut fractures with DESolve or ML8. With ABSORB there were no fractures with mini-kissing balloon inflation at 5 atm or less, which is therefore a safe threshold for postdilatation with the above parameters (Figure 3.2.7).

## VALIDATION OF COMPUTATIONAL MODELS

Computational modeling of blood flow is a common tool for investigation of hemodynamic effects in nonstented and stented vessels with idealized or patient specific shapes [22,23]. These computational fluid dynamic (CFD) simulations can provide superior spatial and temporal resolution compared with other currently used modalities. With sufficient computational resources such as supercomputing facilities with high memory and parallel processing capabilities, computational predictions become increasingly used across many scientific fields. The simplifications and assumptions underlying CFD studies must be validated [24]. One method to validate computationally derived flow and stresses is by measuring flow using phase-contrast magnetic resonance imaging in 3D printed up-scaled models with dimensions derived from a coronary atlas [9,22,23].

## SUMMARY

Bench testing has provided considerable insight into scaffold deployment and optimization, and allowed development of strategies to aid ideal scaffold deployment without scaffold damage. Different stenting strategies can also be assessed that may impact on clinical outcomes. In the future, bench testing will be enhanced by using improved phantoms that are a better representation of human coronary anatomy. This may involve increased use of 3D printing and new phantom materials. All bench tests have limitations because they may not predict clinical behavior.

## REFERENCES

1. Erbel R, Di Mario C, Bartunek J, Bonnier J, de Bruyne B, Erbeli FR, Erne P et al. Temporary scaffolding of coronary arteries with bioabsorbable magnesium stents: A prospective, non-randomized multicentre trial. *Lancet.* 2007;369:1869–1875.
2. Ormiston J, Serruys PW, Regar E, Dudek D, Thuesen L, Webster M, Onuma Y et al. A bioabsorbable everolimus-eluting coronary stent system for patients with single de-novo coronary artery lesions (ABSORB): A prospective open-label trial. *Lancet.* 2008;371:899–907.
3. Ratner B, Hoffman A, Schoen F and Lemons J. Biomaterials Science. An Introduction to Materials in Medicine. San Diego, CA: Academic Press; 1996.
4. Ormiston J, De Vroey F, Serruys PW and Webster M. Bioresorbable polymeric vascular scaffolds: A cautionary tale. *Circ Cardiovasc Interv.* 2011;4:535–538.
5. Ormiston J, Webber B, Ubod B, Darremont O and Webster M. An independent bench comparison of two bioresorbable drug-eluting coronary scaffolds (Absorb and DESolve) with a durable metallic drug-eluting stent (ML8/Expedition). *EuroIntervention.* 2015 May;11(1):60–67.
6. Murray C. The physiology principle of minimum work. I. The vascular system and cost of blood volume. *Proc Natl Acad Sci.* 1926;12:207–214.
7. Huo Y, Finet G, Lefevre T, Louvard Y, Moussa I and Kassab G. Optimal diameter of diseased bifurcation segment: A practical rule for percutaneous intervention. *EuroIntervention.* 2012;7:1310–1316.
8. Finet G and Kassab G. Anatomy and function relation in the coronary tree: From bifurcations to myocardial flow and mass. *EuroIntervention.* 2015;11:V13–V17.
9. Medrano-Gracia P, Ormiston J, Webster M, Beier S, Ellis C, Wang C, Young A et al. *Construction of a Coronary Artery Atlas from CT Angiography,* Springer International Publishing; 2014.
10. Ormiston J, Webster M and Webber B. Percutaneous intervention for coronary lesions: Bench testing in the real world. In Waksman R and Ormiston J, Eds. *Bifurcation Stenting,* Wiley-Blackwell, West Sussex, UK, 2012:83–88.
11. Rogers C, Tseng D, Squire J and Edelman E. Balloon-artery interactions during stent placement. A finite element analysis approach to pressure, compliance, and stent design as contributors to vascular injury. *Circ Res.* 1999;84:378–383.
12. Ormiston J, Webber B, Ubod B, White J and Webster M. Stent longitudinal strength assessed using point compression: Insights from a second-generation, clinically related bench test. *Circ Cardiovasc Interv.* 2013;doi: 10.1161/CIRCINTERVENTIONS.113.000621.
13. Ormiston J, Dixon S, Webster M, Ruygrok P, Stewart J, Minchington I and West T. Stent longitudinal flexibility: A comparison of 13 stent designs before and after expansion. *Catheter Cardiovasc Interv.* 2000;50:120–124.
14. Ormiston J, Webber B, Ubod B, Webster M and White J. Absorb everolimus-eluting bioresorbable scaffolds in coronary bifurcations: A bench study of deployment, side-branch dilatation and post-dilatation strategies. *EuroIntervention.* 2014;pii:20140311–01.
15. Ormiston J, Currie E, Webster M, Kay I, Ruygrok P, Stewart J, Padgett R et al. Drug-eluting stents for coronary bifurcations: Insights into the crush technique. *Catheter Cardiovasc Interv.* 2004;63:332–336.
16. Ormiston J, Webster M, Webber B, Stewart J, Ruygrok P and Hatrick R. The "crush" technique for coronary bifurcation stenting: Insights from micro-computed tomographic imaging of bench deployments. *J Am Coll Cardiol Interv.* 2008;1:351–357.
17. Ormiston J, Blake J, Peebles C, Webster M, Stewart J, Ruygrok P and O'Shaughnessy B. Expanded stent radial strength and flexibility: Benchtop testing of 10 stents. *Am J Cardiol.* 2002;90(Suppl 6A):76H.
18. Iqbal J, Onuma Y, Ormiston J, Abizaid A, Waksman R and Serruys P. Bioresorbable scaffolds: Rationale, current status, challenges and the future. *Eur Heart J.* 2013;35:765–776.
19. Ormiston JA, Webber B, Ben Ubod B, Darremont O and Webster MWI. An independent bench comparison of two bioresorbable drug-eluting coronary scaffolds (Absorb and DESolve) with a durable metallic drug-eluting stent (ML8/Xpedition). *EuroIntervention.* 2015;11:60–67.
20. Ormiston J, Webster M, Ruygrok P, Stewart J, White H and Scott D. Stent deformation following simulated side-branch dilatation: A comparison of five stent designs. *Catheter Cardiovasc Interv.* 1999;47:258–263.
21. Hildick-Smith D, Lassen J, Albiero R, Lefevre T, Darremont O, Pan M, Ferenc M et al. Consensus from the 5th European Bifurcation Club meeting. *EuroIntervention.* 2010;6:34–38.

22. Beier S, Ormiston J, Webster M, Cater J, Norris S, Medrano-Gracia P, Young A et al. Hemodynamics in idealized stented coronary arteries: Important stent design considerations. *Ann Biomed Eng.* 2016;44:315–329.

23. Beier S, Ormiston J, Webster M, Cater J, Norris S, Medrano-Gracia P, Young A et al. Dynamically scaled phantom phase contrast MRI compared to true-scale computational modeling of coronary flow. *J Magn Reson Imaging.* 2016;44:983–992.

24. Antoniadis A, Mortier P, Kassab G, Dubini G, Foin N, Murasato Y, Giannopoulos A et al. Biomechanical modelling to improve coronary artery bifurcation stenting. *J Am Coll Cardiol Interv.* 2015;8:1281–1296.

25. Finet G, Huo Y, Rioufol G, Ohayon J, Guerin P and Kassab G. Structure-function relation in the coronary artery tree: From fluid dynamics to arterial bifurcations. *EuroIntervention.* 2010;6(Suppl. J):J10–J15.

# Bench test for magnesium scaffold

DANIEL LOOTZ, WOLFRAM SCHMIDT, PETER BEHRENS, KLAUS-PETER SCHMITZ, MICHAEL HAUDE, AND RON WAKSMAN

## INTRODUCTION

Intravascular stent implantation is a worldwide accepted minimally invasive procedure to treat cardiac ischemia caused by narrowed coronary arteries since the randomized studies BENESTENT [1] and STRESS [2] showed superiority over plain balloon angioplasty. Today permanent stents, with and without antiproliferative-drug-eluting coatings, are well established for keeping the treated vessel segments open [3,4]. The idea of a bioabsorbable vascular scaffold that alters its mechanical behavior during its lifetime in the human body has been present since the early days [1,3,5,6] of stent development and gaining increasing popularity. Bioabsorbable scaffolds should offer acute implantation properties comparable to permanent stents and subsequently degrade over time. Without the presence of any foreign irritations [7,8], the artery is allowed to return to its natural physiological state and a potential trigger for late restenosis is removed [9].

Most absorbable scaffolds, commercially available or tested in clinical studies, are made of polymers. While they offer cardiovascular outcomes comparable to permanent drug eluting stents, a recent meta-analysis showed a higher incidence of myocardial infarction and scaffold thrombosis [10]. This might be related to the mechanical behavior and the design of the polymeric scaffold.

Magnesium could be considered a better platform material than polymers due to its metal-like behavior. The material has no retardation or relaxation and shows no time-dependent mechanical behavior. The main challenge in designing a magnesium scaffold is to find the right balance between the acute and long-term scaffold performance.

## TECHNICAL REQUIREMENTS FOR STENTS, SCAFFOLDS AND THEIR SYSTEMS

The performance of stents and scaffolds are determined by material and design. Additionally, due to human use biological requirements have to be fulfilled.

Mechanical requirements of stent and scaffold systems were nominated and investigated in detail [10–16]. Research groups [17–20] consider the stent system from the physician's perspective. The most prominent attributes of the stent or scaffold are the radial support, clinically relevant for lumen gain [2,21] and the bending stiffness, supporting the conformability to the vessel. High bending stiffness is linked to provoking vessel trauma resulting in distal or proximal restenosis [12,15,22]. Deliverability, a combination of trackability (passing through tortuous vessels), crossability (passing narrowed lesions), and pushability (rate of force transmitted over the entire catheter length) is also considered as a clinically relevant factor.

The requirements for stent and scaffold systems for the clinical user can be summarized as follows:

- Simple and safe deliverability to the lesion with excellent positioning
- Good trackability with low track forces
- High pushability to ensure a high transmission of force from hub to tip while advancing the system

The requirements for the implant, supporting the healing process, can be summarized as follows:

- Low bending stiffness, to reduce vessel irritation and ensure conformability
- Low shortening during expansion, ensuring lesion covering
- Homogeneous opening
- Optimal strut cross-section to reduce blood flow disturbances
- Good adaption to vessel wall
- Recovery of vessel vasomotion
- High biocompatibility paired with low thrombogenicity
- Appropriate radial strength to support the vessel over healing time

These requirements are essentials for all stents and scaffolds, but because of their complexity not all devices on the market have been able to meet them all to the same degree.

## MECHANICAL BASICS

Designing a stent or scaffold always involves trade-offs between the various performance properties of the implant. For example, helical designs tend to show better bending flexibility than ring designs, but to the cost of lower radial force. Most design variations intended to increase the radial force invariably lead to a lower allowable dilatation diameter. Magnesium makes these trade-offs even more challenging because of major differences in terms of material stiffness, tensile strength, and strain at break (Figure 3.3.1).

The stiffness and tensile strength of a material are linked to the radial force of the scaffold, and the strain at break limits the allowable dilatation diameter. Thanks to a scaffold design specifically tailored to the material properties, current magnesium scaffolds achieve both sufficient radial force and a sufficient allowable dilatation diameter

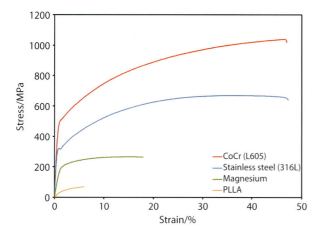

Figure 3.3.1 Exemplary engineering stress–strain curves of various materials used for vascular implants. The graphs compare the mechanical behavior of different commonly used materials. (Note: PLLA curve is reproduced by data of Table 3.3.1.)

compared to current high-performance but durable metals (Table 3.3.1) [23]. To that effect, the most prominent difference to permanent stents is a larger dimension of the strut cross-sections. Polymeric materials, showing a stiffness and tensile strength considerably lower than that of magnesium, require even more efforts in terms of dedicated scaffold designs.

## GENERATION HISTORY OF MAGNESIUM SCAFFOLDS

The evolution of the BIOTRONIK magnesium scaffold is summarized in Table 3.3.2. The refinement of the magnesium alloy, together with changes in the strut dimensions and the addition of a polymer coating helped to slow down the degradation and increased the scaffolding time. All three generations employed ring designs. The increased number of crowns per ring led to more uniform vessel coverage, while a lower number of links between the rings improved the bending flexibility. The incorporation of tantalum composite radioplaque markers added X-ray visibility to the otherwise radiolucent magnesium scaffold. Each generation of the scaffold made better use of the mechanical capabilities of the magnesium alloy, like the material strength or strain rate, to achieve sufficient radial support as well as the possibility of some expansion reserve.

## SYSTEM AND PERFORMANCE OF THE BIOTRONIK MAGNESIUM RESORBABLE SCAFFOLD

The new BIOTRONIK device Magmaris (DREAMS-2G), as shown in Figure 3.3.2, is a Sirolimus-eluting balloon-expandable magnesium resorbable scaffold, mounted on a fast-exchange 0.014 inch guide wire compatible delivery system. The device is a tubular, scaffold laser-cut from a single tube of absorbable magnesium (Mg) alloy. The refined magnesium alloy contains >90% magnesium and additional alloying elements, improving the material homogeneity, corrosion rate, strength, and deformability. The scaffold design consists of radial revolving loops with connectors in the axial direction. The strut thickness and width are both 150 μm (nominal diameter

Table 3.3.1 Material properties of stent and scaffold materials

| Material | Tensile modulus of elasticity (GPa) | Tensile strength (MPa) | Elongation at break (%) |
|---|---|---|---|
| Cobalt chromium | 210–235 | 1449 | ~40 |
| Stainless steel 316L | 193 | 668 | 40+ |
| Magnesium | 40–50 | 220–330 | 2–20 |
| Poly(L-lactide) | 3.1–3.7 | 60–70 | 2–6 |
| Poly(DL-lactide) | 3.1–3.7 | 45–55 | 2–6 |
| Poly(glycolide) | 6.5–7.0 | 90–110 | 1–2 |

*Source:* Serruys PW, Onuma Y, Lafont A, Abizaid A, Waksman R, Ormiston J. Bioresorbable scaffolds in: Eckhout E, Serruys PW, Wijns W, Vahanian A, Van Sambeek M, De Palma R, Eds. *Percutaneous Interventional Cardiovascular Medicine: The PCR-EAPCI Textbook.* Volume II Intervention I, PCR Publishing, Toulouse, France, 2012, pp. 145–177.

Table 3.3.2 Development history of the BIOTRONIK magnesium resorbable scaffold

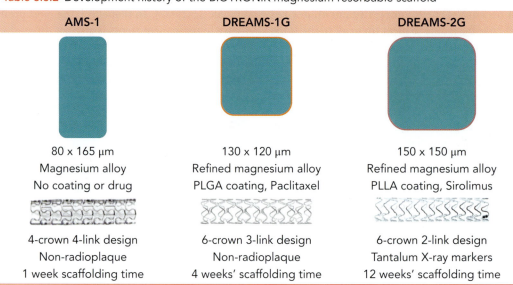

| AMS-1 | DREAMS-1G | DREAMS-2G |
|---|---|---|
| 80 x 165 µm | 130 x 120 µm | 150 x 150 µm |
| Magnesium alloy | Refined magnesium alloy | Refined magnesium alloy |
| No coating or drug | PLGA coating, Paclitaxel | PLLA coating, Sirolimus |
| 4-crown 4-link design | 6-crown 3-link design | 6-crown 2-link design |
| Non-radioplaque | Non-radioplaque | Tantalum X-ray markers |
| 1 week scaffolding time | 4 weeks' scaffolding time | 12 weeks' scaffolding time |

3.0/3.5 mm). At each end two radiopaque markers are placed. The device combines:

- A device component: Resorbable scaffold premounted on balloon-expandable delivery system, a modified platform from Orsiro (BIOTRONIK AG, Bülach, CH)
- An active component: A poly-L-lactic acid (PLLA) polymer eluting Sirolimus at the same rate of the clinically proven Orsiro stent [24] (1.4 µg/mm$^2$ scaffold surface)

## Scaffold deliverability

An essential requirement for a stent or scaffold is the ability to reach the target lesion. Key features in this context are good trackability, pushability, and crossability of the catheter. Crossability is often limited by the profile of the crimped scaffold. Reduction of the profile by crimping to a lower diameter induces higher plastic strains in the crimped scaffold, resulting in reduced strain reserves available for dilatation. Therefore, an improvement of the profile will, in most cases, lead to a lower limit for overexpansion, especially with biodegradable materials that have comparably poor mechanical properties (cf. Figure 3.3.1). This

is the reason why resorbable scaffolds are currently only 6F compatible and have a profile between 1.4 and 1.5 mm compared to 1 and 1.2 mm typical for current permanent DES [18].

With ABSORB (Abbott Vascular, Santa Clara, CA) a few cases of scaffold dislodgement were documented [25], emphasizing the need for sufficient fixation or embedding of the scaffold on the catheter. Balloon shoulders, which further reduce the risk of dislodgement of the scaffold, can often be seen in bioresorbable systems [26].

A low bending stiffness especially in the region of the mounted scaffold is desired for a good accessibility to the stenosis and to reduce trauma during the track. Trackability (the force required to move a stent or scaffold system through a path mimicking the anatomical vasculature [27]) and pushability (the fraction of the proximal push force being transmitted to the distal end of the system) can be measured in bench tests [18]. While the Magmaris and the ABSORB GT1 (Abbott Vascular, Temecula, CA) showed a similar bending stiffness (42.7 N/mm$^2$ vs. 39.2 Nmm$^2$, $p = 0.189$) in bench tests, Magmaris performed better than ABSORB GT1 in terms of pushability (i.e., the force transmitted from the hub to the tip of the device: 45.4% vs. 33.8%, $p < 0.001$) and trackability (i.e., peak force needed to go through a tortuous vessel: 1.7 N vs. 2.4 N, $p < 0.001$, see Figure 3.3.3) [26].

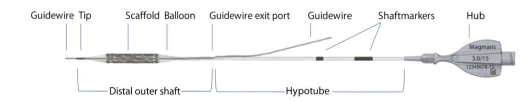

Figure 3.3.2 Schematic representation of the Magmaris device.

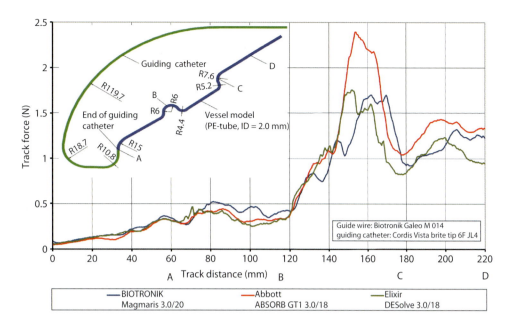

**Figure 3.3.3** Track forces measured while pushing the scaffold systems through the ASTM track model. The ABSORB GT1 showed the highest peak forces between position B and C, when the crimped scaffold is entering the second radius after position B. (Modified from Schmidt W et al., *Cardiovasc Revasc Med.* 2016;17(6):375–83.)

## Acute scaffold performance

The required acute performance of a bioresorbable scaffold is the same as for permanent stents. Also, from a physician's perspective, the implantation procedure should be the same, both in terms of handling and overexpansion. However, a number of special requirements and limitations exist for all the commercially available polymeric bioresorbable products.

According to the ABSORB GT1 IFU deployment of the scaffold should be performed slowly (in increments of 2 atm every 5 s until complete expansion) and the final pressure should be maintained for 30 s. The expansion of the DESolve (Elixir Medical Corp., Sunnyvale, CA) should also be performed slowly (starting with 10 s steps for each atm for the first 2 atm, continuing with 2 s for each atm until complete expansion). For magnesium scaffolds, no such restrictions regarding expansion rate are required.

Limitations also exist related to overdilatation. According to the IFUs, both ABSORB and DESolve should not allowed to be expanded beyond 0.5 mm over the nominal diameter. While the overexpansion limit was 0.3 mm and 0.4 mm for the AMS-1 and the DREAMS-1G, respectively, expansion to 0.6 mm over nominal diameter is allowed for the Magmaris.

Since the overexpansion limit is an important parameter during development, thorough testing is required. The stent or scaffold is gradually dilated, and the balloon diameter at which a fracture occurs is recorded. Similar investigations were done independently by Ormiston et al. [28] and Foin et al. [29]. The allowable dilatation diameter is determined statistically as the diameter where, with a certain probability, the device is still intact (similar to the rated burst pressure of balloons). In a benchtest carried out at BIOTRONIK, the

maximum expansion diameter of the device before fracture was found to be higher than the safety margin reported in the IFUs (see Table 3.3.3).

Another desirable feature of a stent or scaffold is a low bending stiffness of the dilated device, leading to a good adaption to the tortuous geometry of the vessel and causing less irritation of the vessel wall, thereby helping to reduce the risk of restenosis [30]. To evaluate the bending stiffness, the dilated scaffold is fixed at one end, the other end is deflected, and the deflection force is recorded. The procedure is equivalent to the one used for stent systems described by Schmidt et al. [18]. Compared to other scaffolds and permanent stents, Magmaris shows an exceptionally low bending stiffness. This improvement over its predecessors can be attributed to the reduced number of connectors. Also in comparison to current available scaffolds DeSolve and ABSORB GT1, Magmaris has the highest flexibility (up to 80% difference, Table 3.3.3) [26].

The main function of a scaffold, just like that of a stent, is to support the vessel and keep the lumen open. This ability can be characterized by the acute recoil, i.e., the reduction in scaffold diameter between the expanded state (on the pressurized balloon) and after balloon deflation. The amount of acute recoil is governed by two effects: the elastic recoil (load-free spring-back of the structure due to the elastic-plastic material behavior), and the radial load applied by the overstretched vessel balanced by the radial force of the scaffold. Generally, those two effects are investigated by independent *in vitro* tests.

The elastic recoil is determined as the change in diameter of the expanded scaffold during balloon deflation in the absence of external loading. Minimal scaffold recoil is desirable because it reduces the maximum diameter to which

Table 3.3.3 Bench test results in an overview of DREAMS-2G, ABSORB GT-1, and DESolve

| | | Bench test results in summary | | | |
|---|---|---|---|---|---|
| | | Description | Magmaris | Absorb | DESolve |
| Test name | Parameter | – | 3.0/20 | 3.0/18 | 3.0/18 |
| Crimped profile-1[a] | Mean of entire scaffold in (mm) | Unstressed | 1.44 ± 0.00 (n = 6) | 1.38 ± 0.01 (n = 6) | 1.39 ± 0.01 (n = 3) |
| Bending stiffness-1[a] | Mean in (Nmm²) | Crimped scaffold system | 39.2 ± 5.1 (n = 6) | 42.7 ± 3.1 (n = 6) | 21.3 ± 4.1 (n = 3) |
| Trackability-1[a] | Max force (N) | – | 1.70 ± 0.21 (n = 6) | 2.40 ± 0.21 (n = 6) | 1.76 ± 0.24 (n = 3) |
| Trackability-2[a] | Mean force (N) 0–220 mm | – | 0.68 ± 0.09 (n = 6) | 0.75 ± 0.03 (n = 6) | 0.64 ± 0.02 (n = 3) |
| Pushability[a] | Rate of maximum distal force related to the proximal push force (%) | – | 45.41 ± 2.03 (n = 6) | 33.77 ± 1.22 (n = 6) | 36.27 ± 1.30 (n = 3) |
| Elastic recoil-1[a] | Recoil (%) immediatly after expansion | After implantation into rigid Ø 3.0 mm vessel model | 5.57 ± 0.72 (n = 6) | 5.86 ± 0.76 (n = 6) | 7.85 ± 3.45 (n = 3) |
| Elastic recoil-2[a] | Recoil (%) >1 h after expansion | After implantation into rigid Ø 3.0 mm vessel model | 5.62 ± 0.74 (n = 6) | 7.00 ± 0.76 (n = 6) | −3.01 ± 2.23 (n = 3) |
| Acute recoil-1[a] | Recoil (%) shortly after expansion | After implantation into mock vessel (inner Ø 2.7 mm) | 4.94 ± 0.31 (n = 3) | 5.22 ± 0.38 (n = 3) | 9.42 ± 0.21 (n = 3) |
| Acute recoil-2[a] | Recoil (%) >1 h after expansion | After implantation into mock vessel (inner Ø 2.7 mm) | 4.85 ± 0.41 (n = 3) | 7.82 ± 0.47 (n = 3) | 11.41 ± 0.08 (n = 3) |
| Bending stiffness-2[a] | Mean in (Nmm²) | Expanded scaffold | 0.89 ± 0.10 (n = 6) | 4.20 ± 0.58 (n = 6) | 1.50 ± 0.26 (n = 3) |
| Crush resistance[a] | Mean in (kPa) | Of stents with radially applied load (collapse pressure) | 197 ± 5 (n = 3) | 172 ± 2 (n = 3) | – |
| Overexpansion | Mean in (N/mm) | 1st fracture | 4.31 ± 0.47 (n = 6) | 3.75 ± 0.13 (n = 4) | – |
| Inner scaffold area | Mean in (mm²) | After dilatation into mock vessel by µCT (w/o end rings) | 7.02 ± 0.13 (n = 3) | 6.75 ± 0.05 (n = 3) | 6.13 ± 0.08 (n = 3) |

[a]Source: Reproduced from Schmidt W et al., *Cardiovasc Revasc Med.* 2016;17(6):375–83.
Note: Ø = diameter.

a scaffold must be expanded to achieve its final relaxed diameter, and therefore reduces the required overstretching of the vessel. When measuring elastic recoil, the possibly time dependent material behavior of polymers must be considered. The elastic recoil of Magmaris (5.6%) [26] is in the range of permanent stents with 2%–6% [19], it does not change over time. The elastic recoil of the ABSORB scaffold immediately after balloon deflation (5.8%) is comparable to that of the Magmaris, but increases to 7% after 1 h due to relaxation of the polymer [26]. An unusual effect termed "self-correction" [28] is observed for the DESolve scaffold. Immediately after balloon deflation it shows high elastic recoil of nearly 8%, but after 1 h, if the system doesn't have any external loads, DESolve increases its diameter beyond the initial dilated diameter [26].

Approaches to determine the radial force of stents or scaffolds have evolved from crush resistance tests with parallel plates or tests with radially applied hydrostatic load [31] to methods using a sling or a segmented head [32] to apply radial deformation. In all methods the outer diameter of the scaffold is continuously reduced, and diameter and force are recorded synchronously. Literature reports that the radial force of a coronary stent or scaffold, expressed as a pressure, should be at least 200 to 300 mmHg [5,30]. However, while a high radial force can be linked to low acute recoil, a straightforward quantification of its contribution is not possible.

It is more convenient to determine acute recoil directly by implanting the scaffold into a mock vessel with physiological compliance, inducing a clinically reasonable overstretching of the vessel, and measuring the resulting diameter after balloon deflation. This method includes both effects (elastic recoil and vessel load) and closely resembles the physiological situation. As for elastic recoil, the potential time dependence of polymeric material behavior must be considered.

In a bench test [26] using this method (Figure 3.3.4), scaffolds were implanted in mock vessels (Dynatek Labs, Galena, MO, inner diameter 2.7 mm, compliance 5%–7%/100 mmHg) and expanded to their nominal diameter of 3 mm (ca. 10% oversizing). Magmaris showed an acute recoil of 5% and the value did not change over time. The acute recoil of the ABSORB immediately after balloon deflation (5%) was comparable to that of the magnesium scaffold, but increased to nearly 8% after 1 h. A similar phenomenon was shown in a publication by Ormiston et al. [28]. The DESolve scaffold showed high acute recoil of over 9% directly after balloon deflation. However, instead of a diameter increase, as observed under load-free conditions, the recoil further increased to more than 11% after 1 h [26]. This suggests that while the "self-correction" [28] may help to reduce malapposition due to insufficient dilatation, it does not contribute to the scaffolding properties. As shown in Figure 3.3.4, if the three investigated scaffolds are implanted at the same expansion diameter into

comparable vessels, the lumen area of the ABSORB GT1 and especially of the DESolve with –4% and –13% is lower than the lumen area achieved by the Magmaris scaffold.

It is worth noting that, against expectation, there is no statistically significant difference ($p > 0.05$) between the acute recoil and the elastic recoil of the same device. This suggests that the scaffolds are stiff enough, that the expected additional diameter change by the mock-vessel load cannot be detected by the chosen test method. One exception are the values for DESolve >1 h ($p = 0.008$), where the strut self-correction does not contribute to the load bearing.

The overall bench test data are summarized in Table 3.3.3.

## Long-term magnesium scaffold performance

While the characterization of the long-term performance of permanent stents basically means to prove a 10-year resistance against failure due to fatigue, the situation is much more complex for magnesium scaffolds which are intended to be gradually resorbed over time. To achieve a suitable scaffolding time, the interaction between material degradation

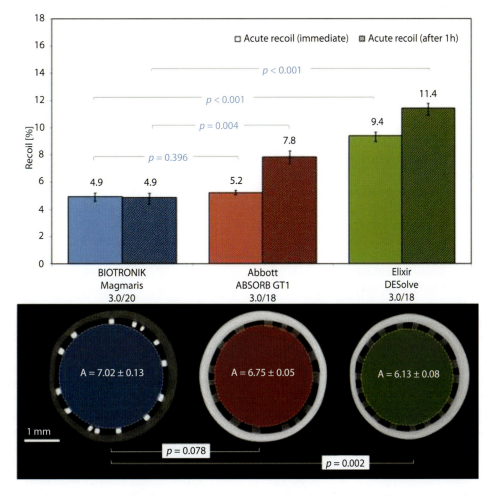

**Figure 3.3.4** Acute recoil of scaffolds immediately and 1 h after implantation into mock vessels. Top: The acute recoil increases over time for the polymer scaffolds, but is stable for the magnesium scaffold. Bottom: Micro-CT scans reveal lumen areas 4% or 13% lower than that of the Magmaris for the Absorb GT1 or the DESolve, respectively. (Modified from Schmidt W et al., *Cardiovasc Revasc Med.* 2016;17(6):375–83.)

and mechanical fatigue, influenced by backbone material, polymeric coating, and scaffold design, must be considered during development.

The predominant mechanism reducing the radial force of an implanted magnesium scaffold over time is the development of strut fractures. Strut fractures occur due to the interplay of corrosion induced by the contact between blood and magnesium, and of oscillating mechanical loading by the pulsing vessel. *In vitro* tests show a direct correlation between the fracture density (i.e., the number of strut fractures per mm scaffold length) and the decrease in radial force.

*In vitro* bench testing to investigate the chronic performance of magnesium scaffolds involve a physiological pulsatile load applied to scaffolds which are implanted into a mock vessel in which a simulated body fluid (SBF) flows. The pH-value of the SBF is controlled to stay in the physiological range, and the integrity of the scaffolds is permanently monitored. The output of the test is the time of the first fracture and the time when the scaffold collapses. Applied to AMS-1, a small increase in scaffolding time was found from uncoated scaffolds to the DREAMS-1G, and the scaffolding time approximately doubled from DREAMS-1G to the latest BIOTRONIK magnesium resorbable scaffold, Magmaris.

Although such tests can show trends, preclinical trials remain essential to characterize the long-term performance of magnesium scaffolds. Moreover, different rankings may occur when comparing the *in vivo* and *in vitro* degradation of different magnesium alloys [3,33].

## CONCLUSION

Magnesium scaffolds are a promising approach to combine the acute performance of a permanent metal stent with the benefits of a degradable device which vanishes after its duty is fulfilled. Bench test results show that the Magmaris scaffold (formerly known as DREAMS-2G) is comparable to established permanent stents regarding acute performance. Furthermore, Magmaris long-term scaffolding ability over at least 3 months is suggested by preclinical data. All these investigations show promising scaffold behavior of the Magmaris device contributing to patient recovery.

## ACKNOWLEDGMENTS

For the assistance and the excellent discussions in manuscript preparation we thank Ludovica Visciola, Christoph Forkmann, and Andre Schoof.

## REFERENCES

1. Sigwart U. Coronary stents. *Z Kardiol.* 1995; 84(2): 65–77.
2. Fischman DL, Leon MB, Baim DS, Schatz RA, Savage MP, Penn I, Detre K et al. A randomized comparison of coronary-stent placement and balloon angioplasty in the treatment of coronary artery disease. *N Engl J Med.* 1994; 331: 496–501.
3. Bowen PK, Drelich J, Goldmann J. A new in vitro–in vivo correlation for bioabsorbable magnesium stents from mechanical behavior. *Mater Sci Eng C.* 2013; 33(8): 5064–5070.
4. Muni NI, Califf RM, Foy JR, Boam AB, Zuckerman BD, Kuntz RE. Coronary drug-eluting stent development: Issues in trial design. *Am Heart J.* 2005; 149(3): 415–433.
5. Agrawal CM, Haas KF, Leopold DA, Clark HG. Evaluation of poly(L-lactic acid) as a material for intravascular polymeric stents. *Biomaterials.* 1992; 13(3): 176–181.
6. Stack RS, Califf RM, Phillips HR, Pryor DB, Quigley PJ, Bauman RP, Tcheng JE, Greenfield JC Jr. Interventional cardiac catheterization at Duke Medical Center. *Am J Cardiol.* 1988; 62(10 Pt 2): 3F–24F.
7. Tsuji T, Tamai H, Igaki K et al. Biodegradable stents as a platform to drug loading. *Int J Cardiovasc Intervent.* 2003; 5: 13–16.
8. Tamai H, Igaki K, Kyo E et al. Initial and 6-month results of biodegradable poly-L-lactic acid coronary stents in humans. *Circulation.* 2000; 102: 399–404.
9. Heublein B, Rohde R, Kaese V et al. Biocorrosion of magnesium alloys: A new principle in cardiovascular implant technology? *Heart.* 2003; 89: 651–656.
10. Lipinski MJ, Escarcega RO, Baker NC, Benn HA, Gaglia MA, Torguson R, Waksman R. Scaffold thrombosis after percutaneous coronary intervention with ABSORB Bioresorbable vascular scaffold a systematic review and meta-analysis. *J Am Coll Cardiol Intv.* 2016; 9: 12–24.
11. Dumoulin C, Cochelin B. Mechanical behaviour modelling of balloon-expandable stents. *J Biomech.* 2000; 33(11): 1461–1470.
12. Gyongyosi M, Yang P, Khorsand A, Glogar D. Longitudinal straightening effect of stents is an additional predictor for major adverse cardiac events. Austrian Wiktor Stent Study Group and European Paragon Stent Investigators. *J Am Coll Cardiol.* 2000; 35(6): 1580–1590.
13. Palmaz JC. Balloon-expandable intravascular stent. *Am J Roentgenol.* 1988; 150(6): 1263–1269.
14. Palmaz JC. Intravascular stenting: From basic research to clinical application. *Cardiovasc Intervent Radiol.* 1992; 15(5): 279–284.
15. Topol EJ. *Textbook of Interventional Cardiology.* 2nd ed., Saunders Company, Philadelphia, 1994; Vol. 1 and 2.
16. Foin N, Lee RD, Torii R, Guitierrez-Chico JL, Mattesini A, Nijjer S, Sen S et al. Impact of stent strut design in metallic stents and biodegradable scaffolds. *Int J Cardiol.* (2014), http://dx.doi.org/10.1016/j.ijcard.2014.09.143.
17. Schmidt W, Behrens P, Behrend D, Andresen R. Experimental study of peripheral, balloon expandable stent systems. *Progr Biomed Res.* 2001; 246–255.

18. Schmidt W, Lanzer P, Behrens P, Topoleski LDT, Schmitz KP. A comparison of the mechanical performance characteristics of seven drug-eluting stent systems. *Catheter Cardiovasc Interv.* 2009; 73: 350–360 (Online 2008).

19. Schmitz KP, Schmidt W, Behrens P, Behrend D, Lootz D, Graf B. In-vitro examination of clinically relevant stent parameters. *Progr Biomed Res.* 2000; 197–203.

20. Lanzer P, Schmidt W. Instrumentation for coronary artery interventions, in Lanzer P (Ed.) *PanVascular Medicine*, 2nd ed., Vol. 3, pp. 1979–2028, Springer, Heidelberg, 2015.

21. Serruys PW, de Jaegere P, Kiemeneij F, Macaya C, Rutsch W, Heyndrickx G, Emanuelsson H et al. A comparison of balloon-expandable-stent implantation with balloon angioplasty in patients with coronary artery disease. *N Engl J Med.* 1994; 331: 489–495.

22. Wentzel JJ, Whelan DM, van der Giessen WJ, van Beusekom HM, Andhyiswara I, Serruys PW, Slager CJ, Krams R. Coronary stent implantation changes 3-D vessel geometry and 3-D shear stress distribution. *J Biomech.* 2000; 33(10): 1287–1295.

23. Serruys PW, Onuma Y, Lafont A, Abizaid A, Waksman R, Ormiston J. Bioresorbable scaffolds in: Eckhout E, Serruys PW, Wijns W, Vahanian A, Van Sambeek M, De Palma R, Eds. *Percutaneous Interventional Cardiovascular Medicine: The PCR-EAPCI Textbook.* Volume II Intervention I, PCR Publishing, Toulouse, France, 2012, pp. 145–177.

24. Windecker S, Haude M, Neumann FJ, Stangl K, Witzenbichler B, Slagboom T, Sabaté M et al. Comparison of a novel biodegradable polymer sirolimus-eluting stent with a durable polymer everolimus-eluting stent results of the randomized BIOFLOW-II trial. *Circ Cardiovasc Interv.* 2015; 8: e001441.

25. Ishibashi Y, Onuma Y, MuramatsuT, Nakatani S, Iqbal J, Garcia-Garcia HM, Bartorelli AL et al. Lessons learned from acute and late scaffold failures in the ABSORB EXTEND trial. *EuroIntervention.* 2014; 10: 449–457, published online ahead of print January 2014.

26. Schmidt W, Behrens P, Brandt-Wunderlich C, Siewert S, Grabow N, Schmitz KP. In vitro performance investigation of bioresorbable scaffolds—Standard tests for vascular stents and beyond. *Cardiovasc Revasc Med.* 2016; 17(6): 375–383.

27. ASTM F2394–07 Standard Guide for Measuring Securement of Balloon Expandable Vascular Stent Mounted on Delivery System, 2013.

28. Ormiston JA, Webber B, Ubod B, Darremont O, Webster M. An independent bench comparison of two bioresorbable drug-eluting coronary scaffolds (Absorb and DESolve) with a durable metallic drug-eluting stent (ML8/Xpedition). *EuroIntervention.* 2015; 11: 60–67.

29. Foin N, Lee R, Mattesini A, Caiazzo G, Fabris E, Kilic D, Chan JN et al. Bioabsorbable vascular scaffold overexpansion: Insights from in vitro post-expansion experiments. *EuroIntervention.* 2016; 11: 1389–1399

30. Schmidt W, Lanzer P. Instrumentation, in: Lanzer P, Ed., *Catheter-Based Cardiovascular Interventions*, Springer-Verlag, Berlin, 2013, pp. 445–472.

31. ISO 25539-2: 2009–08 Cardiovascular implants—Endovascular devices—Part 2: Vascular stents, 2009. http://www.iso.org/iso/isoupdate_march09.pdf. Accessed Nov. 15, 2013.

32. ASTM F3067–14 Guide for Radial Loading of Balloon Expandable and Self Expanding Vascular Stents.

33. Witte F, Fischer J, Nellesen J, Crostack HA, Kaese V, Pisch A, Beckmann F, Windhagen H. In vitro and in vivo corrosion measurements of magnesium alloys. *Biomaterials.* 2006; 27: 1013–1018.

# Simulation of flow and shear stress

NICOLAS FOIN, RYO TORII, JARYL NG, ALESSIO MATTESINI, CARLO DI MARIO,
PHILIP WONG, ERHAN TENEKECIOGLU, TOM CRAKE, CHRISTOS V. BOURANTAS,
AND PATRICK W.J.C. SERRUYS

## IMPORTANCE OF WALL SHEAR STRESS DISTRIBUTION IN RESTENOSIS

The evaluation of wall shear stress (WSS) patterns *in vivo* using computational fluid dynamic (CFD) methods has revealed the important role of WSS distribution in the natural history of atherosclerotic lesion development [1–5]. Low and oscillating WSS are now known to modulate arterial wall biology and in particular endothelial cell function through complex mechano-transduction pathways that regulate gene expression and plaque biology [6,7]. Low WSS has been shown to set the arterial lining cells in a pro-inflammatory mode which accelerates the formation of vulnerable atherosclerotic plaques [6,7]. In stented segments several studies have demonstrated that WSS affects neointima tissue development [8–12]. In particular it has been shown that in bare metal stents the local hemodynamic milieu determines neointima proliferation while in drug eluting stents this effect is attenuated by the antiproliferative drug and it is more obvious in paclitaxel eluting stents than in sirolimus eluting devices [12] (Figures 3.4.1 and 3.4.2).

## IN-VIVO ASSESSMENT OF 3D HEMODYNAMIC ENVIRONMENT AFTER BRSs IMPLANTATION AND INFLUENCE ON NEOINTIMAL RESPONSE

### Implications of the local hemodynamic forces on neointimal formation

Although there are numerous studies investigating the implications of the local hemodynamic forces on neointimal formation in different bare metal and drug eluting stent platforms, only one study has explored the role of WSS on the vessel wall healing process in BRSs [13].

In this report, Bourantas et al. using OCT data reconstructed the coronary anatomy of 12 relatively straight arterial segments implanted with an everolimus eluting bioresorbable scaffold (ABSORB BVSs, Abbott Vascular, Santa Clara, CA). The OCT data acquired at 1-year follow-up were used to reconstruct the luminal surface and the scaffold surface which was assumed that corresponded to the luminal surface at baseline. Blood flow simulation was performed in the scaffolded segment and the estimated WSS on the lumen surface, also referred to as endothelial shear stress (ESS) was compared to the neointimal thickness (NT). A significant negative correlation was found between NT and WSS in all the reconstructed segments (range: −0.662 to −0.140). High WSS was noted on the top of the struts where the NT was minimal and low WSS in between the struts areas where there was increased neointimal formation.

The authors noted that the protruded struts affected the local hemodynamic micro-milieu resulting in flow disturbances and recirculation zones in the areas between the struts that created a low ESS environment which promoted neointimal proliferation. This study was the first to suggest the use of OCT—an imaging modality with a high axial resolution of 10–15 μm—to reconstruct coronary anatomy and examine the association between NT and WSS in treated segments. However, it had a significant limitation as it assumed that the reconstructed arteries were straight vessels and thus did not take into account the effect of vessel curvature on WSS distribution [13,14].

### Toward an optimal reconstruction of scaffolded segments

Bourantas et al. recently modified a well-validated methodology for the reconstruction of coronary anatomy using

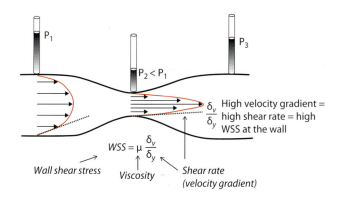

Figure 3.4.1 Wall shear stress definition. Wall shear stress (WSS) is derived from the velocity gradient near the wall (shear rate) multiplied by the viscosity of the blood μ. It has the dimension of a force per unit area and is expressed generally in Pascal or dyne/cm² (1 Pa = 10 dyne/cm²). In a straight cylindrical vessel of a radius r with a developed parabolic laminar flow profile (Poiseuille flow), wall shear stress can be evaluated from the Hagen-Poiseuille equation: WSS = $4Q \cdot \mu/(\pi r^3)$ where Q is the flow-rate, μ is the fluid viscosity, and r is the tube radius.

X-ray angiographic and intravascular ultrasound (IVUS) data acquired during a routine examination. Papafaklis et al. used the modified approach to fuse OCT and X-ray imaging, validated the OCT-derived models using IVUS-based reconstructions, and showed that the fusion of OCT with the angiographic data provides geometrically correct models that allow accurate evaluation of the ESS [15]. This approach was used to compare the efficacy of IVUS-based and OCT-based reconstructions in assessing the implications of the local hemodynamic forces on neointima formation in six segments implanted with an ABSORB BVSs [16,17]. The different resolution of IVUS and OCT affected the morphology of the obtained models and the estimated ESS. IVUS, which has a relatively low axial resolution of 150 μm, did not allow imaging of the protruded struts and thus the IVUS-based models had a smooth luminal surface and a homogenous ESS distribution (Figure 3.4.3). On the other hand, OCT with an axial resolution of 10–15 μm, allowed detailed imaging of the protruded struts and thus the OCT-derived reconstructions had a rugged luminal surface that affected the hemodynamic micro-milieu resulting

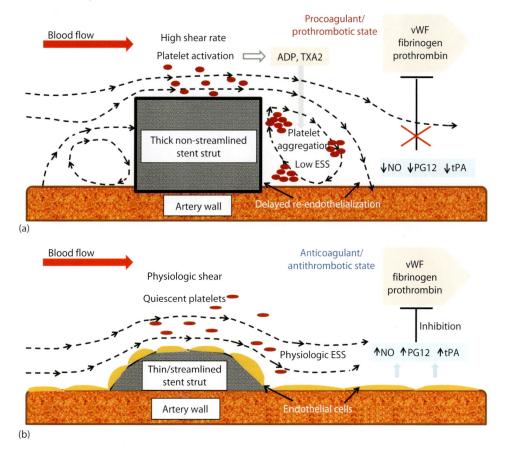

Figure 3.4.2 Effect of strut design on stent thrombogenicity. **(a)** Thicker stent strut designs may promote stent thrombogenicity through: (1) high shear rate induced platelet activation on top of struts; and (2) impaired re-endothelialization, thus attenuating the production of anticoagulants in low-WSS regions downstream of struts. **(b)** Thinner struts produce more physiologic shear distribution, which favors platelet quiescence on top of struts and enhances re-endothelialization and production of antithrombotic factors downstream of struts. Red circle = activated platelet; Red line = quiescent platelet. ESS = endothelial shear stress; NO = nitric oxide; PGI2 = prostacyclin; tPA = tissue plasminogen activator; vWF = von Willebrand factor. (Adapted from Koskinas KC, Chatzizisis YS, Antoniadis AP, Giannoglou GD. *J Am Coll Cardiol.* 2012; 59(15):1337–49.)

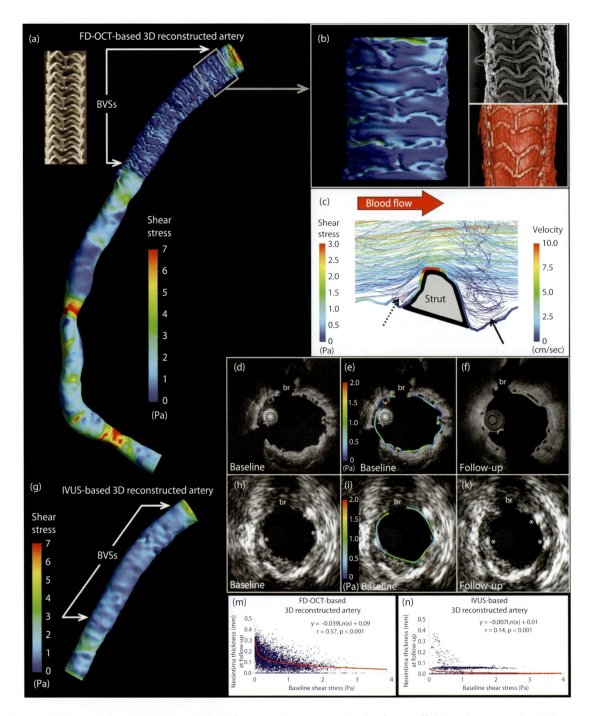

Figure 3.4.3 OCT-based reconstruction and blood flow simulation immediately after scaffold implantation; the ESS are portrayed in a color-coded map **(a)**. A photo of the BVSs Revision 1.1 strut design is also provided. A magnified view of the OCT-derived lumen surface showing the protruded struts that affect the local ESS distribution with higher values noted on top of the struts and lower values in the inter-strut areas **(b)**. There is a good matching between the strut architecture in the OCT-derived lumen surface, the electron microscopy photo (b: top right) acquired from a rabbit iliac artery 14 days post-device implantation and a 3D volume rendered image of a scaffolded patient's artery (b: bottom right) Flow streamlines in a longitudinal cross-section **(c)**; flow disturbance and recirculation regions were noted in between the strut regions (arrow and dotted arrow). Corresponding OCT cross-sectional images (evident by the side branch [br]) at baseline **(d)** and 2-year follow-up **(f)** allows visualization of the struts and the neointima tissue and the heterogeneous ESS distribution **(e)** IVUS-based reconstruction of the scaffolded segment at baseline with the ESS shown in a color-coded map **(g)**. Note the smoother ESS distribution compared to the OCT-based model. IVUS cross-sectional images at baseline **(h)** and 2-year follow-up **(k)** corresponding to the OCT images. The lower IVUS resolution allows a rough assessment of BVSs struts (asterisks) and cannot detect the neointima tissue. The ESS has a homogenous distribution **(i)**. A stronger correlation was noted between the baseline ESS and neointima thickness at 2 years in the OCT-based model (**(m)**, $R^2 = 0.50$) compared to the IVUS-based reconstruction (**(n)**, $R^2 = 0.13$). (Image obtained with permission from Papafaklis MI, Bourantas CV, Farooq V, Diletti R, Muramatsu T, Zhang Y et al. *EuroIntervention*. 2013;9(7):890.)

in flow disturbances, lower ESS, and a heterogeneous WSS distribution (mean WSS: 1.87 ± 0.66 Pa in the IVUS vs. 1.29 ± 0.66 Pa in the OCT-based models, $p = 0.030$). In addition, IVUS appeared less accurate in assessing NT compared to OCT (mean NT: 14 ± 13 μm vs. 102 ± 29 μm). These differences had a significant effect on the estimated association between WSS and NT in the IVUS- and OCT-based models (mean correlation coefficient: –0.10 ± 0.04 vs. –0.52 ± 0.19 respectively, $p = 0.028$).

This study provided robust evidence that OCT-based imaging is superior to IVUS for the study of the hemodynamic implications of implanted endovascular devices, as it allowed for the first time *in vivo* evaluation of the effect of the protruded struts on the local hemodynamic micro-environment. In the past, several *in silico* based studies have been used to examine the implications of different stent designs on the local hemodynamic milieu and the developed neo-intima. These studies have shown that the flow disruption and recirculation zones noted in stented segments depend on the geometrical characteristics of the implanted devices and critically determine vessel wall response (Figure 3.4.3) [18–23]. In particular, thick rectangular shaped struts create larger flow disturbances than the oval-shaped thin struts; moreover, strut connectors that have a parallel alignment to the flow have a smaller effect on the local hemodynamics compared to connectors that are perpendicular to the flow which cause flow disruption. Finally, an increased stent-to-artery ratio has been associated with neointimal proliferation than a smaller stent-to-artery ratio [23,24]. To date, computational modelling has been used to assess the hemodynamic profile of the designed stents. However, it is possible in the future [24] *in vivo* OCT imaging and modelling will be used to assess the impact of different stent designs on WSS distribution and facilitate optimization of their configuration.

## Short- and long-term implications of BRSs implantation on the local hemodynamic forces

Fusion of X-ray angiography and OCT imaging has been used to investigate the long-term implications of ABSORB bioresorbable scaffold implantation on the local hemodynamic forces. In a case report presented by Bourantas et al., it was shown that immediately after device implantation, flow disturbances and recirculation zones were noted that appeared to create an athero-promoting, low WSS environment which facilitated neointima formation in the areas between the struts (Figure 3.4.4) [25]. The developed thick layer of fibro-muscular tissue had features associated with plaque stability, and covered and passivated the underlying high-risk plaques [26]. In parallel, the developed neo-tissue smoothed the luminal morphology and normalized the WSS. As it is shown in Figure 3.4.4, immediately after ABSORB BVSs implantation,

62.6% of the estimated WSS were below 1 Pa, which in the PREDICTION study appeared to predispose atherosclerotic development, while at 2-year follow-up only 16.5% were below 1 Pa. Therefore, it can be speculated that at long-term follow-up, ABSORB BVSs implantation results in the stabilization of high-risk plaques and the restoration of an athero-protective WSS environment. Despite the lack of evidence about the prognostic value of these beneficial implications on vessel physiology and plaque morphology, it has been suggested that these devices may be useful for the invasive sealing of future culprit lesions. Based on this concept, the PROSPECT II study (NCT02171065) has recently commenced and aims to investigate the feasibility of ABSORB BVSs in sealing high-risk non-flow limiting lesions.

## SHEAR RATE: COMPARISON OF DISTRIBUTION IN BRSs AND METALLIC STENTS

Shear rate is defined as the local gradient in velocity between adjacent blood flow streamlines; it can be calculated for any region of the blood stream and is a parameter representative of flow disturbance. Shear rate can affect blood physiology and is a well-known modulator of platelet activation and thrombosis [27–29]. Normal human shear rate (shear rate in large to medium-sized arteries) usually varies from 100 to 1000 $s^{-1}$ [30]. However, protruding and malapposed stent struts create front-facing step and obstacles which disrupt the blood flow stream and produce flow separation and large shear rates [21–24]. In numerical steady simulation of rectangular stent struts, they elicit shear rate values above 3000 $s^{-1}$. As evidenced from *in-vivo* studies, postmortem examinations and *in vitro* experiments, such flow patterns are associated with increased platelet adhesion [23,31], inflammatory response [32,33] and poor re-endothelization [34–37] (Figure 3.4.2). High shear rate (>1000 $s^{-1}$) can activate platelets in a dose-dependent manner through the von Willebrand factor binding to glycoprotein (GP) Ib and GP IIb/IIIa receptors [4,27]. Several experiments have shown *in vitro* the influence of shear on clot formation and high shear rate is actually a prerequisite to reproduce the mechanisms of thrombus formation in both *in-vitro* and *in-vivo* models [28,29].

Strut thickness critically determines shear rate distribution (thicker struts create larger flow disruption and higher shear rate) [21]. Although thinner designs are emerging, currently, most BRSs scaffolds have strut thickness ≥150 μm. The BVS scaffold is based on a poly-L-lactic acid (PLLA) backbone with a 3 μm surface drug coating which gives a total strut thickness of 156 μm. In comparison, the metallic XIENCE Prime drug-eluting stents (DESs) is based on an 81 μm cobalt chromium alloy with a conformable fluorinated polymer coating (thickness of 8 μm). Simulations of flow profile around typical BRSs struts (>150 μm) compared with

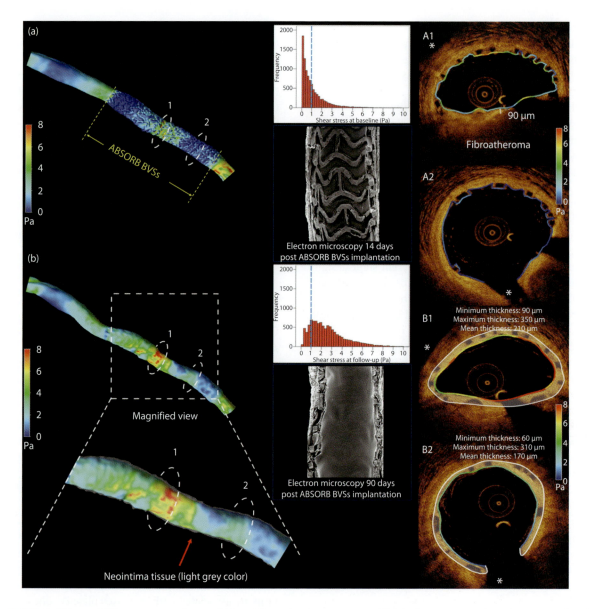

**Figure 3.4.4** OCT-based 3D reconstruction and blood flow simulation in a scaffolded segment at baseline immediately after ABSORB BVSs implantation. The ESS is shown in a color-coded map **(a)**. The rugged surface noted in the scaffolded segment (demonstrated comprehensively by electron microscopy in an animal model) resulted in predominantly low ESS (the histogram of ESS values is provided) that predisposed to neointimal formation. Panels A1 and A2 show the ESS distribution in 2 OCT images; normal ESS noted over a fibroatheroma with a cap thickness of 90μm (A1), whereas in Panel A2 the ESS was low over the vessel and normal over the struts. At follow-up, the ESS was normalized **(b)** whereas the thin layer of the developed neointima (portrayed in semitransparent fashion in the magnified model) covered the underlying plaque and smoothed the luminal surface as shown by electron microscopy in an animal model. The ESS over the fibroatheroma appeared increased, but the neointima has sealed the lipid tissue (B1). (Image obtained with permission from Bourantas CV, Papafaklis MI, Garcia-Garcia HM, Farooq V, Diletti R, Muramatsu T et al. *JACC Cardiovasc Interv.* 2014;7(1):100–1.)

a current thin strut cobalt chrome DESs metallic stent (strut thickness <100 μm) clearly show how local flow patterns, recirculation, and shear rate are affected by strut thickness (Figure 3.4.5) [21].

Apart from the strut size, incomplete stent apposition (ISA) also affects flow and shear profile: immediately after implantation, incompletely apposed struts act as obstacles that disrupt the laminar flow and create areas of high shear

rate [4,22,23]. Multiple clinical, pathological, and model studies have demonstrated an association between stent malapposition (defined as struts detached from the vessel wall) and thrombosis [23,38,39]. In a recent study, we investigated the influence of increased malapposition severity on blood flow disturbances and coverage response and analyzed retrospectively OCT data to confirm *in vivo* the results of the simulation. We computed the shear profile

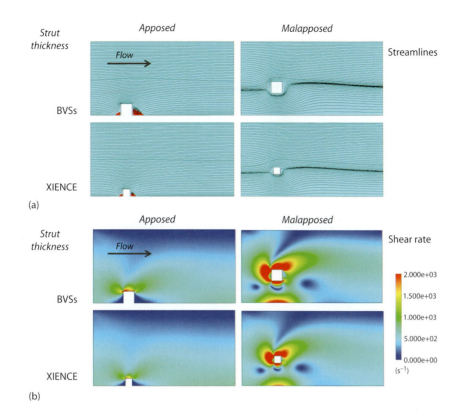

**Figure 3.4.5** Impact of strut thickness on blood flow profiles for model simulating case of well-apposed and malapposed struts. **(a)** Simulated blood flow streamlines (top panel) for the different cases of strut apposition: (1) APPOSED and (2) MALAPPOSED (with strut to wall distance = 300 μm). Models are representative of a 3-mm-diameter straight coronary artery flow with a parabolic upstream velocity profile and a peak velocity of 50 cm/s. The two strut thicknesses are considered to correspond to a total strut thickness (strut + coating) of 156 μm (BVSs) and 97 μm (XIENCE DESs). **(b)** Corresponding shear rate profile in blood around stent strut simulated for each case (lower panel) shows that flow disturbances and high shear rates (red) are increased primarily in thicker and malapposed struts. See also Videos 3.4.1 and 3.4.2. (Adapted from Foin N, Torii R, Mattesini A, Wong P, Di Mario C. *EuroIntervention*. 2015;10(10):1139–42.)

in different strut-wall ISA distances (distance between the strut and the vessel wall), ranging from 100 μm up to 500 μm [22]. Shear rate was shown to increase with malapposition distance; rates over 10,000 s$^{-1}$ were reached for detachment distances >300 μm, while shear rate calculated for embedded or protruding struts remained below 3000 s$^{-1}$ with higher shear values confined to the edge of the struts. The area of the blood stream affected by the highest shear values (over >1000 s$^{-1}$ threshold) was also increased when the ISA detachment distance increased, revealing a critical impact of the extent of malapposition distance on the local hemodynamics [22]. Results from serial OCT studies analyzing cross-sections portraying stented segments with malapposed struts suggest also that most of the struts 98% with ISA detachment distance <300 μm (moderate ISA) are fully endothelialized at 1-year follow-up creating a smooth luminal surface that allows restoration of the smooth laminar flow [22,40,41].

Interestingly, comparison of shear rate for different strut thicknesses in both apposed and malapposed cases showed that strut thickness has a relatively smaller impact on flow disturbances as compared to stent strut malapposition. (Figures 3.4.5 and 3.4.6) [42].

## SHEAR DISTRIBUTION AND STRUT THICKNESS: IMPLICATION FOR FUTURE BRSs DESIGN ITERATION

### Clinical impact of BRSs strut thickness on WSS and restenosis

The impact of strut thickness on restenosis and clinical outcomes has been evidenced in numerous studies in metallic stents [43–48]. Because of the antiproliferative effect of the drug, the impact of strut thickness on outcomes is less obvious in DESs as compared to bare metal stents (BMS) and comparison of DESs with BMS showed that the effect of the antiproliferative drug prevails over stent design characteristics [37,38,49,50]. Irrespective of the neointimal healing response, preclinical evaluation of BMS platforms with thin struts compared to BMS designs with thicker struts showed that smaller strut thickness facilitates re-endothelialization and reduces peri-strut inflammation and fibrin deposition [37,38,50]. It is therefore reasonable to assume that strut thickness will have a similar impact in BRSs technologies as in metallic stent, at least until the scaffold starts to resorb.

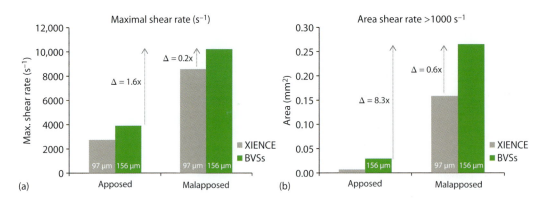

**Figure 3.4.6** Maximal shear rate **(a)** and area of shear rate >1000 s$^{-1}$ **(b)**. Comparison of the shear rate values computed for the two strut thicknesses shows that strut thickness has less impact on high shear flow disturbances as compared to strut malapposition. High shear rate activates platelets in a dose dependent manner through von Willebrand factor binding to glycoprotein (GP) Ib and GP IIb/IIIa receptors. (Adapted with permission from Foin N, Torii R, Mattesini A, Wong P, Di Mario C. *EuroIntervention.* 2015;10(10):1139–42.)

Neointimal hyperplasia and late-loss have been shown to be more extensive in BRSs than in thin-strut metallic DESs [51–54]. However, the mechanisms that regulate vessel wall response in BRSs are different since the scaffold dismantles over time, tends to expand and accommodate the developed neointima [51–54]. Therefore, while the impact of strut thickness on clinical outcome has been largely established for metallic stents, there is still no direct evidence that the same principle is applicable in BRSs. The ABSORB II trial, which is the first randomized controlled trial to directly evaluate a BRSs (ABSORB BVSs, Abbott Vascular, Santa Clara, CA) against a second generation metallic DESs [55] showed comparable results at 1 year in terms of efficacy endpoints [55].

Currently, polymer-based BRSs also require a large strut thickness to provide sufficient radial support. Inadequate scaffold support has been associated with higher risk of late recoil, lumen loss, and restenosis [56]. The principle of "the thinner the better" only applies provided that an effective radial force is maintained. Indeed, biodegradable materials are inherently limited in their strength, and while manufacturing processes can improve mechanical strength, for achieving a radial force comparable to a metallic stent, the current technology still requires an increased strut thickness [21,57]. However, research is focused on the optimization of scaffold devices and it is anticipated that the new revisions would have thinner struts and optimal hemodynamic profiles in the near future (Table 3.4.1).

## BRSs hemodynamic: Clinical implications on scaffold thrombosis

Large strut thickness implies a higher presence of foreign material in the vessel and increases flow disturbances with separation and recirculation zones, which can considerably increase the risk of thrombosis (Figures 3.4.2 and 3.4.3) [4,18,21–24,58]. Kolandaivelu et al. showed the impact of strut thickness on platelet adhesion and early restenosis *in vitro* and *in vivo* in animal models. When perfused with porcine

blood, a thin-strut BMS (81 µm) was shown to be less thrombogenic than an otherwise identical thick-strut (162 µm) stent [23]. Both stents were also shown to rapidly attract clot when left under-deployed in the blood stream [23]. Nevertheless, similar simulation studies are not available in BRSs.

Although BRSs have been available in clinical settings only recently, their use in clinical practice for treating coronary lesions is rapidly expanding.

Recent reports of clinical outcomes with ABSORB BVSs in "real world" patient populations helped to shed light onto the advantages and limitations of this technology in clinical arena [59,60]. In a multicenter retrospective registry published recently [59], Capodanno and colleagues studied 1189 patients treated with ABSORB BVSs (GHOST-EU registry) and found a target lesion failure (TLF) rate of 4.4% at 6 months' follow-up and a considerably high incidence of definite/probable scaffold thrombosis at 30 days' (1.5%) and 6 months' (2.1%) [59] follow-up.

In the ABSORB II trial, the target vessel related myocardial infarction rate was 4.2% in the ABSORB group versus 1.2% in the XIENCE group ($p = 0.07$) at 1-year follow-up; probable and definite stent thrombosis (ST) events were reported in three patients in the ABSORB group (0.9%) and in none of the patients in the XIENCE group [55]. In the ABSORB cohort A and cohort B trial, no scaffold or late scaffold thrombosis was observed at follow-up (up to 5Y for cohort A): a fact that should be attributed to the small number of patients and the low lesion complexity in these studies [61]. Similarly in the first 450 patients enrolled in the ABSORB EXTEND study, the rate of subacute or late scaffold thrombosis was only 0.89% at 12 months [60].

## Incomplete BRSs apposition: A hallmark for thrombosis?

A potential explanation of the discrepancies noted in the abovementioned studies is the differences noted in lesion

**Table 3.4.1** Strut design characteristics of major bioresorbable stent/scaffolds commercially available or currently under development

| Scaffold | Strut material | Strut thickness μm | Drug | Coating | Resorption time, months |
|---|---|---|---|---|---|
| *ReZolve* (REVA Medical) | Poly-tyrosine-derived polycarbonate polymer | 114–228 | Sirolimus | None | 48 |
| IDEAL biostent Gen I (Xenogenics) | Polylactide anhydride | 200 | Sirolimus | Salicilatelinged with adipic acid | 6–9 |
| FORTITUDE BRSs (Amaranth Medical) | PLLA | 150–200 | None | None | 12 |
| IDEAL biostent Gen II (Xenogenics) | Polylactide anhydride | 175 | Sirolimus | Salicilatelinged with adipic acid | 6–9 |
| Igaki-Tamai (Kyoto Medical) | PLLA | 170 | None | None | 24–36 |
| ART 18Z (ART) | PLLA | 170 | None | None | 18 |
| AMS 1.0 (Biotronik) | Mg alloy | 165 | None | None | <4 |
| Xinsorb BRSs (Huaan) | PLLA, PCL, PLGA | 160 | Sirolimus | None | NA |
| ABSORB BVSs 1.0 (Abbott) | PLLA | 150 | Everolimus | PDLLA | 24 |
| ABSORB BVSs 1.1 (Abbott) | PLLA | 150 | Everolimus | PDLLA | 24 |
| DESolve (Elixir Medical) | PLLA | 150 | Novolimus | PLLA | 12–24 |
| On-ABS (OrbusNeich) | PLLA, PDLLA, PCL | 150 | EPC+Sirolimus | None | NA |
| DREAMS 2 (Biotronik) | Mg alloy | 150 | Sirolimus | PLLA | 9 |
| DREAMS 1 (Biotronik) | Mg alloy | 125 | Paclitaxel | PLGA | 9 |
| ZMED (Zorion Medical) | Mg alloy + Polymer | 125 | None | PLLA | 6–9 |
| Fantom (REVA Medical) | Poly-tyrosine-derived polycarbonate polymer | 125 | Sirolimus | na | 12 |
| Mirage (Manli Cardiology) | PDLA fiber | 125 | Sirolimus | PLLA | 6–12 |
| FORTITUDE Next Gen (Amaranth Medical) | PLLA | 120 | Sirolimus | PLLA | 12 |
| Arteriosorb (Arterius) | PLLA | 120 | Sirolimus | PLLA | 12–24 |
| ABSORB BVSs Next Gen (Abbott) | PLLA | 100–120 | Everolimus | PDLLA | 24 |
| MeRes100 (MerilLifescience) | PLLA | 100 | Sirolimus | PDLLA | 6–12 |
| DESolve 100 (Elixir Medical) | PLLA | 100 | Novolimus | PLLA | 12–24 |

complexity and the differences in optimal device expansion. Incomplete stent expansion assessed with intravascular imaging is generally considered a predicator of stent thrombosis and adverse outcomes [22,62–67]. The incidence of ISA has been reported in up to 77% of the cases of very late stent thrombosis (VLST) [62]. Pathological studies have revealed that delayed healing and incomplete re-endothelialization are common findings in fatal cases of LST after DESs implantation [31,68].

There is evidence that malapposed struts create higher shear rate and are more likely to have delayed re-endothelialization and remain uncovered because of the distance to the healthy endothelium and higher ESS [22] while experimental and pathological observations suggest that prolonged exposure of unapposed and non-endothelialized struts to disturbed flow may often lead to stent thrombosis [23,31,68].

Several reports have recently warned about the risk of ISA in BRSs [59,60,69,70]. In a serial analysis of malapposed struts of ABSORB BVS scaffolds using OCT, Gomez

Lara et al. showed that ISA at baseline was related to the presence of uncovered struts and intraluminal masses at 6 months follow-up [71]. Simulations of blood flow in BRSs showed that the shear profile is higher compared to a thin strut metallic stent (Figure 3.4.3) and that the influence of malapposition on shear disturbances is several-fold more important than the effect of strut dimension [42]. Therefore, it is likely that optimal BRSs expansion may be at least as important as what has been shown to be in metallic stents [60,70,72–76]. Of note, in recent reports of clinical outcomes with ABSORB BVSs in broader, more complex "real world" patient populations [59,60,77], the studies with the lowest BVSs thrombosis rates (Costopoulos et al. and Mattesini et al., both with 0% ST) also had the highest postdilatation rates (99.3% and 100%) and the highest postdilatation pressures (>20 ATM in both studies) [77,78]. Intracoronary imaging guidance was almost systematically used in both studies [77,78]. Although these studies were not powered to provide definitive answers, their results underline that appropriate lesion preparation, accurate scaffold sizing, postdeployment optimization, and possibly intracoronary imaging guidance are particularly important for optimizing BVSs implantation and clinical outcomes.

Nevertheless, scaffold thrombosis is still a new phenomenon [42,70,79]. Upcoming data from all-comers studies with longer-term follow-up and large trials including ABSORB III and ABSORB EXTEND are anticipated to shed light on its incidence and the underlying pathophysiological mechanisms leading to these events.

## TAKE-HOME MESSAGE

- BRSs affect WSS distribution and early neointimal response, in a similar way as for metallic stents. However, as the BRSs resorbs, it tends to expand and accommodate the developed neointima, thereby preventing the loss of the lumen area.
- CFD simulations show that BRSs implantation has a clear impact on WSS and shear rate distribution. Incomplete apposition appears to play a more detrimental role on the local hemodynamic milieu than the strut's dimensions. Based on the currently available data, one should ensure a satisfactory final scaffold expansion and postdilate appropriately malapposed struts to minimize the impact of the implanted device on the local hemodynamics.

## CONCLUSION

Understanding the role of flow and the implication of shear distribution on restenosis and thrombosis may provide new insights and recommendations about BRSs implantation. Future *in vitro* and *in vivo* CFD simulations are anticipated to show the clinical value of an optimal hemodynamic profile of the future devices and guide the design of the next BRSs generation.

## VIDEOS

Video 3.4.1 Impact of strut thickness on blood flow profiles for well-apposed and malapposed struts. (Pulsatile flow through cardiac cycle, corresponding to cases in Figure 3.4.5a.): https://youtu.be/37jveoGtyLM

Video 3.4.2 Simulated shear rate profile around stent strut. (Pulsatile flow through cardiac cycle, corresponding to cases in Figure 3.4.5b.): https://youtu.be/I7gYcUS_IBE

## REFERENCES

1. Chatzizisis YS, Coskun AU, Jonas M, Edelman ER, Feldman CL, Stone PH. Role of endothelial shear stress in the natural history of coronary atherosclerosis and vascular remodeling: Molecular, cellular, and vascular behavior. *J Am Coll Cardiol.* 2007;49(25):2379–93.
2. Stone PH. Effect of endothelial shear stress on the progression of coronary artery disease, vascular remodeling, and in-stent restenosis in humans in vivo 6-month follow-up study. *Circulation.* 2003;108(4):438.
3. Wentzel JJ, Gijsen FJH, Stergiopulos N, Serruys PW, Slager CJ, Krams R. Shear stress, vascular remodeling and neointimal formation. *J Biomech.* 2003;36(5):681–8.
4. Koskinas KC, Chatzizisis YS, Antoniadis AP, Giannoglou GD. Role of endothelial shear stress in stent restenosis and thrombosis: Pathophysiologic mechanisms and implications for clinical translation. *J Am Coll Cardiol.* 2012;59(15):1337–49.
5. Stone PH, Saito S, Takahashi S, Makita Y, Nakamura S, Kawasaki T et al. Prediction of progression of coronary artery disease and clinical outcomes using vascular profiling of endothelial shear stress and arterial plaque characteristics: The PREDICTION Study. *Circulation.* 2012;126(2):172–81.
6. Cheng C, Tempel D, van Haperen R, van der Baan A, Grosveld F, Daemen MJAP et al. Atherosclerotic lesion size and vulnerability are determined by patterns of fluid shear stress. *Circulation.* 2006;113(23):2744–53.
7. Chatzizisis YS, Jonas M, Coskun AU, Beigel R, Stone BV, Maynard C et al. Prediction of the localization of high-risk coronary atherosclerotic plaques on the basis of low endothelial shear stress: An intravascular ultrasound and histopathology natural history study. *Circulation.* 2008;117(8):993–1002.
8. Wentzel JJ, Krams R, Schuurbiers JC, Oomen JA, Kloet J, van der Giessen WJ et al. Relationship between neointimal thickness and shear stress after Wallstent implantation in human coronary arteries. *Circulation.* 2001;103(13):1740–5.
9. Carlier SG. Augmentation of wall shear stress inhibits neointimal hyperplasia after stent implantation inhibition through reduction of inflammation? *Circulation.* 2003;107(21):2741.
10. Richter Y. Dynamic flow alterations dictate leukocyte adhesion and response to endovascular interventions. *J Clin Investig.* 2004;113(11):1607.
11. Papafaklis MI, Bourantas CV, Theodorakis PE, Katsouras CS, Naka KK, Fotiadis DI et al. The effect of shear stress on neointimal response following sirolimus- and paclitaxel-eluting stent implantation compared with bare-metal stents in humans. *JACC Cardiovasc Interv.* 2010;3(11):1181–9.
12. Papafaklis MI, Bourantas CV, Theodorakis PE, Katsouras CS, Fotiadis DI, Michalis LK. Relationship of shear stress with in-stent restenosis: Bare metal stenting and the effect of brachytherapy. *Int J Cardiol.* 2009;134(1):25–32.

13. Bourantas CV, Papafaklis MI, Kotsia A, Farooq V, Muramatsu T, Gomez-Lara J et al. Effect of the endothelial shear stress patterns on neointimal proliferation following drug-eluting bioresorbable vascular scaffold implantation: An optical coherence tomography study. *JACC Cardiovasc Interv.* 2014;7(3):315–24.

14. Farooq V, Serruys PW, Heo JH, Gogas BD, Onuma Y, Perkins LE et al. Intracoronary optical coherence tomography and histology of overlapping everolimus-eluting bioresorbable vascular scaffolds in a porcine coronary artery model: The potential implications for clinical practice. *JACC Cardiovasc Interv.* 2013;6(5):523–32.

15. Papafaklis MI, Bourantas CV, Yonetsu T, Vergallo R, Kotsia A, Nakatani S et al. Anatomically correct three-dimensional coronary artery reconstruction using frequency domain optical coherence tomographic and angiographic data: Head-to-head comparison with intravascular ultrasound for endothelial shear stress assessment in humans. *EuroIntervention.* 2015;11(4):407–15.

16. Bourantas CV, Papafaklis MI, Lakkas L, Sakellarios A, Onuma Y, Zhang YJ et al. Fusion of optical coherence tomographic and angiographic data for more accurate evaluation of the endothelial shear stress patterns and neointimal distribution after bioresorbable scaffold implantation: Comparison with intravascular ultrasound-derived reconstructions. *Int J Cardiovasc Imaging.* 2014;30(3):485–94.

17. Papafaklis MI, Bourantas CV, Farooq V, Diletti R, Muramatsu T, Zhang Y et al. In vivo assessment of the three-dimensional haemodynamic microenvironment following drug-eluting bioresorbable vascular scaffold implantation in a human coronary artery: Fusion of frequency domain optical coherence tomography and angiography. *EuroIntervention.* 2013;9(7):890.

18. Jiménez J, Davies P. Hemodynamically driven stent strut design. *Ann Biomed Eng.* 2009;37(8):1483–94.

19. Balossino R, Gervaso F, Migliavacca F, Dubini G. Effects of different stent designs on local hemodynamics in stented arteries. *J Biochem.* 2008;41(5):1053–61.

20. LaDisa J, Jr., Guler I, Olson L, Hettrick D, Kersten J, Warltier D et al. Three-dimensional computational fluid dynamics modeling of alterations in coronary wall shear stress produced by stent implantation. *Ann Biomed Eng.* 2003;31(8):972–80.

21. Foin N, Lee RD, Torii R, Guitierrez-Chico JL, Mattesini A, Nijjer S et al. Impact of stent strut design in metallic stents and biodegradable scaffolds. *Int J Cardiol.* 2014;177(3):800–8.

22. Foin N, Gutiérrez-Chico JL, Nakatani S, Torii R, Bourantas CV, Sen S et al. Incomplete stent apposition causes high shear flow disturbances and delay in neointimal coverage as a function of strut to wall detachment distance: Implications for the management of incomplete stent apposition. *Circ Cardiovasc Interv.* 2014;7(2):180–9.

23. Kolandaivelu K, Swaminathan R, Gibson WJ, Kolachalama VB, Nguyen-Ehrenreich KL, Giddings VL et al. Stent thrombogenicity early in high-risk interventional settings is driven by stent design and deployment and protected by polymer-drug coatings. *Circulation.* 2011;123(13):1400–9.

24. Duraiswamy N, Schoephoerster RT, Moreno MR, Moore JE. Stented artery flow patterns and their effects on the artery wall. *Ann Rev Fluid Mech.* 2006;39(1):357–82.

25. Bourantas CV, Papafaklis MI, Garcia-Garcia HM, Farooq V, Diletti R, Muramatsu T et al. Short- and long-term implications of a bioresorbable vascular scaffold implantation on the local endothelial shear stress patterns. *JACC Cardiovasc Interv.* 2014;7(1):100–1.

26. Bourantas CV, Serruys PW, Nakatani S, Zhang YJ, Farooq V, Diletti R et al. Bioresorbable vascular scaffold treatment induces the formation of neointimal cap that seals the underlying plaque without compromising the luminal dimensions: A concept based on serial optical coherence tomography data. *EuroIntervention.* 2014.

27. Holme PA, Orvim U, Hamers MJ, Solum NO, Brosstad FR, Barstad RM et al. Shear-induced platelet activation and platelet microparticle formation at blood flow conditions as in arteries with a severe stenosis. *Arterioscl Throm Vasc Biol.* 1997;17(4):646–53.

28. Strony J, Beaudoin A, Brands D, Adelman B. Analysis of shear stress and hemodynamic factors in a model of coronary artery stenosis and thrombosis. *Am J Physiol.* 1993;265(5 Pt 2):H1787–H96.

29. Badimon L, Badimon JJ, Turitto VT, Vallabhajosula S, Fuster V. Platelet thrombus formation on collagen type I. A model of deep vessel injury. Influence of blood rheology, von Willebrand factor, and blood coagulation. *Circulation.* 1988;78(6):1431–42.

30. Hanson SR, Sakariassen KS. Blood flow and antithrombotic drug effects. *Am Heart J.* 1998;135(5 Pt 2 Su):S132–S45.

31. Nakazawa G, Yazdani SK, Finn AV, Vorpahl M, Kolodgie FD, Virmani R. Pathological findings at bifurcation lesions: The impact of flow distribution on atherosclerosis and arterial healing after stent implantation. *J Am Coll Cardiol.* 55(16):1679–87.

32. Nagel T, Resnick N, Dewey CF, Gimbrone MA. Vascular endothelial cells respond to spatial gradients in fluid shear stress by enhanced activation of transcription factors. *Arterioscl Throm Vasc Biol.* 1999;19(8):1825–34.

33. Finn AV. Differential response of delayed healing and persistent inflammation at sites of overlapping sirolimus- or paclitaxel-eluting stents. *Circulation.* 2005;112(2):270.

34. Sprague EA, Luo J, Palmaz JC. Human aortic endothelial cell migration onto stent surfaces under static and flow conditions. *J Vasc Interv Radiol.* 1997;8(1):83–92.

35. Simon C, Palmaz JC, Sprague EA. Influence of topography on endothelialization of stents: Clues for new designs. *J Long-Term Eff Med Implants.* 2000;10(1–2):143–51.

36. Finn AV, Joner M, Nakazawa G, Kolodgie F, Newell J, John MC et al. Pathological correlates of late drug-eluting stent thrombosis: Strut coverage as a marker of endothelialization. *Circulation.* 2007;115(18):2435–41.

37. Joner M, Nakazawa G, Finn AV, Quee SC, Coleman L, Acampado E et al. Endothelial cell recovery between comparator polymer-based drug-eluting stents. *J Am Coll Cardiol.* 2008;52(5):333–42.

38. Finn AV, Nakazawa G, Joner M, Kolodgie FD, Mont EK, Gold HK et al. Vascular responses to drug eluting stents: Importance of delayed healing. *Arterioscl Throm Vasc Biol.* 2007;27(7):1500–10.

39. Guagliumi G, Sirbu V, Musumeci G, Gerber R, Biondi-Zoccai G, Ikejima H et al. Examination of the in vivo mechanisms of late drug-eluting stent thrombosis: Findings from optical coherence tomography and intravascular ultrasound imaging. *JACC Cardiovasc Interv.* 2012;5(1):12–20.

40. Gutierrez-Chico JL, Wykrzykowska JJ, Nesch E, van Geuns RJ, Koch KT, Koolen JJ et al. Vascular tissue reaction to acute malapposition in human coronary arteries: Sequential assessment with optical coherence tomography. *Circ Cardiovasc Interv.* 2012;5(1):20–9.

41. Ozaki Y, Okumura M, Ismail TF, Naruse H, Hattori K, Kan S et al. The fate of incomplete stent apposition with drug-eluting stents: An optical coherence tomography-based natural history study. *Eur Heart J.* 2010;31(12):1470–6.

42. Foin N, Torii R, Mattesini A, Wong P, Di Mario C. Biodegradable vascular scaffold: Is optimal expansion the key to minimising flow disturbances and risk of adverse events? *EuroIntervention.* 2015;10(10):1139–42.

43. Kastrati A, Mehilli J, Dirschinger J, Pache J, Ulm K, Schühlen H et al. Restenosis after coronary placement of various stent types. *Am J Cardiol.* 2001;87(1):34–9.

44. Kastrati A, Mehilli J, Dirschinger J, Dotzer F, Schühlen H, Neumann F-J et al. Intracoronary stenting and angiographic results: Strut thickness effect on restenosis outcome (ISAR-STEREO) trial. *Circulation.* 2001;103(23):2816–21.

45. Yoshitomi Y, Kojima S, Yano M, Sugi T, Matsumoto Y, Saotome M et al. Does stent design affect probability of restenosis? A randomized trial comparing

Multilink stents with GFX stents. *Am Heart J.* 2001;142(3):445–51.

46. Dibra A, Kastrati A, Mehilli J, Pache J, von Oepen R, Dirschinger J et al. Influence of stent surface topography on the outcomes of patients undergoing coronary stenting: A randomized double-blind controlled trial. *Cathet Cardiovasc Interv.* 2005;65(3):374–80.

47. Pache Jü, Kastrati A, Mehilli J, Schühlen H, Dotzer F, Hausleiter Jö et al. Intracoronary stenting and angiographic results: Strut thickness effect on restenosis outcome (ISAR-STEREO-2) trial. *J Am Coll Cardiol.* 2003;41(8):1283–8.

48. Briguori C, Sarais C, Pagnotta P, Liistro F, Montorfano M, Chieffo A et al. In-stent restenosis in small coronary arteries: Impact of strut thickness. *J Am Coll Cardiol.* 2002;40(3):403–9.

49. Pache J, Dibra A, Mehilli J, Dirschinger J, Schömig A, Kastrati A. Drug-eluting stents compared with thin-strut bare stents for the reduction of restenosis: A prospective, randomized trial. *Eur Heart J.* 2005;26(13):1262–8.

50. Soucy NV, Feygin JM, Tunstall R, Casey MA, Pennington DE, Huibregtse BA et al. Strut tissue coverage and endothelial cell coverage: A comparison between bare metal stent platforms and platinum chromium stents with and without everolimus-eluting coating. *EuroIntervention. Journal of EuroPCR in collaboration with the Working Group on Interventional Cardiology of the European Society of Cardiology.* 2010;6(5):630–7.

51. Bourantas CV, Onuma Y, Farooq V, Zhang Y, Garcia-Garcia HM, Serruys PW. Bioresorbable scaffolds: Current knowledge, potentialities and limitations experienced during their first clinical applications. *Int J Cardiol.* 2013;167(1):11–21.

52. Serruys PW, Onuma Y, García-García HM, Muramatsu T, van Geuns R-J, de Bruyne B et al. Dynamics of vessel wall changes following the implantation of the Absorb everolimus-eluting bioresorbable vascular scaffold: A multi-imaging modality study at 6, 12, 24 and 36 months. *EuroIntervention.* 2014;9(11):1271–84.

53. Ormiston JA, Serruys PW, Onuma Y, van Geuns RJ, de Bruyne B, Dudek D et al. First serial assessment at 6 months and 2 years of the second generation of absorb everolimus-eluting bioresorbable vascular scaffold: A multi-imaging modality study. *Circ Cardiovasc Interv.* 2012;5(5):620–32.

54. Otsuka F, Pacheco E, Perkins LEL, Lane JP, Wang Q, Kamberi M et al. Long-term safety of an everolimus-eluting bioresorbable vascular scaffold and the cobalt-chromium XIENCE V stent in a porcine coronary artery model. *Circ Cardiovasc Interv.* 2014;7(3):330–42.

55. Serruys PW, Chevalier B, Dudek D, Cequier A, Carrié D, Iniguez A et al. A bioresorbable everolimus-eluting scaffold versus a metallic everolimus-eluting stent for ischaemic heart disease caused by de-novo native coronary artery lesions (ABSORB II): An interim 1-year analysis of clinical and procedural secondary outcomes from a randomised controlled trial. *Lancet.* 2014.

56. Onuma Y, Serruys PW, Gomez J, de Bruyne B, Dudek D, Thuesen L et al. Comparison of in vivo acute stent recoil between the bioresorbable everolimus-eluting coronary scaffolds (revision 1.0 and 1.1) and the metallic everolimus-eluting stent. *Cathet Cardiovasc Interv.* 2011;78(1):3–12.

57. Onuma Y, Serruys PW. Bioresorbable Scaffold: The advent of a new era in percutaneous coronary and peripheral revascularization? *Circulation.* 2011;123(7):779–97.

58. Bourantas CV, Papafaklis MI, Kotsia A, Farooq V, Muramatsu T, Gomez-Lara J et al. Effect of the endothelial shear stress patterns on neointimal proliferation following drug-eluting bioresorbable vascular scaffold implantation: An optical coherence tomography study. *JACC Cardiovasc Interv.* 2014;7(3):315–24.

59. Capodanno D, Gori T, Nef H, Latib A, Mehilli J, Lesiak M et al. Percutaneous coronary intervention with everolimus-eluting bioresorbable vascular scaffolds in routine clinical practice: Early and midterm outcomes from the European multicentre GHOST-EU registry. *EuroIntervention.* 2014.

60. Ishibashi Y, Onuma Y, Muramatsu T, Nakatani S, Iqbal J, García-García HM et al. Lessons learned from acute and late scaffold failures in the ABSORB EXTEND trial. *EuroIntervention.* 2014;10(4):449–57.

61. Serruys PW, Onuma Y, Ormiston JA, de Bruyne B, Regar E, Dudek D et al. Evaluation of the second generation of a bioresorbable everolimus drug-eluting vascular scaffold for treatment of de novo coronary artery stenosis: Six-month clinical and imaging outcomes. *Circulation.* 2010;122(22):2301–12.

62. Cook S, Wenaweser P, Togni M, Billinger M, Morger C, Seiler C et al. Incomplete stent apposition and very late stent thrombosis after drug-eluting stent implantation. *Circulation.* 2007;115(18):2426–34.

63. Holme PA, Orvim U, Hamers MJAG, Solum NO, Brosstad FR, Barstad RM et al. Shear-induced platelet activation and platelet microparticle formation at blood flow conditions as in arteries with a severe stenosis. *Arterioscl Throm Vasc Biol.* 1997;17(4):646–53.

64. Ormiston JA. Stent deformation following simulated side-branch dilatation: A comparison of five stent designs. *Cathet Cardiovasc Interv.* 1999;47(2):258.

65. Uren NG, Schwarzacher SP, Metz JA, Lee DP, Honda Y, Yeung AC et al. Predictors and outcomes of stent thrombosis. An intravascular ultrasound registry. *Eur Heart J.* 2002;23(2):124–32.

66. Cook S, Ladich E, Nakazawa G, Eshtehardi P, Neidhart M, Vogel R et al. Correlation of intravascular ultrasound findings with histopathological analysis of thrombus aspirates in patients with very late drug-eluting stent thrombosis. *Circulation.* 2009;120(5):391–9.

67. Ozaki Y, Okumura M, Ismail TF, Naruse H, Hattori K, Kan S et al. The fate of incomplete stent apposition with drug-eluting stents: An optical coherence tomography-based natural history study. *Eur Heart J.* 2010;31(12):1470–6.

68. Joner M, Finn AV, Farb A, Mont EK, Kolodgie FD, Ladich E et al. Pathology of drug-eluting stents in humans: Delayed healing and late thrombotic risk. *J Am Coll Cardiol.* 2006;48(1):193–202.

69. Ormiston JA, De Vroey F, Serruys PW, Webster MWI. Bioresorbable polymeric vascular scaffolds: A cautionary tale. *Circ Cardiovasc Interv.* 2011;4(5):535–8.

70. Di Mario C, Caiazzo G. Biodegradable stents: The golden future of angioplasty? *Lancet.* 2014.

71. Gomez-Lara J, Radu M, Brugaletta S, Farooq V, Diletti R, Onuma Y et al. Serial analysis of the malapposed and uncovered struts of the new generation of everolimus-eluting bioresorbable scaffold with optical coherence tomography. *JACC Cardiovasc Interv.* 2011;4(9):992–1001.

72. Hur S-H, Kitamura K, Morino Y, Honda Y, Jones M, Korr KS et al. Efficacy of postdeployment balloon dilatation for current generation stents as assessed by intravascular ultrasound. *Am J Cardiol.* 2001;88(10):1114–9.

73. Russo RJ, Silva PD, Teirstein PS, Attubato MJ, Davidson CJ, DeFranco AC et al. A randomized controlled trial of angiography versus intravascular ultrasound-directed bare-metal coronary stent placement (The AVID Trial)/Clinical Perspective. *Circ Cardiovasc Interv.* 2009;2(2):113–23.

74. Gerber RT, Latib A, Ielasi A, Cosgrave J, Qasim A, Airoldi F et al. Defining a new standard for IVUS optimized drug eluting stent implantation: The PRAVIO study. *Cathet Cardiovasc Interv.* 2009;74(2):348–56.

75. Fujii K, Carlier SG, Mintz GS, Yang Y-m, Moussa I, Weisz G et al. Stent underexpansion and residual reference segment stenosis are related to stent thrombosis after sirolimus-eluting stent implantation: An intravascular ultrasound study. *J Am Coll Cardiol.* 2005;45(7):995–8.

76. Doi H, Maehara A, Mintz GS, Yu A, Wang H, Mandinov L et al. Impact of post-intervention minimal stent area on 9-month follow-up patency of paclitaxel-eluting stents: An integrated intravascular ultrasound analysis from the TAXUS IV, V,

and VI and TAXUS ATLAS workhorse, long lesion, and direct stent trials. *JACC Cardiovasc Interv.* 2009;2(12):1269–75.

77. Mattesini A, Secco GG, Dall'Ara G, Ghione M, Rama-Merchan JC, Lupi A et al. ABSORB Biodegradable stents versus second-generation metal stents: A comparison study of 100 complex lesions treated under OCT guidance. *JACC Cardiovasc Interv.* 2014;7(7):741–50.

78. Costopoulos C, Latib A, Naganuma T, Miyazaki T, Sato K, Figini F et al. Comparison of early clinical outcomes between absorb bioresorbable vascular scaffold and everolimus-eluting stent implantation in a real-world population. *Cathet Cardiovasc Interv.* 2014.

79. Ishibashi Y, Nakatani S, Onuma Y. Definite and probable bioresorbable scaffold thrombosis in stable and ACS patients. *EuroIntervention.* 2014.

# Preclinical assessment of bioresorbable scaffolds and regulatory implication

TOBIAS KOPPARA, ERIC WITTCHOW, RENU VIRMANI, AND MICHAEL JONER

## INTRODUCTION

Bioresorbable stents (BRSs) represent an intuitively appealing technology with potential to solve some of the issues associated with the use of metallic drug eluting stents (DESs) over the last few years. Currently, three BRSs with distinct design properties have received CE (Conformité Européene) mark approval for use in Europe (Figure 3.5.1). Despite the early adoption of this technology in clinical practice after achieving favorable initial clinical results, some concerns remain with respect to acute thrombogenicity and sustainability of clinical efficacy especially when targeting atherosclerotic coronary lesions with greater complexity [1]. In addition to bench testing of material characteristics and toxicological evaluation of device components, preclinical studies represent an important milestone in the safety evaluation of BRSs. *In vivo* testing in preclinical animals followed by histologic assessment at various time points for vascular response during biodegradation is key in the understanding of the safety profile of BRSs.

A significant body of knowledge has been accumulated by investigations describing multiple features of BRSs biocompatibility in preclinical animal studies to date. Intravascular imaging techniques, such as intravascular ultrasound (IVUS) and optical coherence tomography (OCT), were utilized to characterize BRSs *in vivo* and revealed valuable insights of vascular healing after BRSs implantation. This chapter reviews existing literature and its major objective is to describe the key experiments essential for preclinical investigation of BRSs with special focus on regulatory requirements, *in vivo* degradation analysis, and responses that can be monitored via the use of intravascular imaging.

## OVERVIEW OF PRECLINICAL EVALUATION OF BRSs WITH FOCUS ON REGULATORY SUBMISSION

In general, the emphasis of all preclinical testing is to determine the safety profile of a device by implanting it in the appropriate vascular bed for which it is indicated. An ideal animal model that is most representative of human coronary disease does not exist today. Currently used animal models provide mechanistic insights into fundamental biological processes reflecting biocompatibility and safety of coronary stents. With respect to efficacy testing, several hypercholesterolemic preclinical animal models have been described [2–6] to overcome the limitations of healthy animals with non-diseased arteries. However, none of them have proven to truly reflect the efficacy of coronary stents for human clinical applications to date. Nonetheless, preclinical research studies have been helpful in proving safety and to deliver valuable insights into the vascular healing responses after stent implantation. Current standards for preclinical and clinical evaluation of coronary stents in Europe have recently been reported in an executive summary report by the European Society of Cardiology–European Association of Percutaneous Cardiovascular Interventions task force on the evaluation of coronary stents in Europe [7].

Since a vast amount of knowledge exists about metallic bare metal (BMS) and drug eluting stents (DESs), these must be used as comparators in preclinical studies when evaluating BRSs with or without drug coating in animal models. Comparative investigation of these novel devices versus metallic stents with known efficacy and safety may help to facilitate appreciation of their future clinical performance. BRSs are markedly different from metallic stents as

| | Elixir medical | Abbott vascular | Kyoto medical |
|---|---|---|---|
| Market name | DESolve | ABSORB BVSs | Igaka-Tamai |
| Platform | PLLA | PLLA | PLLA |
| Drug | Novolimus | Everolimus | None |
| Approved application | Coronary | Coronary | Peripheral |
| Stent design | 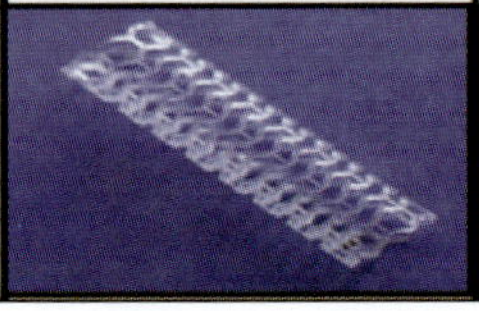 | 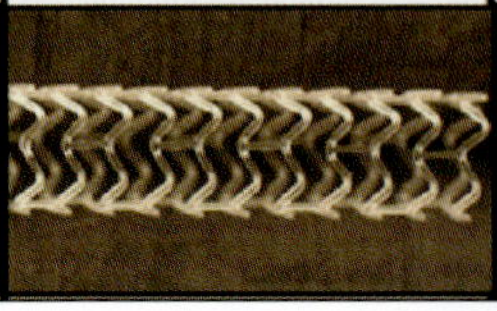 | 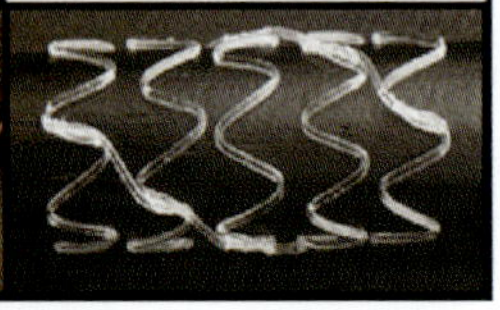 |

Figure 3.5.1 Current BRSs with CE-mark approval.

they degrade over time and lose their structural integrity. Thus, the demands for preclinical assessment of BRSs are different from those of metallic DESs, as they require thorough investigation of biodegradation. Vascular remodeling may be observed after BRSs implantation as a consequence of biodegradation and inflammation. Thus, it is imperative that animals are sacrificed at regular intervals to monitor such effects. Most published preclinical studies have been performed in healthy porcine coronary arteries, a widely accepted animal model for the evaluation of coronary stents because of similarities to human coronary size and device requirements [8]. The traditional follow-up included early, intermediate, and long-term time-points in order to understand the bioresorption characteristics and the responses elicited [9–18]. Controlling animal growth is of particular importance when studying long-term effects of cardiovascular devices and needs to be carefully monitored over time. Therefore, miniature swine models have been preferred over landrace pigs to study long-term effects of bioresorption.

The rabbit iliac artery model is also recognized as a reliable model to assess safety and biocompatibility for coronary stents. However, as the devices are not placed in the location intended for use in humans, it is not universally accepted [19]. The advantage of the rabbit iliac artery model is less variability of injury to the vessel wall at the time of stent implantation and more consistent and predictable inflammatory responses. Therefore, it is a valuable addition for the evaluation of biocompatibility and safety of investigational devices. It has also been used for studies focusing on endothelialization of stents because the rate of endothelial regrowth in the rabbit is slower as compared to swine [20,21].

Overall, clinico-pathological observations, include blood work-up (Table 3.5.1), daily monitoring of animal health, investigation of embolic or ischemic events in the myocardium that the stent supplies, and thorough examination of all organs for untoward or toxic effects. Standard contemporary

antiplatelet therapy that is advocated in humans should be utilized in all animal models. Adjustment of dosing and duration should be employed in the animal studies according to the labeling for the clinical indication of the product. As a general rule, preclinical testing should be performed within the intended vascular territory (i.e., stents designated for use in coronary arteries should be tested in coronary arteries). There may be instances in which a switch to a different vascular location may provide valuable information about the biological behavior of stents owing to the differences in reaction to vascular injury and inflammation among species and vascular territories, but it needs to be justified. Contemporary standards for BRSs evaluation in preclinical animal models are listed in Table 3.5.2.

Special attention is required for safety assessment of multicomponent devices employing bioresorbable stent backbones with either permanent or biodegradable coatings of different origin compared to the stent backbone. In these instances, it is strongly recommended to investigate each component individually on the stent backbone and also as a complete device. The interaction of degradation processes among the different stent components needs to be characterized as clearly as possible. For example, when the degradation of a polymer influences the breakdown of metallic biodegradable components, and vice versa, specifically designed experimental and preclinical investigations are required to provide sufficient reassurance of vascular safety.

According to Oberhauser et al., the life cycle of a bioresorbable scaffold can be divided into three periods (Figure 3.5.2): (1) revascularisation; (2) restoration; and (3) resorption [22]. In the revascularization phase during the first three months after deployment the bioresorbable scaffold should perform similar to a metallic drug-eluting stents (DESs) in terms of deliverability, radial strength, recoil, and neointimal thickening. The importance of this crucial time period for the assessment of vascular healing, neointimal growth, and device stability has been documented in a multitude of

Table 3.5.1 Checklist of bloodwork for clinical pathology

| Time points | Prior to implantation | 1 day after implantation | 7 days after implantation | 28 days after implantation | Every 6 months for study periods beyond 6 months | Prior to sacrifice |
|---|---|---|---|---|---|---|
| Blood work | Hematology Coagulation Serum Chemistry | Hematology Coagulation Serum Chemistry | Hematology Coagulation Serum Chemistry | Hematology Coagulation Serum Chemistry | Hematology Coagulation Serum Chemistry | Hematology Coagulation Serum Chemistry |

Hematology, coagulation and serum chemistry

- Hematology
  - Red blood cell (RBC) count
  - Hemoglobin (HGB)
  - Hematocrit (HCT)
  - Mean corpuscular volume (MCV)
  - Mean corpuscular haemoglobin (MCH)
  - Mean corpuscular haemoglobin concentration (MCHC)
  - Platelet count (PLT count)
  - White blood cells (WBC)
  - WBC differential count
  - Cell morphology
  - Reticulocyte count
- Coagulation
  - Fibrinogen

- Serum chemistry
  - Alanine aminotransferase (ALT)
  - Albumin
  - Alkaline aminotransferase (ALP)
  - Aspartate aminotransferase (AST)
  - Calcium (Ca)
  - Chloride (Cl)
  - Cholesterol (Chol)
  - Creatine kinase (CK)
  - Creatinine (Crea)
  - Gamma-glutamyl transferase (GGT)
  - Globulins (Glob)
  - Glucose (Gluc)
  - Inorganic phosphorus (IP)
  - Potassium (K)
  - Sodium (Na)
  - Total protein (TP)
  - Triglycerides (Trig)
  - Urea nitrogen (Urea)

preclinical studies [12,19,23–25]. The restoration phase is characterized by gradual reduction of radial strength with loss of device structural integrity, where the pace of these processes is determined by basic biochemical reactions such as hydrolysis in the biodegradation of polyesters and corrosion in metallic biodegradable devices. Finally, in the resorption phase, the implant is sequentially resorbed by the body using natural biochemical pathways [22].

## Revascularization phase

To date, only a few dedicated preclinical studies have been reported for the investigation of the early phase responses following implantation of BRSs in animals [12,14,18]. First and foremost, one needs to determine the extent of thrombosis that occurs early following implantation of BRSs in preclinical animal models, usually at 1–3 days. The optimal time point to assess re-endothelialization after BRSs implantation is determined from comparative assessment of DESs and BMS [26], which is classically considered to be at 1 month. However, endothelial coverage must also be assessed at a later time-point to confirm the absence of adverse effects of biodegradation on endothelial integrity. A recent preclinical study in juvenile healthy swine from our institute compared ABSORB BVSs (Version 1.1) and XIENCE V with

respect to their differential rates of re-endothelialization [10]. By scanning electron microscopy, both ABSORB BVSs and XIENCE V showed complete stent strut coverage with mild neointimal growth and presence of full coverage by endothelial cells at 1 and 3 months, which was maintained at the final SEM follow-up of 12 months [10]. However, it needs to be recognized that these data were acquired in healthy juvenile swine, which have been shown to exhibit a more rapid healing response compared to other species and humans [27]. It has also been reported that ABSORB's preceding version (ABSORB BVSs Version 1.0) showed substantially less endothelial coverage at 28 days when investigated in rabbit iliac arteries [19] as compared to what was reported in swine.

Inflammation must be assessed in the early, intermediate, and late phases after implantation of a BRSs. Inflammation should be judged on the basis of acute and chronic inflammatory cells, which mostly consist of neutrophils/monocytes as an acute response to injury or the foreign material and lymphocytes/macrophages/giant cells chronically for clearing of biodegradation products. Minimal inflammation is an expected phenomenon as foreign material is being implanted inside the artery. Granulomatous response in pigs is not unusual and is observed in up to 10% of implants. Anything more than 10% must be regarded as a

Table 3.5.2 Checklist of standards and references for BRSs evaluation in preclinical animal models

| Test modalities | References |
|---|---|
| <ul><li>Procedural and histopathology standards<ul><li>Angiography</li><li>Device deployment procedures</li><li>Device acute performance</li><li>Complications</li><li>Final angiography and intravascular imaging at follow-up</li><li>Necropsy information</li><li>Histomorphometry</li><li>Assessment of inflammation</li><li>Assessment of thrombus formation</li><li>Characterization of strut degradation in BRSs</li><li>Characterization of tissue composition during degradation in BRSs</li></ul></li><li>Intravascular imaging<ul><li>Morphometric assessment</li><li>Judgement of strut coverage</li><li>Characterization of strut degradation in BRSs</li><li>Assessment of thrombus formation</li></ul></li></ul> | <ul><li>EMEA/CHMP/EWP/110540/2007: Guideline on the clinical and non-clinical evaluation during the consultation procedure on medicinal substances contained in drug-eluting</li><li>MEDDEV 2.1/3 rev 3</li><li>ANSI/AAMI/ISO 25539-2:2012: Cardiovascular implants—Endovascular devices—Part 2: Vascular stents</li><li>FDA Coronary Drug-Eluting Stents—Nonclinical and Clinical Studies (March 2008)</li><li>FDA Coronary Drug-Eluting Stents: Companion Document—Nonclinical and Clinical Studies (March 2008)</li><li>FDA Guidance for Industry and FDA Staff: General Considerations for Animal Studies for Cardiovascular Devices (2010)</li><li>Consensus standards for acquisition, measurement, and reporting of intravascular optical coherence tomography studies: a report from the International Working Group for Intravascular Optical Coherence Tomography Standardization and Validation. Tearney GJ et al. *J Am Coll Cardiol.* 2012;59(12):1058–72.</li><li>Expert review document on methodology, terminology, and clinical applications of optical coherence tomography: physical principles, methodology of image acquisition, and clinical application for assessment of coronary arteries and atherosclerosis. Prati F et al. *Eur Heart J.* 2010;31(4):401–15.</li></ul> |

*Source:* Modified and reproduced with permission from Byrne RA, Serruys PW, Baumbach A, Escaned J, Fajadet J, James S, Joner M et al. *Report of a European Society of Cardiology-European Association of Percutaneous Cardiovascular Interventions Task Force on the Evaluation of Coronary Stents In Europe: Executive Summary.* 2015.

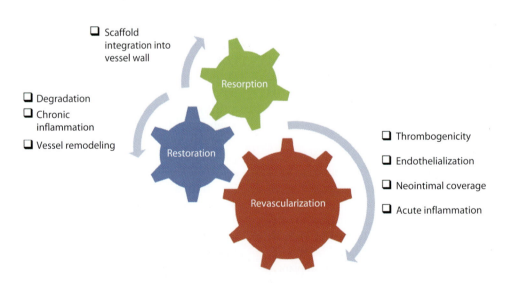

Figure 3.5.2 The life cycle of a bioresorbable scaffold: Revascularization, restoration, and resorption. In the revascularization phase during the first 3 months after deployment of the bioresorbable scaffold, thrombogenicity, endothelialization, neointimal hyperplasia, and acute inflammation determine device safety. In the restoration phase, scaffold degradation, chronic inflammatory response, and vessel remodeling are important topics during this intermediate phase. In the resorption phase, the vascular scaffold undergoes complete integration into the vessel wall. (Modified and reproduced with permission from Oberhauser JP, Hossainy S, Rapoza RJ. Design principles and performance of bioresorbable polymeric vascular scaffolds. *EuroIntervention.* 2009;5 Suppl F:F15–22.)

consequence of non-germfree animals or toxic effects of the device. Similarly, standard injury scores may be misleading at long-term follow-up as destruction of the internal elastic lamina may result from inflammation rather than reflecting vascular residues of acute injury at the time of stent implantation.

## Restoration phase

While main features of polymer degradation can be established *in vitro*, preclinical studies play an important role in the assessment of polymer biodegradation as certain aspects of biological interactions can only be determined *in vivo*. Otsuka et al. reported on the degradation profile of ABSORB BVSs in a preclinical study with follow-up of 4 years [10]. Polymer number–average molecular weight decreased slowly within the first 6 months but rapidly thereafter with 93% drop at 24 months. Percent mass loss was not significant until 18 months following implantation, with rapid mass loss occurring thereafter. On the other hand, histological signs of dismantling stent struts were only apparent after 12 months, with complete resorption of stent struts observed between 36 and 42 months. Interestingly, there were important differences observed in the inflammatory reactions between BRSs and metallic DESs. Inflammation is largely determined by the rate of polymer breakdown and is biphasic as the surface and base polymer degrades at different rates. Metallic DESs show an increase in inflammatory reaction in the surrounding of stent struts following the complete release of drug, while there is a biphasic inflammatory response in most drug-eluting BRSs, with a somewhat dampened inflammation reaction arising from surface polymer degradation during active drug release and

a second deferred peak resulting from base polymer mass loss in the absence of antiproliferative drug (Figure 3.5.3). It is therefore important to clearly characterize inflammatory reactions in each individual BRSs as the exact timing of these reactions will depend on the rate of biodegradation, which is dependent on the nature of the polymer and is substantially different among devices. Metal-based BRSs, such as the absorbable magnesium stent, react substantially different from polymeric BRSs. The magnesium stent exhibits greater foreign body response including giant cell reaction likely from the replacement of stent struts by amorphous calcium phosphate conjugations [15]. There appears to be an important link between BRSs-related inflammatory reactions and the onset of lumen enlargement, which has been reported in a number of different BRSs technologies to date [10,28].

In the study by Otsuka et al., morphometric analysis showed expansive vessel remodeling in ABSORB-implanted arteries starting at 12 months when compared to XIENCE V, which showed no changes in internal or external elastic lamina areas [10]. Similar findings of positive vessel remodeling and lumen enlargement have been reported by Strandberg et al. in histological assessment obtained from a preclinical study evaluating a tyrosine-derived polycarbonate polymer-based BRSs over a 4-year period in a porcine model [16]. These ground-breaking pathological observations reinforce the notion that arterial microenvironment and plaque-associated inflammatory responses may have a profound impact on vascular remodeling after implantation of a BRSs. In keeping with this, it has been reported that vascular remodeling involves a complex interplay of shear-stress induced molecular pathways inducing changes in vessel composition in native

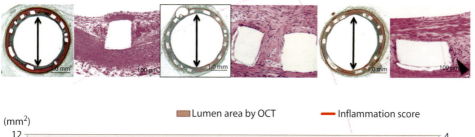
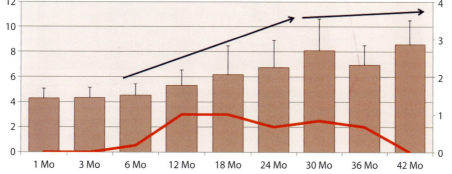

**Figure 3.5.3** Biphasic inflammatory response in BRSs with an early peak of inflammation as a result of polymer degradation when active drug release is exhausted and a second and somewhat deferred peak after initiation of polymer mass loss in the absence of antiproliferative drug.

and diseased arteries [29]. High shear stress regions show reduction in plaque size and larger lumen without changes in vessel size. In contrast, regions of low shear stress are the predominant areas of positive remodeling with maintenance of lumen size secondary to compensatory enlargement of vessel size.

Another potential advantage of BRSs over permanent metallic DESs seems to be the restoration of vasomotor function within the stented segment, which has been reported in preclinical and in clinical surveillance imaging investigations [30,31]. ABSORB BVSs was previously investigated at 12 months' follow-up with respect to its ability to allow vasomotion in response to administration of vasoactive substances in porcine coronary arteries, which showed a small but remarkable lumen gain in ABSORB BVSs stented arteries relative to nonstented control arteries [11]. In addition, Lane et al. provided further evidence of vasomotion after ABSORB BVSs implantation utilizing IVUS-based investigation of vessel pulsatility [11]. These promising preclinical results were ultimately corroborated in small clinical studies applying vasomotion testing in a subgroup of patients, with evidence for improved vasomotion in BRSs [30,31].

## Resorption phase

The resorption phase is characterized by complete disintegration of the BRSs and slow replacement of degradation products by arterial tissue. In the study by Otsuka et al., there were two time-dependent aspects recognized with resorption sites of stent struts in ABSORB BVSs. There was an increasing frequency of strut discontinuities and basophilic staining of resorption sites by hematoxylin and eosin (H&E) (Figure 3.5.4), blue-green staining by Movat Pentachrome, and blue with alcian stains (Figure 3.5.5), which is consistent with the presence of proteoglycans. Discontinuities were defined as sites where the conventional box shape appearance of stent struts was lost, with integration of arterial tissue. At later time points (i.e., 18–24 months), resorption sites showed positive staining for Alcian blue and increasing basophilia with H&E (Figures 3.5.4 and 3.5.5) [18]. It is important to carefully monitor inflammation during this phase of resorption as smaller fragments of polymeric material may provoke untoward reactions, eventually resulting in delayed catchup of neointimal growth. Degradation occurs much faster in metallic BRSs, what has been described by Wittchow et al.

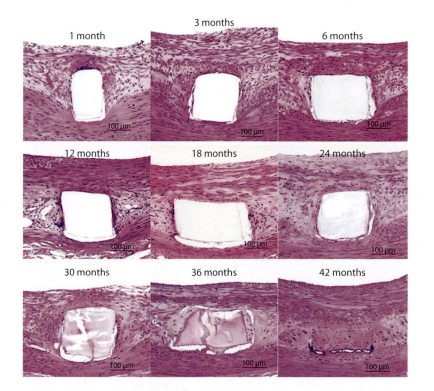

Figure 3.5.4 Histological images showing the scaffold appears intact without histological signs of degradation at 1 month and 3 months when stained by hematoxylin and eosin stains. Increasing frequency of strut discontinuities and basophilic staining of resorption sites due to active polymer resorption is observed at 18–24 months. At 36 months, partial replacement of struts with provisional matrix is shown, while images at 42 months depict provisional matrix maturation and connective tissue replacement [10]. Mild inflammatory infiltrate was observed from 12–36 months (black arrows at 12 and 18 months) and consisted mostly of macrophages and a few lymphocytes. At 42 months, inflammation was not readily observed. Giant cells were occasionally observed at 1 month; however, they were uncommon after 3 months. Peak fibrin deposition was noted at 1 month with rapid decrease at 3 months and becoming absent or minimal thereafter. Minor areas of calcification were observed around struts/resorption sites after 3 months. (Modified and reproduced with permission from Otsuka F, Pacheco E, Perkins LE, Lane JP, Wang Q, Kamberi M, Frie M et al. *Cir Cardiovasc Interv.* 2014;7:330–342.)

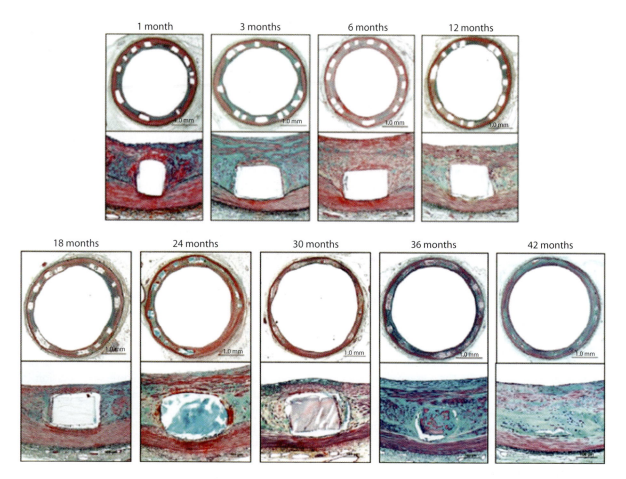

**Figure 3.5.5** Histology of BRSs degradation and integration into arterial vessel wall. Representative histological images of ABSORB bioresorbable vascular scaffold in porcine coronary arteries from 1–42 months (Movat penta-chrome). Color changes are appreciated at resorption sites beginning at 18 months, in that resorption sites are increasingly alcian blue positive from 18–24 months. Thereafter, resorption sites undergo further changes, and there is progressive dismantling with corresponding integration of proteoglycans and collagen with few smooth muscle cells. The resorption sites are almost completely replaced by connective tissue at 42 months. (Modified and reproduced with permission from Otsuka F, Pacheco E, Perkins LE, Lane JP, Wang Q, Kamberi M, Frie M et al. *Cir Cardiovasc Interv.* 2014;7:330–342.)

in a porcine model employing the AMS magnesium 3.0 generation stent [15]. The bioresorption process was complete at 180 days in the AMS 3.0 as established by histology and spectroscopical analysis leaving an amorphous conversion product behind.

## CHEMICAL ANALYSIS OF DRUG LEVELS AND POLYMER DEGRADATION

In contrast to permanent metallic implants, which are nearly chemically inert within the biological environment of arterial tissue [32], fully bioresorbable devices are subject to structural and chemical alterations caused by degradation processes. The dismantling of a mechanically stable structure into smaller molecules and biologic products allows the body to metabolize degradation products using natural pathways [33]. However, these reactions are all dependent on the compounds used. In order to assess the biocompatibility of BRSs, it is necessary to identify the physicochemical structure and biological behavior of all chemical products liberated during bioresorption, including substances, which occur only in small amounts or even in traces. It is likely that the chemical decomposition of bioresorbable polymers is connected to an inherent acidification of the environment [34], whereas degrading bioresorbable metals provoke a shift toward higher pH-values [35]. Monitoring the tissue concentration of degradation products may be helpful to understand the biological response of the arterial microenvironment, but is limited by the existing analytical technologies.

*In vitro* degradation tests are supportive to elucidate degradation mechanisms and kinetics, even if it is difficult to mimic the complex *in vivo* environment occurring during bioresorption of BRSs. Nonetheless, *in vitro* degradation tests may not necessarily reflect *in vivo* degradation kinetics adequately in all cases. During the course of an *in vivo–in vitro* correlation (IVIVC), the suitability and the limitations of the *in vitro* degradation test to predict *in vivo* degradation kinetics should be critically acknowledged [36,37].

Bioresorbable metals or alloys degrade by erosion of the surface. Therefore, *in vivo* degradation processes can be monitored by morphometric assessment of tissue blocks embedded in methacrylate polymer [38]. The degradation analysis of polymeric material is more complex as degradation occurs by reduction of the length of the respective polymer chains, which is not accompanied by any macroscopic change. Mass loss can only be recognized during the final stage of degradation when the molecular mass of the produced oligomers is low enough to result in complete clearance of polymer residues. The onset of degradation can be detected by pH sensitive stains (e.g., May Grunwald staining), which results in colorimetric recognition of the polymer after generation of the first acidic degradation products [39]. Mass loss can be monitored by homogenizing the entire vessel including the stent, followed by complete chemical depolymerization of the stent into its monomers and quantitative analysis of the degradation product by HPLC [40]. The most versatile analysis method is GPC (gel permeation chromatography), which reveals important information to characterize the polymer by molecular weight distribution and polydispersity index (PDI) and is helpful to explain the observed biological behavior [41].

The individual degradation kinetics of the respective BRSs system should be taken into account when designing preclinical studies to assess safety in order to cover the time points of peak degradation and loss of structural integrity. Surrogate parameters such as change in stent diameter and histologic analysis can be used to estimate the remaining stability as well as a count of fractures based on Faxitron or microCT imaging. Fatigue tests *in vitro* should be performed with fully processed systems (including potential drug coating) in the same medium as the degradation tests are carried out.

The demands for pharmacokinetic studies of bioresorbable systems are comparable to those of permanent systems regarding time points of evaluation and sample size calculations. After onset of fragmentation, the separation of stent and tissue may be challenging or even impossible. In this case, analysis of the complete homogenized vessel segment including the BRSs should be considered. Pharmacokinetic determination of drug tissue levels should be performed until drug tissue concentrations drop below detection limit of the applied methodology. Standards for pharmacokinetic studies and biochemical analysis of degradation products of BRSs are listed in Table 3.5.3.

## THE ROLE OF INTRAVASCULAR IMAGING IN PRECLINICAL ASSESSMENT OF BRSs

Intracoronary imaging can provide useful information for the evaluation of BRSs in preclinical analysis; nevertheless it cannot replace histologic examination owing to the inability to mirror basic vascular reactions such as inflammation or endothelialization. Substantial recoil of the stented arterial segment may be observed in histology even after physiologic arterial pressure fixation. Vessels and scaffolds undergo shrinkage during fixation, due to dehydrating procedures, which are inevitable for histological processing. This precludes from deriving vessel dimensions by histological analysis alone to truly reflect device performance under *in vivo* conditions. Therefore, *in vivo* imaging has become an integral part during the preclinical assessment of BRSs.

A quantitative coronary analysis (QCA) should be performed in a core laboratory to study angiographic outcomes in preclinical studies. The principal angiographic endpoints of interest are in-stent late lumen loss (defined as the difference between the minimal lumen diameter

Table 3.5.3 Checklist of standards and references for pharmacokinetic studies and biochemical analysis of degradation products of BRSs

| Pharmacokinetic studies | |
| --- | --- |
| • *In vitro* pharmacokinetics<br>• *In vivo* pharmacokinetics<br>• Establishment of *in vitro–in vivo* correlations | • EMEA/CHMP/EWP/110540/2007: Guideline on the clinical and non-clinical evaluation during the consultation procedure on medicinal substances contained in drug-eluting (medicinal substance-eluting) coronary stents<br>• MEDDEV 2.1/3 rev 3<br>• FDA Coronary Drug-Eluting Stents—Nonclinical and Clinical Studies (March 2008)<br>• FDA Coronary Drug-Eluting Stents: Companion Document—Nonclinical and Clinical Studies (March 2008) |
| **Biochemical Analysis of Degradation Products in BRSs** | |
| • Definition of Degradation Products<br>• *In vitro* degradation profile<br>• *In vivo* degradation profile<br>• Establishment of *in vitro–in vivo* correlations | • Use of International Standard ISO-10993, "Biological Evaluation of Medical Devices Part 1: Evaluation and Testing"<br>• ISO/TS 12417:2011<br>• ISO/DIS 12417-1<br>• ISO/TR 37137:2014<br>• ISO/TS 17137:2014 |

*Source:* Modified and reproduced with permission from Byrne RA, Serruys PW, Baumbach A, Escaned J, Fajadet J, James S, Joner M et al. *Report of a European Society of Cardiology-European Association of Percutaneous Cardiovascular Interventions Task Force on the Evaluation of Coronary Stents In Europe: Executive Summary.* 2015.

[MLD] immediately post-stent implantation and the MLD at follow-up), percentage diameter stenosis at follow-up angiography, and in-segment binary restenosis (renarrowing ≥50% diameter stenosis within the body and margins of the stent) at follow-up angiography. The use of these standardized parameters of device performance facilitates comparative assessment of BRSs along with other stent-based technologies, such as nonbioresorbable metallic DESs.

Other intravascular imaging techniques, such as ultrasound (IVUS) and optical coherence tomography (OCT) are also broadly used in preclinical studies evaluating BRSs. IVUS is an ultrasound-based imaging technique with an axial resolution of 150–200 μm [42,43]. Relevant endpoints of IVUS-based analysis are stent area (mm²), mean lumen area (mm²), minimal lumen area (mm²), external elastic lamina area (mm²), plaque area (mm²), and neointima area (mm²) [44]. In preclinical studies, intravascular ultrasound imaging was utilized to evaluate everolimus-eluting polymeric bioabsorbable stents in porcine coronary arteries [11]. Lane et al. showed a progressive increase in luminal area of arteries after implantation of ABSORB BVSs and a corresponding increase in the reference vessel luminal area in a porcine model by means of IVUS imaging [11]. Intravascular ultrasound was also used to corroborate rapid bioabsorbable metallic scaffold degradation as a precursor of the current fully bioresorbable metallic DREAMS stent [43].

OCT represents a catheter-based imaging technique based on near-infrared light that can detect stent strut coverage and malapposition with an axial resolution of 10–20 μm [42,45]. OCT has a resolution nearly 10 times greater than IVUS [46]. Its resolution in relationship to dimensions of vascular structures relevant for preclinical evaluation of BRSs is shown in Figure 3.5.6. The accuracy of both IVUS and OCT has been broadly corroborated in histological analysis of preclinical and autopsy studies [21,28,47–50] and in clinical application [44,51–53]. The main advantage of these intravascular imaging modalities over angiography is a consequence of higher resolution. Most accurate visualization and measurement of neointimal formation within stented vessel segments and an appreciation of the arterial wall changes is achieved using OCT. Relevant endpoints for OCT analysis include lumen area (mm²), stent area (mm²), neointimal thickness (mm), neointimal area (mm²), percent volume obstruction (%), percentage of uncovered stent struts (%), and malapposed stent struts, percentage as well as incomplete stent apposition (ISA) distance (mm) and area (mm²). An important limitation of IVUS is that although it enables direct visualization of neointimal tissue within the stented segment, the limited axial resolution (150–200 μm) does not allow determination of the type of neointimal tissue coverage of individual stent struts, which is detectable by OCT owing to its higher resolution [46]. Nonetheless, OCT has clear limitations in visualizing deeper vascular morphologies due to the limited penetration depth of OCT laser light. Therefore, a combination of IVUS and OCT imaging may be useful to completely delineate vascular reactions following BRSs implantation.

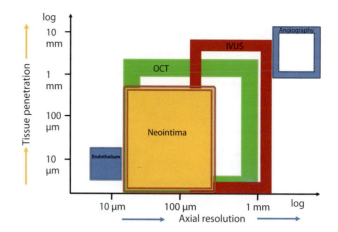

**Figure 3.5.6** Comparison of OCT and IVUS imaging resolution in relationship to vessel structure dimensions. Graphic representation of tissue penetration versus spatial resolution of optical coherence tomography (OCT) compared with other imaging methods. The open boxes represent the maximal resolution and tissue penetration achieved with angiography, OCT, and IVUS. The solid boxes represent the range of selected arterial vessel structures that are relevant for preclinical evaluation of BRSs. The requirements to accurately detect neointimal hyperplasia observed after BRSs implantation exceed the capabilities of intravascular ultrasound (IVUS). However, current OCT systems are not suitable to assess tissue at depths beyond 2 mm. Currently, evaluation of single cell endothelial layers cannot be assessed by OCT systems. (Modified and reproduced with permission from Bezerra HG, Costa MA, Guagliumi G, Rollins AM, Simon DI. *JACC. Cardiovasc Interv.* 2009;2:1035–1046.)

The morphological changes of everolimus eluting fully bioresorbable scaffolds over time have been examined in preclinical follow-up investigations and assessed by histology up to 48 months [18]. In this study, Onuma et al. proposed an approach toward characterization of degrading BRSs by OCT by classifying the morphological appearance of stent struts and resorption sites into four different categories (preserved box, open box, dissolved black box, dissolved white box) in a healthy porcine model (Figure 3.5.7). However, it has to be considered that a large number of stent struts were not discernible at late time points and could not be correlated to histopathology. This methodology is based on the findings derived from observations with the ABSORB BVSs, and it has yet to be validated, whether these categories can be applied to BRSs of differential compositions [18]. Apart from characterization of morphological changes of BRS struts, the high resolution of OCT facilitates *in vivo* determination of strut coverage, apposition, and area measurements. Despite their complementary features, neither IVUS nor OCT nor their combination are able to accurately detect endothelial or smooth muscle cell presence after stent implantation, nor individual type of inflammatory cell. Thus, intravascular imaging techniques warrant further improvement to decipher these important features of vascular healing.

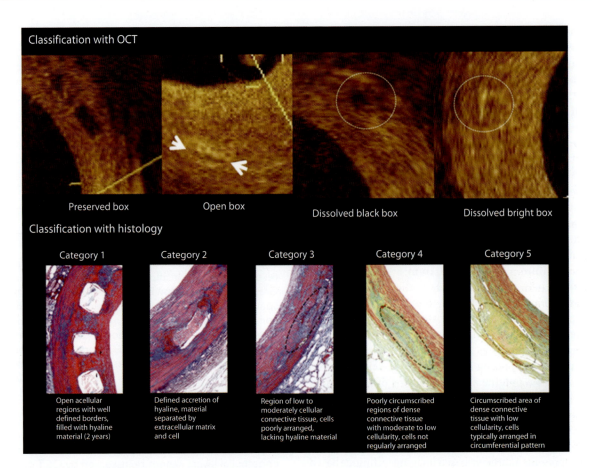

**Figure 3.5.7** Serial preclinical assessment of an everolimus-eluting BRSs (ABSORB BVSs) at 6–42 months after implantation in a porcine model. OCT images and corresponding histology stained with Movat Pentachrome exhibited "preserved box" appearance as visible by OCT (6–24 months) and corresponding histological view of struts at high magnification. Open box appearance of BRSs struts at 30 months and corresponding histology showing tinctorial change in strut at high magnification. ABSORB BVSs struts showed "dissolved black box" appearance at 36 months and dissolved white box appearance at 42 months, while histology showed progressive integration of the scaffold into arterial tissue. (Reproduced with permission from Onuma Y, Serruys PW, Perkins LE, Okamura T, Gonzalo N, Garcia-Garcia HM, Regar E et al. *Circulation.* 2010;122:2288–2300.)

# REFERENCES

1. Capodanno D, Gori T, Nef H, Latib A, Mehilli J, Lesiak M, Caramanno G et al. Percutaneous coronary intervention with everolimus-eluting bioresorbable vascular scaffolds in routine clinical practice: Early and midterm outcomes from the European multicentre ghost-EU registry. *EuroIntervention. Journal of EuroPCR in Collaboration with the Working Group on Interventional Cardiology of the European Society of Cardiology.* 2015;10:1144–1153.

2. Kolodgie FD, Katocs AS, Jr., Largis EE, Wrenn SM, Cornhill JF, Herderick EE, Lee SJ et al. Hypercholesterolemia in the rabbit induced by feeding graded amounts of low-level cholesterol. Methodological considerations regarding individual variability in response to dietary cholesterol and development of lesion type. *Arterioscler Throm Vasc Biol.* 1996;16:1454–1464.

3. Muller DW, Ellis SG, Topol EJ. Experimental models of coronary artery restenosis. *J Am Coll Cardiol.* 1992;19:418–432.

4. Rosenfeldt FL, Chi L, Black AJ, Waugh JR, Pedersen JS, Levatter J. Excimer laser angioplasty in the atherosclerotic rabbit: Comparison with balloon angioplasty. *Am Heart J.* 1992;124:349–355.

5. Tellez A, Seifert PS, Donskoy E, Sushkova N, Pennington DE, Milewski K, Krueger CG et al. Experimental evaluation of efficacy and healing response of everolimus-eluting stents in the familial hypercholesterolemic swine model: A comparative study of bioabsorbable versus durable polymer stent platforms. *Coron Artery Dis.* 2014.

6. Wanibuchi H, Dingemans KP, Becker AE, Ueda M, Naruko T, Tanizawa S, Nakamura K. Is the watanabe heritable hyperlipidemic rabbit a suitable experimental model for percutaneous transluminal coronary angioplasty in humans? A light microscopic,

immunohistochemical and ultrastructural study. *J Am Coll Cardiol.* 1993;21:1490–1496

7. Byrne RA, Serruys PW, Baumbach A, Escaned J, Fajadet J, James S, Joner M et al. *Report of a European Society of Cardiology-European Association of Percutaneous Cardiovascular Interventions Task Force on the Evaluation of Coronary Stents In Europe: Executive Summary.* 2015.

8. Schwartz RS, Edelman ER, Carter A, Chronos N, Rogers C, Robinson KA, Waksman R et al. Drug-eluting stents in preclinical studies: Recommended evaluation from a consensus group. *Circulation.* 2002;106:1867–1873.

9. Campos CM, Ishibashi Y, Eggermont J, Nakatani S, Cho YK, Dijkstra J, Reiber JH et al. Echogenicity as a surrogate for bioresorbable everolimus-eluting scaffold degradation: Analysis at 1-, 3-, 6-, 12-, 18, 24-, 30-, 36- and 42-month follow-up in a porcine model. *Int J Cardiovasc Imaging.* 2015;31:471–482.

10. Otsuka F, Pacheco E, Perkins LE, Lane JP, Wang Q, Kamberi M, Frie M et al. Long-term safety of an everolimus-eluting bioresorbable vascular scaffold and the cobalt-chromium xience v stent in a porcine coronary artery model. *Circ Cardiovasc Interv.* 2014;7:330–342.

11. Lane JP, Perkins LE, Sheehy AJ, Pacheco EJ, Frie MP, Lambert BJ, Rapoza RJ et al. Lumen gain and restoration of pulsatility after implantation of a bioresorbable vascular scaffold in porcine coronary arteries. *JACC Cardiovasc Interv.* 2014;7:688–695.

12. Durand E, Sharkawi T, Leclerc G, Raveleau M, van der Leest M, Vert M, Lafont A. Head-to-head comparison of a drug-free early programmed dismantling polylactic acid bioresorbable scaffold and a metallic stent in the porcine coronary artery: Six-month angiography and optical coherence tomographic follow-up study. *Circ Cardiovasc Interv.* 2014;7:70–79.

13. Zopf DA, Flanagan CL, Wheeler M, Hollister SJ, Green GE. Treatment of severe porcine tracheomalacia with a 3-dimensionally printed, bioresorbable, external airway splint. *JAMA Otolaryngol Head Neck Surg.* 2014;140:66–71

14. Farooq V, Serruys PW, Heo JH, Gogas BD, Onuma Y, Perkins LE, Diletti R et al. Intracoronary optical coherence tomography and histology of overlapping everolimus-eluting bioresorbable vascular scaffolds in a porcine coronary artery model: The potential implications for clinical practice. *JACC Cardiovasc Interv.* 2013;6:523–532.

15. Wittchow E, Adden N, Riedmuller J, Savard C, Waksman R, Braune M. Bioresorbable drug-eluting magnesium-alloy scaffold: Design and feasibility in a porcine coronary model. *EuroIntervention. Journal of EuroPCR in Collaboration with the Working Group on Interventional Cardiology of the European Society of Cardiology.* 2013;8:1441–1450

16. Strandberg E, Zeltinger J, Schulz DG, Kaluza GL. Late positive remodeling and late lumen gain contribute to vascular restoration by a non-drug eluting bioresorbable scaffold: A four-year intravascular ultrasound study in normal porcine coronary arteries. *Circ Cardiovasc Interv.* 2012;5:39–46.

17. Gogas BD, Radu M, Onuma Y, Perkins L, Powers JC, Gomez-Lara J, Farooq V et al. Evaluation with in vivo optical coherence tomography and histology of the vascular effects of the everolimus-eluting bioresorbable vascular scaffold at two years following implantation in a healthy porcine coronary artery model: Implications of pilot results for future pre-clinical studies. *Int J Cardiovasc Imaging.* 2012;28:499–511.

18. Onuma Y, Serruys PW, Perkins LE, Okamura T, Gonzalo N, Garcia-Garcia HM, Regar E et al. Intracoronary optical coherence tomography and histology at 1 month and 2, 3, and 4 years after implantation of everolimus-eluting bioresorbable vascular scaffolds in a porcine coronary artery model: An attempt to decipher the human optical coherence tomography images in the absorb trial. *Circulation.* 2010;122:2288–2300.

19. Vorpahl M, Nakano M, Perkins LE, Otsuka F, Jones R, Acampado E, Lane JP et al. Vascular healing and integration of a fully bioresorbable everolimus-eluting scaffold in a rabbit iliac arterial model. *EuroIntervention. Journal of EuroPCR in Collaboration with the Working Group on Interventional Cardiology of the European Society of Cardiology.* 2014;10:833–841.

20. Faxon DP, Balelli LA, Sandborn T, Haudenschild C, Valeri R, Ryan TJ. The effect of antiplatelet therapy on platelet accumulation after experimental angioplasty in the rabbit iliac model. *Int J Cardiol.* 1992;36:41–47.

21. Malle C, Tada T, Steigerwald K, Ughi GJ, Schuster T, Nakano M, Massberg S et al. Tissue characterization after drug-eluting stent implantation using optical coherence tomography. *Arterioscler Throm Vasc Biol.* 2013;33:1376–1383.

22. Oberhauser JP, Hossainy S, Rapoza RJ. Design principles and performance of bioresorbable polymeric vascular scaffolds. *EuroIntervention. Journal of EuroPCR in Collaboration with the Working Group on Interventional Cardiology of the European Society of Cardiology.* 2009;5 Suppl F:F15–22.

23. Taylor AJ, Gorman PD, Kenwood B, Hudak C, Tashko G, Virmani R. A comparison of four stent designs on arterial injury, cellular proliferation, neointima formation, and arterial dimensions in an experimental porcine model. *Cathet Cardiovasc Interv. Official Journal of the Society for Cardiac Angiography & Interventions.* 2001;53:420–425.

24. Hietala EM, Salminen US, Stahls A, Valimaa T, Maasilta P, Tormala P, Nieminen MS et al. Biodegradation of the copolymeric polylactide stent. Long-term follow-up in a rabbit aorta model. *J Vasc Res.* 2001;38:361–369.

25. Koppara T, Joner M, Bayer G, Steigerwald K, Diener T, Wittchow E. Histopathological comparison of biodegradable polymer and permanent polymer based sirolimus eluting stents in a porcine model of coronary stent implantation. *Thromb Haemost.* 2012;107:1161–1171.

26. Joner M, Nakazawa G, Finn AV, Quee SC, Coleman L, Acampado E, Wilson PS et al. Endothelial cell recovery between comparator polymer-based drug-eluting stents. *J Am Coll Cardiol.* 2008;52:333–342.

27. Llano R, Winsor-Hines D, Patel DB, Seifert PS, Hamamdzic D, Wilson GJ, Wang H et al. Vascular responses to drug-eluting and bare metal stents in diabetic/hypercholesterolemic and nonathero-sclerotic porcine coronary arteries. *Circ Cardiovasc Interv.* 2011;4:438–446.

28. Onuma Y, Dudek D, Thuesen L, Webster M, Nieman K, Garcia-Garcia HM, Ormiston JA et al. Five-year clinical and functional multislice computed tomography angiographic results after coronary implantation of the fully resorbable polymeric everolimus-eluting scaffold in patients with de novo coronary artery disease: The absorb cohort a trial. *JACC Cardiovasc Interv.* 2013;6:999–1009.

29. Korshunov VA, Schwartz SM, Berk BC. Vascular remodeling: Hemodynamic and biochemical mechanisms underlying glagov's phenomenon. *Arterioscler Throm Vasc Biol.* 2007;27:1722–1728.

30. Brugaletta S, Heo JH, Garcia-Garcia HM, Farooq V, van Geuns RJ, de Bruyne B, Dudek D et al. Endothelial-dependent vasomotion in a coronary segment treated by absorb everolimus-eluting bioresorbable vascular scaffold system is related to plaque composition at the time of bioresorption of the polymer: Indirect finding of vascular reparative therapy? *Eur Heart J.* 2012;33:1325–1333.

31. Sarno G, Bruining N, Onuma Y, Garg S, Brugaletta S, De Winter S, Regar E et al. Morphological and functional evaluation of the bioresorption of the bioresorbable everolimus-eluting vascular scaffold using ivus, echogenicity and vasomotion testing at two year follow-up: A patient level insight into the absorb a clinical trial. *Int J Cardiovasc Imaging.* 2012;28:51–58.

32. Halwani DO, Anderson PG, Brott BC, Anayiotos AS, Lemons JE. Clinical device-related article surface characterization of explanted endovascular stents: Evidence of in vivo corrosion. *J Biomed Mater Res B Appl Biomater.* 2010;95:225–238.

33. Waksman R. Biodegradable stents: They do their job and disappear. *J Invasive Cardiol.* 2006;18:70–74.

34. Taylor M, Daniels A, Andriano K, Heller J. Six bioabsorbable polymers: In vitro acute toxicity of accumulated degradation products. *J Appl Biomater.* 1994;5:151–157.

35. Song G. Recent progress in corrosion and protection of magnesium alloys. *Adv Eng Mater.* 2005;7:563–586.

36. Hou L, Li Z, Pan Y, Du L, Li X, Zheng Y, Li L. In vitro and in vivo studies on biodegradable magnesium alloy. *Prog Nat Sci Mater Int.* 2014;24:466–471.

37. Tracy M, Ward K, Firouzabadian L, Wang Y, Dong N, Qian R, Zhang Y. Factors affecting the degradation rate of poly (lactide-co-glycolide) microspheres in vivo and in vitro. *Biomaterials.* 1999;20:1057–1062.

38. Wittchow E, Adden N, Riedmueller J, Savard C, Waksman R, Braune M. Bioresorbable drug-eluting magnesium-alloy scaffold: Design and feasibility in a porcine coronary model. *EuroIntervention. Journal of EuroPCR in Collaboration with the Working Group on Interventional Cardiology of the European Society of Cardiology.* 2013;8:1441–1450.

39. Schwach G, Vert M. In vitro and in vivo degradation of lactic acid-based interference screws used in cruciate ligament reconstruction. *Int J Biol Macromol.* 1999;25:283–291.

40. Ghaffar A, Verschuren PG, Geenevasen JA, Handels T, Berard J, Plum B, Dias AA et al. Fast in vitro hydrolytic degradation of polyester urethane acrylate biomaterials: Structure elucidation, separation and quantification of degradation products. *J Chromatogr A.* 2011;1218:449–458.

41. Weidner SM, Trimpin S. Mass spectrometry of synthetic polymers. *Anal Chem.* 2010;82:4811–4829.

42. Kim BK, Ha J, Mintz GS, Kim JS, Shin DH, Ko YG, Choi D, Jang Y, Hong MK. Randomised comparison of strut coverage between nobori biolimus-eluting and sirolimus-eluting stents: An optical coherence tomography analysis. *EuroIntervention. Journal of EuroPCR in Collaboration with the Working Group on Interventional Cardiology of the European Society of Cardiology.* 2014;9:1389–1397.

43. Slottow TL, Pakala R, Okabe T, Hellinga D, Lovec RJ, Tio FO, Bui AB, Waksman R. Optical coherence tomography and intravascular ultrasound imaging of bioabsorbable magnesium stent degradation in porcine coronary arteries. *Cardiovasc Revasc Med: Including Molecular Interv.* 2008;9:248–254.

44. American College of Cardiology Clinical Expert Consensus Document on Standards for Acquisition, Measurement and Reporting of Intravascular Ultrasound Studies (IVUS). A report of the American College of cardiology task force on clinical expert consensus documents developed in collaboration with the European Society of Cardiology endorsed by the Society of Cardiac Angiography and Interventions. *Eur J Echocardiogr: The Journal of the Working*

Group on Echocardiography of the European Society of Cardiology. 2001;2:299–313.

45. Prati F, Cera M, Ramazzotti V, Imola F, Giudice R, Giudice M, Propris SD, Albertucci M. From bench to bedside: A novel technique of acquiring OCT images. *Circ J Official Journal of the Japanese Circulation Society.* 2008;72:839–843.

46. Bezerra HG, Attizzani GF, Sirbu V, Musumeci G, Lortkipanidze N, Fujino Y, Wang W et al. Optical coherence tomography versus intravascular ultrasound to evaluate coronary artery disease and percutaneous coronary intervention. *JACC Cardiovasc Interv.* 2013;6:228–236.

47. Murata A, Wallace-Bradley D, Tellez A, Alviar C, Aboodi M, Sheehy A, Coleman L et al. Accuracy of optical coherence tomography in the evaluation of neointimal coverage after stent implantation. *JACC Cardiovasc Interv.* 2010;3:76–84.

48. Virmani R, Otsuka F, Prati F, Narula J, Joner M. Matching human pathology is essential for validating OCT imaging to detect high-risk plaques. *Nat Rev Cardiol.* 2014;11:638.

49. Kang SJ, Mintz GS, Pu J, Sum ST, Madden SP, Burke AP, Xu K et al. Combined IVUS and NIRS detection of fibroatheromas: Histopathological validation in human coronary arteries. *JACC Cardiovasc Interv.* 2015;8:184–194.

50. Burke AP, Joner M, Virmani R. IVUS-VH: A predictor of plaque morphology? *Eur Heart J.* 2006;27:1889–1890.

51. Klersy C, Ferlini M, Raisaro A, Scotti V, Balduini A, Curti M, Bramucci E et al. Use of ivus guided coronary stenting with drug eluting stent: A systematic review and meta-analysis of randomized controlled clinical trials and high quality observational studies. *Int J Cardiol.* 2013;170:54–63.

52. Maehara A, Mintz GS, Stone GW. OCT versus IVUS: Accuracy versus clinical utility. *JACC Cardiovasc Interv.* 2013;6:1105–1107.

53. Meredith IT, Verheye S, Weissman NJ, Barragan P, Scott D, Valdes Chavarri M et al. Six-month IVUS and two-year clinical outcomes in the evolve FHU trial: A randomised evaluation of a novel bioabsorbable polymer-coated, everolimus-eluting stent. *EuroIntervention. Journal of EuroPCR in Collaboration with the Working Group on Interventional Cardiology of the European Society of Cardiology.* 2013;9:308–315.

54. Bezerra HG, Costa MA, Guagliumi G, Rollins AM, Simon DI. Intracoronary optical coherence tomography: A comprehensive review clinical and research applications. *JACC Cardiovasc Interv.* 2009;2:1035–1046.

# PART 4

# Lessons learned from preclinical assessment

# PLA scaffold

KAZUYUKI YAHAGI, SHO TORII, ERICA PACHECO, FRANK D. KOLODGIE, ALOKE V. FINN, AND RENU VIRMANI

Coronary artery disease (CAD) is the leading cause of death worldwide and percutaneous coronary intervention (PCI) is the dominant treatment modality for patients with obstructive coronary disease. Although the treatment with bare metal stents (BMSs) was hampered by high rates of restenosis, these limitations have been largely addressed with metallic drug-eluting stents (DESs) such that metallic DESs are currently used as the first choice devices for PCI. On the other hand, there are several important limitations to metallic DESs implantation including a risk for hypersensitivity reaction from chronic exposure to durable polymers, late/very late stent thrombosis due to uncovered stent struts, and the development of neoatherosclerosis (atherosclerosis developing within stent-induced neointima) as well as an impaired coronary vasomotion and preclusion of bypasses to stented segments [1–3].

Drug eluting bioresorbable scaffolds (BRSs) have emerged as a novel technology that is proposed to overcome these issues. One of the unique features of BRSs is the resorption of fully polymeric struts, with the expectation that the long-term absence of a rigid scaffold would restore the vessel to a natural state allowing for coronary vasomotion and avoiding future complications caused by permanent metal devices [4,5]. The Igaki-Tamai bioabsorbable scaffold (Kyoto Medical Planning Co. Ltd., Kyoto, Japan) was the first BRSs used in humans, which was made of poly-L-lactic acid (PLLA) without drug coating [4]. Nishio et al. reported the acceptable long-term safety with Igaki-Tmai scaffold in the first-in-man study which included 50 patients [6]. As expected, intravascular ultrasound (IVUS) studies showed that most of scaffolds disappeared within 3 years. Following on this novelty, many BRSs devices have been developed and have currently either completed clinical trials or are reaching the phase of clinical testing and two devices have received CE-Mark approval in Europe (ABSORB BVSs, Abbott Vascular, CA) [7] and the DESolve stent (Elixir Medical, CA) [8,9] while the former has already reported the FDA-initiated large, multicenter, randomized clinical trial against XIENCE (Abbott Vascular, CA) DESs,

showing noninferiority with respect to target lesion failure at 1 year [10].

In this chapter, we focus on the histopathology of different poly-lactic acid (PLA) scaffolds including ABSORB, DESolve, Amaranth-BRSs, and ART-BRSs in animal models and the pathological changes that take place over time in relation to findings by intravascular imaging.

## PRECLINICAL EVALUATION OF BIORESORBABLE SCAFFOLD IN ANIMAL MODELS

### Histopathology

Preclinical studies with histopathological evaluation of biological responses to medical devices are a mandatory requirement for U.S. Food and Drug Administration (FDA) approval. Such studies are used to predict safety of device performance in clinical practice because important vascular reactions consequent to device degradation can only be examined in animal studies [11]. In addition to similar techniques of standard measurements for the preclinical assessment of DESs [12], characterization of degradation kinetics of the scaffold including molecular weight loss, strength, and mass loss are important for assessment of BRSs. The degree of inflammation should be assessed at various time-points based on the extent of acute and chronic inflammatory cell infiltration and the time of evaluation can be adjusted according to the *in vitro* kinetics of scaffold degradation. The evaluation of histological changes at middle- and long-term follow-up is essential. In general, if the duration of complete strut biodegradation of BRSs is 2 years, it is necessary to fully capture device safety beyond 2 years. Following bioresorption, inflammation, patency of the vessel especially late lumen gain should be evaluated at late phase. Attention must be devoted to longer-term inflammation that may result in destruction of the internal elastic lamina which is an indication of inflammation related effects rather than reflecting vascular injury during the device deployment at implantation.

## Intravascular imaging

Intravascular imaging modalities such as intravascular ultrasound (IVUS) and optical coherence tomography (OCT) are valuable tools for the assessment of coronary devices (Figure 4.1.1) [13–15]. High intensity grayscale quantification by IVUS is correlated to PLA residual molecular weight loss and can be used as a surrogate for the monitoring of the degradation of the semicrystalline polymers scaffolds [16]. OCT has been more effectively used not only for the evaluation of *in vivo* healing parameters such as stent strut coverage, neointima formation, presence of malapposition, and extent of thrombus, but also as a surrogate for monitoring the integrity of PLA scaffolds that could provide a greater understanding of the characteristics of *in vivo* bioresorption of polylactide scaffolds in preclinical and clinical trials [17].

It is important to realize that almost all the data published to date almost exclusively apply to ABSORB BVSs and are not necessarily applicable to other scaffolds made of PLA because the latter have dissimilar molecular weights and manufacturing processes. Moreover, each device will also have distinct histologic responses and degradation characteristics. Therefore, it is very important to evaluate each scaffold on its own with intravascular imaging during first-in-man (FIM) studies and trials.

## Biochemical analysis of degradation products

Biochemical analysis is also mandatory for the temporal determination of physiochemical structure along with *in vivo* biological responses. In addition to *in vitro* and *in vivo* degradation analysis, gel permeation chromatography (GPC) for assessing molecular weight and polydispersity index indicate the exact timing of the expected degradation and potential untoward effects of the scaffold during *in vivo* human studies may be predicted. It is also important to correlate results of bioengineering tests (e.g., radial strength, recoil, and fracture rates) with those determined from *in vivo* degradation analysis to facilitate understanding of BRSs integrity. For the assessment of BRSs devices, other techniques such as biochemical analysis, micro CT, scanning electron microscopy (SEM) and, in case of metallic biodegradation scaffolds, elemental analysis may also have to be applied to appropriately examine the effects of various degradation products.

## ABSORB BVSs 1.0 AND 1.1 (ABBOTT VASCULAR, SANTA MONICA, CA)

ABSORB BVSs is a balloon-expandable, bioresorbable scaffold that consists of a poly (L-lactide) (PLLA) backbone

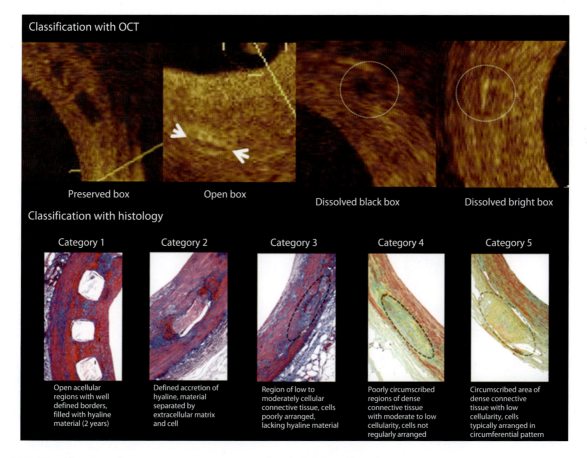

**Figure 4.1.1** Classification of strut appearances assessed with OCT and histology in porcine coronary arteries. (Reproduced with permission from Onuma Y et al., *Circulation*. 2010;122:2288–2300.)

coated with a poly (D, L-lactide) (PDLLA) eluting everolimus applied at similar concentration and release kinetics as on the XIENCE stent. The cohort A preclinical study using BVSs 1.0, with zig-zag hoops linked directly and by straight bridges, in porcine coronary arteries showed the safety, efficacy, and complete integration of the struts into the arterial wall at 3 and 4 years, as confirmed by histology and OCT (Figure 4.1.2) [13]. However, a clinical trial using ABSORB BVSs 1.0 observed shrinkage of scaffold at 6 months, which suggesting the insufficient radial strength following scaffold implantation [5,18]. The late lumen loss (0.44 mm) caused by scaffold shrinkage was observed at 6 months. In a preclinical study, GPC analysis demonstrated that the weight-average molecular weight (Mw) and number-average molecular weight (Mn) of PLLA dropped by ≈100%, from 200 kDa (Mw) and 100 kDa (Mn) at T0 to below the limit of detection by 2 years following ABSORB BVSs 1.0 implantation. The molecular percentage mass loss weight loss increased by ≈20%, 60%, and 90% at 1, 1.5, and 2 years, respectively, and became undetectable by 3 years [13].

ABSORB BVSs (ABSORB BVSs 1.1) was optimized to maintain stronger radial strength for at least the initial 3 months after implant, whereas material, coating, and backbone were unchanged. Recently, we conducted a preclinical study (Cohort B) comparing ABSORB BVSs (ABSORB BVSs 1.1) and everolimus eluting metallic stent XIENCE V in porcine coronary arteries [19]. The polymer number-average molecular weight dropped to below the measurement limit (4.7 kDa) at 30 months after implantation.

## Imaging studies including angiography, IVUS, and OCT

In the above-mentioned preclinical ABSORB BVSs 1.1 preclinical study coronary angiography showed mild to moderate luminal narrowing up to 3 months for both ABSORB BVSs and XIENCE; however, the degree of luminal narrowing became less thereafter, and smooth lumen contours were observed in both devices at 42 months (Table 4.1.1) [19]. Both ABSORB BVSs and XIENCE tended to show larger follow-up mean luminal diameter at later time points as compared with earlier time points with the exception of 36 months at which time both ABSORB and XIENCE were of similar size as compared to less than 18 months. Late lumen loss and percent diameter stenosis (% DS) were greater in ABSORB BVSs than XIENCE at 1 to 6 months, followed by comparable late lumen loss and % DS between the groups at 12–24 months. ABSORB BVSs exhibited lower late lumen loss and smaller % DS as compared with XIENCE from 30 to 42 months, where the difference was statistically significant at 36 months. Late lumen loss and % DS were maximal at 3 months for both ABSORB BVSs and XIENCE but decreased thereafter for both implants up to 12 months, and the decrease was more remarkable for ABSORB BVSs than XIENCE beyond 12 months (Table 4.1.1).

Lane et al. evaluated the potential of progressive lumen gain and a return of pulsatility after implantation of ABSORB BVSs and XIENCE in healthy porcine coronary arteries [20]. From 1 to 6 months, lumen area by IVUS was stable in both ABSORB BVSs and XIENCE; however, lumen

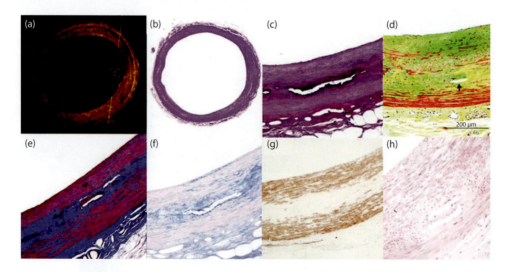

Figure 4.1.2 OCT image and histology at 4 years after implantation. Struts are no longer discernible by either OCT **(a)** or histology using hematoxylin and eosin (**b** and **c**) and Alcian Blue staining **(f)**. Locations in the arterial wall suggestive of prior strut location are minimally discernible with Movat pentachrome staining **(d)**, which are illustrated by focal regions of low smooth muscle cell density and circumscribed with connective tissue (**e**, trichrome staining). As at 3 years, there is a paucity of cells within the connective tissue replacing the preexisting strut that stain positively with SMA **(g)**. Scant remnant calcification (**d**, arrow), now less notable compared with that observed at 2 and 3 years, is the solitary evidence remaining of the prior strut. With von Kossa staining **(h)**, negative staining was consistently obtained on multiple sections at 4 years, suggesting the minimal amount of calcification relative to the control section. (Reproduced with permission from Onuma Y et al., *Circulation.* 2010;122:2288–2300.)

Table 4.1.1 Quantitative coronary angiography (QCA)

| | | 1 month | 3 months | 6 months | 12 months | 18 months | 24 months | 30 months | 36 months | 42 months | p value[a] | p value for interaction[b] |
|---|---|---|---|---|---|---|---|---|---|---|---|---|
| Balloon: artery ratio | ABSORB | 1.03 ± 0.06 | 1.06 ± 0.03 | 1.07 ± 0.04 | 1.08 ± 0.06 | 1.05 ± 0.05 | 1.05 ± 0.07 | 1.05 ± 0.03 | 1.05 ± 0.04 | 1.07 ± 0.06 | 0.46 | 0.35 |
| | XIENCE V | 1.11 ± 0.06 | 1.12 ± 0.05 | 1.10 ± 0.04 | 1.15 ± 0.05 | 1.19 ± 0.06 | 1.13 ± 0.02 | 1.11 ± 0.05 | 1.11 ± 0.03 | 1.14 ± 0.04 | 0.079 | |
| | p value[c] | 0.089 | 0.013 | 0.085 | 0.058 | 0.019 | 0.015 | 0.021 | 0.025 | 0.063 | | |
| Pre-implant mean luminal diameter (mm) | ABSORB | 2.81 ± 0.19 | 3.00 ± 0.10 | 2.91 ± 0.20 | 2.70 ± 0.15 | 2.71 ± 0.17 | 2.73 ± 0.18 | 2.85 ± 0.18 | 2.74 ± 0.11 | 2.71 ± 0.13 | 0.008 | 0.46 |
| | XIENCE V | 2.77 ± 0.19 | 2.85 ± 0.12 | 2.86 ± 0.21 | 2.68 ± 0.16 | 2.63 ± 0.07 | 2.67 ± 0.09 | 2.87 ± 0.20 | 2.79 ± 0.18 | 2.69 ± 0.15 | 0.006 | |
| | p value[c] | 0.89 | 0.024 | 0.51 | 0.68 | 0.046 | 0.35 | 0.83 | 0.42 | 0.50 | | |
| Post-implant mean luminal diameter (mm) | ABSORB | 2.89 ± 0.22 | 3.11 ± 0.10 | 2.98 ± 0.16 | 2.78 ± 0.19 | 2.84 ± 0.18 | 2.81 ± 0.20 | 2.95 ± 0.15 | 2.81 ± 0.10 | 2.80 ± 0.11 | 0.006 | 0.59 |
| | XIENCE V | 2.92 ± 0.20 | 3.09 ± 0.09 | 3.09 ± 0.19 | 3.01 ± 0.15 | 2.91 ± 0.14 | 2.92 ± 0.18 | 3.06 ± 0.17 | 2.97 ± 0.22 | 2.88 ± 0.21 | 0.098 | |
| | p value[c] | 0.59 | 0.62 | 0.092 | 0.024 | 0.13 | 0.24 | 0.19 | 0.14 | 0.42 | | |
| Follow-up mean luminal diameter (mm) | ABSORB | 2.31 ± 0.19 | 2.24 ± 0.18 | 2.29 ± 0.19 | 2.49 ± 0.18 | 2.82 ± 0.32 | 2.84 ± 0.32 | 3.19 ± 0.37 | 2.65 ± 0.29 | 3.20 ± 0.40 | <0.001 | 0.010 |
| | XIENCE V | 2.67 ± 0.23 | 2.34 ± 0.42 | 2.71 ± 0.26 | 2.77 ± 0.23 | 2.78 ± 0.13 | 3.03 ± 0.26 | 3.08 ± 0.32 | 2.58 ± 0.32 | 3.05 ± 0.29 | 0.004 | |
| | p value[c] | 0.067 | 0.26 | 0.013 | 0.058 | 0.59 | 0.20 | 0.44 | 0.27 | 0.13 | | |
| Late lumen loss (mm) | ABSORB | 0.58 ± 0.21 | 0.87 ± 0.17 | 0.69 ± 0.18 | 0.29 ± 0.17 | 0.02 ± 0.36 | −0.03 ± 0.33 | −0.26 ± 0.40 | 0.15 ± 0.31 | −0.42 ± 0.35 | <0.001 | <0.001 |
| | XIENCE V | 0.28 ± 0.11 | 0.74 ± 0.41 | 0.38 ± 0.15 | 0.24 ± 0.18 | 0.13 ± 0.17 | −0.11 ± 0.25 | −0.001 ± 0.22 | 0.39 ± 0.26 | −0.12 ± 0.31 | <0.001 | |
| | p value[c] | 0.023 | 0.23 | 0.010 | 0.44 | 0.24 | 0.42 | 0.10 | 0.033 | 0.059 | | |
| Percent diameter stenosis (%) | ABSORB | 19.85 ± 6.40 | 28.06 ± 5.46 | 22.96 ± 5.56 | 10.23 ± 5.82 | 0.34 ± 12.31 | −1.39 ± 11.77 | −8.76 ± 13.54 | 5.35 ± 11.10 | −14.82 ± 12.26 | <0.001 | <0.001 |
| | XIENCE V | 9.54 ± 3.86 | 24.12 ± 13.49 | 12.44 ± 4.92 | 8.03 ± 6.10 | 4.41 ± 6.00 | −3.91 ± 7.97 | −0.16 ± 7.21 | 13.00 ± 8.85 | −4.57 ± 10.50 | <0.001 | |
| | p value[c] | 0.022 | 0.23 | 0.009 | 0.37 | 0.23 | 0.45 | 0.093 | 0.034 | 0.062 | | |

a  p value for the comparison across all time points.
b  p value for interaction with time and device.
c  p value for ABSORB versus XIENCE V at each time point.

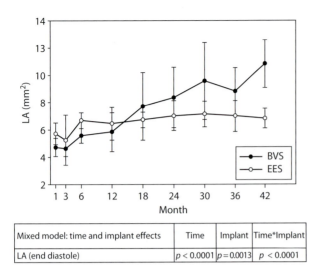

| Mixed model: time and implant effects | Time | Implant | Time*Implant |
|---|---|---|---|
| LA (end diastole) | $p < 0.0001$ | $p = 0.0013$ | $p < 0.0001$ |

**Figure 4.1.3** IVUS-obtained LA for BVS- and EES-implanted porcine coronary arteries from 1 to 42 months. From 1 to 12 months, EES and BVS implanted arteries follow similar trends in LA as the arteries stabilize after implantation. From 12 to 42 months, the LA of EES-implanted arteries remains relatively stable, whereas a progressive increase in LA occurs for BVS-implanted arteries. As illustrated in Figure 4.1.2, the lower LA at 36 months for BVS-implanted arteries is related to the smaller RLA of these arteries at this time point. BVS = bioresorbable vascular scaffold(s); EES = everolimus-eluting stent(s); IVUS = intravascular ultrasound; LA = lumen area. (Reproduced with permission from Lane JP, *J Am Coll Cardiol Intv* 2014;7:688–695.)

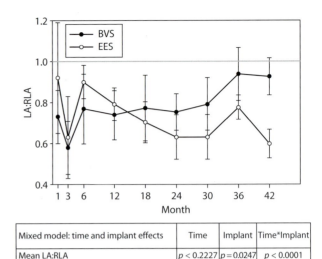

| Mixed model: time and implant effects | Time | Implant | Time*Implant |
|---|---|---|---|
| Mean LA:RLA | $p < 0.2227$ | $p = 0.0247$ | $p < 0.0001$ |

**Figure 4.1.4** Normalization of in-segment LA (LA:RLA) of BVS- and EES-implanted porcine coronary arteries as assessed by IVUS. An LA:RLA ratio of 1.0 (gray line) indicates uniformity in the LA between the reference vessel and the implanted region. From 1 to 6 months, EES- and BVS-implanted arteries illustrate similar trends in the LA:RLA ratio that is related to the peak neointimal thickness typical of this model at 3 months. For BVS-implanted arteries, the LA:RLA ratio remains relatively stable from 6 to 30 months and increases thereafter, approaching 1.0, indicating a normalization of the in-segment LA. BVS = bioresorbable vascular scaffold(s); EES = everolimus-eluting stent(s); IVUS = intravascular ultrasound; LA = lumen area; RLA = reference vessel lumen area. (Reproduced with permission from Lane JP, *J Am Coll Cardiol Intv* 2014;7:688–695.)

area progressively increased in ABSORB BVSs from 12 to 24 months, whereas lumen area in XIENCE remained relatively stable throughout this time period (Figure 4.1.3) [20].

Normalized lumen area by reference lumen area was also evaluated for lumen enlargement since reference vessel lumen area increased over time in both ABSORB BVSs and XIENCE groups, illustrating normal growth of the porcine coronary arteries which occurs as the animal gains weight over the period of the study. The ratio of the lumen area to reference lumen area approached 1.0 at 36 and 42 months, indicating that the lumen area of the implanted segment reached that of the reference vessel (Figure 4.1.4). On the other hand, this ratio decreased in XIENCE (0.60 at 42 months). Restoration of pulsatility was assessed as the differences of lumen area between the end-diastolic and end-systolic state, which was observed in only ABSORB BVSs starting at 12 months [20]. Recently, Nakatani et al. analyzed intracoronary imaging studies using IVUS and OCT from the same preclinical study, which also showed similar findings [17]. Mean lumen area by IVUS and OCT significantly increased over time, indicating lumen enlargement following implantation of ABSORB BVSs (IVUS: $4.59 \pm 0.88$ mm$^2$ at 3 months, $9.45 \pm 1.18$ mm$^2$ at 48 months, $p < 0.001$, OCT: $4.04 \pm 0.62$ mm$^2$ at 3 months, $9.69 \pm 1.61$ mm$^2$ at 48 months, $p < 0.001$). Furthermore, the relationship between the integration process and luminal enlargement with OCT was

investigated [17]. The normalized light intensity, defined as the light intensity value of strut cores normalized by the median light intensity value of the interstrut neointima in the vicinity of each strut, was used for the assessment. The normalized light intensity increased over time (0.17 [0.15–0.19] at 3 months, 0.82 [0.79–0.83] at 48 months, $p < 0.001$), and resulted in a significant increase beyond 24 months compared to 3 months.

## Histological morphometric analysis

Histological assessment by light microscopy revealed that vascular responses to ABSORB BVSs were comparable to XIENCE at all time points (Figure 4.1.5 and 4.1.6) with patent stents/scaffold and near (1 month) to complete (>1 month) sequestration of struts within the neointimal tissue [19]. Any significant thrombus in the main or the side branch arterial lumens was not seen in both ABSORB BVSs and XIENCE groups. Morphometric analysis showed vessel positive remodeling in ABSORB BVSs implanted arteries starting at 12 months. On the other hand, XIENCE showed no changes in external elastic lamina (EEL) or internal elastic lamina (IEL) areas (Figure 4.1.7 and Table 4.1.2) [19]. Increased vessel area in ABSORB BVSs was observed beyond

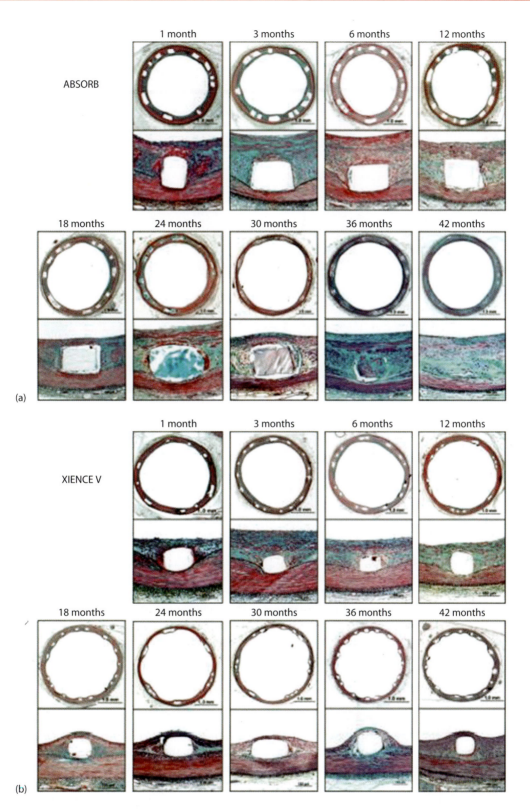

Figure 4.1.5 Representative histologic images of Absorb bioresorbable vascular scaffold (ABSORB BVSs) (a) and XIENCE V (b) in porcine coronary arteries from 1 to 42 months (Movat pentachrome). Color changes are appreciated at resorption sites beginning at 18 months in that resorption sites are increasingly alcian blue positive from 18 to 24 months. Thereafter, resorption sites undergo further changes, and there is progressive dismantling with corresponding integration of proteo-glycans and collagen with few smooth muscle cells. The resorption sites are almost completely replaced by connective tissue at 42 months. (Reproduced with permission from Otsuka F et al., *Circ Cardiovasc Interv* 2014;7:330–342.)

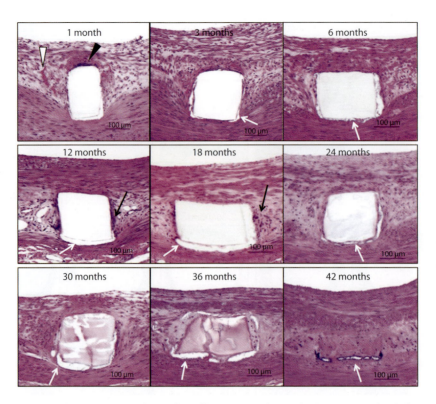

**Figure 4.1.6** Histologic images showing minimal to mild inflammation, fibrin deposition, and calcification around ABSORB struts/resorption sites (hematoxylin and eosin stains). Mild inflammatory infiltrate was observed from 12 to 36 months (black arrows at 12 and 18 months) and consisted mostly of macrophages and a few lymphocytes. At 42 months, inflammation was not readily observed. Giant cells were occasionally observed at 1 month (black arrowheads); however, they were uncommon beyond 3 months. Peak fibrin deposition was noted at 1 month (white arrowheads) with rapid decrease at 3 months and becoming absent or minimal thereafter. Minor areas of calcification (white arrows) were observed around struts/resorption sites beyond 3 months. (Reproduced with permission from Otsuka F et al., *Circ Cardiovasc Interv* 2014;7: 330–342.)

12 months, which was markedly increased at 18 months and followed by a slower rate of enlargement beyond 18 months. On the other hand, significant lumen enlargement was not observed in XIENCE throughout the period of observation almost certainly because of metallic caging of the vessel. The lumen area paralleled the changes observed in IEL (lumen area = $4.9 \pm 0.6$ mm$^2$ at 1 month, $8.3 \pm 1.5$ mm$^2$ at 42 months, $p < 0.001$; IEL area = $6.7 \pm 0.8$ mm$^2$ at 1 month, $10.9 \pm 1.4$ mm$^2$, $p < 0.001$). Interestingly, the lumen area enlarged beyond 12 months and the difference in lumen area between the devices reached statistical significance at 36 and 42 months. At 36 and 42 months, ABSORB BVSs showed greater percentage area stenosis ($26.4 \pm 6.1\%$ and $24.5 \pm 4.9\%$, respectively) as compared with XIENCE ($19.4 \pm 8.8\%$ and $16.0 \pm 1.6\%$, respectively); however, the effective lumen area was larger in ABSORB BVSs as compared with XIENCE [19], thus suggesting vessel remodeling due to the breakdown of the BVSs which was not present in the metallic DESs.

## Histological assessment

Inflammation was overall mild to moderate for both devices, with absence of inflammation at 1 month in ABSORB BVSs and XIENCE. Inflammation scores were greater for ABSORB BVSs than XIENCE beyond 6 months; however, the scores progressively declined beyond 18 months in ABSORB BVSs ($p < 0.001$ for the comparison across time [18–42 months]). Both devices exhibited absent or minimal inflammation at 42 months. Overall the inflammatory infiltrate was minimal to mild and consisted mostly of macrophages and a few lymphocytes (Figure 4.1.6) [19]. Giant cells were the most frequently observed at 1 month in both devices; however, they were uncommon beyond 3 months, and there were no significant differences observed between the devices (Figure 4.1.6). Injury scores were generally low and comparable within the groups up to 30 months, although the score was greater for ABSORB BVSs as compared with XIENCE despite lower balloon-to-artery ratio in the former, and the difference was statistically significant at 12 months (Figure 4.1.7, Table 4.1.2). The extent of fibrin deposition was similar between both groups with peak fibrin deposition observed at 1 month and rapidly decreasing by 3 months and becoming absent or minimal at 6 months and beyond. Minor areas of calcification were identified around struts/resorption sites of ABSORB BVSs at all time points; these likely represent pre-existing PDLLA coating and is an inconsequential feature (Figure 4.1.6).

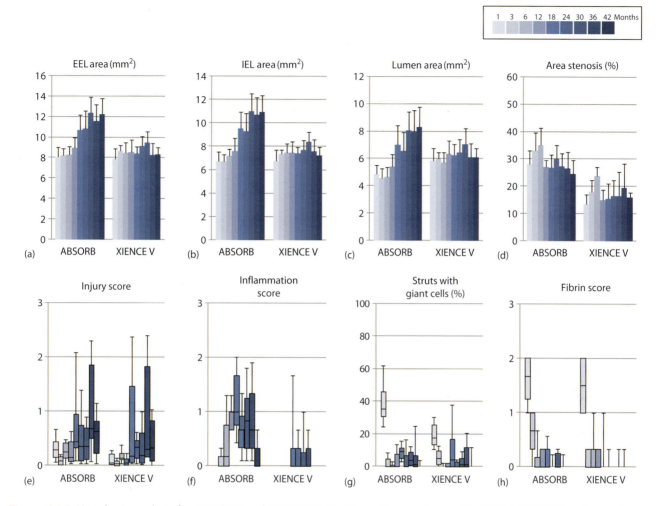

**Figure 4.1.7** Histologic analysis for ABSORB and XIENCE V. Devices with granulomas (3 of 102 ABSORB [1 at 3 months and 2 at 12 months] and 4 of 67 XIENCE V [3 at 3 months and 1 at 12 months]) were excluded. **(a–d)** Bar graphs showing external elastic lamina (EEL) **(a)**, internal elastic lamina (IEL) **(b)**, and lumen areas **(c)** as well as percentage area stenosis **(d)**. Bars represent mean values and T-bars indicate SD. Note late vessel and lumen enlargement observed for ABSORB beyond 12 months. **(e–h)** Box-and-whisker plots showing injury score **(e)**, inflammation score **(f)**, giant cell reaction **(g)**, and fibrin score **(h)**. Lines within boxes represent median values; the upper and lower lines of the boxes represent the 75th and 25th percentiles, respectively; and the upper and lower bars outside the boxes represent the 90th and 10th percentiles, respectively. (Reproduced with permission from Otsuka F et al., *Circ Cardiovasc Interv* 2014;7:330–342.)

## Discontinuity following ABSORB implantation

Discontinuity is defined as sites of struts/resorption that are different from the conventional box shape with integration of arterial derived tissue. Onuma et al. reported the incidence of strut discontinuity following ABSORB BVSs implantation from the ABSORB cohort B trial including 51 patients with OCT analysis (Figure 4.1.8) [21]. Of 51 patients, acute scaffold disruption was observed in 2 patients (3.9%), whereas 21 out of 49 patients (42.9%) did not have acute scaffold disruption but had late discontinuities (Figure 4.1.9). Of 21 patients, only one patient had non-ischemia-driven target lesion revascularization. Histologically, there were two time-dependent aspects appreciated with struts/resorption sites of ABSORB BVSs, both of which are a

reflection of the scaffold's transience. We have observed increasing discontinuities with time, and they appear as pink staining of the scaffold resorption sites by H&E and blue staining by Movat stain. Otsuka et al. showed that discontinuities increased with time, especially at time points beyond 12 months [19]. Furthermore, beginning at 18 months, resorption sites undergo color changes that included alcian blue positive staining at 18 and 24 months with Movat pentachrome and increasing eosinophilia with H&E thereafter. When both of these chronological changes are occurring there is increasing integration of arterial tissue into resorption sites such that by 42 months the previous sites of the scaffold are mostly replaced by collagen and proteoglycans with sparse infiltration by spindle cells (e.g., smooth muscle cells [SMC]) and rare as previously reported remnants of calcification near the resorption sites. Thus,

Table 4.1.2  Histologic analysis

| | | 1 month | 3 months | 6 months | 12 months | 18 months | 24 months | 30 months | 36 months | 42 months | p value[a] | p value for interaction[b] |
|---|---|---|---|---|---|---|---|---|---|---|---|---|
| EEL (mm²) | ABSORB | 8.1 ± 0.9 | 8.3 ± 0.7 | 8.3 ± 0.8 | 9.5 ± 1.9 | 10.7 ± 1.5 | 10.8 ± 1.7 | 12.3 ± 1.5 | 11.6 ± 1.6 | 12.2 ± 1.5 | <0.001 | <0.001 |
| | XIENCE V | 7.9 ± 1.0 | 9.3 ± 2.2 | 8.5 ± 1.0 | 8.7 ± 1.2 | 8.4 ± 0.6 | 9.2 ± 0.9 | 9.5 ± 1.0 | 8.3 ± 1.1 | 8.3 ± 0.7 | 0.13 | |
| | p value[c] | 0.77 | 0.12 | 0.86 | 0.14 | 0.014 | 0.052 | 0.014 | 0.010 | 0.007 | | |
| IEL (mm²) | ABSORB | 6.7 ± 0.8 | 6.7 ± 0.5 | 7.2 ± 0.6 | 8.1 ± 1.8 | 9.5 ± 1.5 | 9.3 ± 1.5 | 11.0 ± 1.5 | 10.7 ± 1.4 | 10.9 ± 1.4 | <0.001 | <0.001 |
| | XIENCE V | 6.8 ± 0.9 | 7.1 ± 0.6 | 7.4 ± 0.8 | 7.5 ± 0.9 | 7.4 ± 0.6 | 7.7 ± 0.8 | 8.4 ± 0.8 | 7.6 ± 1.0 | 7.2 ± 0.7 | 0.21 | |
| | p value[c] | 0.84 | 0.16 | 0.60 | 0.22 | 0.017 | 0.030 | 0.015 | 0.010 | 0.008 | | |
| Media (mm²) | ABSORB | 1.35 ± 0.22 | 1.56 ± 0.31 | 1.14 ± 0.22 | 1.43 ± 0.32 | 1.17 ± 0.30 | 1.55 ± 0.54 | 1.33 ± 0.30 | 0.85 ± 0.32 | 1.30 ± 0.31 | 0.038 | 0.82 |
| | XIENCE V | 1.10 ± 0.08 | 2.25 ± 2.08 | 1.05 ± 0.20 | 1.20 ± 0.38 | 1.02 ± 0.11 | 1.47 ± 0.34 | 1.10 ± 0.21 | 0.72 ± 0.28 | 1.09 ± 0.18 | 0.056 | |
| | p value[c] | 0.057 | 0.28 | 0.26 | 0.025 | 0.067 | 0.80 | 0.083 | 0.024 | 0.025 | | |
| Lumen (mm²) | ABSORB | 4.9 ± 0.6 | 4.3 ± 0.9 | 4.7 ± 0.7 | 5.6 ± 1.1 | 7.0 ± 1.4 | 6.5 ± 1.4 | 8.0 ± 1.4 | 7.9 ± 1.6 | 8.3 ± 1.5 | <0.001 | 0.002 |
| | XIENCE V | 5.9 ± 0.9 | 4.8 ± 1.8 | 5.7 ± 0.8 | 6.2 ± 0.9 | 6.3 ± 0.8 | 6.5 ± 1.0 | 7.0 ± 1.2 | 6.1 ± 1.0 | 6.1 ± 0.6 | 0.15 | |
| | p value[c] | 0.10 | 0.26 | 0.045 | 0.19 | 0.18 | 0.97 | 0.16 | 0.020 | 0.014 | | |
| % Stenosis | ABSORB | 27.9 ± 5.1 | 35.9 ± 10.8 | 35.1 ± 6.1 | 29.2 ± 5.3 | 26.8 ± 4.8 | 30.1 ± 5.0 | 27.2 ± 4.7 | 26.4 ± 6.1 | 24.5 ± 4.9 | 0.021 | 0.10 |
| | XIENCE V | 13.5 ± 3.5 | 32.9 ± 22.2 | 23.8 ± 3.2 | 17.1 ± 6.9 | 15.4 ± 5.6 | 16.4 ± 5.9 | 16.5 ± 8.6 | 19.4 ± 8.8 | 16.0 ± 1.6 | 0.008 | |
| | p value[c] | 0.022 | 0.44 | 0.011 | 0.012 | 0.033 | 0.010 | 0.018 | 0.023 | 0.015 | | |
| Neointimal thickness (mm) | ABSORB | 0.10 ± 0.04 | 0.18 ± 0.09 | 0.15 ± 0.05 | 0.14 ± 0.08 | 0.13 ± 0.04 | 0.15 ± 0.03 | 0.14 ± 0.04 | 0.16 ± 0.06 | 0.15 ± 0.04 | 0.031 | 0.006 |
| | XIENCE V | 0.07 ± 0.04 | 0.27 ± 0.23 | 0.14 ± 0.03 | 0.08 ± 0.05 | 0.06 ± 0.04 | 0.07 ± 0.05 | 0.06 ± 0.07 | 0.07 ± 0.05 | 0.04 ± 0.01 | 0.006 | |
| | p value[c] | 0.016 | 0.56 | 0.015 | 0.013 | 0.014 | 0.012 | 0.006 | 0.007 | 0.006 | | |
| Injury score | ABSORB | 0.29 (0.15, 0.44) | 0.09 (0.02, 0.18) | 0.25 (0.14, 0.42) | 0.19 (0.08, 0.63) | 0.44 (0.32, 0.95) | 0.35 (0.09, 0.74) | 0.35 (0.11, 0.69) | 0.68 (0.50, 1.85) | 0.63 (0.22, 0.82) | 0.32 | 0.34 |
| | XIENCE V | 0.05 (0.02, 0.21) | 0.08 (0.01, 1.30) | 0.14 (0.11, 0.22) | 0.05 (0, 0.23) | 0.18 (0.06, 1.46) | 0.34 (0.14, 0.46) | 0.19 (0.05, 0.60) | 0.30 (0.16, 1.83) | 0.32 (0.08, 0.83) | 0.24 | |
| | p value[c] | 0.070 | 0.87 | 0.51 | 0.045 | 0.77 | 0.51 | 0.32 | 0.60 | 0.23 | | |

(Continued)

Table 4.1.2 (Continued) Histologic analysis

| | | 1 month | 3 months | 6 months | 12 months | 18 months | 24 months | 30 months | 36 months | 42 months | p value[a] | p value for interaction[b] |
|---|---|---|---|---|---|---|---|---|---|---|---|---|
| Inflammation score | ABSORB | 0 (0, 0) | 0 (0, 0.33) | 0.17 (0, 0.75) | 1.00 (0.67, 1.33) | 1.00 (0.75, 1.67) | 0.67 (0.33, 0.92) | 0.83 (0.33, 1.25) | 0.67 (0.33, 1.33) | 0 (0, 0.33) | <0.001 | 0.013 |
| | XIENCE V | 0 (0, 0) | 0 (0, 4.00) | 0 (0, 0) | 0 (0, 0) | 0 (0, 0.33) | 0 (0, 0.33) | 0 (0, 0.25) | 0 (0, 0.33) | 0 (0, 0) | 0.17 | |
| | p value[c] | 0.79 | 0.52 | 0.031 | 0.012 | 0.032 | 0.090 | 0.034 | 0.038 | 0.062 | | |
| Strut with giant cells | ABSORB | 35.1 (30.6, 46.0) | 1.3 (0, 6.6) | 0 (0, 0.6) | 2.6 (0, 13.3) | 9.3 (5.1, 11.4) | 0 (0, 6.8) | 3.5 (0.6, 8.7) | 1.2 (0, 6.6) | 0 (0, 0) | <0.001 | 0.24 |
| | XIENCE V | 17.6 (13.4, 25.4) | 6.7 (2.9, 23.1) | 0 (0, 0) | 0 (0, 2.2) | 4.2 (0, 16.6) | 0 (0, 2.8) | 1.1 (0, 4.9) | 1.1 (0, 11.7) | 0 (0, 0) | 0.031 | |
| | p value[c] | 0.16 | 0.15 | 0.47 | 0.18 | 0.12 | 0.99 | 0.16 | 0.66 | 0.45 | | |
| (%) Fibrin score | ABSORB | 1.67 (1.25, 2.00) | 0.50 (0.25, 1.00) | 0 (0, 0.17) | 0 (0, 0.33) | 0 (0, 0.33) | 0 (0, 0) | 0 (0, 0.25) | 0 (0, 0) | 0 (0, 0) | 0.006 | 0.30 |
| | XIENCE V | 1.50 (1.00, 2.00) | 0 (0, 0.33) | 0 (0, 0.33) | 0 (0, 0.33) | 0 (0, 0) | 0 (0, 0) | 0 (0, 0) | 0 (0, 0) | 0 (0, 0) | 0.042 | |
| | p value[c] | 0.81 | 0.083 | 0.21 | 0.82 | 0.34 | 0.82 | 0.12 | 0.66 | 0.33 | | |

Note: The analyses include devices with granulomas which were observed in 3 of 102 Absorb (2.9%, 1 at 3 months and 2 at 12 months) and 4 of 67 XIENCE V (6.0%, 3 at 3 months and 1 at 12 months). Eosinophil infiltration was absent in both devices except in stents/scaffolds that have a granulomatous reaction, and in these the number of eosinophils per high power field varied from 2 to 50 cells which were observed along with lymphocytes and macrophages. Values are expressed as mean ± SD or median (25th percentile, 75th percentile).

Abbreviations: EEL = external elastic lamina; IEL = internal elastic lamina.

[a] p value for the comparison across all time points.
[b] p value for interaction with time and device.
[c] p value for ABSORB versus XIENCE V at each time point.

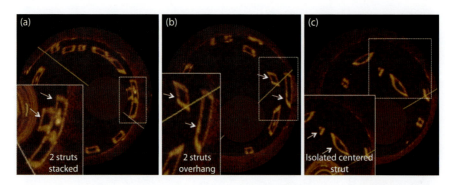

Figure 4.1.8 OCT criteria to diagnose acute scaffold disruption (phantom assessment). In a silicon phantom, a 3.0-mm ABSORB BVS scaffold was disrupted through inflation of a semicompliant balloon up to 4.3 mm in diameter. Optical coherence tomography (OCT) showed the following: more than two struts in the same angular sector with close contact (two struts stacked) **(a)** or without any contact (overhung struts) **(b)**. The other presentation of disrupted scaffold is the detection of an isolated malapposed strut located at the center of the lumen with loss of circularity of the scaffold **(c)**. The distance from the abluminal side of the strut to the luminal border should be more than one-third of the distance from the center of gravity to the lumen border in the corresponding angular sector. (Reproduced with permission from Onuma Y et al. *J Am Coll Cardiol Interv* 2014;7:1400–11.)

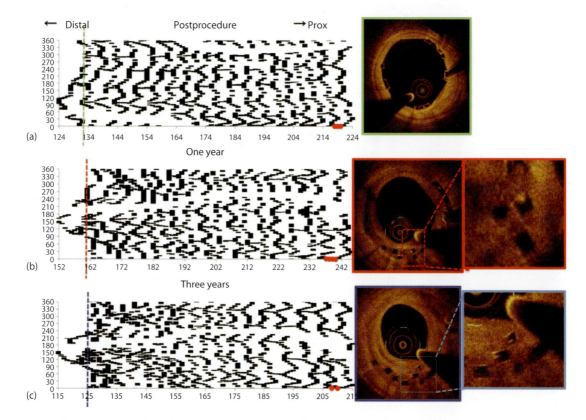

Figure 4.1.9 Serial assessment of late discontinuities using spread-out-vessel graphics. **(a–c)** The foldout views represent spread-out vessel graphics created by correlating the longitudinal distance from the distal scaffold edge to the individual struts detected in a single cross-section (abscissa) on the ordinate the angle where the individual strut was located in the circular cross-section with respect to the center of gravity of the vessel (ordinates). In each cross-section (axial resolution of 200 μm), the circumferential length of each individual strut was depicted in an angular fashion. The resultant graphic represented the scaffolded vessel, as if it had been cut longitudinally along the reference angle and spread out on a flat surface. The spread-out view postprocedure **(a)** showed that the scaffold consisted of 19 rings interconnected by 3 links. At 1 year **(b)** and 3 years **(c)**, mechanical integrity has gradually subsided and the distal part of the scaffold was starting to show signs of dismantling, along which late discontinuities were observed. At baseline, in the distal edge of the scaffold (green dotted line in the foldout view), 2-dimensional optical coherence tomography (OCT) (green frame) revealed well-apposed struts. At 1 year, in the distal edge (red dotted line in the foldout view), 2-dimensional OCT (red frame) showed overhung and apposed struts. At 3 years, these struts remained overhung (blue line in the foldout view, corresponding to 2-dimensional OCT with a blue frame). The phenomenon is considered benign because the struts are mostly covered at 1 and 3 years. Red dots represent the proximal metallic markers. (Reproduced with permission from Onuma Y et al. *J Am Coll Cardiol Interv* 2014;7:1400–11.)

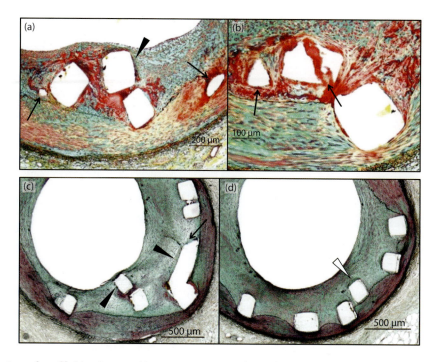

**Figure 4.1.10** Disruption of scaffolds observed in two arteries implanted with ABSORB. **(a)** and **(b)** are histologic images showing strut irregularity (arrows) and overlaid struts (black arrowhead) observed in the left anterior descending coronary artery (LAD) with ABSORB at 1 month. **(c)** and **(d)** are histologic images showing strut irregularity (arrow) in the LAD with ABSORB at 3 months with overlaid struts (black arrowheads) and atypical strut alignment (white arrowhead). Note complete neointimal coverage of all struts in both arteries with increased neointimal growth; however, in both arteries, the lumens remained patent. (Reproduced with permission from Otsuka F et al., *Circ Cardiovasc Interv* 2014;7:330–342.)

discontinuities should be observed as a normal finding as the scaffold degrades. On the other hand, we have observed rare acute scaffold disruption (one each at 1 and 3 months). Disruption appears as strut overlap and/or strut deformation and it occurs at the time of implant. Overlapped struts, which are incompletely apposed to the IEL, may also be observed (Figure 4.1.10). The maximum percentage stenosis seen at 1 month and 3 months was 39% and 65%, respectively, which was likely from increased neointimal proliferation that occurred in relation to the overlapped struts. No thrombus was seen at the site of implant. However, neither excess neointimal or adventitial inflammation nor injury to the artery wall was observed. However, fibrin was seen at these sites, which related to the presence of drug and delayed healing.

## Scanning electron microscopy (SEM)

SEM study at 1 month for both ABSORB BVSs and XIENCE in the porcine coronary model showed almost complete strut coverage by endothelial cells and mild neointimal growth so that the underlying outline of the struts was clearly visible. The luminal endothelial cells had a cobblestone morphology and generally showed tight and well-formed cell-to-cell contacts (Figure 4.1.11) [19]. Endothelial coverage for both ABSORB BVSs and XIENCE observed at 1 month was also observed at all other time points and at the final SEM follow-up at 12 months (Figure 4.1.11).

## Pharmacokinetics of the drug release

By 28 days the mean cumulative percentage of everolimus release was 79%, with 35% being released in the first 24 hours. Overall everolimus release peaked at 90 days (96%) postimplantation (Figure 4.1.12a) [19]. On the other hand, everolimus maximum concentration in the tissue around the scaffolded arterial segments was observed at 3 hours following implantation with a mean of 16.2 ng/mg (Figure 4.1.12b). The everolimus arterial concentrations ranged from 4.6 ng/mg to 2.3 ng/mg from 1 day to 28 days, which is greater than the $IC_{50}$ for SMC. The levels were significantly less at 90 days (0.6 ng/mg). The blood concentration ($C_{max}$) of everolimus is low 3.75 ± 0.96 ng/mL at 15 minutes. It has been reported that the desirable systemic safety levels in blood are below 3 ng/mL, which is the minimally effective concentration for immunosuppression in organ transplant patients [22]. Nevertheless blood levels of everolimus quickly declined to below the limit of quantification (<0.1 ng/mL) after 168 hours (7 days) (Figure 4.1.12c). Everolimus in the lungs, kidneys, spleen, and liver are only measurable (0.01–0.02 ng/mg) at 3 hours.

## Gel permeation chromatography

As previously described, ABSORB BVSs 1.0 demonstrated relatively early degradation [13], leading to the shrinkage. In the recent animal study with ABSORB BVSs 1.1, the GPC

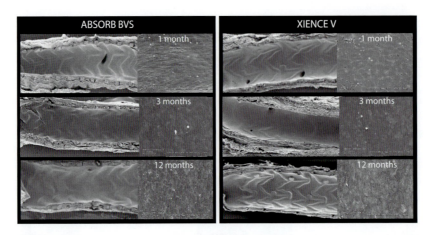

**Figure 4.1.11** Representative scanning electron microscopy images of ABSORB bioresorbable vascular scaffold (ABSORB BVS) and XIENCE V at 1, 3, and 12 months following device placement in porcine coronary arteries. The low power images acquired at 15× magnification show complete strut coverage by mildly thickened neointima at 1 month in both ABSORB and XIENCE V, which are maintained at 3 and 12 months. High power images acquired at 600× magnification show completely endothelialized luminal surface with cells arranged in cobblestone morphology and showing well-formed cell-to-cell contacts that indicate the mature nature of the endothelium in both ABSORB and XIENCE V at 1, 3, and 12 months. Both devices show infrequent adherent inflammatory cells and scattered red blood cells on luminal surfaces with no evidence of luminal thrombus. (Reproduced with permission from Otsuka F et al., *Circ Cardiovasc Interv* 2014;7:330–342.)

results indicated the polymer Mn decreased slowly by about 18% during the first 6 months of scaffold implantation, suggesting good integrity of the device. There is a period of more rapid decline thereafter (by 49, 72, and 93% at 12, 18, and 24 months, respectively). Therefore, we can expect less shrinkage and/or recoil of the current device as compared to ABSORB BVSs 1.0, especially within 6 months following implantation (Figure 4.1.13a). The polymer Mn dropped to below the measurement limit of detection (4.7 kDa) at 30 months. The percentage mass loss of the BVSs polymer is 10% during the first 18 months, with a rapid decline occurring at 24, 30, and 36 months (31, 74, and 97%, respectively), and is undetectable at 42 months (Figure 4.1.13b). Thirty-six month chromatograms show only a very small peak below the limit of quantification of polymer (0.3 mg/mL) (Figure 4.1.13c), thus suggesting that the polymer is completely resorbed at 36 months.

## Vasomotion studies in the porcine model

Although vasomotion studies in patients implanted with ABSORB cohort A and B have shown endothelium dependent and independent vasodilatation following acetycholine and nitroglycerine, respectively at 12 and 24 months, however, the percentage responders was under 50% [23,24]. Recently, Gogas et al. have reported appropriate vasoconstriction with acetylcholine in the porcine model along with vasodilation with nitroglycerine at 1 and 2 years, with the in-segment response being similar to that observed at proximal and distal edges in BVSs but not in XIENCE [25]. *Ex vivo* assessment with prostaglandin F2-α was associated with greater constriction in BVSs than XIENCE. Similarly vasorelaxation with substance P was greater with BVSs than XIENCE. From these small studies performed

prior to complete dissolution of the scaffold, it is difficult to make long-term predictions of vessel behavior.

## DESOLVE (ELIXIR MEDICAL CORPORATION, SUNNYVALE, CA)

The DESolve scaffold is composed of a PLLA-based polymer with 150 µm strut thickness and 2 platinum radio-opaque markers. The scaffold is coated with a matrix of polylactide-based polymer with the drug novolimus (5 µg/mm), a metabolite of sirolimus. However, the drug coating in the preclinical animal study and in the FIM trial published by Verheye et al. was myolimus (3 µg/mm) with more than 85% of the drug released in 4 weeks (Figure 4.1.14) [8]. The system has a crossing profile of 1.47 mm and is 6-F catheter compatible. Novolimus, the drug used in the current generation, has a release kinetic so that 80% of the drug is released over 4 weeks. The polymer coating is said to degrade within 6 to 9 months and the scaffold degrades within 12 months and resorbs within 24 months. However, the preclinical data is based on OCT images shown in the porcine model [8]; however, no table or figure of the actual data is available. Preclinical *in vivo* study results assessing the bioresorption profile of the DESolve scaffold (with myolimus) where molecular weight measurements by gel permeation chromatography have demonstrated bioresorption of the DESolve scaffold with molecular weight reduction of >95% taking more than 1 year (Figure 4.1.14) and mass loss occurring over 24 months. *In vitro* degradation studies appear to track closely with those carried out *in vivo*. Results show that the scaffold maintains structural integrity and radial support to the vessel wall for at least 3 months. However, to our knowledge no actual percentage stenosis or lumen or vessel areas nor any histologic studies have been published.

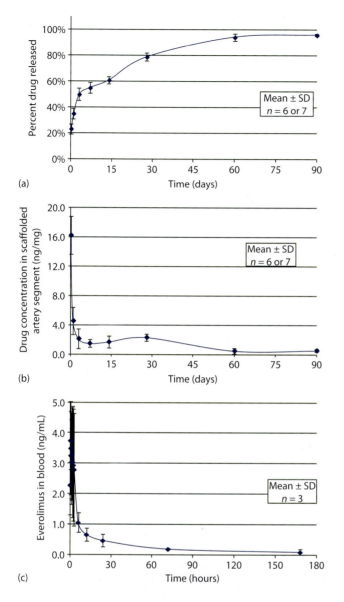

(a)

(b)

(c)

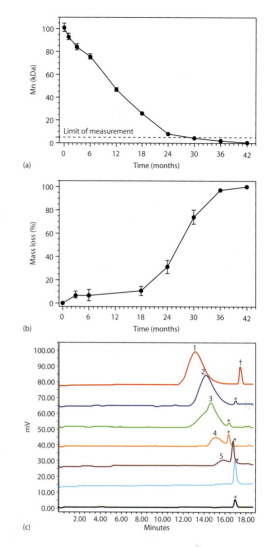

(a)

(b)

(c)

**Figure 4.1.12** Pharmacokinetics showing drug release profile **(a)**, drug concentrations in implanted vessel segment **(b)**, and drug concentrations in whole blood **(c)** following ABSORB implantation. **(a)** The mean cumulative percentage of everolimus released during the first 28 days was 79% and drug release peaked at 90 days (96%). **(b)** Everolimus concentration in scaffolded arterial segments was the greatest at 3 hours following implantation with a mean concentration being 16.2 ng/mg. Arterial everolimus concentrations ranged from 2.3 to 4.6 ng/mg in 1 to 28 days, which were greater than $IC_{50}$ of smooth muscle cell (SMC) that is required for the inhibition of human SMC proliferation. **(c)** The concentration of everolimus in blood peaked at 15 minutes following ABSORB implantation with a mean value being 3.75 ng/mL, and quickly declined to below the limit of quantification (<0.1 ng/mL) after 168 hours (7 days). (Reproduced with permission from Otsuka F et al., *Circ Cardiovasc Interv* 2014;7:330–342.)

**Figure 4.1.13** Gel permeation chromatography (GPC) for the assessment of degradation of ABSORB. **(a)** The *in vivo* degradation of polymer of ABSORB over time. The lower limit of measurement for the number-average molecular weight (Mn) is 4.7 kDa. **(b)** The *in vivo* mass loss of polymer of ABSORB over time. The limit of detection for the mass loss is 0.1 mg/mL (0.1 mg of average initial mass of 5.2 mg, equivalent to 1.9% of initial mass), and the limit of quantification is 0.3 mg/mL (0.3 mg of average initial mass of 5.2 mg, equivalent to 5.8% of initial mass). The polymer mass loss values at 1 month and 12 months were not reported since they were likely overestimated due to incomplete polymer recovery. **(c)** Top to bottom: Representative chromatograms of polymer samples before ABSORB implantation and at 18, 24, 30, 36, and 42 months after implantation, and of tissue blank. Peaks 1 to 5 represent PLLA polymer peaks obtained before ABSORB implantation and at 18, 24, 30, and 36 months, respectively, following scaffold implantation. The shift of these peaks to the right (lower *Mw* range) relative to the polymer peak on the chromatogram from samples at T0 is consistent with polymer degradation. *Trace tissue species. †Everolimus peak. (Reproduced with permission from Otsuka F et al., *Circ Cardiovasc Interv* 2014;7:330–342.)

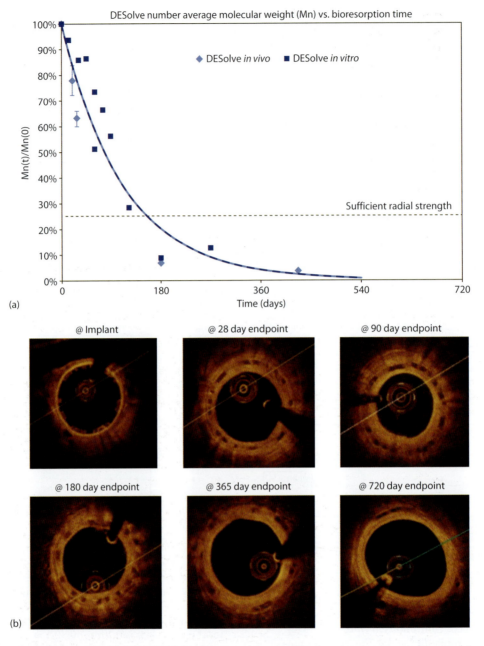

**Figure 4.1.14** DESolve bioresorption. **(a)** The DESolve bioresorption profile showing *in vitro* and *in vivo* bioresorption at about 1 year. Molecular weight measurements by gel permeation chromatography were made *in vivo* and *in vitro*. **(b)** *In vivo* OCT analysis in a porcine model shows scaffold bioresorption over time, from implant to 720 days. OCT = optical coherence tomography. (Reproduced with permission from Verheye S et al. *JACC Cardiovasc Interv.* 2014;7(1):89–99.)

The scaffold has some differentiating features as compared to BVSs. First, the scaffold can self-correct to the vessel wall especially in early malapposition to fill the empty spaces soon after implantation when expanded to the nominal diameter. In bench experiments, the self-correcting characteristic of the DESolve scaffold has been demonstrated by expanding a DESolve scaffold inside a rigid plastic block with a rod along the length. The rod was removed, creating an intentional 0.3-mm "gap" or malapposition. In the *in vitro* studies at 20 min, the strut malapposition was observed to resolved (Figure 4.1.15). Second, the scaffold has

a wide safety margin for expansion where a 3.0-mm scaffold can be expanded to 4.5 mm in diameter without strut fracture (Figure 4.1.16).

Clinical prospective nonrandomized studies carried out in multiple centers in patients with silent ischemia (*n* = 8), stable (*n* = 95) and unstable (*n* = 16) angina and asymptomatic postmyocardial infarction (*n* = 7) to determine the safety and efficacy of the DESolve novolimus eluting bioabsorbable scaffold with complex and noncomplex coronary lesions demonstrated a high device success rate at implantation. At 24 months there was a low thrombosis rate of 0.8%,

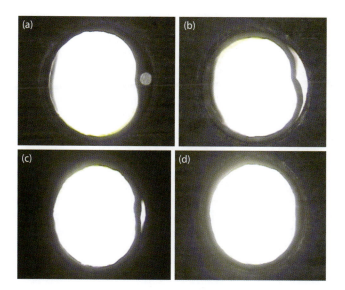

**Figure 4.1.15** Self-resolution of apposition. Intentionally created suboptimal strut apposition of a DESolve scaffold was made, and progression over time until the condition self-resolved is shown. **(a)** Expanding a DESolve scaffold inside a rigid plastic block with a rod along the length. **(b)** The rod was removed, creating an intentional 0.3-mm "gap" or malapposition. **(c, d)** After approximately 20 min, the strut malapposition was resolved. (Reproduced with permission from Verheye S et al. *JACC Cardiovasc Interv.* 2014;7(1):89–99.)

and major adverse event rate of 7.4% [26]. At 6 months, the angiographic late loss was 0.20 ± 0.32 mm. A preclinical study for the next generation scaffold named DESolve 100 with significantly reduced strut thickness (100 μm) is ongoing; however, special attention especially in the calcified lesions is required because radial strength is still one of the major concerns of BRSs [27].

## AMARANTH BIORESORBABLE SCAFFOLD (AMARANTH MEDICAL INC., CA)

The Amaranth Fortitude™ BRSs is made of PLLA, from a proprietary tube fabrication [28]. The company claims that the high molecular weight PLLA bioresorbable polymer carries a high amount of crystalline and amorphous domains and the combination delivers strength and resistance to fracture. The structural integrity of the Amaranth scaffold lasts 3–6 months, and the resorption process of scaffold requires roughly 1–2 years.

In preclinical animal studies assessed by OCT at 28, 90, and 180 days following the Amaranth Fortitude scaffold with 120 μm thickness implantation in porcine arteries, the scaffold showed a relatively smaller percentage area stenosis (Amaranth BRSs 21%, 31%, and 34% vs. ABSORB 31%, 37%, and 35%, respectively) and neointimal area (Amaranth BRSs 1.68 mm², 2.23 mm², and 2.08 mm² vs. ABSORB 2.57 mm², 2.64 mm², and 2.40 mm², respectively) compared with ABSORB BRSs. According to the histopathological analysis, which presented fibrin deposition and neointimal maturity grade, Amaranth Fortitude showed favorable trends with healing observed from 28 to 90 days.

MEND-II (South America) and RENASCENT-I (Italy), which assessed Amaranth's FORTITUDE sirolimus-eluting bioresorbable scaffold with 150 micron scaffold in patients with symptomatic coronary artery disease is expected to conclude enrolment by mid-2016. In addition, patient enrolment of RENASCENT- II, a study of a new 120-micron scaffold, has also started in several centers in Italy and Colombia to apply for a CE Mark after the conclusion of the 9-month patient follow-up.

## ART BIORESORBABLE SCAFFOLD (ARTERIAL REMODELING TECHNOLOGIES, NOISY LE ROI, FRANCE)

The arterial remodeling technologies (ART)-BRSs is made of PLA98, a stereocopolymer composed of 98% L-lactic acid and 2% D-lactic acid with strut thickness of 170 μm without a drug, and a design that is flexible resulting in a stent-to-luminal surface area ratio of <25% (Figure 4.1.17) [29]. The ART-BRSs with the distinguishing feature of early programmed dismantling, starting at 3 months after implantation, allows for rapid vascular restoration with progressive lumen enlargement [29,30]. A previous 6-month preclinical study, which compared ART-BRSs and BMS in porcine coronary arteries, provided insights into the performance of the ART-BRSs [31]. Acute recoil following implantation of ART-BRSs was minimal and similar to that of BMS (4.6 ± 6.7% vs. 4.6 ± 5.1%, *p* = 0.98) (Figure 4.1.18) [31]. QCA

3.0 mm DESolve™ scaffold expansion capability

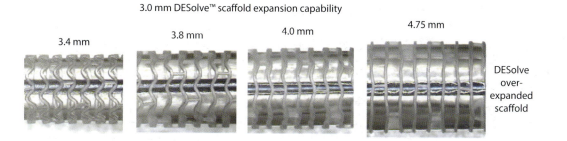

**Figure 4.1.16** Scaffold expansion properties. Bench testing demonstrated the expansion properties and fracture resistance of the DESolve scaffold. (Reproduced with permission from Verheye S et al. *JACC Cardiovasc Interv.* 2014;7(1):89–99.)

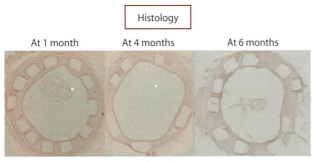

Figure 4.1.17 Hemalin eosin staining of stented iliac rabbit arteries at 1, 4, and 6 months with well-embedded stents showing a satisfactory healing process without neointimal hyperplasia, despite PLA resorption. (Reproduced with permission from Lafont A, *EuroIntervention* 2009;5 Suppl F:F83–87.)

analysis demonstrated that the minimal lumen diameter in ART-BRSs was significantly increased from 1 to 6 months ($p < 0.0001$), whereas BMS remained constant ($p = 0.159$)

(Figure 4.1.18). In this study, micro-CT was performed which showed that the dismantling of struts starts at 3 months (Figure 4.1.19). GPC analysis showed that Mw of ART-BRSs was 20% and 14% of their initial values at 3 and 6 months, respectively. Therefore, ART-BRSs showed a more rapid degradation relative to established results of approved devices during the first 6 months after implantation [29,32].

## THROMBOGENICITY AND EARLY VASCULAR HEALING RESPONSE IN BRSs COMPARED TO DESs

Delayed vascular healing following DESs implantation has been shown to be an important determinant of stent thrombosis in preclinical and autopsy studies [33,34] and is a key contributing mechanism of stent failure including restenosis [35]. Protection against acute thrombogenicity has been shown in select second generation permanent polymer DESs as compared to first generation DESs and BMSs in recent preclinical and clinical studies [36–38]. Overall it appears that thrombogenicity is associated with thickness of scaffold struts as well as polymer coating. The thickness of ABSORB BVSs is

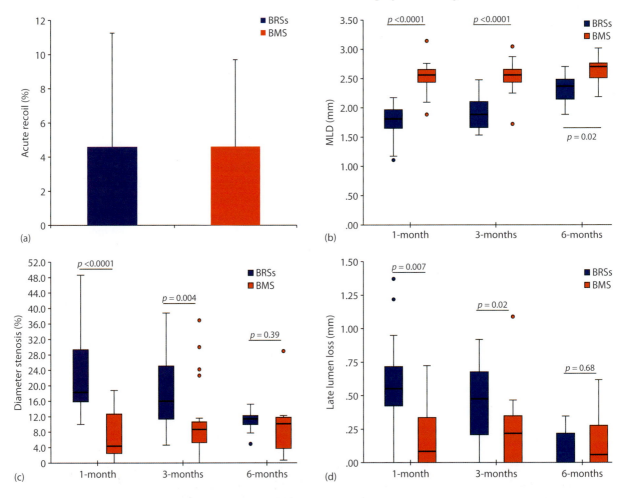

Figure 4.1.18 Quantitative coronary angiography analysis. **(a)** Bar graph analysis of acute recoil in bioresorbable scaffolds (BRSs; blue) and bare metal stent (BMS; red) stents. **(b–d)** Box plot analysis of minimal luminal diameter (MLD, **b**), diameter stenosis **(c)**, and late lumen loss **(d)** in BRSs (blue) and BMS (red) groups. (Reproduced with permission from Durand E et al., *Circ Cardiovasc Interv* 2014;7:70–79.)

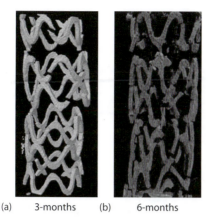

(a)  3-months    (b)  6-months

Figure 4.1.19 Microcomputed tomographic (μCT) analysis. Examples of μCT images of bioresorbable scaffolds (BRSs) at 3 (a) and 6 (b) months. BRSs dismantling was seen at 3 months with the presence of strut discontinuity at 3–6 months. (Reproduced with permission from Durand E et al., *Circ Cardiovasc Interv* 2014;7:70–79.)

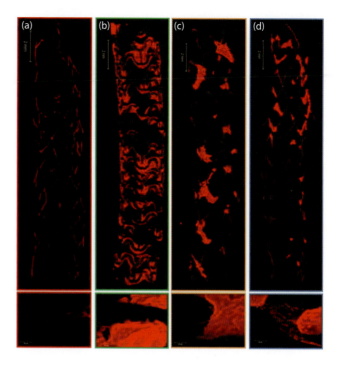

Figure 4.1.20 *Ex-vivo* arteriovenous porcine shunt model. Representative images derived from confocal microscopy after 1 hour in a swine *ex vivo* shunt model at low (10×) and high (20×) magnification. (a) Shows biodegradable polymer metallic everolimus eluting stent (EES) (n = 6). (b) Shows fully bioabsorbable everolimus eluting stent (bEES) (n = 6). (c) Shows biodegradable polymer metallic biolimus eluting stent (n = 6). (d) Shows bare metal stent (BMS) (n = 6). (Reproduced with permission from Koppara T et al., *Circ Cardiovasc Interv* 2015;8:e002427.)

157 μm, which is definitely thicker than contemporary DESs. We conducted a swine shunt model study to address these clinically relevant endpoints with thin strut biodegradable polymer metallic everolimus eluting stents (Synergy, Boston Scientific, Marlborough, MA; 74 μm strut thickness) against thick strut fully bioresorbable everolimus eluting scaffold (ABSORB BVSs; 150 μm strut thickness), thick strut biodegradable polymer metallic biolimus eluting stents (BioMatrix Flex, Biosensors, Newport Beach, CA; 120 μm strut thickness), and control bare metal stents (Omega, Boston Scientific, Marlborough, MA; 81 μm strut thickness) [39]. We also examined endothelial restoration and inflammatory reaction in the rabbit iliofemoral artery model using those four devices.

Platelet aggregation as detected by confocal microscopy (CD61 and CD42b) demonstrated a significantly lower mean percentage of fluorescent positive area in Synergy as compared to ABSORB BVSs, BioMatrix, and Omega (Figure 4.1.20) [39]. Linear mixed-effects model procedures demonstrated biologically relevant and statistically significant differences in percentage and absolute positive fluorescence area between Synergy versus ABSORB BVSs ($p < 0.001$), BioMatrix ($p = 0.002$), and Omega ($p = 0.014$), respectively. Percentage acute inflammatory cell adhesion on the stents based on fluorescent staining against monocyte marker CD14 and neutrophil marker PM1 showed significantly less positive cell counts in Synergy compared to ABSORB BVSs.

We also reported that the endothelial coverage above struts by SEM was numerically greater in Synergy compared to ABSORB BVSs at 14 days ($p = 0.15$); however, it was lower when compared to control Omega ($p = 0.27$). The percentage of endothelial coverage by confocal microscopy evaluating CD31/PECAM-1 staining was also numerically higher in Synergy when compared to ABSORB BVSs ($p = 0.55$) and lower when compared to Omega ($p = 0.15$) at 14 days. No differences were observed between Synergy and BioMatrix [39].

At 28 days, SEM revealed significantly greater endothelial coverage above struts in Synergy as compared to ABSORB BVSs ($p = 0.05$). No differences were observed between Synergy and BioMatrix. For control Omega, endothelial coverage was near complete above struts. Confocal microscopy performed following CD31/PECAM-1 staining showed endothelial coverage above struts was numerically greater in Synergy as compared to ABSORB BVSs ($p = 0.20$). However, no significant differences were observed among the four devices.

Adhesion of RAM-11 positive macrophages was predominantly visualized in the surrounding of stent struts, where coverage with CD31/PECAM-1 positive endothelial cells was absent. Overall RAM-11 positive macrophage adhesion was lower in Synergy at 14 and 28 days compared to ABSORB BVSs (14 days, $p = 0.05$; 28 days, $p = 0.11$) without significant differences to BioMatrix or Omega.

## EARLY AND LATE/VERY LATE SCAFFOLD THROMBOSIS FOLLOWING BRSs IMPLANTATION

Recently, a large randomized noninferiority clinical trial showed the safety and efficacy in ABSORB BVSs as compared

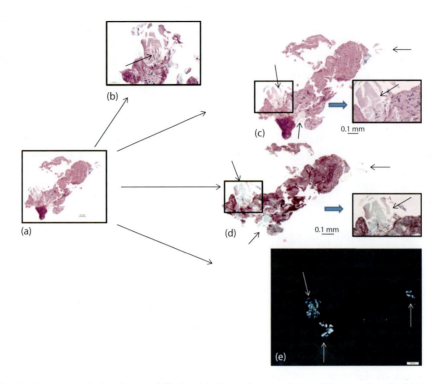

**Figure 4.1.21** Histological images of platelet- and fibrin-rich thrombus aspirate. When stained with hematoxylin and eosin, fibrin stains pink and platelets stain grayish at 10× and 20× magnification (**a** and **c**). Glycoproteins and proteoglycans within foreign material appear purple magenta with periodic acid–Schiff stain at 20× magnification (**b**). Foreign material stains green when assessed in Movat pentachrome staining (**d**). Polarized light shows birefringence within foreign material at 10× magnification (**e**). Arrows point to foreign material within aspirated thrombus. (Reproduced with permission from Räber L, *J Am Coll Cardiol* 2015;66:1901–14.)

to XIENCE in patients with stable coronary artery disease at 1 year [10]. On the other hand, more recently, meta-analysis of six clinical trials including ABSORB II, ABSORB III, ABSORB Japan, ABSORB China, EVERBIO II, and TROFI II showed higher risk of definite or probable stent thrombosis in ABSORB BVSs compared to everolimus-eluting metallic stent (OR 1.99 [95% CI 1.00 to 3.98, $p = 0.05$]), with the highest risk between 1 and 30 days following implantation of ABSORB BVSs (OR 3.11 [95% CI 1.24 to 7.82], $p = 0.02$) [40]. As previously described, our swine shunt model study demonstrated higher thrombogenicity in ABSORB BVSs than thin-strut DESs (Synergy) [39], which also suggests that thick struts lead to higher incidence of stent thrombosis, especially in the early time-point before the strut coverage with endothelial cells.

Räber et al. reported four cases with very late scaffold thrombosis following ABSORB BVSs implantation [41]. OCT was performed following aspiration of thrombus and showed malapposed struts with and without scaffold thrombus in all four cases, occurring at 44, 19, 22, and 19 months after scaffold implantation and one case also showed scaffold strut discontinuity with malapposition (44 months). Two of the four cases (44 and 19 months) showed the presence of neoatherosclerosis consisting of macrophage accumulation by OCT. All four patients were on aspirin therapy and two were also receiving prasugrel [41]. Basically, thrombus aspirates showed a platelet and/or fibrin-rich thrombus and mononuclear cell infiltration.

In the one case, foreign materials were observed within the thrombus, which were identified as positive birefringence by polarized light. Interestingly, spectroscopic thrombus aspirate analysis showed foreign materials consistent with persistent remnants of ABSORB BVSs (Figure 4.1.21) [41]. Therefore, the discontinuity resulting from the intended degradation of scaffold might lead to scaffold thrombosis; however, more studies are needed to understand the mechanisms and the relationship between the discontinuity and scaffold thrombosis.

## CONCLUSIONS

The preclinical studies with ABSORB BVSs made of PLLA demonstrated comparable safety and efficacy compared to XIENCE in the normal porcine coronary arteries up to 48 months. Furthermore, ART-BRSs device made of PDLLA also showed favorable results up to 36 months. Lumen enlargement is a unique feature of BRSs including both PLLA and PDLLA, which was associated with inflammatory reactions during degradation. BRSs made of PDLLA showed faster degradation (within 3 years) than that observed for BVSs PLLA (3–4 years). However, currently, the only bioabsorbable scaffold with long-term clinical data in nearly 4000 patients is BVSs which has shown comparable results to XIENCE for target vessel revascularization in randomized trial although early stent thrombosis was higher. Our preclinical studies suggest greater likelihood of thrombosis and delayed endothelialization as compared to contemporary metallic second generation DESs. Nevertheless, this technology may hold great promise as the vessel returns to its native state with vasomotion and perhaps less neoatherosclerotic change.

# REFERENCES

1. Nakazawa G, Finn AV, Vorpahl M, Ladich ER, Kolodgie FD, Virmani R. Coronary responses and differential mechanisms of late stent thrombosis attributed to first-generation sirolimus- and paclitaxel-eluting stents. *J Am Coll Cardiol.* 2011;57:390–8.

2. Nakazawa G, Otsuka F, Nakano M et al. The pathology of neoatherosclerosis in human coronary implants: Bare-metal and drug-eluting stents. *J Am Coll Cardiol.* 2011;57:1314–22.

3. Serruys PW, Garcia-Garcia HM, Onuma Y. From metallic cages to transient bioresorbable scaffolds: Change in paradigm of coronary revascularization in the upcoming decade? *Eur Heart J.* 2012;33:16–25b.

4. Tamai H, Igaki K, Kyo E et al. Initial and 6-month results of biodegradable poly-l-lactic acid coronary stents in humans. *Circulation.* 2000;102:399–404.

5. Ormiston JA, Serruys PW, Regar E et al. A bioABSORBable everolimus-eluting coronary stent system for patients with single de-novo coronary artery lesions (ABSORB): A prospective open-label trial. *Lancet.* 2008;371:899–907.

6. Nishio S, Kosuga K, Igaki K et al. Long-term (>10 years) clinical outcomes of first-in-human biodegradable poly-l-lactic acid coronary stents: Igaki-Tamai stents. *Circulation.* 2012;125:2343–53.

7. Gogas BD, Farooq V, Onuma Y, Serruys PW. The ABSORB bioresorbable vascular scaffold: An evolution or revolution in interventional cardiology? *Hellenic J Cardiol.* 2012;53:301–9.

8. Verheye S, Ormiston JA, Stewart J et al. A next-generation bioresorbable coronary scaffold system: From bench to first clinical evaluation: 6- and 12-month clinical and multimodality imaging results. *JACC Cardiovasc Interv.* 2014;7:89–99.

9. de Ribamar Costa JVS, Webster M, Stewart J, Abizaid A, Costa R, Staico R, Chamie DBV et al. Six-month intravascular ultrasound analysis of the DESOLVE FIM trial with a novel PLLA–based fully biodegradable drug-eluting scaffold. *J Am Coll Cardiol.* 2013;61:E1646.

10. Ellis SG, Kereiakes DJ, Metzger DC et al. Everolimus-eluting bioresorbable scaffolds for coronary artery disease. *New Eng J Med.* 2015;373:1905–15.

11. Byrne RA, Serruys PW, Baumbach A et al. Report of a European Society of Cardiology-European Association of Percutaneous Cardiovascular Interventions task force on the evaluation of coronary stents in Europe: Executive summary. *Eur Heart J.* 2015;36:2608–20.

12. Schwartz RS, Edelman ER, Carter A et al. Drug-eluting stents in preclinical studies: Recommended evaluation from a consensus group. *Circulation.* 2002;106:1867–73.

13. Onuma Y, Serruys PW, Perkins LE et al. Intracoronary optical coherence tomography and histology at 1 month and 2, 3, and 4 years after implantation of everolimus-eluting bioresorbable vascular scaffolds in a porcine coronary artery model: An attempt to decipher the human optical coherence tomography images in the ABSORB trial. *Circulation.* 2010;122:2288–300.

14. Nissen SE, Gurley JC, Grines CL et al. Intravascular ultrasound assessment of lumen size and wall morphology in normal subjects and patients with coronary artery disease. *Circulation.* 1991;84:1087–99.

15. Mintz GS, Kent KM, Pichard AD, Satler LF, Popma JJ, Leon MB. Contribution of inadequate arterial remodeling to the development of focal coronary artery stenoses. An intravascular ultrasound study. *Circulation.* 1997;95:1791–8.

16. Campos CM, Ishibashi Y, Eggermont J et al. Echogenicity as a surrogate for bioresorbable everolimus-eluting scaffold degradation: Analysis at 1-, 3-, 6-, 12- 18, 24-, 30-, 36- and 42-month follow-up in a porcine model. *Int J Cardiovasc Imaging.* 2015;31:471–82.

17. Nakatani S, Ishibashi Y, Sotomi Y et al. Bioresorption and Vessel Wall Integration of a Fully Bioresorbable Polymeric Everolimus-Eluting Scaffold: Optical Coherence Tomography, Intravascular Ultrasound, and Histological Study in a Porcine Model With 4-Year Follow-Up. *JACC Cardiovasc Interv.* 2016;9:838–51.

18. Serruys PW, Ormiston JA, Onuma Y et al. A bioABSORBable everolimus-eluting coronary stent system (ABSORB): 2-year outcomes and results from multiple imaging methods. *Lancet.* 2009;373:897–910.

19. Otsuka F, Pacheco E, Perkins LE et al. Long-term safety of an everolimus-eluting bioresorbable vascular scaffold and the cobalt-chromium XIENCE V stent in a porcine coronary artery model. *Circ Cardiovasc Interv.* 2014;7:330–42.

20. Lane JP, Perkins LE, Sheehy AJ et al. Lumen gain and restoration of pulsatility after implantation of a bioresorbable vascular scaffold in porcine coronary arteries. *JACC Cardiovasc Interv.* 2014;7:688–95.

21. Onuma Y, Serruys PW, Muramatsu T et al. Incidence and imaging outcomes of acute scaffold disruption and late structural discontinuity after implantation of the ABSORB Everolimus-Eluting fully bioresorbable vascular scaffold: Optical coherence tomography assessment in the ABSORB cohort B Trial (A Clinical Evaluation of the Bioabsorbable Everolimus Eluting Coronary Stent System in the Treatment of Patients With De Novo Native Coronary Artery Lesions). *JACC Cardiovasc Interv.* 2014;7:1400–11.

22. Kovarik JM, Kaplan B, Tedesco Silva H et al. Exposure-response relationships for everolimus in de novo kidney transplantation: Defining a therapeutic range. *Transplantation.* 2002;73:920–5.

23. Gori T, Schulz E, Hink U et al. Clinical, angiographic, functional, and imaging outcomes 12 months after implantation of drug-eluting bioresorbable vascular scaffolds in acute coronary syndromes. *JACC Cardiovasc Interv.* 2015;8:770–7.

24. Brugaletta S, Heo JH, Garcia-Garcia HM et al. Endothelial-dependent vasomotion in a coronary segment treated by ABSORB everolimus-eluting bioresorbable vascular scaffold system is related to plaque composition at the time of bioresorption of the polymer: Indirect finding of vascular reparative therapy? *Eur Heart J.* 2012;33:1325–33.

25. Gogas BD, Benham JJ, Hsu S et al. Vasomotor function comparative assessment at 1 and 2 years following implantation of the Absorb everolimus-eluting bioresorbable vascular scaffold and the Xience V everolimus-eluting metallic stent in porcine coronary arteries: Insights from in vivo angiography, ex vivo assessment, and gene analysis at the stented/scaffolded segments and the proximal and distal edges. *JACC Cardiovasc Interv.* 2016;9:728–41.

26. Abizaid A, Costa RA, Schofer J et al. Serial multimodality imaging and 2-year clinical outcomes of the novel desolve novolimus-eluting bioresorbable coronary scaffold system for the treatment of single de novo coronary lesions. *JACC Cardiovasc Interv.* 2016;9:565–74.

27. D'Ascenzo F, Frangieh AH, Templin C. Radial strength and expansion of scaffold struts remain a concern when considering a PCI with bioresorbable vascular scaffold. *Int J Cardiol.* 2015;191:254–5.

28. Zhang Y, Bourantas CV, Farooq V et al. Bioresorbable scaffolds in the treatment of coronary artery disease. *Med Devices.* (Auckland, NZ) 2013;6:37–48.

29. Lafont A, Durand E. A.R.T.: Concept of a bioresorbable stent without drug elution. *EuroIntervention. Journal of EuroPCR in Collaboration with the Working Group on Interventional Cardiology of the European Society of Cardiology* 2009;5 Suppl F:F83–7.

30. Onuma Y, Serruys PW. Bioresorbable scaffold: The advent of a new era in percutaneous coronary and peripheral revascularization? *Circulation.* 2011;123:779–97.

31. Durand E, Sharkawi T, Leclerc G et al. Head-to-head comparison of a drug-free early programmed dismantling polylactic acid bioresorbable scaffold and a metallic stent in the porcine coronary artery: Six-month angiography and optical coherence tomographic follow-up study. *Circ Cardiovasc Interv.* 2014;7:70–9.

32. Schwach G, Vert M. In vitro and in vivo degradation of lactic acid-based interference screws used in cruciate ligament reconstruction. *Int J Biol Macromol.* 1999;25:283–91.

33. Joner M, Finn AV, Farb A et al. Pathology of drug-eluting stents in humans: Delayed healing and late thrombotic risk. *J Am Coll Cardiol.* 2006;48:193–202.

34. Finn AV, Joner M, Nakazawa G et al. Pathological correlates of late drug-eluting stent thrombosis: Strut coverage as a marker of endothelialization. *Circulation.* 2007;115:2435–41.

35. Byrne RA, Joner M, Tada T, Kastrati A. Restenosis in bare metal and drug-eluting stents: Distinct mechanistic insights from histopathology and optical intravascular imaging. *Minerva Cardioangiol.* 2012;60:473–89.

36. Palmerini T, Biondi-Zoccai G, Della Riva D et al. Stent thrombosis with drug-eluting and bare-metal stents: Evidence from a comprehensive network meta-analysis. *Lancet.* 2012;379:1393–402.

37. Sabate M, Cequier A, Iniguez A et al. Everolimus-eluting stent versus bare-metal stent in ST-segment elevation myocardial infarction (EXAMINATION): 1 year results of a randomised controlled trial. *Lancet.* 2012;380:1482–90.

38. Kolandaivelu K, Swaminathan R, Gibson WJ et al. Stent thrombogenicity early in high-risk interventional settings is driven by stent design and deployment and protected by polymer-drug coatings. *Circulation.* 2011;123:1400–9.

39. Koppara T, Cheng Q, Yahagi K et al. Thrombogenicity and early vascular healing response in metallic biodegradable polymer-based and fully bioabsorbable drug-eluting stents. *Circ Cardiovasc Interv.* 2015;8:e002427.

40. Cassese S, Byrne RA, Ndrepepa G et al. Everolimus-eluting bioresorbable vascular scaffolds versus everolimus-eluting metallic stents: A meta-analysis of randomised controlled trials. *Lancet.* 2016;387:537–44.

41. Raber L, Brugaletta S, Yamaji K et al. Very late scaffold thrombosis: Intracoronary imaging and histopathological and spectroscopic findings. *J Am Coll Cardiol.* 2015;66:1901–14.

# Iron

RUNLIN GAO, DEYUAN ZHANG, HONG QIU, CHAO WU, YING XIA, AND GUI ZHANG

The excellent mechanical properties, wide body distribution, and important physiological functions of the biocorrodible metal iron [1] render it a promising candidate as a building block for a biocorrodible metal scaffold. To this end, pure iron scaffolds appear safe and demonstrate outstanding biocompatibility in rabbit and porcine abdominal aortas and porcine coronary arteries [2–4], and Fe(II) and Fe(III) inhibit vascular smooth muscle cell proliferation *in vitro* by reducing proliferation-related gene expression [5–7]. However, studies on a biodegradable iron scaffold have been scarce, and an iron scaffold is currently not commercially available.

We summarize here the results of preclinical studies on safety, efficacy, and biocompatibility of the iron-based bioresorbable coronary scaffold (IBS™) which was independently developed by Lifetech Scientific (Shenzhen) Co., Ltd., China, using the vacuum plasma nitriding technology; the scaffold features thin struts, high radial force, high resistance to fracture, and accelerated corrosion.

## METHODOLOGY

The animal studies described herein involved a bare (i.e., without drug or polymer) nitrided iron-based scaffold with strut thickness of 70 microns, and the widely used overexpansion model of porcine coronary artery; the Vision™ cobalt-chromium stent (Abbott Vascular, Santa Clara, CA) was selected as a control. All scaffolds/stents were implanted with a scaffold/stent-to-artery (diameter) ratio of 1.1–1.2:1 in the left anterior descending (LAD) and right coronary artery (RCA) of healthy mini-swine. The left circumflex artery (LCX) was used if the LAD or RCA was not suitable for scaffold/stent implantation.

Follow-up observations were conducted at 1, 3, 6, and 12 months after scaffold/stent implantation, and histopathological changes also were evaluated at 9, 18, and 33 months. At each follow-up time point, quantitative coronary angiography (QCA) and optical coherence tomography (OCT) were performed. Animals were then sacrificed by rapid intravenous injection of 0.1 g/kg potassium chloride or by cutting the ascending aorta to remove the blood under deep anesthesia. The heart was harvested and placed into precooled normal saline solution with 25,000 IU heparin and 60 mg papaverine per 1000 mL. A 6Fr dilator was inserted from the ascending aorta into the ostium of the left and right coronary artery, respectively. After enhanced perfusion under 100 mmHg pressure for 5 minutes with the aforementioned solution, the target vessels were carefully dissected from the epicardial surface of the heart (retaining the 5 mm distal and proximal segments to the stented segment) and flushed once with special stationary liquid or 4% paraformaldehyde solution. The vessels then were divided into 3–4 segments and prepared for plastic and paraffin-embedded sections and sectioning for evaluation by scanning or transmission electron microscopy (SEM or TEM). The plastic-embedded sections samples with the scaffold/stent struts in situ were prepared for histomorphometric measurement [8]. The embedded vascular tissue was treated as described by Rippstein et al. [9]. The Buehler IsoMet 5000 high-speed precision saw (Buehler, Dusseldorf, Germany) was used to slice the tissue into 150 μm sections. These slices were then ground into 10–20 μm sections using a variety of silicon carbide sandpapers from coarse to fine. Harris hematoxylin-eosin (HE) and Weigert resorcin fuchsin (ET+VG) staining were used. After quickly dissolving or carefully removing the scaffold/stent struts, paraffin-embedded sections were prepared for histopathological and immunohistochemical analyses [2] using HE, ET+VG, or immunohistochemical staining. Conventional SEM sampling with the scaffold/stent struts *in situ* was made for SEM observation. TEM sampling in which scaffold/stent struts were carefully removed under microscopy was conducted according to conventional methods.

Both aforementioned conventional methods for preparing sections have limitations. Mechanical scaffold/stent strut removal during conventional paraffin-embedded section preparation may result in damage to the vessel wall, while the scaffold promptly suffers corrosion *in vitro* on contact with water during conventional plastic-embedded section preparation. Furthermore, when an iron-based biocorrodible scaffold is studied, the yellow corrosion products will permeate and deposit into adjacent tissue, which may significantly affect section staining and sample quality for examination. We explored two methods of preparing tissue sections containing iron-based scaffold for histomorphologic and histopathological analysis. The first method involves quickly dissolving the iron-based scaffold in the tissue using a mixture of ethanol, formaldehyde, glacial acetic acid, and nitric acid prior to paraffin-embedded section preparation. The latter process does not damage the vessel wall or neointima and does not impact tissue antigenic properties, allowing subsequent successful conventional paraffin-section and immunohistochemical analysis. Using a chemical solvent to dissolve the iron-based scaffold in the vascular tissue can preserve tissue structure and staining capacity; the staining methods and histomorphologic findings for the sections prepared using this new technique are the same as those used for conventional paraffin sections. The second method involves an improved plastic-embedded section preparation method using an ethanol, formaldehyde, and vitamin C combination stationary liquid that reduces contact time between iron scaffold and water in the stationary liquid, thus minimizing the chance of scaffold corrosion *in vitro*.

## VASCULAR HISTOMORPHOMETRY AND HISTOLOGY

One month after implantation, histomorphometric measurements, namely mean neointimal thickness (0.46 ± 0.17 mm vs. 0.45 ± 0.18 mm, $p = 0.878$), neointimal area (2.55 ± 0.91 mm² vs. 3.04 ± 1.15 mm², $p = 0.360$), and area stenosis percentage (44.50 ± 11.40% vs. 46.00 ± 17.95%, $p = 0.845$), were not significantly different between the iron based scaffold and the VISION stent control groups (Figure 4.2.1) [10]. Neointimal coverage percentage by SEM examination was numerically higher in iron-based scaffolds than in VISION stents (84.38 ± 14.50% vs. 65.00 ± 22.04%, $p = 0.057$), however the difference did not achieve statistical significance (Figure 4.2.2) [10].

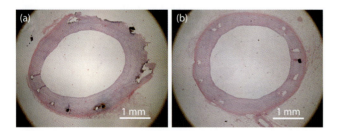

Figure 4.2.1 Light microscopic findings of stented segments of coronary arteries in the two groups at 28 days (conventional plastic-embedded sections, HE, 40×). **(a)** Iron scaffold: mild intimal hyperplasia is apparent, and a brownish tinge in the vascular wall adjacent to the iron scaffold struts is detected. **(b)** VISION stent: only mild intimal hyperplasia is seen. (Reproduced with permission from authors including Runlin Gao, Deyuan Zhang, Hong Qiu, Chao Wu, Ying Xia, and Gui Zhang.)

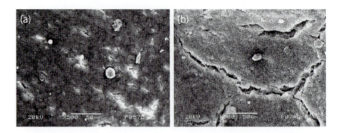

Figure 4.2.2 SEM view of coronary artery re-endothelialization at 28 days (500×). **(a)** Iron scaffold: complete endothelial coverage is apparent. **(b)** VISION stent: a few intimal peels and incomplete endothelial coverage are apparent. (Reproduced with permission from authors including Runlin Gao, Deyuan Zhang, Hong Qiu, Chao Wu, Ying Xia, and Gui Zhang.)

At 3, 6, and 12 months, neointimal hyperplasia and all measured parameters did not differ significantly between iron-based scaffold and Vision control groups (Figure 4.2.3), with neointimal proliferation reaching its highest volume at 6 months in both groups. The restenosis rate at 6 months was comparable between the two groups (37% vs. 33%). No thrombosis was observed in either group.

## INFLAMMATION SCORE

Inflammatory reaction is one of the main causes of intimal hyperplasia. Inflammation score [8] for each individual strut was graded as 0–3: 0, no inflammatory cells surrounding the strut; 1, light, noncircumferential lymphohistiocytic infiltrate surrounding the strut; 2, localized, moderate to dense cellular aggregate surrounding the strut noncircumferentially; and 3, circumferential dense lymphohistiocytic cell infiltration of the strut. The average inflammation score for each cross-section was calculated by dividing the sum of inflammation scores by the total number of struts at the examined section [9]. The inflammatory reaction in the vessel wall of the stented segment was mild in both groups. The average inflammation score was approximately 1 at each time point with only a few infiltrating inflammatory cells surrounding the scaffold/stent struts; no thrombosis or tissue necrosis was observed. At each time point, inflammation scores did not differ statistically between groups. Although inflammation scores demonstrated no temporal variation within groups, inflammatory reaction tended to decrease over time.

## IMMUNOHISTOCHEMICAL STUDIES

### Endothelial cell functional examination

The recovery of endothelial cell function can be measured by immunohistochemical staining for eNOS protein expression. At 1 month after implantation, immunoreactivity for eNOS protein in endothelial cells was weak (+), even when the neointima was completely formed. Only a

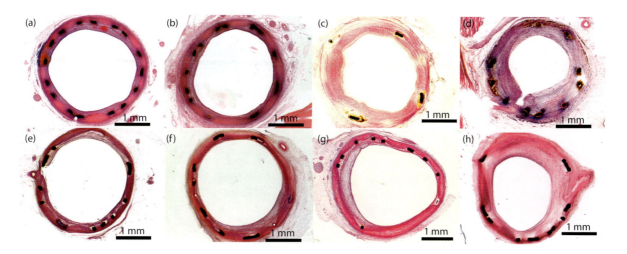

**Figure 4.2.3** Histomorphometric temporal variation after scaffold/stent implantation (modified plastic-embedded sections, H&E, 25×). **(a)–(d)** 1, 3, 6, and 12 months, respectively, after iron-based scaffold implantation; **(e)–(h)** 1, 3, 6, and 12 months, respectively, after Vision stent implantation. (Reproduced with permission from authors including Runlin Gao, Deyuan Zhang, Hong Qiu, Chao Wu, Ying Xia, and Gui Zhang.)

few endothelial cells demonstrated light immunoreactivity. Immunoreactivity for eNOS protein markedly increased over time. After 3 months, eNOS immunoreactivity reached "+++," forming a clear brown line pattern on the vessel wall indicating functional recovery of the endothelial cells covering the neointima.

## Proliferating cell nuclear antigen (PCNA) analysis

PCNA plays an important role in promoting cell division and proliferation, and its expression level is directly proportional to cell proliferation activity. At each time point, PCNA expression positivity did not differ significantly between the iron scaffold and control groups, indicating similar cell proliferative activity between the two groups.

## HISTOPATHOLOGICAL TEMPORAL VARIATION AFTER IRON-BASED SCAFFOLD IMPLANTATION

At 1 month after iron-based scaffold implantation, the neointima was thin with mild proliferation (Figure 4.2.4a), and mostly contained disorganized and loosely aligned smooth muscle cells and fibroblasts and abundant extracellular matrix (Figure 4.2.4b). The media, composed of compact circularly arranged smooth muscle cells, demonstrated obvious compression without atrophy around scaffold struts. Stent endothelialization was complete, with neointima clearly apparent on surface areas with and without scaffold struts. There was no obvious inflammatory cell or macrophage infiltration around scaffold struts, in-stent thrombosis, or tissue necrosis.

At 3 months after implantation, neointimal proliferation was active with mostly mucus and collagens, cell alignment

remained disorganized, and there was no obvious inflammatory reaction. Although a few macrophages containing corroded iron particles were observed surrounding the scaffold struts, no foreign-body giant cells were found (Figure 4.2.4c,d).

At 6 months postprocedure, the neointima was thick, and smooth muscle cells were aligned, with more cells than at 3 months. The neointimal tissue was compact. Significant strut corrosion and macrophages were observed, however, no foreign-body giant cells were apparent. Iron staining was positive in the tissue surrounding iron scaffold struts. A slight inflammatory reaction was apparent in the media around struts. In neointimal areas surrounding struts, missing smooth muscle was apparent as cavities harboring small erythrocyte-containing vessels (Figure 4.2.4e) and displaying intensive collagen and peak inflammatory reactions. Numerous macrophages containing corrosion products surrounded some significantly corroded struts. The media was intact without obvious injury. In the intima surrounding scaffold struts, a few lymphocytes could be found close to the media.

At 9 months postprocedure, the scaffolds were obviously corroded and formed a band of iron staining positive substances (blue) (Figure 4.2.4f). The media showed obvious atrophy, the intima moderately proliferated, and the internal and external elastic laminae were intact (Figure 4.2.4g).

By 12 months postprocedure, the inflammatory and collagen reactions had stabilized. Many macrophages containing corrosion products were present around scaffold struts. The number of cavities caused by scaffold corrosion had not increased, and some had started to show signs of repair with intercellular substance filling. New small vessel formation had ceased in the arterial wall. In some samples, macrophages containing corrosion products were found far from the adventitia, aligning regularly among muscle fibers

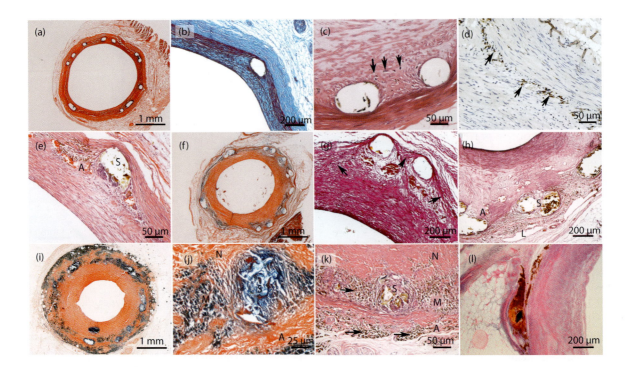

**Figure 4.2.4** Histopathological temporal variation after iron-based scaffold implantation. **(a)** By Perls iron staining at 1 month after scaffold implantation, no corrosion of the iron-based scaffold is detected; the intima is slightly proliferated and the lumen is patent. **(b)** In Masson staining at 1 month after scaffold implantation, neointima appears thin and immature, with sparse cells and abundant extracellular matrix. **(c)** In HE staining at 3 months after scaffold implantation, a few macrophages containing corroded iron particles are observed in the intima near the scaffold struts (shown by arrow). No acute inflammatory cells (granulocytic neutrophils), chronic inflammatory cells (lymphocytes), or allergic inflammatory cells (eosinophilic granulocytes) are observed. **(d)** In immunohistochemical staining at 3 months, the macrophages containing corroded iron particles are labelled with CD68 antibody. The arrow points to macrophages that are apparent as brown particles. **(e)** In HE staining at 6 months after scaffold implantation, neoangiogenesis and macrophages containing corroded iron particles (see the arrow) are found in the intima. A = new vessel; S = scaffold. **(f)** In Perls iron staining at 9 months after scaffold implantation, the scaffold appears obviously corroded forming a band of iron staining positive substances (blue). There is obvious media atrophy, and the intima shows moderate proliferation without restenosis. **(g)** In elastic tissue + Van Gieson staining at 9 months after scaffold implantation, the media has obvious atrophy, while the internal elastic lamina (shown by the arrow) and external elastic lamina are intact. **(h)** In HE staining at 12 months after scaffold implantation, the macrophages containing corroded iron particles accumulate in the media and adventitia of the vessel wall surrounding the stent struts. The neointima is relatively mature, containing many smooth muscle cells in dense array (on the luminal side). Scant extracellular matrix is observed. L = lymphatic in adventitia; A = new vessel in intima; S = scaffold. **(i)** In Perls iron staining at 33 months after scaffold implantation, the scaffold is obviously corroded and forms a band of iron staining positive substances (blue). Some scaffold struts are completely corroded. **(j)** In Perls iron staining at 33 months after scaffold implantation, struts are broken and irregularly shaped (S), and massive iron staining positive substances are observed at the site of struts or outside the surrounding tissues. N = neointima; M = media; A = adventitia. **(k)** In HE staining at 33 months after scaffold implantation, the strut is completely corroded (S) and replaced by histiocytes and fibroblasts. There is substantial accumulation of macrophages containing corroded iron particles in the surrounding tissues. N = neointima; M = media; A = adventitia. **(l)** In HE staining of plastic-embedded sections at 33 months after scaffold implantation, struts are almost totally corroded. There is extensive accumulation of macrophages containing corroded iron particles in the adventitia. (Reproduced with permission from authors including Runlin Gao, Deyuan Zhang, Hong Qiu, Chao Wu, Ying Xia, and Gui Zhang.)

without an apparent adverse effect on smooth muscle cells (Figure 4.2.4h).

At 18 months postprocedure, scaffold strut corrosion was obvious. More corrosion products had been engulfed by macrophages and transferred to the adventitia. The media was markedly atrophied. The smooth muscle cells in the neointima were aligned in a loose, circular arrangement.

At 33 months after implantation, some scaffold struts were broken or had become smaller and irregular (Figure 4.2.4i,j), and some had completely corroded and had been replaced by histiocytes and fibroblasts (Figure 4.2.4k,l). Corrosion products arising from the iron-based scaffold were extensive and continually transferred to the adventitia by macrophages (Figure 4.2.4l). Iron staining revealed a high iron level in the vessel wall. No lymphocytes were present in the neointima at this time point.

## TRANSMISSION ELECTRON MICROSCOPE ANALYSIS AT 12 MONTHS

The ultrastructure of the cells was normal, and no necrocytosis appeared. A complete layer of endothelial cells was apparent by TEM. In the neointimal layer, some corrosion particles had been engulfed by macrophages, and some were extracellular. The cells containing particles had normal membranes and abundant intranuclear euchromatin without intranuclear particles, broken nuclei, or nucleolysis. Extracellular matrix and collagenous fibers were abundant.

## CONCLUSION

The preliminary preclinical studies summarized in this chapter indicate biocompatibility, safety, and efficacy of an iron-based scaffold. Neointima proliferation and tissue reactions were similar after iron-based scaffold or Vision stent implantation. Re-endothelialization was complete at 1 month after scaffold implantation, without significant inflammation or thrombosis. Corrosion of iron-based scaffold struts was first apparent after 3 months, obvious after 12 months, and complete, i.e., replaced by histiocytes and fibroblasts with corroded particles relocated to the vessel wall adventitia by macrophages, by 33 months. No obvious inflammation was observed around macrophages that had phagocytized corroded products.

## REFERENCES

1. Hermosilla D, Cortijo M, Huang CP. The role of iron on the degradation and mineralization of organic compounds using conventional Fenton and photo-Fenton processes. *Chem Eng J.* 2009; 155:637–646.

2. Peuster M, Wohlsein P, Brugmann M, Ehlerding M, Seidler K, Fink C, Brauer H et al. A novel approach to temporary stenting: Degradable cardiovascular stents produced from corrodible metal—Results 6-18 months after implantation into New Zealand white rabbits. *Heart.* 2001;86:563–569.

3. Peuster M, Hesse C, Schloo T, Fink C, Beerbaum P, von Schnakenburg C. Long-term biocompatibility of a corrodible peripheral iron stent in the porcine descending aorta. *Biomaterials.* 2006;27: 4955–4962.

4. Waksman R, Pakala R, Baffour R, Seabron R, Hellinga D, Tio FO. Short-term effects of biocorrodible iron stents in porcine coronary arteries. *J Interv Cardiol.* 2008;21:15–20.

5. Mueller PP, May T, Perz A, Hauser H, Peuster M. Control of smooth muscle cell proliferation by ferrous iron. *Biomaterials.* 2006; 27:2193–2200.

6. Drynda A, Hoehn R, Peuster M. Influence of Fe(II) and Fe(III) on the expression of genes related to cholesterol- and fatty acid metabolism in human vascular smooth muscle cells. *J Mater Sci Mater Med.* 2010;21:1655–1663.

7. Wu C, Qiu H, Xu LJ, Ye J, Yang ZH, Qian X, Meng XM et al. Inhibitory effect of iron on in vitro proliferation of smooth muscle cells. *Chin Med J (Engl).* 2013;126:3728–3731.

8. Kornowski R, Hong MK, Tio FO, Bramwell O, Wu H, Leon MB. In-stent restenosis: Contributions of inflammatory responses and arterial injury to neointimal hyperplasia. *J Am Coll Cardiol.* 1998;31:224–230.

9. Rippstein P Black MK, Boivin M, Veinot JP, Ma X, Chen YX, Human P et al. Comparison of processing and sectioning methodologies for arteries containing metallic stents. *J Histochem Cytochem.* 2006;54:673–681.

10. Wu C, Qiu H, Hu XY, Ruan YM, Tian Y, Chu Y, Xu XL et al. Short-term safety and efficacy of the biodegradable iron stent in mini swine coronary arteries. *Chin Med J (Engl).* 2013;126:4752–4757.

# PART 5

# Imaging to evaluate the bioresorbable scaffold: A core lab perspective: Methodology of measurement and assessment

# Quantitative coronary angiography of bioresorbable vascular scaffold: A core lab perspective

YOHEI SOTOMI, PATRICK W.J.C. SERRUYS, AND YOSHINOBU ONUMA

## INTRODUCTION

Invasive quantitative coronary angiography (QCA) is one of the most commonly used methods for the assessment of coronary vessels with bioresorbable scaffolds (BRSs) or metallic stents. The same QCA parameters can be used for the assessment of the performance of BRSs as used in the metallic stents. Nonetheless, in contrast to metallic stents, some of the polymeric scaffolds are partially translucent and radiolucent to gamma radiation with the exception of the radiopaque platinum markers at the edges, which could affect the QCA measurements. In addition, BRSs have their unique property as compared to metallic stents, which could make the interpretation of the conventional parameters complicated. In this chapter, we present the summary of QCA parameters for the assessment of the performance of BRSs and differential impact of BRSs and metallic stents on QCA measurements.

## BIORESORBABLE SCAFFOLD

As the stent itself represents a foreign body in the vasculature with prothrombogenic and inflammatory potential, employment of an entirely bioresorbable scaffolds appears to be a logical and attractive approach. The potential drawback to BRSs is the reduced radial strength compared to metallic stents as the polymers are more flexible. The optimum duration for the need for scaffolding is not clear and premature stent bioresorption can lead to recoil and subsequent restenosis. Moreover, biodegradation, in some examples, has been shown to elicit intense inflammatory reaction which can lead to an increase in the risk of restenosis. Some of the BRSs are radiolucent, and can therefore be technically challenging for accurate placement, accurate postdilatation, and placement of additional overlapping stents without gaps or long overlap. In addition, the strut thickness of these stents is larger (150–200 μm) and vessel coverage by struts is greater compared to contemporary durable stents. For BRSs, strut thickness and vessel coverage by struts could be a problem earlier on, eliciting a greater inflammatory reaction and greater propensity for restenosis in the few months after implantation.

Thus, the interaction of the mechanical and biological forces in BRSs differs from permanent metallic stents. To understand and assess the behavior of BRSs comprehensively, various QCA parameters have been precisely employed and evaluated to date.

## GENERAL METHOD FOR QCA

### Contour detection

The contour detection technique is based on resampling the image perpendicular to a model (pathline), computing a cost coefficient matrix representing for each point in the resampled matrix the edge strength defined by the weighted sum of the first and second derivative values in the brightness levels computed along the pathline, and applying the minimal cost contour detection technique to the cost coefficient matrix. This first iteration of the contour detection procedure provides a first approximation of the arterial boundaries. The contour detection algorithms are applied to the original, white-compressed images. As a next step, an automatic defined region of interest of size centered around the defined arterial segment is digitally magnified by a factor of two with bilinear interpolation. The contours detected in the first iteration function as models for the contour detection in the second iteration. To correct for the limited resolution of the X-ray imaging system, the first- and second-derivative functions, which are used for the calculation of the edge strength for each pixel, are modified in the second iteration based on an analysis of the point spread function of the imaging chain. This is of particular importance for the accurate measurement of small vessels. The finally detected contours are subsequently transformed back to the original images [1].

## ESTIMATION OF LUMINAL AREA USING VIDEODENSITOMETRY AND EDGE DETECTION

In edge detection, the calculation of luminal diameter is obtained by direct comparison with the diameter of the filmed catheter, which is used to calibrate the system. Videodensitometry yields a densitometric profile which has to be compared with a segment of known luminal area. This is achieved by automatic selection of a reference site where it is assumed that no occlusive atheromatous disease is present and that the lumen is circular. From the reference diameter (calculated from direct comparison with the coronary catheter as described above), a geometric circular cross-sectional area at the reference site is calculated and compared with the densitometric profile at the same site. In this way, density units are transformed into area units. By direct comparison of the densitometric area thus calculated at the reference site and the smallest densitometric profile in the stenotic segment, minimal luminal cross-sectional area is derived [2].

## QCA PARAMETERS FOR THE ASSESSMENT OF BRSs PERFORMANCE

The treated segment (in-scaffold) and the peri-scaffold segments (defined by a length of 5 mm proximal and distal to the scaffold edge: in-segment) should be analyzed by QCA. In case of polymeric scaffolds, the metallic markers at the proximal and distal ends of the device are the only visible structures for QCA analysis. All QCA parameters are analyzed in paired matched angiographic views after the procedure and at follow-up. The following QCA parameters can be computed: mean lumen diameter, minimal lumen diameter (MLD), reference vessel diameter (RVD), percentage diameter stenosis, D$_{max}$, lumen area by edge detection and videodensitometry, acute gain, acute recoil, late loss, late luminal gain, net gain, curvature, angulation, and vasomotion. Definitions and formulas of QCA parameters for assessment of BRSs are summarized in Table 5.1.1.

## REFERENCE VESSEL DIAMETER

Several quantitative angiography systems, including the Cardiovascular Angiography Analysis System (CAAS), can perform automated stenosis detection in a given coronary segment. With the use of information obtained from computerized analysis of the entire segment, automated analysis not only detects the proximal and distal boundaries of the stenosis but also interpolates the expected dimensions of

the coronary vessel at the point of obstruction (interpolated RVD). In another approach, average diameter of proximal and distal healthy segments by QCA is defined as RVD. Either 5 mm or 10 mm normal reference segments are commonly selected proximal and distal to the stenosis and averaged to define the RVD.

In the ABSORB III trial (2008 patients randomized at 193 centers), the ABSORB bioresorbable vascular scaffold was noninferior to the XIENCE stent for target lesion failure (TLF) at 1 year [3]. In the meanwhile, in a subgroup analysis of the ABSORB III trial [4], outcomes according to whether a lesion was treated with RVD <2.25 mm by QCA was analyzed. 375/1998 patients (18.8%) had treatment of lesion(s) with QCA RVD <2.25 mm (median RVD 2.09 mm). One-year TLF and device thrombosis tended to be higher for ABSORB compared to XIENCE in very small vessels (QCA RVD <2.25 mm), but was similar in not very small vessels (QCA RVD ≥2.25 mm). The ABSORB 2.5 mm scaffold tended to have worse results than a 2.5 mm XIENCE stent in very small vessels, but good outcomes in not very small vessels. These findings have important implications for device selection (and potentially technique) to optimize clinical outcomes when considering ABSORB use.

## DMAX ASSESSMENT

QCA guidance of BRSs implantation relies on the angiographic diameter function curve of the pretreatment vessel segment that contains three nonambiguous data points; namely, the MLD and the D$_{max}$ with respect to the MLD of the proximal (proximal D$_{max}$) and distal (distal D$_{max}$) vessel segments of interest (Figure 5.1.1). In the preprocedural angiography, the landing zone where the scaffold will be implanted needs to be defined as a first step. Within the landing zone, the peak of the diameter function curve proximal to the MLD is defined as proximal D$_{max}$, whereas the peak diameter function curve distal to the MLD is defined as distal D$_{max}$.

Clinical utility of D$_{max}$ assessment for guidance of ABSORB implantation was demonstrated by Ishibashi et al. [7]. Scaffold oversize and nonoversize was compared in a pooled database from ABSORB Cohort B, ABSORB II, and ABSORB EXTEND trials (n = 1232 patients). The selection of device size was considered "oversized" (scaffold oversize) when the patient received one or more devices in vessels in which both the proximal and the distal D$_{max}$ were smaller than the nominal size of the device. Patients who received ABSORB scaffolds in vessels with either a proximal or a distal D$_{max}$ or both D$_{max}$ larger than the nominal size of the device constituted the "scaffold nonoversize." The rates of major adverse cardiac event (MACE) and myocardial infarction (MI) at 1 year were significantly higher in the scaffold oversize group than in the scaffold nonoversize group (MACE 6.6% vs. 3.3%; log-rank $p < 0.01$, all MI: 4.6% vs. 2.4%; log-rank $p = 0.04$), mainly driven by a higher MI rate within 1 month postprocedure (3.5% vs. 1.9%; $p = 0.08$).

**Table 5.1.1** Definitions and formulas of QCA parameters for assessment of BRSs

| Parameters | Formula | Definition and notes |
|---|---|---|
| Reference vessel diameter | Expected dimension of the coronary vessel at the point of MLD interpolated based on the proximal and distal boundaries of the stenosis | In another approach, average diameter of proximal and distal healthy segments is defined as RVD. Either 5 mm or 10 mm normal reference segments are commonly selected proximal and distal to the stenosis and averaged to define the RVD. |
| Percentage diameter stenosis | $100 \times (1 - MLD/RVD)$ | The mean values from two orthogonal views (when possible). |
| $D_{max}$ (proximal and distal) | The peak of the diameter function curve proximal to the MLD is defined as proximal $D_{max}$, whereas the peak diameter function curve distal to the MLD is defined as distal $D_{max}$. | |
| Acute gain | MLD (postprocedure) – MLD (preprocedure) | |
| Acute recoil | 1. Without postdilation: mean diameter (delivery balloon at the highest pressure) – mean luminal diameter (after implantation)<br>2. With postdilation: mean diameter (postdilation balloon at the highest pressure) – mean luminal diameter (after postdilation) | Two specific views need to be analyzed: one is an image of complete expansion of the last balloon (either the device delivery balloon or the postdilation balloon) at the highest pressure and the other is a cine frame immediately after the last balloon deflation and subsequent nitrate injection; these two images are analyzed in the same angiographic projection selected to minimize foreshortening |
| Late loss/ late luminal gain | MLD (postprocedure) – MLD (follow-up) | For a lumen diameter reduction, this will be a positive number; for a late increase in lumen size, this will be a negative number |
| Net gain | Sum of the offsetting effects of acute gain and late loss | |
| Curvature | $1$/radius of the circle in $cm^{-1}$<br>Defined as the infinitesimal rate of change in the tangent vector at each point of the center line; this measurement has a reciprocal relationship with the radius of the perfect circle defined by the curve at each point | End-diastole curvature is assessed in the still angiographic view corresponding to the peak of the QRS complex of the electrocardiogram; and end-systole curvature is assessed in the still angiographic view corresponding with the peak of the T wave of the electrocardiogram [5,6]. |
| Angulation | Defined as the angle in degrees that the tip of an intracoronary guidewire would need to reach the distal part of a coronary bend | End-diastole and end-systole angulations are assessed at the same timing as curvature. The tangents of the centerlines defined by the 5-mm proximal and distal parts of the analyzed region at the end-diastolic angiographic frame determine the angle [5,6]. |
| Vasomotion | 1. Vasoconstriction: Δmean lumen diameter (post-pre) $\leq -3\%$<br>2. Vasodilation: Δmean lumen diameter (post-pre) $\geq 3\%$ | Vasoconstriction/vasodilation are defined as at least 3% change in the mean lumen diameter after infusion of the maximal dose of Ach/nitrates, respectively |

*Abbreviations:* RVD = reference vessel diameter; MLD = minimum lumen diameter.

## PERCENTAGE DIAMETER STENOSIS

The percentage diameter stenosis is calculated as $100 \times (1 - MLD/RVD)$ using the mean values from two orthogonal views (when possible) by QCA. Coronary restenosis as an efficacy parameter of BRSs performance is defined as percentage diameter stenosis >50%. A clear understanding of the coronary restenotic mechanics of BRSs needs a thorough understanding of the interplay of acute gain, late loss, and net gain [8,9].

### Acute gain

Figure 5.1.2 summarizes the lumen size changes of BRSs. Acute gain is defined as the difference between MLD at

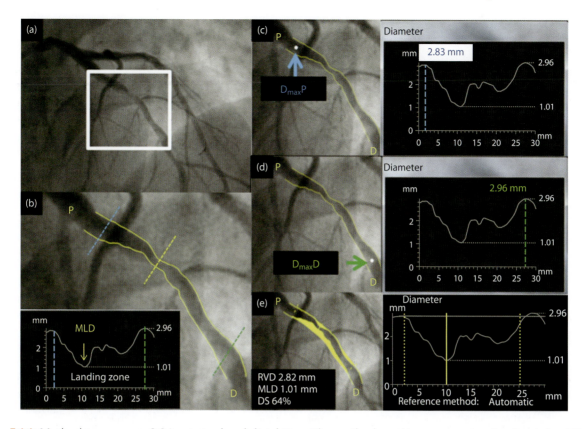

**Figure 5.1.1** Method to measure QCA proximal and distal D$_{max}$. The method used to measure proximal and distal D$_{max}$ with QCA is shown. In the preprocedural angiography **(a)**, the operator has to define the landing zone where the scaffold will be implanted **(b)**. Within the landing zone, the peak of the diameter function curve proximal to the minimal lumen diameter is defined as proximal **(P)** D$_{max}$ **(c)**, whereas the peak diameter function curve distal **(d)** to the minimal lumen diameter is defined as distal D$_{max}$ **(d)**. In this case, the proximal and distal D$_{max}$ of 2.83 and 2.96 mm led to the correct sizing of the ABSORB (3.0 mm) with regard to the vessel diameter **(e)**. D$_{max}$D = maximal lumen diameter distal; D$_{max}$P = maximal lumen diameter proximal; MLD = minimal lumen diameter; QCA = quantitative coronary angiography; RVD = reference vessel diameter.

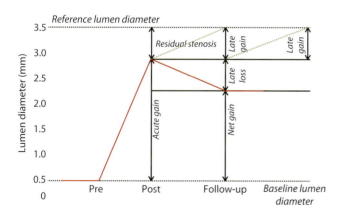

**Figure 5.1.2** Angiographic parameters for bioresorbable scaffold assessment. Immediately after scaffold implantation, there is an important luminal increase (acute gain); at follow-up, there could be either a reduction in lumen size in comparison with the luminal size after implantation (late loss) or a further increase in lumen size (late gain). The latter is a unique angiographic finding following the use of bioresorbable scaffolds.

pre- and post-scaffold implantation. In the ABSORB II trial, angiographic acute gain was lower in the ABSORB arm than in the XIENCE arm (1.15 mm vs. 1.46 mm, $p < 0.0001$) [10]. The main difference in acute gain in MLD by QCA was observed at the time of device implantation (ABSORB vs. XIENCE, Δ+1.23 mm vs. Δ+1.50 mm, respectively), whereas the gain from postdilation was similar between the two arms (Δ+0.16 mm vs. Δ+0.16 mm) when patients underwent postdilation (Figure 5.1.3) [11].

## Acute recoil

For acute recoil assessment, two specific views are analyzed. One is an image of complete expansion of the last balloon (either the device delivery balloon or the postdilation balloon) at the highest pressure. The other is a cine frame immediately after the last balloon deflation and the subsequent nitrate injection. These two images should be analyzed in the same angiographic projection selected to minimize foreshortening.

Acute stent/scaffold recoil is calculated as follows: (1) When a stent/scaffold delivery balloon is used for stent/scaffold

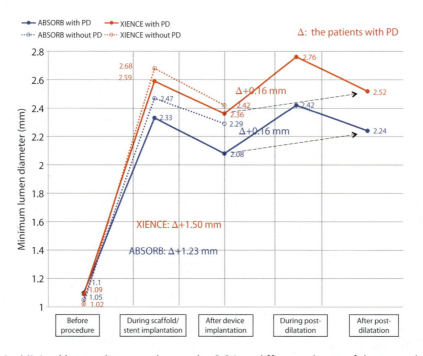

**Figure 5.1.3** Acute gain: Minimal lumen diameter changes by QCA at different phases of the procedure. Change of MLD by QCA of the ABSORB and the XIENCE in the ABSORB II trial are depicted by blue and red, respectively [9]. Dotted lines show minimal lumen diameter changes for those lesions that were not postdilated, whereas solid lines show minimal lumen diameter change of the lesions that underwent postdilation. Differences in acute gains were mainly observed at the time of device implantation (Δ+1.50 mm vs. Δ+1.23 mm), whereas the gain from postdilation was similar between the two arms (Δ+0.16 mm vs. Δ+0.16 mm) when patients underwent postdilation. MLD = minimum lumen diameter; QCA = quantitative coronary angiography.

expansion, acute absolute stent/scaffold recoil is defined as the difference between the mean diameter of the stent/scaffold delivery balloon at the highest pressure at implantation of stent/scaffold (X) and mean luminal diameter of stented/scaffolded segment after implantation (Y). Absolute acute stent/scaffold recoil is calculated as X – Y, whereas relative acute stent/scaffold recoil is defined as (X – Y)/X and is expressed as a percentage; (2) when a postdilation balloon is used in the procedure, acute absolute recoil is defined as the difference between the mean diameter of the postdilation balloon at the highest pressure in the postdilated segment (X′) and mean luminal diameter after postdilation (Y′). Relative acute recoil is defined as (X′ – Y′)/X′ and is expressed as a percentage.

The same methodology was used throughout the ABSORB Cohort A and Cohort B trials. The absolute acute recoil in ABSORB 1.1 was 0.19 ± 0.18 mm (6.7 ± 6.4%), which was not statistically different from that in ABSORB 1.0 (0.20 ± 0.21 mm; 6.9 ± 7.0%) or the metallic everolimus-eluting stent (0.13 ± 0.21 mm; 4.3 ± 7.1%). In multivariable models of the three pooled populations, the balloon/artery ratio was an independent predictor of acute recoil, whereas the type of device (scaffold or stent) was not [12]. In the ABSORB II randomized trial, acute recoil during device implantation was similar in both devices (XIENCE vs. ABSORB, 0.20 ± 0.18 mm vs. 0.19 ± 0.19 mm, respectively; $p = 0.716$), whereas acute recoil during postdilation was larger in the XIENCE than in the ABSORB (0.21 ± 0.21 mm vs. 0.13 ± 0.20 mm, respectively;

$p = 0.006$) [9]. The DESolve novolimus-eluting bioresorbable scaffold (Elixir Medical Corporation, Sunnyvale, CA) and the ART stent (ART, Noisy le Roi, France) have acute recoils of 6.4 ± 4.6% and 4.0% (data on file, ART), respectively [13,14].

## Late loss, late luminal gain, and net gain

Late loss and/or late luminal gain are defined as the difference between MLD at postprocedure minus MLD at follow-up. For lumen diameter reduction, this will be a positive number; for late increase in lumen size, this will be a negative number. The net gain is the sum of the offsetting effects of acute gain and late loss.

For contemporary permanent metallic stents (both bare metal stent and drug eluting stent), the negative constrictive remodeling is minimal and thus late loss is a good indicator of neointimal hyperplasia. For BRSs, both negative constrictive remodeling and neointimal hyperplasia could contribute toward restenosis. Nonetheless, the unique expectation of the BRSs technology is the maintenance of the lumen area, or even occurrence of late lumen enlargement, associated with wall thinning and adaptive remodeling [15,16]. This luminal gain starts when BRSs start to lose their mechanical integrity.

Figure 5.1.4 summarizes late loss of several BRSs in clinical scenarios. In the ABSORB first-in-man trial (ABSORB Cohort B trial), late loss of ABSORB at 5 years was 0.26 ± 0.42 mm ($n = 63$) and the MLD was 2.02 ± 0.45 mm ($n = 64$) [16]. Late loss of DESolve at 6 months was 0.20 ± 0.32 mm

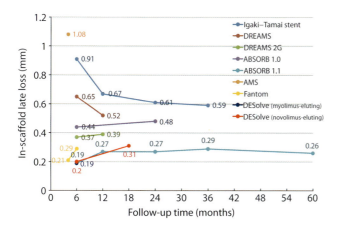

**Figure 5.1.4** Time-related late loss of bioresorbable vascular scaffolds. Serial changes of in-scaffold late loss in various bioresorbable vascular scaffolds in clinical trials are illustrated.

($n$ = 113, DESolve Nx trial) [17]. In the first-in-man trial of magnesium scaffold (DREAMS 2G; Biotronik AG, Buelach, Switzerland), the late loss at 6 months was 0.27 ± 0.37 mm ($n$ = 123, BIOSOLVE-II study) [18].

## CONFORMABILITY

Coronary geometry changes after stenting might result in wall shear stress changes and adverse events. These changes in 3-dimensional vessel geometry are associated with decreased and increased shear stress zones close to the stent edges. These changes were found to be related to the asymmetrical patterns of in-stent restenosis [19]. Angiographically, the geometric changes can be assessed by measuring the curvature and angulation [5,6]. Curvature is defined as the infinitesimal rate of change in the tangent vector at each point of the center line (Figure 5.1.5). This measurement has a reciprocal relationship with the radius of the perfect circle defined by the curve at each point. The curvature value is calculated as 1/radius of the circle in $cm^{-1}$. Angulation is defined as the angle in degrees that the tip of an intracoronary guidewire would need to reach the distal part of a coronary bend. The tangents of the centerlines defined by the 5-mm proximal and distal parts of the analyzed region at the end-diastolic angiographic frame determine the angle. End-diastole curvature/angulation is assessed in the still angiographic view corresponding to the peak of the QRS complex of the electrocardiogram; and end-systole curvature/angulation is assessed in the still angiographic view corresponding with the peak of the T wave of the electrocardiogram. Relative differences, before and after device implantation, are estimated at the end-diastole as (absolute difference in curvature or angulation between pre- and postimplantation/curvature or angulation at preimplantation) ×100 [5,6].

For the Absorb scaffold, from postimplantation to follow-up, curvature increased by 8.4% ($p$ < 0.01) with Absorb and decreased 1.9% ($p$ = 0.54) with the metallic platform stents

($p$ = 0.01) [6]. Angulation increased 11.3% with Absorb ($p$ < 0.01) and 3.8% with metallic stents ($p$ = 0.01); $p$ < 0.01. From preimplantation to follow-up, the artery curvature decreased 3.4% with Absorb ($p$ = 0.05) and the artery angulation decreased 3.9% ($p$ = 0.16), whereas metallic stents presented with 26.1% decrease in curvature ($p$ < 0.01) and 26.9% decrease in angulation ($p$ < 0.01) (both $p$ < 0.01 for the comparison between BRSs and metallic stents) [5]. For drug-eluting absorbable magnesium scaffolds (DREAMS), the vessel curvature decreased 40.5% postimplantation ($p$ < 0.01), but the difference between baseline and 12-month follow-up was reduced to 7.4% ($p$ = 0.03) [20]. This means that the BRSs tended to restore the coronary configuration and systolodiastolic movements to those seen before implantation, whereas the coronary geometry remained similar to that seen after implantation with metallic stents.

## VASOMOTION

Vasomotor testing, using nitroglycerin, methylergometrine (endothelium-independent vasoconstrictor), and acetylcholine (Ach) (endothelium-dependent vasoactive agent), can be performed at various time points. Vasoconstriction/vasodilation are defined as at least 3% change in the mean lumen diameter after infusion of the maximal dose of drugs, respectively.

Vasomotion of the scaffolded segment following intraluminal administration of Ach suggests that: (1) the scaffolding function of the struts has completely disappeared and the scaffolded segment can now exhibit vasomotion; (2) the endothelial lining (coverage) is coalescent; (3) the ciliary function of the endothelial cell is functional; and (4) the biochemical process through which nitric oxide is released properly works. A positive Ach test with vasodilation of the scaffold is indirect proof that the endothelium is functional [21]. Mean lumen diameters in the scaffolded proximal and distal segments are measured by QCA after a baseline infusion of saline and subselective intra-coronary administration of Ach, infused through a microcatheter at increasing doses up to a maximum of $10^{-6}$ M. In particular, a 2-min selective infusion of Ach ($10^{-8}$, $10^{-7}$, and $10^{-6}$ mol/L) is administered with a washout period of at least 5 min between each dose. Nitrate (200 mg) is administrated following Ach. Vasoconstriction to Ach is defined as a 3% change in the mean lumen diameter, beyond the variability of the method of analysis, after infusion of the maximal dose of Ach ($10^{-6}$ M).

In the ABSORB Cohort A and B trials, patients at 24 months ($n$ = 8) exhibited a significant increase in the mean lumen diameter after Ach administration compared with patients at 12 months ($n$ = 18) [+2.14% (−2.58, +8.80) vs. −5.46% (−8.25, +1.86); $p$ = 0.038] [22]. In particular, 11 patients (42.3%) exhibited a vasodilatory response to Ach (6/18 at 12 and 5/8 at 24 months; $p$ = 0.390), whereas 14 patients (54.2%) had an abnormal response to Ach with vasoconstriction, with only 1 patient not exhibiting any changes in the mean lumen diameter. Overall, the change in

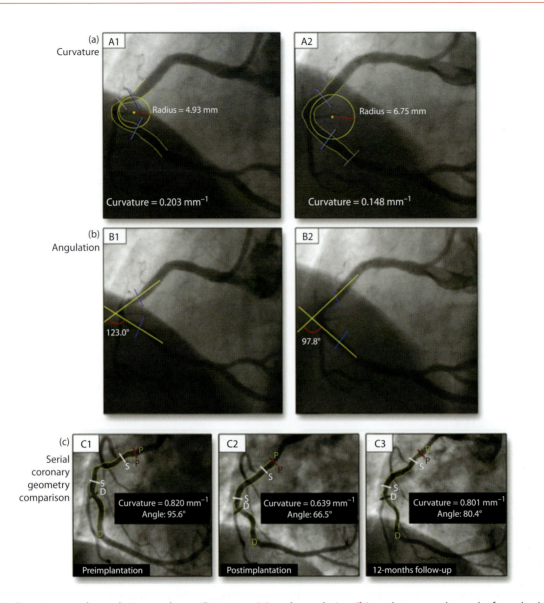

**Figure 5.1.5** Curvature and angulation analyses. Curvature **(a)** and angulation **(b)** analyses are shown before deployment (**A1** and **B1**) and after deployment (**A2** and **B2**). Curvature is estimated as 1/radius (0.203 mm⁻¹ in **A1** and 0.148 mm⁻¹ in **A2**). Angulation is defined by the tangents of the center lines. BRSs tends to allow restoration of the coronary geometry and systo-diastolic movements of the coronary arteries similar to that seen before implantation (**C1** to **C3**).

the mean lumen diameter after nitrate administration compared with baseline was +0.41% (−3.77, +5.52; $p = 0.494$). Patients at 24 months demonstrated a higher increase in the mean lumen diameter to nitrates compared with the 12-month group [+5.79 (+1.41, +12.0) vs. −0.60% (−5.46, +3.91); $p = 0.032$] [22]. In the ABSORB Japan randomized trial comparing ABSORB and XIENCE, an angiographic vasomotion test before and after nitrate administration was performed and unexpectedly demonstrated no significant differences between the two arms in vasodilatation (ABSORB $0.06 \pm 0.14$ mm vs. XIENCE $0.07 \pm 0.17$ mm, $p = 0.89$) at 2-year follow-up [23].

The timing of restored vasomotion after BRSs is a surrogate for loss of structural integrity of the device and an indication when the vessel may respond to normal and exercise-induced changes in coronary blood flow and pressure. For the ABSORB scaffold, the time seems to be 12 months; for the DREAMS scaffold, the time seems to be 6 months [20].

## DIFFERENTIAL IMPACT OF POLYMERIC SCAFFOLDS AND METALLIC STENTS ON QCA MEASUREMENTS

Sotomi et al. reported that in the ABSORB Japan randomized trial comparing ABSORB and XIENCE, QCA underestimated lumen diameter as compared to OCT immediately after stent/scaffold implantation by 9.1%, 4.9%, and 9.8% in the native (nonstented, nonscaffolded), stented, and scaffolded segments, respectively (Figure 5.1.6). In the stented vessel, laminar flow of contrast is disturbed by the protruded struts and cannot get into close contact with the vessel wall compared

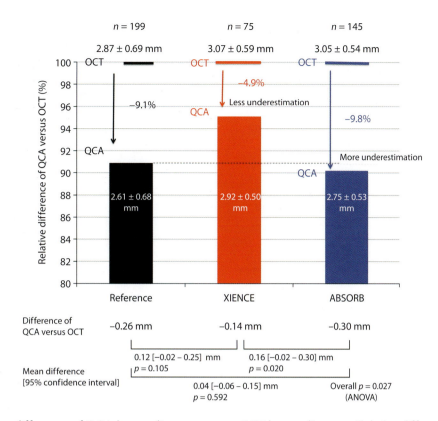

**Figure 5.1.6** Relative difference of QCA-lumen diameter versus OCT-lumen diameter. Relative difference of QCA-lumen diameter versus OCT-lumen diameter was assessed in ABSORB Japan trial. In the reference segments (native coronary: black), QCA underestimated LD by 9.1% compared to OCT; in the stented segments (red), QCA underestimated LD less (4.9%), whereas in the scaffolded segments (blue), QCA underestimated LD more severely (9.8%) compared to OCT. OCT = optical coherence tomography; QCA = quantitative coronary angiography; LD = lumen diameter.

to the native unstented/unscaffolded vessels. However, high radiopacity of metallic struts could cause an artifactual outward enlargement of the lumen contours (blooming artifact of metal), resulting in less underestimation in the stented vessels than in the scaffolded vessels. A radiolucent polymeric strut does not cause any inherent X-ray artifact in the brightness function and analysis by QCA. However, in the scaffolded vessels, the laminar flow disturbance is larger than in the stented vessels due to more strut protrusions, resulting in less close contact of the contrast medium with the vessel wall. Thereby, scaffolded vessels generate possibly a more severe underestimation of the lumen dimension on QCA than the one observed in the native vessels.

The study would imply the unfairness of the assessment for ABSORB compared to XIENCE, which could raise a question whether the commonly used acute gain analysis by QCA for the comparison of ABSORB with XIENCE is appropriate and accurate. The QCA acute gain data from previous trials comparing ABSORB and XIENCE might be critically reconsidered.

## CONCLUSIONS

Quantitative coronary angiography is one of the most commonly used methods in the interventional field. In the present chapter, we introduced detailed descriptions of the QCA

parameters, methodologies for the assessment of BRSs, and clinical utility of QCA for the guidance of BRSs implantation. We also presented the artifactual difference of the impact of radiopaque metallic stents and radiolucent polymeric scaffolds on the QCA assessments. The unique features of BRSs as compared to metallic stents could have some concomitant unknown impacts on the assessment of the conventional QCA parameters. This point requires considerable attention especially in the future trials comparing BRSs and metallic stents.

## REFERENCES

1. Reiber JH, van der Zwet PM, Koning G, von Land CD, van Meurs B, Gerbrands JJ, Buis B et al. Accuracy and precision of quantitative digital coronary arteriography: Observer-, short-, and medium-term variabilities. *Cathet Cardiovasc Diagn.* 1993;28:187–98.
2. Escaned J, Haase J, Foley DP, Di Mario C, Den Boer A, Van Swijndregt EM, and Serruys PW. Videodensitometry in percutaneous coronary interventions: A critical appraisal of its contributions and limitations. In: Serruys PW, Foley DP, and De Feyter PJ, Eds. *Quantitative Coronary Angiography in Clinical Practice,* Dordrecht: Springer Netherlands; 1994: 69–87.

3. Ellis SG, Kereiakes DJ, Metzger DC, Caputo RP, Rizik DG, Teirstein PS, Litt MR et al. Everolimus-eluting bioresorbable scaffolds for coronary artery disease. *New Engl J Med.* 2015;373:1905–15.

4. Stone GW, Ellis S, Simonton C, Metzger D, Caputo R, Rizik D, Teirstein PS et al. Outcomes of the Absorb bioresorbable vascular scaffold in very small and not very small coronary arteries: The Absorb III randomized trial. *J Am Coll Cardiol.* 2016;67:35–35.

5. Gomez-Lara J, Brugaletta S, Farooq V, van Geuns RJ, De Bruyne B, Windecker S, McClean D et al. Angiographic geometric changes of the lumen arterial wall after bioresorbable vascular scaffolds and metallic platform stents at 1-year follow-up. *JACC Cardiovasc Interv.* 2011;4:789–99.

6. Gomez-Lara J, Garcia-Garcia HM, Onuma Y, Garg S, Regar E, De Bruyne B, Windecker S et al. A comparison of the conformability of everolimus-eluting bioresorbable vascular scaffolds to metal platform coronary stents. *JACC Cardiovasc Interv.* 2010;3:1190–8.

7. Ishibashi Y, Nakatani S, Sotomi Y, Suwannasom P, Grundeken MJ, Garcia-Garcia HM, Bartorelli AL et al. Relation between bioresorbable scaffold sizing using QCA-$D_{max}$ and clinical outcomes at 1 year in 1,232 patients from 3 study cohorts (ABSORB Cohort B, ABSORB EXTEND, and ABSORB II). *JACC Cardiovasc Interv.* 2015;8:1715–26.

8. Meijboom WB, Van Mieghem CA, van Pelt N, Weustink A, Pugliese F, Mollet NR, Boersma E et al. Comprehensive assessment of coronary artery stenoses: Computed tomography coronary angiography versus conventional coronary angiography and correlation with fractional flow reserve in patients with stable angina. *J Am Coll Cardiol.* 2008;52:636–43.

9. Bangalore S and Mauri L. Late loss in a disappearing frame of reference: Is it still applicable to fully absorbable scaffolds? *EuroIntervention. Journal of EuroPCR in Collaboration with the Working Group on Interventional Cardiology of the European Society of Cardiology.* 2009;5:F43–F48.

10. Serruys PW, Chevalier B, Dudek D, Cequier A, Carrie D, Iniguez A, Dominici M et al. A bioresorbable everolimus-eluting scaffold versus a metallic everolimus-eluting stent for ischaemic heart disease caused by de-novo native coronary artery lesions (ABSORB II): An interim 1-year analysis of clinical and procedural secondary outcomes from a randomised controlled trial. *Lancet (London, England).* 2015;385:43–54.

11. Sotomi Y, Ishibashi Y, Suwannasom P, Nakatani S, Cho YK, Grundeken MJ, Zeng Y et al. Acute gain in minimal lumen area following implantation of everolimus-eluting ABSORB biodegradable vascular scaffolds or Xience metallic stents: Intravascular ultrasound assessment from the ABSORB II trial. *JACC Cardiovasc Interv.* 2016;9:1216–27.

12. Onuma Y, Serruys PW, Gomez J, de Bruyne B, Dudek D, Thuesen L, Smits P et al. Comparison of in vivo acute stent recoil between the bioresorbable everolimus-eluting coronary scaffolds (revision 1.0 and 1.1) and the metallic everolimus-eluting stent. *Cathet Cardiovasc Interv. Official Journal of the Society for Cardiac Angiography & Interventions.* 2011;78:3–12.

13. Verheye S, Ormiston JA, Stewart J, Webster M, Sanidas E, Costa R, Costa JR, Jr. et al. A next-generation bioresorbable coronary scaffold system: From bench to first clinical evaluation: 6- and 12-month clinical and multimodality imaging results. *JACC Cardiovasc Interv.* 2014;7:89–99.

14. Garcia-Garcia HM, Serruys PW, Campos CM, Muramatsu T, Nakatani S, Zhang YJ, Onuma Y et al. Assessing bioresorbable coronary devices: Methods and parameters. *JACC Cardiovasc Imaging.* 2014;7:1130–48.

15. Serruys PW, Ormiston JA, Onuma Y, Regar E, Gonzalo N, Garcia-Garcia HM, Nieman K et al. A bioabsorbable everolimus-eluting coronary stent system (ABSORB): 2-year outcomes and results from multiple imaging methods. *Lancet (London, England).* 2009;373:897–910.

16. Serruys PW, Ormiston J, van Geuns RJ, de Bruyne B, Dudek D, Christiansen E, Chevalier B et al. A poly-lactide bioresorbable scaffold eluting everolimus for treatment of coronary stenosis: 5-year follow-up. *J Am Coll Cardiol.* 2016;67:766–76.

17. Abizaid A, Costa RA, Schofer J, Ormiston J, Maeng M, Witzenbichler B, Botelho RV et al. Serial multi-modality imaging and 2-year clinical outcomes of the novel DESolve novolimus-eluting bioresorbable coronary scaffold system for the treatment of single de novo coronary lesions. *JACC Cardiovasc Interv.* 2016;9:565–74.

18. Haude M, Ince H, Abizaid A, Toelg R, Lemos PA, von Birgelen C, Christiansen EH et al. Safety and performance of the second-generation drug-eluting absorbable metal scaffold in patients with de-novo coronary artery lesions (BIOSOLVE-II): 6 month results of a prospective, multicentre, non-randomised, first-in-man trial. *Lancet (London, England).* 2016;387:31–9.

19. Wentzel JJ, Whelan DM, van der Giessen WJ, van Beusekom HM, Andhyiswara I, Serruys PW, Slager CJ et al. Coronary stent implantation changes 3-D vessel geometry and 3-D shear stress distribution. *J Biomech.* 2000;33:1287–95.

20. Waksman R, Prati F, Bruining N, Haude M, Bose D, Kitabata H, Erne P et al. Serial observation of drug-eluting absorbable metal scaffold: Multi-imaging modality assessment. *Circ Cardiovasc Interv.* 2013;6:644–53.

21. Holzmann S. Endothelium-induced relaxation by ace-tylcholine associated with larger rises in cyclic GMP in coronary arterial strips. *J Cyclic Nucleotide Res.* 1982;8:409–19.

22. Brugaletta S, Heo JH, Garcia-Garcia HM, Farooq V, van Geuns RJ, de Bruyne B, Dudek D et al. Endothelial-dependent vasomotion in a coronary segment treated by ABSORB everolimus-eluting bioresorbable vascular scaffold system is related to plaque composition at the time of bioresorption of the polymer: Indirect finding of vascular reparative therapy? *Eur Heart J.* 2012;33:1325–33.

23. Onuma Y, Sotomi Y, Shiomi H, Ozaki Y, Namiki A, Yasuda S, Ueno T et al. Two-year clinical, angio-graphic, and serial optical coherence tomographic follow-up after implantation of an everolimus-eluting bioresorbable scaffold and an everolimus-eluting metallic stent: Insights from the randomised ABSORB Japan trial. *EuroIntervention. Journal of EuroPCR in Collaboration with the Working Group on Interventional Cardiology of the European Society of Cardiology.* 2016;12.

# Assessment of bioresorbable scaffolds by IVUS: Echogenicity, virtual histology, and palpography

CARLOS M. CAMPOS AND HECTOR M. GARCIA-GARCIA

## INTRODUCTION

Bioresorbable devices have gradually matured and there are numerous devices available for preclinical or clinical evaluation. This technology has required new imaging methodology for the assessment of bioresorbable scaffolds (BRSs) since their design, degradation rate, loss of mechanical properties, coating, and drug deliverability may affect safety and efficacy [1,2].

Intravascular ultrasound (IVUS)—and its derived parameters—may contribute to the BRSs assessment from procedural planning to acute/late vascular response and scaffold degradation rate [1]. The aim of this chapter is to revisit IVUS imaging acquisition, basic concepts, to describe its derived parameters and the dedicated methodology on BRSs appraisal. The main focus will be related to grayscale, virtual histology, echogenicty, and palpography since these methods have been largely used for BRSs assessment.

## Imaging formation

The IVUS image is the result of reflected ultrasound waves that are converted to electrical signals. Ultrasound transmitted from the transducer will "rebound" whenever it encounters an interface of different acoustic impedance. Acoustic impedance is primarily dependent on tissue density: ultrasound emitted from the transducer traverses the blood with minimal reflection and is highly reflected when it meets the calcium. These signals are sent to an external processing system for filtering, amplification, and scan conversion.

The IVUS equipment consists of a catheter incorporating a miniaturized transducer and a console to reconstruct and display the image. Two different approaches to transducer design have emerged: mechanically rotated devices and multielement electronic arrays. Mechanical probes use a drive cable to rotate a single piezoelectric transducer. In electronic systems, multiple transducer elements in an annular array are activated sequentially to generate the image [3].

Grayscale IVUS imaging is formed by the amplitude of the radiofrequency signal [4] (Figure 5.2.1). Differential echogenicity uses the conventional grayscale acquired image to classify tissue according to use as a reference the mean level of the adventitia brightness [5]; i.e., brighter or darker than adventitia (Figure 5.2.1).

Autoregressive spectral analysis of IVUS backscattered data has been incorporated into conventional IVUS systems to identify different tissue components. The first commercially available IVUS backscattering image analysis, named virtual histology™ (VH® IVUS; Volcano Corporation, San Diego, CA), was built on the electronic 20 MHz IVUS platform (Eagle Eye® Catheter, Volcano Corporation, San Diego, CA) [6]. More recently, a rotational mechanical 45 MHz IVUS system has also integrated the classification tree for virtual histology tissue characterization [7] (Figure 5.2.1).

Another approach is to assess the deformability of coronary plaque using also the radiofrequency signals analysis at different diastolic pressure levels using palpography. This method creates a "strain" image in which harder (low strain) and softer (high strain) regions of the coronary arteries can be identified, with radial strain values ranging between 0 and 2% (Figure 5.2.1).

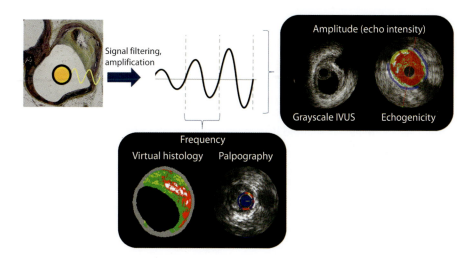

**Figure 5.2.1** Intravascular ultrasound signal is obtained from the vessel wall. Grayscale intravascular ultrasound imaging is formed by the envelope (amplitude) of the radiofrequency signal. Echogenicity classifies the tissue components intensity in comparison with the mean value of adventitia. The frequency and power of the signal commonly differ between tissues, regardless of similarities in the amplitude. From the backscatter radiofrequency data different types of information can be retrieved: virtual histology and palpography.

## GRAYSCALE IVUS

Table 5.2.1 summarizes IVUS parameters used in BRSs assessment. Treated coronary arteries are examined after the procedure and at follow-up with IVUS catheters. The scaffolded segment and its 5-mm distal and proximal segments are also examined. The vessel area, scaffold area, lumen area, intrascaffold neointimal area, and luminal area stenosis are measured using a computer-based contour detection program [1].

### Percentage of lumen area stenosis

The percentage of lumen area stenosis is calculated as 100 times the mean lumen cross-sectional area minus the minimal lumen area divided by mean lumen cross-sectional area within the scaffolded segment.

### Eccentricity/symmetry

The eccentricity and symmetry is easily detectable by IVUS. These parameters have demonstrated to be related to either favorable or adverse clinical outcomes [8,9]. With the transition from a metallic stent to different bioresorbable platforms, the need for the re-evaluation of these geometrical parameters is required at short- and long-term follow-up.

The symmetry index is calculated as (maximum scaffold diameter in a single frame–minimum stent/scaffold diameter in a single frame) divided by the maximum scaffold diameter. Note that the maximum and the minimum stent/scaffold diameters in this calculation are possibly located in two different frames over the length of the device implanted. Eccentricity index is defined as a ratio between the minimum and maximum diameters in each frame;

thereafter, the average of all eccentricity indices is calculated (Figure 5.2.2).

### IVUS assessment of BRSs efficacy

Grayscale IVUS provides a comprehensive assessment of BRSs efficacy since it is the only method that allows the measurement of vessel, scaffold, lumen, and hyperplasia areas. A BRSs restenosis may be the result of device recoil, extra-scaffold neointimal formation, and intra-stent hyperplasia (Figure 5.2.3).

Assessment of the neointima hyperplasia by IVUS is similar to the methodology used for metallic devices. Neointimal hyperplasia area is defined as scaffold area minus lumen area if all struts are apposed. Percentage volume obstruction is defined as neointima hyperplasia volume divided by scaffold volume.

Although the term of late recoil has been used frequently in interventional cardiology to describe the constrictive remodeling of the external elastic membrane area, in the present case, it relates more specifically to the area reduction of the scaffolded segment, a phenomenon not previously observed in metallic stents. Attributed to the early alteration of the mechanical integrity of the scaffold, this phenomenon can be controlled by material processing or modifying the device design [10]. Late absolute stent recoil is defined as scaffold area postprocedure–scaffold area at follow-up. Late percentage scaffold recoil is defined as (scaffold area postprocedure–scaffold area at follow-up)/scaffold area postprocedure ×100.

The use of IVUS helped to clarify the reasons for the suboptimal performance of the first generation magnesium scaffold. For the AMS-1 late recoil was responsible for 42% of luminal obstruction due to its rapid scaffold degradation and led to its design modification [10,11].

**Table 5.2.1** IVUS definitions and formulas of parameters for the assessment of BRSs

| Parameter | Imaging modality | Formula | Definition and notes |
|---|---|---|---|
| Percentage lumen area stenosis | Grayscale IVUS | [(Mean lumen area − minimum lumen area)/mean lumen area] × 100 | |
| Eccentricity index | Grayscale IVUS | Minimum scaffold diameter/maximum scaffold diameter in a frame | The average of all eccentricity indices of each frame within scaffolded segment is calculated. |
| Symmetry index | Grayscale IVUS | (Minimum scaffold diameter − maximum scaffold diameter)/maximum scaffold diameter within a scaffolded segment | The maximum and the minimum stent/scaffold diameters in this calculation were possibly located in two different frames over the length of the device implanted. |
| Neointima hyperplasia area | Grayscale IVUS | Scaffold area − lumen area | Applicable in the frames where all struts are apposed. |
| Percentage area obstruction | Grayscale IVUS | Neointima hyperplasia area/scaffold area ×100 | |
| Late recoil | Grayscale IVUS | Scaffold area at postprocedure − scaffold area at follow-up | |
| Incomplete apposition/ late incomplete apposition | Grayscale IVUS | | Defined as one or more scaffold struts separated from the vessel wall; acquired late incomplete apposition is defined as incomplete apposition at follow-up that is not present after the procedure. |
| Compositional area | Virtual histology (VH) | | The necrotic core, dense calcium, fibrofatty, and fibrous area are analyzed. Of note, polymeric struts are usually recognized as dense calcium. |
| Compositional area | iMAP | | The fibrotic, lipidic, necrotic, and calcified tissue are analyzed. |
| Compositional area | IB-IVUS | | The lipid, fibrous, dense fibrous, and calcified tissue are analyzed. |
| Strain value | Palpography | | Radiofrequency data obtained at different pressure levels are compared to determine the local tissue deformation. The strain value is normalized to a pressure difference of 2.5 mmHg per frame: this allows the construction of a "strain" image in which hard (low strain/compliance) and soft (high strain/compliance) values range between 0% and 2%. |
| Hyper/upper echogenicity | Echogenicity | % Differential echogenicity = (% hyper follow-up − % hyper preimplantation) − (% hyper postimplantation − % hyper preimplantation)/(% hyper postimplantation − % preimplantation) | IVUS grayscale data is used to classify tissue according to the adventitia echogenicity. Scaffold struts are identified as tissue areas brighter than adventitia (hyper/upper echogenicity). Echogenicity has been used to assess BRSs degradation as they become less bright as they degrade. |

*Source:* Garcia-Garcia HM, Campos CM, Muramatsu T, Nakatani S, Zhang YJ, Onuma Y, Stone GW. *JACC Cardiovasc Imaging.* 2014;7:1130–48.

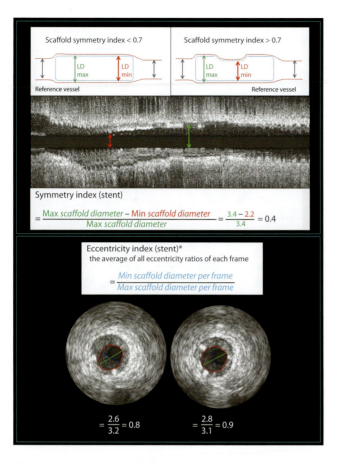

**Figure 5.2.2** Definition of the symmetry and eccentricity indices according to IVUS.

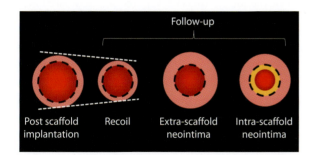

**Figure 5.2.3** Mechanisms of bioresorbable scaffolds restenosis according to IVUS. (Modified from Waksman R, Erbel R, Di Mario C, Bartunek J, de Bruyne B, Eberli FR, Erne P et al. *JACC Cardiovasc Interv.* 2009;2:312–20.)

Late absolute and percentage recoil of the ABSORB BVSs 1.0 was $0.65 \pm 1.71$ mm$^2$ (95% confidence interval [CI]: 0.49–0.80 mm$^2$) and $7.60 \pm 23.3\%$ (95% CI: 5.52–9.68%) [12]. In the newer generation, ABSORB BVSs 1.1, the mean scaffold area increased from baseline to 3 years by IVUS (6.3–7.1 mm$^2$) and by OCT (7.8–8.6 mm$^2$) [13]. Similarly, the Elixir DESolve Nx BRSs showed an increase in mean scaffold area by IVUS (5.4–5.6 mm$^2$) and OCT (6.6–6.8 mm$^2$) [14].

In addition, the other critical observation made by IVUS between 6-month and 3-year follow-up was a late luminal enlargement (from $6.39 \pm 1.08$ to $6.79 \pm 1.61$ mm$^2$) with significant plaque media reduction (from $8.13 \pm 2.70$ to $7.75 \pm 1.72$ mm$^2$) and without significant change in the vessel wall area (EEM) [13]. Still today, it is unknown whether this "plaque media regression" on IVUS is a true atherosclerotic regression, with change in vessel wall composition and plaque morphology (from thin-cap atheroma to thick-cap atheroma) or a pseudo-regression due to bioresorption of the polymeric struts. True atherosclerotic regression could only be hypothesized based on animal and *in vitro* experiments, showing that mammalian target of rapamycin can trigger a complex chain of biological reactions that leads finally to activation of genes related to autophagy of macrophages. Systemic application of everolimus decreases atherosclerotic plaque formation in low-density lipoprotein-receptor (LDL-R-/-) knockout mice [15].

## Incomplete scaffold apposition (ISA)

Incomplete apposition is defined as one or more scaffold struts separated from the vessel wall. It is classified as acquired late incomplete apposition when incomplete apposition at follow-up is not present after the procedure.

Using BVSs 1.1, at baseline, four patients showed incomplete scaffold apposition. One ISA persisted at follow-up, and three ISAs resolved. At 6 months' follow-up, three patients developed a late acquired ISA [16]. In the other group followed up to 1 year, at baseline, there were five patients with ISA and at follow-up there were only four [17]. At 2 years, incomplete appositions by IVUS were only observed in two patients. At 3 years, three patients presented late acquired malapposition [13]. The Elixir DESolve Nx BRSs had only one patient with malapposition at 6 months by OCT [14].

## Edge effects

The edge effect was introduced in the era of endovascular brachytherapy utilizing radioactive stents to describe the tissue proliferation at the nonirradiated proximal and distal edges. During the advent of first generation drug-eluting stents (DESs), it was also found that when in-segment (stent and 5 mm proximal and distal margins) restenosis occurred, it was most commonly focal and located at the proximal edge.

In the ABSORB Cohort B trial, the edges effects by IVUS was assessed in 101 patients at either 6 months (B1) or 1 year (B2). The adjacent (5-mm) proximal and distal vessel segments to the implanted ABSORB BVSs were investigated. At the 5-mm proximal edge, the only significant change was modest constrictive remodeling at 6 months ($\Delta$ vessel cross-sectional area: $-1.80\%$ [$-3.18$; 1.30], $p < 0.05$), with a tendency to regress at 1 year ($\Delta$ vessel cross-sectional area: $-1.53\%$ [$-7.74$; 2.48], $p = 0.06$). The relative change of the fibrotic and fibrofatty (FF) tissue areas at this segment were not statistically significant at either time point. At the 5-mm distal edge, a significant increase in the FF tissue of 43.32% [−19.90; 244.28], ($p < 0.05$) 1-year postimplantation was evident. Changes in dense calcium areas were also observed, which need to be interpreted with caution. The polymeric struts are detected as "pseudo" dense calcium structures with the VH-IVUS imaging modality and the edges of the polymeric scaffold are not sharply demarcated since the vessels surrounding the imaging device are affected by the "to and fro" motion of the cardiac contraction, causing a longitudinal displacement of the IVUS catheter related to the arterial wall [18].

## VIRTUAL HISTOLOGY (VH)

Ultrasound backscattered signals are acquired using either a 20-MHz (electronic) or 45-MHz (mechanical) IVUS catheters [6,7]. Backscattering of radiofrequency signals provides information on vessel wall tissue composition with autoregressive classification systems identifying four tissue components: necrotic core, red; dense calcium, white; fibrous, green; and fibrofatty, light green (Figure 5.2.4a–c).

In each cross-section, polymeric scaffold struts are detected as areas of apparent dense calcium and necrotic core resulting from the strong backscattering properties of the polymer (Figure 5.2.4d). We use the change in quantitative analyses of these areas between implantation and follow-up as a surrogate assessment of the chemical and structural alterations of the polymeric struts.

The most recent data of the ABSORB cohort B trial showed that the mean dense calcium areas were 29.84 mm$^2$ (postimplantation), 28.16 mm$^2$ (6 month), 24.25 mm$^2$ (1 year); 27.74 mm$^2$ (2 year) and 21.52 mm$^2$ (3 year follow-up). The average necrotic core areas, at the same aforementioned time points, were: 31.31 mm$^2$, 30.11 mm$^2$, 30 mm$^2$, 31.67 mm$^2$, and 26.49 mm$^2$. The sharp decrease in dense calcium and necrotic core between 24 and 36 months may also reflect the end of the inflammatory process with regression of the plaque behind the struts and not only scaffold degradation [13].

## ECHOGENICITY

Echogenicity aims to classify the vessel wall components located between the luminal boundary and the external elastic membrane into categories based on their gray-level intensity. The mean gray value of the adventitia—defined as a 0.2–0.3 mm layer outside the external elastic membrane—is used as a reference. All pixels representing gray-level intensity values lower than the reference gray-level intensity are characterized as hypoechogenic, and all pixels with higher gray-level intensity as hyperechogenic. Additionally, lower and upper discrimination values are set. The lower discrimination value serves as a lower limit of the hypoechogenic region, to exclude truly shadowed

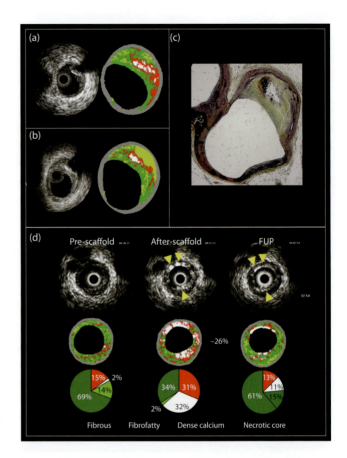

**Figure 5.2.4** IVUS derived virtual histology (IVUS VH). IVUS VH is able to detect four tissue types: necrotic core, fibrous, fibrofatty, and dense calcium. **(a)** 20 MHz and **(b)** 45 MHz IVUS VH representation of an atherosclerotic plaque **(c)**. **(d)** IVUS VH pre- and post-ABSORB BVSs implantation. Scaffold struts are misrepresented as necrotic core or dense calcium (yellow arrowheads) and are less apparent as the scaffold degrades.

or artifact-pixels. The upper discrimination value serves as an upper limit of the hyperechogenic region, and is set to exclude all matter in the dataset that does not account for regular tissue, e.g., metallic structures. Calcified tissue is typically identified in B-mode IVUS images as a highly echogenic area creating an acoustic shadow (Figure 5.2.5).

The software calculates the echogenicity as a volume and percentage for each scaffolded segment. The percentage differential echogenicity may be calculated for each scaffolded coronary segment, as follows [5,19].

Echogenicity parameters have shown to be able to detect temporal changes in the gray level intensities for polymeric and metallic BRSs, being putatively correlated to scaffold degradation over time. More recently, in a porcine model, the decrease in hyperechogenic volumes has been directly correlated with the decrease of poly-l-lactide-acid molecular weight of ABSORB BVS, being thus far, the gold standard method for *in vivo* detection of polymeric scaffold degradation [20].

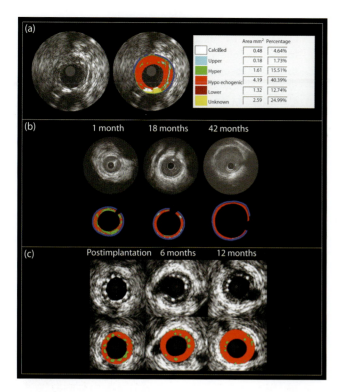

**Figure 5.2.5** Echogenicity. **(a)** Echogenicity classifies the tissue components according to the grayscale intensity as compared with the mean value of adventitia (blue contour). **(b)** Echogenicity and ABSORB BVSs degradation. Echogenicity has been validated with the residual scaffold molecular weight in a porcine model of percutaneous coronary intervention. Notice as the struts are less bright along the time (upper panels) and echogenity is able to quantify these changes. **(c)** Echogenicity and drug-eluting absorbable metal scaffold degradation (DREAMS). (Modified from Campos CM, Ishibashi Y, Eggermont J, Nakatani S, Cho YK, Dijkstra J, Reiber JH et al. *Int J Cardiovasc Imaging.* 2015;31:471–82; and Waksman R, Prati F, Bruining N, Haude M, Bose D, Kitabata H, Erne P et al. *Circ Cardiovasc Interv.* 2013;6:644–53.)

## PALPOGRAPHY

Palpography assesses the local mechanical properties of the coronary plaque. It measures the relative displacements of backscattered radiofrequency signals, recorded during IVUS acquisition with a commercially available catheter (20 MHz Jovus Avanar, Volcano, Rancho Cordova, CA). This technique detects differences in deformability or strain of various plaque components. As such, lipid-rich plaques will deform more and thus show a higher strain value compared with calcified or fibrous plaques [21]. In coronary arteries, the tissue of interest is the vessel wall, whereas the blood pressure, with its physiological changes during the heart cycle, is used as the excitation force. Radiofrequency data obtained at different pressure levels are compared to determine the local tissue deformation. The strain value is normalized to a pressure difference of 2.5 mmHg per frame:

this allows the construction of a "strain" image in which hard (low strain/compliance) and soft (high strain/compliance) values range between 0% and 2%. In postmortem coronary arteries, the sensitivity and specificity of palpography to detect high strain values have previously been reported as 88% and 89%, respectively [22]. Plaque strain values are classified according to the Rotterdam classification (ROC) score in a range from I to IV (ROC I: 0–0.6%; ROC II: 0.6–0.9%; ROC III: 0.9–1.2%; ROC IV: 1.2%) [23]. A region is defined as a high-strain spot when it had high strain (ROC III–IV) that spanned an arc of at least 12° at the surface of a plaque (identified on the IVUS recording) adjacent to low-strain regions (<0.5%), as previously reported [24]. The highest value of strain in the cross-section is taken as the strain level of the spot. The compliance of each segment is

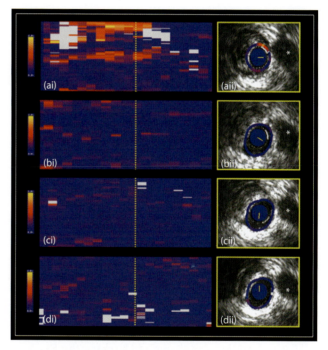

**Figure 5.2.6** Palpography. Spread out plot of the vessel wall strain at baseline before ABSORB BVSs implantation **(ai)**, immediate after scaffold deployment **(bi)**, at short-term **(ci)**, and mid-term follow-up **(di)**. The blue color indicates low strain values where the red/yellow indicates a high strain. It is apparent that the incidence of the high strain values decreased immediately after scaffold deployment and it is even lower at short- and mid-term follow-up. Panels **aii**, **bii**, **cii**, and **dii** portray corresponding IVUS cross-sections acquired at baseline before and immediately after scaffold deployment, at short-term, and at mid-term follow-up, respectively. The position of these frames in the spread-out vessel plots is indicated with a yellow line. High strain values are noted at the shoulders of an echolucent plaque before scaffold implantation **(aii)**; however, immediately after device deployment the strain values are low in the entire circumference of the lumen **(bii)**. (From Bourantas CV, Garcia-Garcia HM, Campos CA, Zhang YJ, Muramatsu T, Morel MA, Nakatani S et al. *Int J Cardiovasc Imaging.* 2014;30:477–84.)

calculated per segment (proximal edge, scaffold segment, and distal edge) and defined as the mean of the maximum strain values per cross-section in ROC I/II/III/IV spots, expressed as ROC/mm.

Palpography has been used to evaluate postimplantation effect of ABSORB BVSs [25]. Fifty-three patients implanted with an ABSORB BVSs that had palpographic evaluation at any time point (before device implantation, immediately after treatment, at short-term [6–12 months] or mid-term follow-up [24–36 months]) were analyzed (Figure 5.2.6). Scaffold implantation led to a significant decrease of the vessel wall strain in the treated segment (0.35 [0.20, 0.38] vs. 0.19 [0.09, 0.29]; $p = 0.005$) but it did not affect the proximal and distal edges.

# REFERENCES

1. Garcia-Garcia HM, Campos CM, Muramatsu T, Nakatani S, Zhang YJ, Onuma Y, Stone GW. Assessing bioresorbable coronary devices: Methods and parameters. *JACC Cardiovasc Imaging.* 2014;7:1130–48.

2. Campos CM, Lemos PA. Bioresorbable vascular scaffolds: Novel devices, novel interpretations, and novel interventions strategies. *Cathet Cardiovasc Interv. Official Journal of the Society for Cardiac Angiography & Interventions.* 2014;84:46–7.

3. Nissen SE, Yock P. Intravascular ultrasound: Novel pathophysiological insights and current clinical applications. *Circulation.* 2001;103:604–16.

4. Garcia-Garcia HM, Costa MA, Serruys PW. Imaging of coronary atherosclerosis: Intravascular ultrasound. *Eur Heart J.* 2010;31:2456–69.

5. Bruining N, Verheye S, Knaapen M, Somers P, Roelandt JR, Regar E, Heller I et al. Three-dimensional and quantitative analysis of atherosclerotic plaque composition by automated differential echogenicity. *Catheter Cardiovasc Interv.* 2007;70:968–78.

6. Nair A, Margolis MP, Kuban BD, Vince DG. Automated coronary plaque characterisation with intravascular ultrasound backscatter: Ex vivo validation. *EuroIntervention. Journal of EuroPCR in Collaboration with the Working Group on Interventional Cardiology of the European Society of Cardiology.* 2007;3:113–20.

7. Campos CM, Fedewa RJ, Garcia-Garcia HM, Vince DG, Margolis MP, Lemos PA, Stone GW et al. Ex vivo validation of 45 MHz intravascular ultrasound backscatter tissue characterization. *Eur Heart J Cardiovasc Imaging.* 2015.

8. de Jaegere P, Mudra H, Figulla H, Almagor Y, Doucet S, Penn I, Colombo A et al. Intravascular ultrasound-guided optimized stent deployment. Immediate and 6 months clinical and angiographic results from the Multicenter Ultrasound Stenting in Coronaries Study (MUSIC Study). *Eur Heart J.* 1998;19:1214–23.

9. Otake H, Shite J, Ako J, Shinke T, Tanino Y, Ogasawara D, Sawada T et al. Local determinants of thrombus formation following sirolimus-eluting stent implantation assessed by optical coherence tomography. *JACC Cardiovasc Interv.* 2009;2:459–66.

10. Campos CM, Muramatsu T, Iqbal J, Zhang YJ, Onuma Y, Garcia-Garcia HM, Haude M et al. Bioresorbable drug-eluting magnesium-alloy scaffold for treatment of coronary artery disease. *Int J Mol Sci.* 2013;14:24492–500.

11. Erbel R, Di Mario C, Bartunek J, Bonnier J, de Bruyne B, Eberli FR, Erne P et al. Temporary scaffolding of coronary arteries with bioabsorbable magnesium stents: A prospective, non-randomised multicentre trial. *Lancet.* 2007;369:1869–75.

12. Tanimoto S, Bruining N, van Domburg RT, Rotger D, Radeva P, Ligthart JM, Serruys PW. Late stent recoil of the bioabsorbable everolimus-eluting coronary stent and its relationship with plaque morphology. *J Am Coll Cardiol.* 2008;52:1616–20.

13. Serruys PW, Onuma Y, Garcia-Garcia HM, Muramatsu T, van Geuns RJ, de Bruyne B, Dudek D et al. Dynamics of vessel wall changes following the implantation of the Absorb everolimus-eluting bioresorbable vascular scaffold: A multi-imaging modality study at 6, 12, 24 and 36 months. *EuroIntervention.* 2014;9:1271–84.

14. Verheye S, Ormiston JA, Stewart J, Webster M, Sanidas E, Costa R, Costa JR, Jr. et al. A next-generation bioresorbable coronary scaffold system: From bench to first clinical evaluation: 6- and 12-month clinical and multimodality imaging results. *JACC Cardiovasc Interv.* 2014;7:89–99.

15. Mueller MA, Beutner F, Teupser D, Ceglarek U, Thiery J. Prevention of atherosclerosis by the mTOR inhibitor everolimus in LDLR-/- mice despite severe hypercholesterolemia. *Atherosclerosis.* 2008;198:39–48.

16. Serruys PW, Onuma Y, Ormiston JA, de Bruyne B, Regar E, Dudek D, Thuesen L et al. Evaluation of the second generation of a bioresorbable everolimus drug-eluting vascular scaffold for treatment of de novo coronary artery stenosis: Six-month clinical and imaging outcomes. *Circulation.* 2010;122:2301–12.

17. Serruys PW, Onuma Y, Dudek D, Smits PC, Koolen J, Chevalier B, de Bruyne B et al. Evaluation of the second generation of a bioresorbable everolimus-eluting vascular scaffold for the treatment of de novo coronary artery stenosis: 12-month clinical and imaging outcomes. *J Am Coll Cardiol.* 2011;58:1578–88.

18. Gogas BD, Serruys PW, Diletti R, Farooq V, Brugaletta S, Radu MD, Heo JH et al. Vascular response of the segments adjacent to the proximal and distal edges of the ABSORB everolimus-eluting bioresorbable vascular scaffold: 6-month and 1-year follow-up assessment: A virtual histology

intravascular ultrasound study from the first-in-man ABSORB cohort B trial. *JACC Cardiovasc Interv.* 2012;5:656–65.

19. Bruining N, de Winter S, Roelandt JR, Regar E, Heller I, van Domburg RT, Hamers R et al. Monitoring in vivo absorption of a drug-eluting bioabsorbable stent with intravascular ultrasound-derived parameters a feasibility study. *JACC Cardiovasc Interv.* 2010;3:449–56.

20. Campos CM, Ishibashi Y, Eggermont J, Nakatani S, Cho YK, Dijkstra J, Reiber JH et al. Echogenicity as a surrogate for bioresorbable everolimus-eluting scaffold degradation: Analysis at 1-, 3-, 6-, 12- 18, 24-, 30-, 36- and 42-month follow-up in a porcine model. *Int J Cardiovasc Imaging.* 2015;31:471–82.

21. de Korte CL, Sierevogel MJ, Mastik F, Strijder C, Schaar JA, Velema E, Pasterkamp G et al. Identification of atherosclerotic plaque components with intravascular ultrasound elastography in vivo: A Yucatan pig study. *Circulation.* 2002;105:1627–30.

22. Schaar JA, De Korte CL, Mastik F, Strijder C, Pasterkamp G, Boersma E, Serruys PW et al. Characterizing vulnerable plaque features with intravascular elastography. *Circulation.* 2003;108:2636–41.

23. Van Mieghem CA, McFadden EP, de Feyter PJ, Bruining N, Schaar JA, Mollet NR et al. Noninvasive detection of subclinical coronary atherosclerosis coupled with assessment of changes in plaque characteristics using novel invasive imaging modalities: The Integrated Biomarker and Imaging Study (IBIS). *J Am Coll Cardiol.* 2006;47:1134–42.

24. Schaar JA, Regar E, Mastik F, McFadden EP, Saia F, Disco C et al. Incidence of high-strain patterns in human coronary arteries: Assessment with three-dimensional intravascular palpography and correlation with clinical presentation. *Circulation.* 2004;109:2716–9.

25. Bourantas CV, Garcia-Garcia HM, Campos CA, Zhang YJ, Muramatsu T, Morel MA, Nakatani S et al. Implications of a bioresorbable vascular scaffold implantation on vessel wall strain of the treated and the adjacent segments. *Int J Cardiovasc Imaging.* 2014;30:477–84.

26. Waksman R, Erbel R, Di Mario C, Bartunek J, de Bruyne B, Eberli FR, Erne P et al. Early- and long-term intravascular ultrasound and angiographic findings after bioabsorbable magnesium stent implantation in human coronary arteries. *JACC Cardiovasc Interv.* 2009;2:312–20.

27. Waksman R, Prati F, Bruining N, Haude M, Bose D, Kitabata H, Erne P et al. Serial observation of drug-eluting absorbable metal scaffold: Multi-imaging modality assessment. *Circ Cardiovasc Interv.* 2013;6:644–53.

# Optical coherence tomography analysis of bioresorbable vascular scaffolds in comparison with metallic stents: A core lab perspective

YOHEI SOTOMI, PANNIPA SUWANNASOM, JOUKE DIJKSTRA, CARLOS COLLET, SHIMPEI NAKATANI, PATRICK W.J.C. SERRUYS, AND YOSHINOBU ONUMA

## INTRODUCTION

The implantation of a bioresorbable scaffolds (BRSs) is a new approach that provides transient vessel support with drug delivery capability, potentially without the limitations of permanent metallic implants [1]. The potential short- and long-term performance of this technology has been repeatedly investigated with optical coherence tomography (OCT) [2–7]. However, images acquired by OCT after implantation of BRSs are different from those with metallic stents due to the translucency of polymeric materials compared to the opacity of metallic compounds (Figure 5.3.1). Metallic struts appear on OCT as a reflective leading structure with abluminal shadowing, while polymeric struts appear as a "black box" area surrounded by bright reflecting frames without abluminal shadowing. As a consequence, in polymeric scaffolds the vessel wall behind the struts and the luminal area can easily be imaged and assessed, contributing to several advantages in quantitative analysis: (1) capability of measuring the lumen vessel wall interface at baseline; (2) accurate assessment of malapposed struts; (3) measurement of strut/strut core area; (4) precise measurements of flow area; and (5) measurement of neointimal area between and on top of the struts.

In previous ABSORB studies of polymeric scaffolds without comparison with metallic stents, OCT methods were developed to take advantage of the optical properties of poly-L-lactic-acid (PLLA); however, some of these were not applicable to metallic stents. For example, strut core area is not directly measurable in metallic stents. To evaluate the performance of polymeric scaffolds and metallic stents fairly and comparably, it is important to use a standardized and comparative method for quantitative analysis on OCT rather than the conventional methods used in the metallic stent era.

In this chapter, we present the potential bias of conventional methodology and the consensus of multiple core labs and expert researchers of OCT on a standard methodology that enables us to compare two different devices using an almost identical, methodological language [8]. Additional specific analyses for BRSs are also summarized.

## POTENTIAL BIASES CAUSED BY APPLICATION OF CONVENTIONAL METHODS

The basic differences in the two OCT measurement methods for polymeric struts and metallic stents stem from the translucency of the polymeric device. The conventional bioresorbable methodology provides more parameters than metallic methods: the area occupied by the struts and tracing of the back of struts. These parameters influence the measurement and calculation of the scaffold area, lumen area, total strut area, flow area, and malapposition area. In some parameters (e.g., flow area), the conventional metallic methods are incomplete in that the strut area is ignored. When the conventional methods are applied for the comparison of the polymeric bioresorbable scaffold and the permanent metallic stents, the following methodological discrepancies lead to biased results postprocedure and at follow-up (Table 5.3.1).

### Stent (endoluminal)/scaffold (abluminal) area

Postprocedure (Figure 5.2.2), in metallic stents, the stent area is typically measured by interpolated contours connecting the endoluminal edge of the reflective border. In polymeric scaffolds, the scaffold area is measured by interpolated contours connecting the abluminal side of black

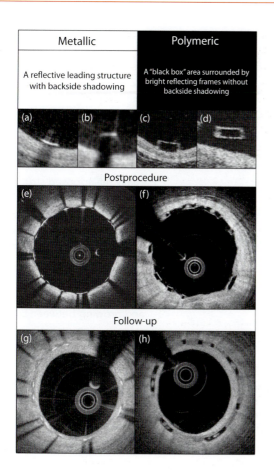

**Figure 5.3.1** The inherent differences between metallic stents and polymeric scaffolds on OCT. Representative appearance of metallic and polymeric struts is shown in **a–d**. Cross-sections postprocedure with well-apposed strut (**e** and **f**) and those at follow-up (**g** and **h**) are illustrated.

strut cores. The scaffold area of polymeric devices (abluminal) is expected to be systematically larger than the stent area of metallic devices (endoluminal).

Theoretically speaking, when a 3.0 mm ABSORB device with a strut thickness of 150 μm is deployed perfectly at the nominal size, endoluminal device area and abluminal device area are 7.07 mm² and 8.54 mm², respectively. In the clinical cases where the endoluminal stent area and endoluminal scaffold area are identical (7.07 mm²), the conventional stent area is measured on OCT as 7.07 mm², while the abluminal scaffold area is measured as 8.98 mm² (Figure 5.3.2). This causes the difference in reporting the stent/scaffold area of approximately 2 mm². The same is applicable to the follow-up up to 3 years. At a very long-term follow-up (>4 years), the scaffold area becomes difficult to measure due to the complete integration (disappearance) of the polymeric struts. In addition, this is not the case when the compared devices have the same struts thickness.

## Lumen area

The lumen area measured with BRSs methods includes the entire strut area, while the lumen area with metallic methods excludes some of the strut area. Therefore, the lumen area by BRSs methods tends to be larger than that by metallic methods (0.42 mm² on average).

Postprocedure (Figure 5.3.3), the luminal contour of metallic stents is generally traced somewhat behind the apposed strut and interpolated through the struts virtually. The embedded part of the metallic strut is excluded from the lumen area measurement. In polymeric devices, the embedded part of the polymeric strut (struts not buried) is fully included in the lumen area measurement.

At follow-up (Figure 5.3.4), the two methods do not cause discrepancy as long as all struts are apposed and covered. In the presence of uncovered metallic struts, the metallic lumen area tends to be smaller since the uncovered struts are excluded from the lumen.

## Total strut area

The abluminal edge of metallic struts cannot be visualized on OCT imaging due to the outer shadow. Therefore, the area occupied by metallic struts has not been quantified and taken into account in any measurements. In polymeric scaffolds, two areas have been measured for individual struts: (1) total strut area (tracing the outer boundary of the bright reflective frame), and (2) strut core area (tracing the black core). This inconsistency affects the lumen and flow area measurement both postprocedure (Figure 5.3.3) and at follow-up (Figure 5.3.4).

## Flow area

The flow area of metallic methods tends to be larger than that of BRS methods in the presence of malapposed struts. Flow area is defined as the cross-sectional area where the blood flows. This excludes any intraluminal structures (such as thrombus, malapposed struts, and their surrounding neointimal tissue). In metallic struts, due to the lack of direct measurement of metallic strut areas, the malapposed struts and surrounding tissues are typically included (Figure 5.3.3).

## Malapposed strut assessment

Postprocedure (Figure 5.3.3) and at follow-up (Figure 5.3.4), the frequency of malapposed struts is potentially overestimated with the metallic methods compared to BRSs methods. In the metallic stents, the struts are judged as malapposed when the distance from the midpoint of the bright leading edge to the interpolated lumen contour exceeds the strut thickness (including polymer, if present) as provided by the manufacturer. In this method, partially malapposed struts (a part of the strut is in contact with the vessel wall, which is invisible due to outer shadow) are counted as malapposed struts. In polymeric devices, the contact of struts with the vessel wall is directly visible. When any part of the strut is touching the vessel wall, the struts are judged as apposed.

**Table 5.3.1** Biased results postprocedure and at follow-up caused by methodological discrepancies

| | Metallic stent | Bias | Bioresorabable scaffold |
|---|---|---|---|
| **Postprocedure** | | | |
| Stent/scaffold area | Endoluminal | < | Abluminal |
| Lumen area | Embedded area of the struts is excluded | < | Total area of struts are included |
| Strut area | Not measured | < | Measured |
| Flow area | Protruding and malapposed area of struts are included | > | The area occupied by struts are excluded |
| Malapposed strut assessment | Partially malapposed struts are defined as malapposed struts | > | Partially malapposed struts are defined as apposed struts |
| Incomplete stent apposition area | Difference between endoluminal stent contour and lumen contour at malapposed struts | > | Difference between abluminal scaffold contour and lumen contour at malapposed struts |
| **At follow-up** | | | |
| Stent/scaffold area | Endoluminal | < | Abluminal |
| Neointimal area | Neointimal area on top of struts | < | Neointimal area on top of struts and growing between struts |
| Lumen area | Protruding part of the uncovered struts is included | < | Total area of struts are excluded |
| Strut (core) area | Not measured | < | Measured |
| Flow area | Area of struts without any tissue are included | > | Area of struts is excluded |
| Malapposed strut assessment | Struts with reflective bridge to vessel wall are defined as malapposed struts when the distance from the midpoint of bright leading edge to the lumen contour exceeds the strut thickness | > | Struts with reflective bridge to vessel wall are defined as apposed struts |
| Incomplete stent apposition area | Difference between endoluminal stent contour and lumen contour at malapposed struts | > | Difference between abluminal scaffold contour and lumen contour at malapposed struts |

At follow-up (Figure 5.3.4), with polymeric devices, when any part of the struts is connected to the vessel wall by an abluminal connecting bridge, a lateral connecting bridge, or a bilateral connecting bridge (directly visible), the struts are judged as apposed. With metallic stents, the back of the struts is invisible, so that, in the presence or absence of an abluminal connecting bridge, the struts are always judged as malapposed.

## Incomplete stent apposition area

Due to the discrepancy of the methods, the incomplete stent apposition (ISA) area in the polymeric scaffold is expected to be systematically smaller than that in the metallic stent both postprocedure (Figure 5.3.3) and at follow-up (Figure 5.3.4). Postprocedure, in metallic stents, the ISA area is defined as the area between the endoluminal leading edge of the metallic struts and the lumen contour at the site of malapposed struts. In polymeric scaffolds, this is defined as the area between the scaffold (abluminal) and the lumen contour.

## Neointimal area

The neointimal area measurement in metallic stents is expected to be systematically smaller than that of polymeric scaffolds (Figure 5.3.4). Metallic methods quantify the neointima on top of the struts, but ignore the neointima growing between the struts as well as the neointima surrounding the malapposed strut. In polymeric devices, the neointima growing between the strut and the neointima surrounding the malapposed strut are included in the neointimal area measurement.

## COMPARATIVE MEASUREMENT METHODS

To minimize/eliminate the discrepancy in measurement and reporting due to the difference in measurement, the following measurement methods are created in consensus among core labs and expert researchers. The most important changes are: standardization of device area measurement (abluminal or endoluminal) and the direct or virtual measurement of the area occupied by struts.

## Stent/scaffold area

### ABLUMINAL STENT/SCAFFOLD AREA

The measurement of abluminal device area represents the area of the device that interacts with the vessel wall. Furthermore, it will give the baseline landmark in measurement of a neointimal hyperplasia between and on top of the struts. In polymeric scaffolds, the abluminal scaffold contour is drawn by joining the midpoint of the abluminal side

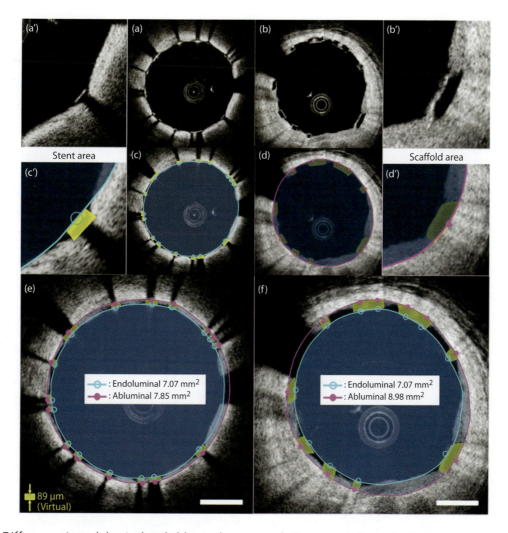

**Figure 5.3.2** Differences in endoluminal and abluminal stent area between metallic and polymeric struts. Metallic struts and polymeric struts postprocedure are shown in **(a)** and **(b)**. Conventional measurements of stent/scaffold area are indicated in **(c)** and **(d)**. **(a'–d')** Show magnified views of **(a–d)**. In the cases where the endoluminal stent area and endoluminal scaffold area are identical (7.07 mm$^2$), conventional stent area is measured as 7.07 mm$^2$ **(e)**, while abluminal scaffold area is measured as 8.98 mm$^2$ **(f)**.

of the black core in the apposed struts (Figures 5.3.5 and 5.3.6), or the abluminal edge of the reflective frame borders of malapposed struts (Figure 5.3.7).

Postprocedure (Figure 5.3.5) and at follow-up (Figure 5.3.6), in metallic stents, the abluminal stent contour cannot be directly delineated. Therefore, simulation of virtual strut contours is mandatory to delineate the abluminal stent contours. The automatic delineation of virtual struts and abluminal stent contour is currently possible only in custom-built research software. After identifying all struts in a cross-section, the abluminal stent contour is delineated by a curvilinear interpolation connecting the middle points of the abluminal edge of virtual metallic struts.

## ENDOLUMINAL STENT/SCAFFOLD AREA

Measurement of the endoluminal device area enables a direct comparison of the internal dimensions of the device. The endoluminal metallic stent contour is delineated by a curvilinear interpolation connecting the midpoints of the

endoluminal leading edge of the reflective border (Figure 5.3.5). At follow-up, the bright leading edge of the metallic strut is generally still detectable in the neointima (Figure 5.3.6).

The endoluminal polymeric scaffold contour is delineated by a curvilinear interpolation connecting the midpoint of the endoluminal side of the reflective frame. Whenever the polymeric reflective frame is not discernible, such as with buried struts in the vessel wall postprocedure or struts at follow-up, there is no other alternative and the leading edge of the black box in polymeric struts has to be compared with the bright leading edge of the metallic struts (Figure 5.3.6).

## Lumen area

Lumen contour is defined as the continuous interface between a blood and non-blood structure. Since any intraluminal structures isolated in the blood area are measured separately, the lumen area does not primarily exclude them

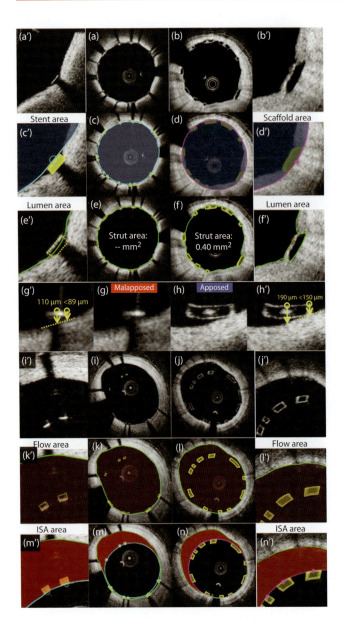

**Figure 5.3.3** Potential biases caused by application of conventional methods postprocedure. Representative cross-sections of apposed struts, stent/scaffold area measurement, lumen area measurement, apposition of struts, ISA, flow area measurement, and ISA area measurement are shown in **(a)**, **(c)**, **(e)**, **(g)**, **(i)**, **(k)**, **(m)** (metallic stents) and **(b)**, **(d)**, **(f)**, **(h)**, **(j)**, **(l)**, **(n)** (polymeric struts), respectively. **(a'–n')** are magnified views of **(a–n)**.

(intraluminal mass and isolated malapposed struts not connected to the vessel wall by a bridge) (Figures 5.3.7 and 5.3.8).

At follow-up, when the side-to-side bridge divides the vessel into a double channel lumen, the second lumen behind the bridge should be included in lumen area measurement (Figure 5.3.9c, d, m, n).

## Malapposed struts

In general, when the distance between the endoluminal surfaces of struts with respect to the interpolated lumen contour

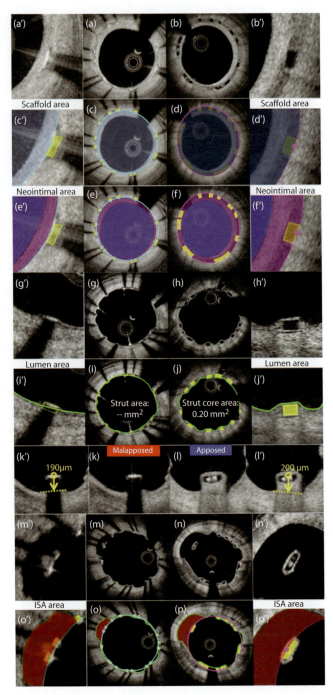

**Figure 5.3.4** Potential biases caused by application of conventional methods at follow-up. Representative cross-sections of covered struts, stent/scaffold area measurement, neointimal area measurement, uncovered struts, strut area or strut core area measurement, apposition of struts, ISA, ISA area measurement are shown in **(a)**, **(c)**, **(e)**, **(g)**, **(i)**, **(k)**, **(m)**, **(o)** (metallic stents) and **(b)**, **(d)**, **(f)**, **(h)**, **(j)**, **(l)**, **(n)**, **(p)** (polymeric struts), respectively. **(a'–p')** are magnified views of **(a–p)**.

is more than the strut thickness, either metallic or polymeric, the strut is considered a malapposed strut. It is measured at the midpoint of the endoluminal reflective border of metallic stents or the endoluminal side of the reflective frame of polymeric scaffolds (endoluminal ISA distance) (Figure 5.3.9).

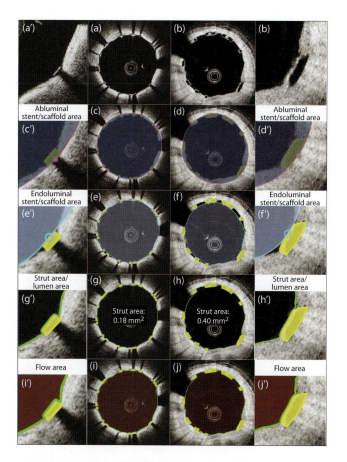

**Figure 5.3.5** Comparative analysis methods postprocedure in the cross-section without malapposed struts. Representative cross-sections with well-apposed metallic struts and polymeric struts are shown in **(a)** and **(b)**. Comparative methods of abluminal stent/scaffold area, endoluminal stent/scaffold area, strut area/lumen area, and flow area are illustrated in **(c)**, **(e)**, **(g)**, **(i)** (metallic strut), and **(d)**, **(f)**, **(h)**, **(j)** (polymeric strut), respectively. **(a'–j')** are the magnified views of **(a–j)**.

Postprocedure, the malapposition distance can also be measure as abluminal ISA distance which is the distance between the interpolated lumen contour and the back of the completely malapposed metallic or polymeric struts (abluminal reflective frame in polymeric struts and virtual back [= 89 μm from the bright leading edge] in metallic [XIENCE®; Abbott Vascular] struts) at the mid-point of the abluminal edge of the strut. An abluminal ISA distance greater than zero is the criterion of malapposition. When only part of the abluminal strut surface is in contact with the lumen contour, the malapposition is characterized as "partial malapposition." Even in case of partial malapposition, the abluminal and endoluminal ISA distance can be measured.

At follow-up, in polymeric scaffolds, the abluminal and endoluminal sides of the black core are used for the measurement of abluminal and endoluminal ISA distance, since the reflective bright frame cannot be distinguished from the neointima coverage.

In recent core lab experiences, we have observed on follow-up OCT that malapposed struts are sometimes

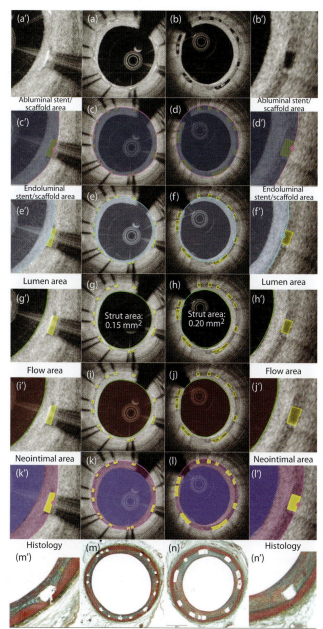

**Figure 5.3.6** Comparative analysis methods at follow-up in the cross-section of covered struts without malapposed struts. Representative cross-sections with well-covered metallic and polymeric struts at follow-up are shown in **(a)** and **(b)**, respectively. Abluminal stent/scaffold area, endoluminal stent/scaffold area, lumen area, flow area, and neointimal area are shown in **(c)**, **(e)**, **(g)**, **(i)**, **(k)** (metallic strut), and **(d)**, **(f)**, **(h)**, **(j)**, **(l)** (polymeric strut), respectively. Histomorphometric analyses of the animal models are shown in **(m)** (metallic strut) and **(n)** (polymeric strut). **(a'–n')** are the magnified views of **(a–n)**.

connected with the vessel wall by tissue created behind the struts or between the struts and vessel wall unilaterally or bilaterally. This aspect should be described and classified according to the type of connecting bridge (Figure 9): (1) malapposed struts without connecting bridge (isolated malapposed strut), (2) malapposed struts with a potentially thin abluminal connecting bridge, which could be masked by the shadow in metallic struts, (3) malapposed struts with an abluminal connecting bridge, (4) malapposed struts with a lateral connecting bridge, and (5) malapposed struts with a bilateral connecting bridge.

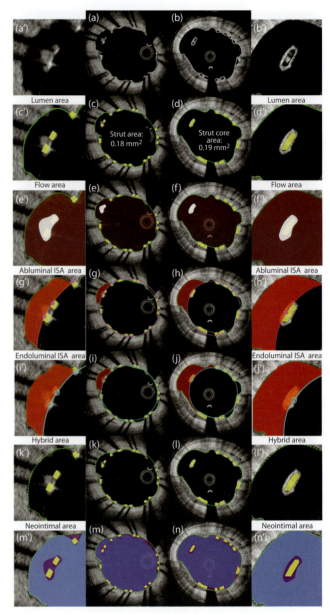

**Figure 5.3.8** Comparative analysis methods at follow-up in the presence of malapposed struts. Representative cross-sections with malapposed metallic and polymeric struts at follow-up are shown in **(a)** and **(b)**, respectively. Lumen area, flow area, abluminal ISA area, endoluminal ISA area, hybrid area, and neointimal area are shown in **(c)**, **(e)**, **(g)**, **(i)**, **(k)**, **(m)** (metallic strut) and **(d)**, **(f)**, **(h)**, **(j)**, **(l)**, **(n)** (polymeric strut), respectively. **(a'–n')** are the magnified views of **(a–n)**.

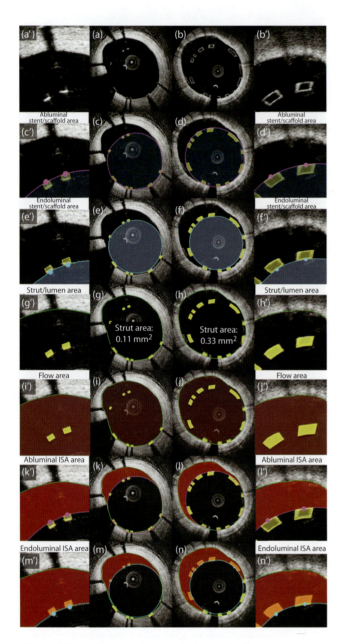

**Figure 5.3.7** Comparative analysis methods post-procedure in the presence of malapposed struts. Representative cross-sections with malapposed metallic struts and polymeric struts are shown in **(a)** and **(b)**. Comparative methods of abluminal stent/scaffold area, endoluminal stent/scaffold area, strut area/lumen area, flow area, endoluminal ISA area, and abluminal ISA area are illustrated in **(c)**, **(e)**, **(g)**, **(i)**, **(k)**, **(m)** (metallic strut), and **(d)**, **(f)**, **(h)**, **(j)**, **(l)**, **(n)** (polymeric strut), respectively. **(a'–n')** are the magnified views of **(a–n)**.

## Incomplete stent apposition area

The incomplete stent apposition (ISA) area is a part of the blood flow area located behind the malapposed struts. As described above, when the scaffold/stent area is drawn using the endoluminal and/or abluminal contours, the same principle should be applied for measurement of the ISA area.

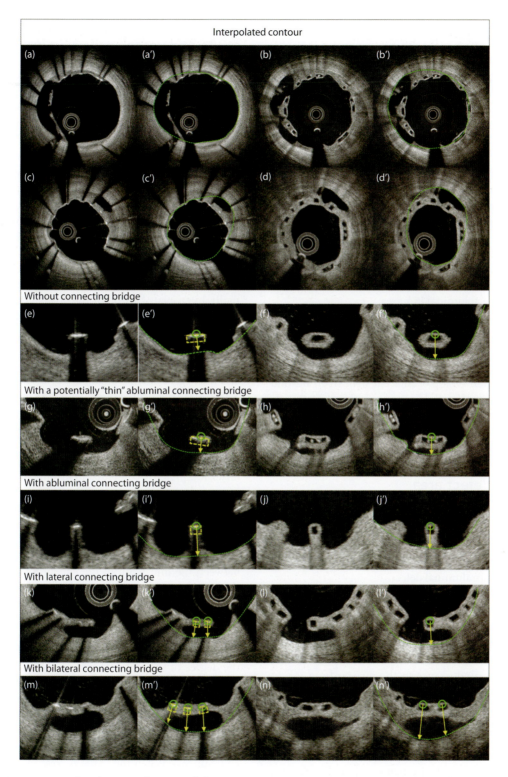

**Figure 5.3.9** Assessment of malapposed strut at follow-up. Representative cross-sections with malapposed metallic and polymeric struts at follow-up are shown in **(a)** and **(b)**, respectively. Classifications of malapposed struts are displayed in **(e–n)**. Malapposed struts without connecting bridge, those with a potentially thin backside connecting bridge, those with backside connecting bridge, those with lateral connecting bridge, and those with bilateral connecting bridge are shown in **(e)**, **(g)**, **(i)**, **(k)**, **(m)** (metallic strut), and **(f)**, **(h)**, **(j)**, **(l)**, **(n)** (polymeric strut), respectively. **(a'–n')** Display interpolated contour of **(a–n)**.

## ABLUMINAL INCOMPLETE STENT APPOSITION AREA

The abluminal ISA area is the difference between the abluminal stent/scaffold area and the lumen area at the site of malapposed metallic/polymeric struts (Figure 5.3.7). Although we could use endoluminal/abluminal ISA area, we favor the use of abluminal ISA area for consistency with the measurement of the flow area.

## ENDOLUMINAL INCOMPLETE STENT APPOSITION AREA

The endoluminal ISA area is the difference between the endoluminal scaffold/stent area and the lumen area at the site of malapposed polymeric/metallic struts (Figure 5.3.7). This parameter was used for the studies evaluating the metallic stents. However, as show in Figure 5.3.7, this area includes the malapposed strut itself in delineation, and therefore overestimates the malapposition area. It is recommended to use the abluminal ISA area.

## Prolapse area

Postprocedure, prolapse is a protrusion of the vessel wall structure between or on top of adjacent stent struts beyond the endoluminal stent/scaffold contour without disruption of the continuity of the lumen vessel surface [9] (modified from the previously published methodology [10]). At follow-up, this area is measured as a part of the neointima.

## Intraluminal defect area

An irregularly shaped structure in contact with the luminal contour is defined as an intraluminal defect attached to the vessel wall. The area of defect can be measured. An isolated structure in the lumen distant from the vessel wall is defined as a free intraluminal defect.

## Flow area

The flow area concept was introduced in 2010 to describe the vessel lumen filled by circulating blood, which reflects the blood supply conductance to the myocardium [6]. In order to exclude systematically the intraluminal structures attached to or free from the vessel wall, the measurement of malapposed struts with surrounding tissue is mandatory, either with direct measurement or by virtual simulation of the metallic strut area. The flow area can be calculated using the following formula: (lumen area [see the previous definition]) (second lumen area [if any]) − (intraluminal structures area [e.g., isolated intraluminal defect area, strut area of malapposed strut without surrounding tissue and malapposed strut with surrounding tissues not connected to the vessel wall including strut area, if any]) (Figures 5.3.5 through 5.3.8).

## Assessment of the interaction between the struts and vessel wall using interpolated lumen contour

In order to assess the strut–vessel wall interaction, the interpolated contour should be drawn at the site where the metallic or polymeric struts are embedded inside the vessel wall level. In case of a single protruding or malapposed strut, a short linear interpolation between the two edges should be used. In case of multi-strut extensive malapposition, a curvilinear interpolation should be used (Figure 5.3.9).

Postprocedure, this contour interpolates through the protruding metallic or polymeric struts. At follow-up, this contour should keep circularity and interpolate through the uncovered struts and the connecting reflective bridge of malapposed struts. However, it should be noted that the interpolated contour is the line of the lumen vessel wall virtually interpolated through the struts. Therefore, the area measurement according to this contour has no meaning from the biological point of view, but reflects the vessel wall injury.

Using the interpolated lumen contour, malapposition and the degree of embedment are assessed per strut (Figure 5.3.10) [11]. The degree of embedment could be the parameter of the vessel injury caused by the implantation of the scaffold/stent struts. Notably, the current BRSs has a larger surface (ABSORB: 26%) area compared to metallic stents (XIENCE: 12%). When the same force is applied, BRSs struts create less pressure compared to metallic struts, which could result in less embedment of BRSs struts [12]. Therefore, the reporting of the degree of embedment could be important to describe the difference in device-vessel interaction [11].

The degree of embedment (in percentage) could be calculated using the following formula: (1 − [the distance between the mid-point of the endolumnal strut surface to the interpolated lumen contour]/[the thickness of the strut (as indicated by the manufacturer)]) × 100 (%). Complete protruding is defined as the (virtual) abluminal surface of metallic or polymeric struts being aligned with the interpolated lumen contour line (i.e., 0% embedment). When the degree of the embedment is between 0% and 50%, the strut is classified as partially protruding. When the degree is between 50% and 100%, such struts are categorized as partially embedded. Complete embedment is defined as the endoluminal surface of metallic or polymeric struts being aligned with the interpolated lumen contour line (i.e., 100% embedment). When the tissue is covering the endoluminal surface of struts, the struts are considered buried. The algorithm and semi-automatic program for embedment analysis is reproducible and appear to be feasible to use in future studies [11].

The vessel wall lumen contour implicates the whole vessel wall which consists of a three-layer structure (intima, media, adventitia); these structures are deformed during stent/scaffold implantation, and therefore the vessel wall lumen contour should be drawn behind the abluminal side of metallic struts (virtual contour, taking into account the strut thickness) or the scaffold strut (visible contour of black core) at the site of apposed struts.

## Neointimal area

After an implantation of a coronary device, neointimal tissue grows not only on top of the struts but also between the struts as a response to the acute injury. In histomorphometry, the amount of neointimal tissue between the struts is quantified using the internal elastic membrane (IEM). On OCT, the abluminal scaffold/stent contour measured directly or virtually could serve as a landmark indicating the original lumen border (surrogate for an IEM), which enables quantification of a neointimal hyperplasia as in histomorphometry (Figure 5.3.6).

When all struts are apposed, the neointimal area is calculated as: (abluminal stent/scaffold area) − (lumen area + strut/strut core area). With this comparative method, the areas occupied by the metallic or polymeric struts are excluded, and the neointima between and on top of the struts is quantified. In the presence of any malapposed struts, there is a need to introduce the concept of a hybrid area, consisting of a combination of scaffold contour and lumen contour (Figure 5.3.8). The hybrid area is delineated by the abluminal side of the struts (abluminal stent/scaffold contour) of the apposed struts and by the interpolated lumen contour at malapposed struts (interpolated contour). According to these measurements, the neointimal area is calculated as: ([hybrid area] − [lumen area] − [apposed strut/strut core area]) + ([isolated malapposed strut with surrounding tissues area] − [malapposed strut/strut core area]).

The presence of neointima between struts could be described as: covered strut with complete inter-strut

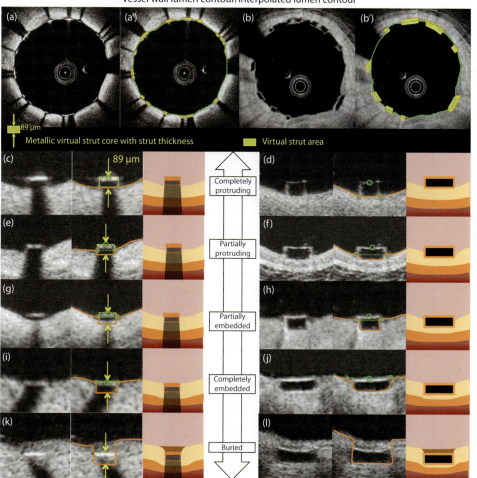

**Figure 5.3.10** Assessment of the interaction between the struts and vessel wall. Representative cross-sections with well-apposed metallic struts and polymeric struts are shown in **(a)** and **(b)**. **(a')** and **(b')** show the strut area measurement and interpolated lumen contour. Definitions of embedment based on the distance between strut and interpolated lumen contour are shown in **(c–l)**. Completely protruding, partially protruding, partially embedded, completely embedded, and buried struts are shown in **(c)**, **(e)**, **(g)**, **(i)**, **(k)** (metallic strut), and **(d)**, **(f)**, **(h)**, **(j)**, **(l)** (polymeric struts), respectively.

neointima, covered strut with incomplete inter-strut neo-intima, uncovered strut with complete inter-strut neo-intima, and uncovered strut with incomplete inter-strut neointima (Figure 5.3.11).

## Strut coverage

Coverage of polymeric struts and metallic stents should be assessed using different criteria (Figure 5.3.11). Typically, on OCT the polymeric struts look like black boxes surrounded by a bright frame, which is the interface between the blood and PDLLA/PLLA. Immediately after the implantation *in vivo* of BRSs, the thickness of the endoluminal bright border is measured as 30 μm on average [4]. The light intensity of neointimal tissue is similar to the bright border, and they are indistinguishable on visual assessment. Any tissue coverage on top of the struts should result in an increase of the thickness of the bright border: therefore, the threshold of coverage thickness ≥30 μm should be used to assess the coverage of the polymeric struts.

Regarding metallic struts, the coverage thickness of >0 μm (tissue can be identified above the struts) should be used to classify covered and uncovered struts.

In malapposed struts without an abluminal connecting bridge (Figure 5.3.9e, f, k–n), the coverage of the abluminal strut side should be assessed. The neointimal abluminal coverage at the back of the metallic or polymeric strut does not reflect the initial degree of malapposition, but reflects a biological attempt to create a connecting bridge between the struts and the lumen interface (Figure 5.3.9g, i, k, m).

The coverage thickness (neointimal thickness on top of struts) is defined as the distance between the luminal surface of the covering tissue and endoluminal reflective edge in metallic struts or endoluminal side of the black core in polymeric struts. In malapposed struts, it is possible to measure the thickness of the abluminal neointima.

In malapposed struts without an abluminal connecting bridge, the neointimal thickness should be measured on both the abluminal and endoluminal sides. The endoluminal neointimal thickness is defined as the distance from the

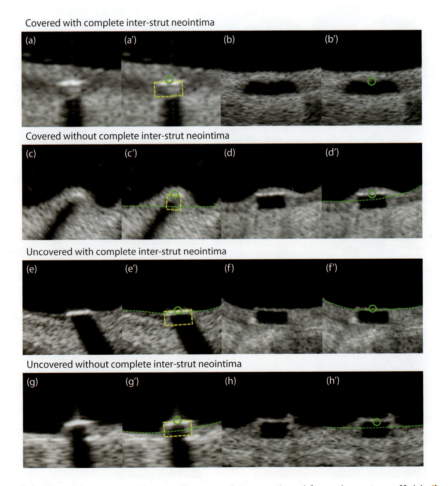

**Figure 5.3.11** Assessment of strut coverage. For metallic stents **(a, c, e, g)** and for polymeric scaffolds **(b, d, f, h)**, covered strut with complete inter-strut neointima **(a)** and **(b)**, covered strut with incomplete inter-strut neointima **(c)** and **(d)**, uncovered with complete inter-strut neointima **(e)** and **(f)**, and uncovered strut with incomplete inter-strut neointima **(g)** and **(h)** are displayed. Regarding metallic struts, the coverage thickness of >0 μm (tissue can be identified above the struts) should be used to classify covered **(a, c)** and uncovered struts **(e, g)**. As for polymeric scaffolds, any tissue coverage on top of the struts should result in an increase of the thickness of the bright border: therefore, thickness of bright border ≥30 μm is defined as covered **(b, d)** whereas the thickness <30 μm is defined as uncovered **(f, h)**. **(a'–h')** displays interpolated contour of **(a–h)**.

abluminal side of the strut (abluminal side of the black core in a polymeric strut or that of a virtual strut in a metallic stent) to the neointima-lumen interface, following a straight line connecting the midpoint of the longitudinal axis of the strut with the center of gravity of the lumen. We use the back of metallic or polymeric struts to take into account the initial degree of malapposition postprocedure.

## LIMITATIONS OF THE CURRENT COMPARATIVE METHOD

The comparative OCT method is applicable specifically for the ABSORB scaffolds, and in general for metallic stents. Among PLLA-based scaffolds, there is considerable variance in the initial molecular weight, the presence of a copolymer, the purity of PLLA (monomer, solvent) and postprocessing methods (extrusion, annealing, microbraiding, etc.), which could influence the bioresorption time and optical properties of struts (OCT imaging). For example, the same methods could be used at baseline for the other PLLA devices such as ART® BRSs (Arterial Remodeling Technologies, Noisy-le-Roi, France), Amaranth FORTITUDE® (Amaranth Medical, Inc., CA), and DESolve® (Elixir Medical, Sunnyvale, CA) but not for the Mirage PLLA scaffold (ManLi Cardiology, Singapore). OCT appearances of different types of bioresorbable scaffold are summarized in Figure 5.3.12. On OCT, the strut of the Mirage scaffold is bright at implantation, and therefore OCT cannot measure its dimensions. Regarding

the ART, Amaranth, and DESolve scaffolds, the proposed methods may not be applicable at follow-up due to the different resorption times. The general concept of measuring endoluminal and abluminal scaffold contours and strut area should be applied for the other PLLA technologies, but the details of analysis (follow-up method) should be fine-tuned for each individual device.

After the integration of a bioresorbable scaffold to the vessel wall, we can no longer use the measurement of scaffold area, neointimal area, and ISA area (if present), and at long-term follow-up we can only compare the flow area between metallic stents and bioresorbable scaffolds. We therefore emphasize the accurate measurement of flow area in the currently proposed methods.

In metallic stents, it could be challenging to simulate the area occupied by a strut and the location of the abluminal surface of the strut by drawing a virtual square with a length that is equivalent to the known strut plus polymer (if present) thickness. To the best of our knowledge, we do not have commercially available software that enables us to depict the abluminal metallic stent contour with the strut thickness automatically, which could result in limited reproducibility in the measurements. In addition, the virtual metallic struts should be drawn considering the limitations of OCT images in the following cross-sections: (1) in the cross-section with suboptimal flushing, the stent struts are illustrated as blurred and enlarged due to the low lateral resolution, (2) in the cross-section when the OCT catheter is

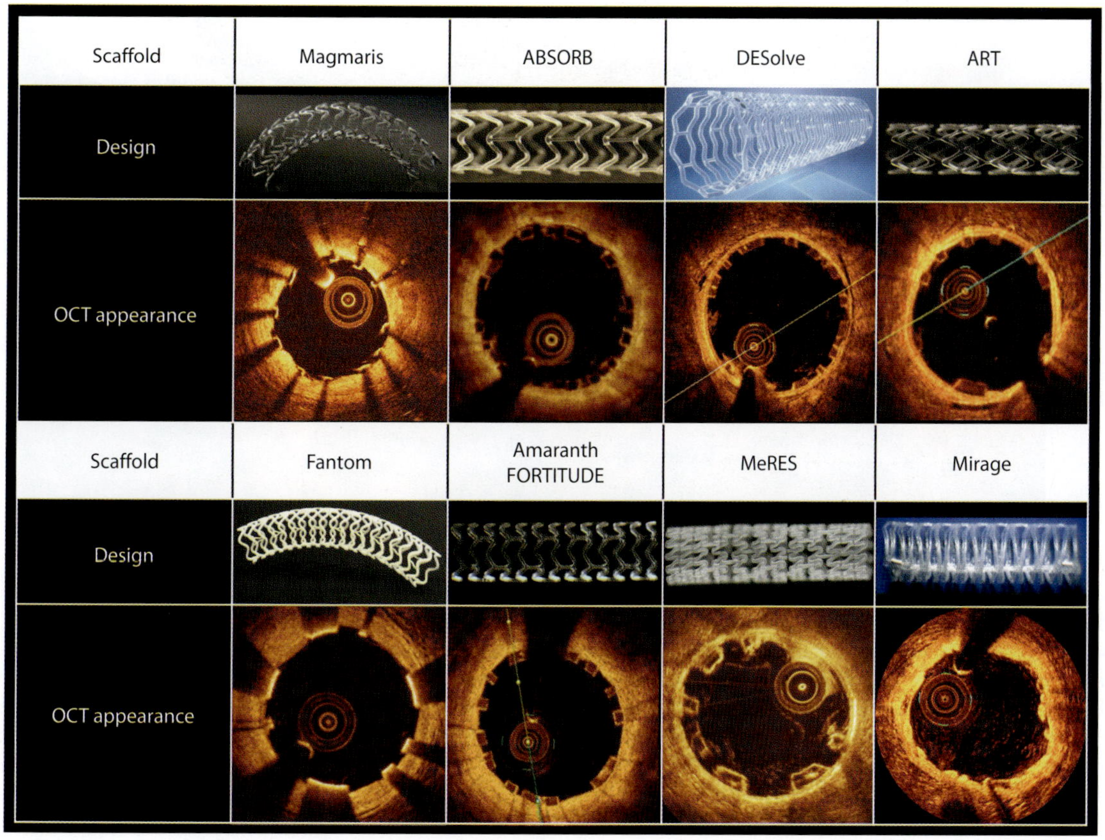

**Figure 5.3.12** OCT appearances of different types of bioresorbable scaffolds.

located toward one side of the vessel, the stent struts appear to face the catheter (strut orientation artifact) [13].

## ADDITIONAL SPECIFIC ANALYSIS FOR BRSs

### Light intensity analysis

The relationship between OCT findings and histology focusing on the bioresorption and integration process was evaluated visually, resulting in a fair reproducibility (the value of interobserver agreement was 0.58) [14]. The representative images of histology and OCT are illustrated in Figure 5.3.13 [15]. Compared to the qualitative visual assessment, the light intensity analysis is a quantitative assessment of the strut cores on OCT with a high reproducibility (interobserver intraclass correlation coefficient = 0.92) [16]. Nakatani et al. demonstrated the clear relationship between the normalized light intensity on OCT and integration process using the 73 nonatherosclerotic swine models that received 112 BRSs (Figure 5.3.14) [17]. The quantitative light intensity analysis of strut cores on OCT can be used as a surrogate method for monitoring the matrix infiltration and integration of

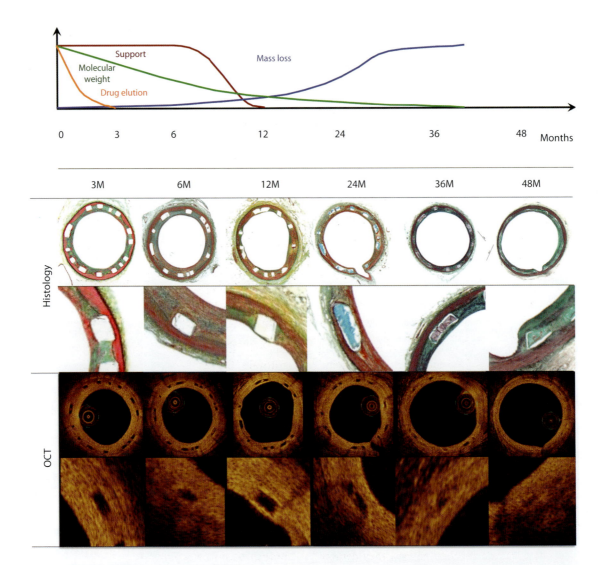

**Figure 5.3.13** Phases of bioresorbable scaffold functionality. The three phases of BRSs functionality include mechanical support and drug delivery functions during the revascularization phase; the loss of radial rigidity and mechanical restraint during the restoration phase, during which cyclic pulsatility and vasomotion return; and resorption caused by mass loss with return of adaptive vascular remodeling responses. The time course for phases/changes noted on the top is specific for the ABSORB bioresorbable vascular scaffold. Molecular weight starts to decrease immediately after implantation, and drug elution is almost complete at 3 months. Radial support decreases at ≈6 months and is minimal at 12 months. Representative histology and optical coherence tomography (OCT) images are from Yucatan swine. On OCT, the struts are sequestered from the lumen by fibromuscular neointima at 3 to 6 months. At 24 months, with progressive mass loss, the strut footprints begin to be replaced by provisional matrix (histology) while still discernible as black cores (OCT). At 36 months, mass loss is complete, and infiltration of connective tissue into strut voids makes the struts invisible on OCT between 36 and 48 months.

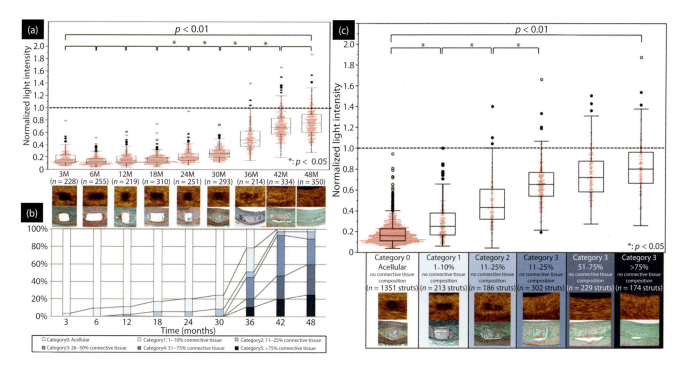

**Figure 5.3.14** Normalized light intensity and histological findings in matched strut cores. Panel **(a)** illustrates whisker plots combined with scatter plots of matched strut cores in normalized light intensity (dimensionless) overtime. The normalized light intensity increased graduall y between 18 and 30 months, then surged between 30 and 42 months, and approached close to 1.0 at 48 months. Panel **(b)** demonstrates the changes in histological categories of struts over time. The rate of acellular struts decreased gradually during the first 30 months, and then abruptly decreased 75.5% at 30 months to 13.6% at 36 months. Spontaneously, the frequency of moderately to highly integrated struts (histological grade ≥3) increased from 0.7% to 94% between 30 and 42 months. After 42 months, there was no strut without integration. Panel **(c)** represents the correlation between normalized light intensity on OCT and histological categorization in whisker plots in combination with scatter plots. The normalized light intensity was significantly different between category 0 and 1 ($p < 0.05$), between category 1 and 2 ($p < 0.05$), and between category 2 and 3 ($p < 0.05$). There were no significant differences in normalized light intensity between category 3, 4, and 5. M = months.

collagen-rich connective tissue within the polymeric struts that coincides with the time of the late lumen enlargement.

## Light attenuation analysis

Karanasos et al. reported the light attenuation analysis for quantitative tissue characterization of the signal-rich layer and the neoplaque 5 years after BRSs implantation (ABSORB Cohort A) [2]. In *ex vivo* validation experiments, highly attenuating regions (attenuation coefficient $\mu_t \geq 8$ mm$^{-1}$) have been associated with necrotic core or macrophages. Conversely, $\mu_t < 6$ mm$^{-1}$ was associated with healthy vessel, intimal thickening, or calcified plaque [18,19]. Using the light attenuation analysis, they demonstrated the developed endoluminal signal-rich layer which showed remarkable homogeneity in the attenuation analysis, with low attenuation values hinting at the absence of high-risk wall components such as necrotic core and macrophages (Figure 5.3.15).

## Three-dimensional side branch analysis

Jailed side branch by BRSs can be analyzed qualitatively and quantitatively with the recently validated "cut-plane"

method in 3D-OCT analysis with the QAngioOCT software (Medis Specials BV, Leiden, the Netherlands) (Figure 5.3.16) [20].

The position and orientation of the cut-plane was set using the cross-sectional and longitudinal images as follows: (1) In the cross-sectional image, the cut-plane line was oriented in such way that it was perpendicular to the lumen center, through the center of the struts (Figure 5.3.16b). (2) In the longitudinal image, the cut-plane was arranged in such a way that it was in parallel to the longitudinal strut line (Figure 5.3.16c). The "depth" of the cut-plane was set to 200 pixels (Figure 5.3.16d). In the created cut-plane, the number of compartments in which the side branch ostium was separated was qualitatively assessed (Figure 5.3.16e, middle panel). Contours of these compartments were drawn manually after which the surface area of the compartment was calculated automatically by the software (Figure 5.3.16e, right panel). The "ostium free from struts area" was defined as the sum of the surface areas of all compartments (Figure 5.3.16e, right panel).

Onuma et al. evaluated the fate of jailed side branches by BRSs in the ABSORB Cohort B data using this methodology. The study showed that the relatively new cut-plane

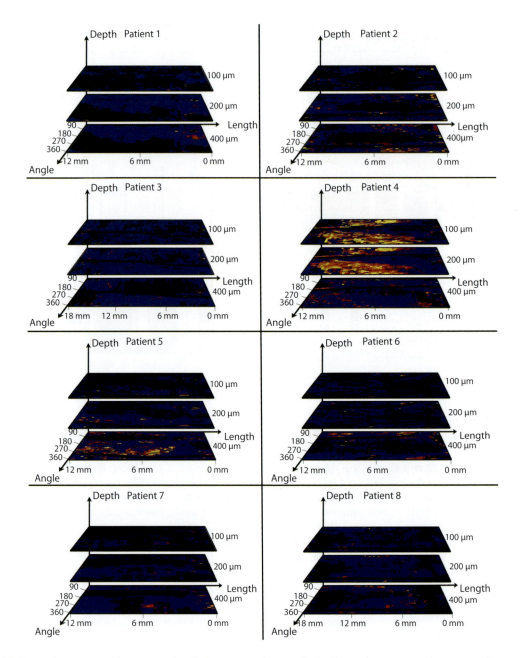

**Figure 5.3.15** Spread-out maps demonstrating light attenuation analysis. Spread-out maps demonstrating attenuation coefficient in predefined depths from the vessel surface (100, 200, and 400 µm) per patient (#1–8). In most patients, there was a low-attenuating layer of 200 µm separating the underlying plaque (starting at ~400 µm) from the lumen. In Patient #4, this layer was absent, and attenuating areas were close to the lumen.

methodology is feasible and reproducible to assess side branch ostium free from strut areas at different follow-up time points. Furthermore, the study showed that in most cases, the ostium area free from struts initially decreases from postprocedure to subsequent follow-up time points, with a coinciding decrease in the number of compartments due to compartment closure. However, after full bioresorption of the scaffold, the surface of the compartments that remained patent gradually increased from 2/3 years to 5 years in the vast majority. Several patterns of the fate of jailed side branches are demonstrated in Figure 5.3.17. Understanding the differential mechanisms of the different

fate of the jailed side branches would be important and essential for future bifurcation treatment using BRSs. The "cut-plane" method in 3D-OCT analysis would be helpful for the precise analysis on this matter.

## SUMMARY

Compared to metallic stents, BRSs have different optical properties. Therefore, the comparative methodology for OCT assessment needs to be employed. In comparison with the conventional OCT measurement method, the comparative OCT method is summarized as follows: (1) Both

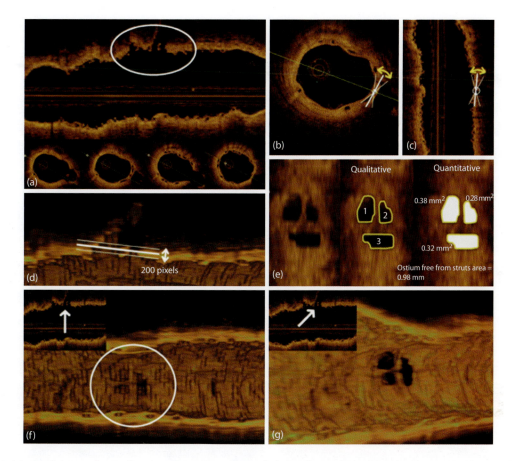

**Figure 5.3.16** Methodology of cut-plane analysis. First, the side branch was located using the cross-sectional and longitudinal images **(a)**. Then, the appropriate orientation for the cut-plane was set in the cross-sectional **(b)** and longitudinal **(c)** image. Then, the cut-plane thickness was set to 200 pixels to capture both the struts as well as the side branch ostium in one plane **(d)**. Two analyses were performed on the cut-plane: a qualitative (number of compartments) and a qualitative (surface areas of compartments) **(e)**. Panels **f** and **g** show the benefit of cut-plane analysis over the 3D-OCT analysis in which the orientation toward the side branch determines the ostial areas: when having a perpendicular viewing angle, it seems there is not even a side branch **(f)**; however, when taking a more oblique view, it is clear there is a side branch separated in three ostia **(g)**.

endoluminal and abluminal scaffold/stent contours should be traced. (2) Consistently, endoluminal and abluminal ISA area should be measured. (3) The area occupied by scaffold/stent struts should be quantified directly or virtually. (4) The strut area should be systematically excluded from the flow area as well as the neointimal area. (5) Additional information on the degree of the embedment could be reported using the interpolated lumen contour. Additional OCT analyses (light intensity analysis, light attenuation analysis, and 3D-OCT side branch analysis) would be helpful to understand the mechanisms of the fate of BRSs more accurately and comprehensively.

# REFERENCES

1. Serruys PW, Garcia-Garcia HM and Onuma Y. From metallic cages to transient bioresorbable scaffolds: Change in paradigm of coronary revascularization in the upcoming decade? *Eur Heart J*. 2012;33:16–25b.

2. Karanasos A, Simsek C, Gnanadesigan M, van Ditzhuijzen NS, Freire R, Dijkstra J, Tu S et al. OCT assessment of the long-term vascular healing response 5 years after everolimus-eluting bioresorbable vascular scaffold. *J Am Coll Cardiol*. 2014;64:2343–56.

3. Ormiston JA, Serruys PW, Onuma Y, van Geuns RJ, de Bruyne B, Dudek D, Thuesen L et al. First serial assessment at 6 months and 2 years of the second generation of absorb everolimus-eluting bioresorbable vascular scaffold: A multi-imaging modality study. *Circ Cardiovasc Interv*. 2012;5:620–32.

4. Serruys PW, Onuma Y, Dudek D, Smits PC, Koolen J, Chevalier B, de Bruyne B et al. Evaluation of the second generation of a bioresorbable everolimus-eluting vascular scaffold for the treatment of de novo coronary artery stenosis: 12-month clinical and imaging outcomes. *J Am Coll Cardiol*. 2011;58:1578–88.

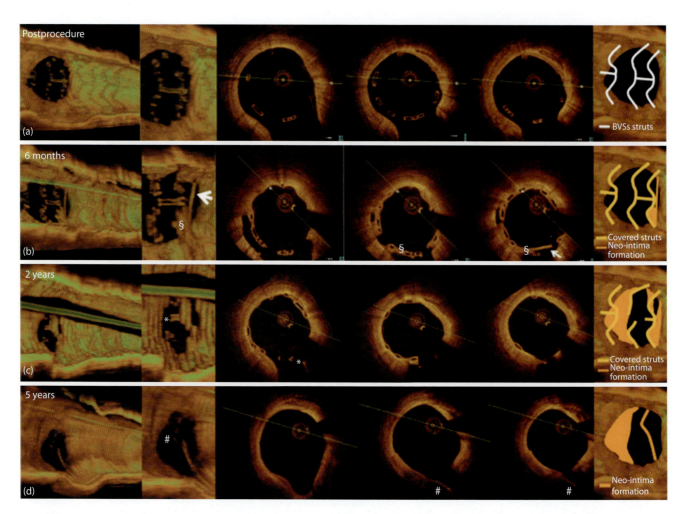

**Figure 5.3.17** Fate of BRS struts jailing a large septal branch. Panels **a–d** show the 2D and 3D optical coherence tomography (OCT) findings after placement of a bioresorbable vascular scaffolds (BVSs) jailing a large septal branch. The panels on the outer right indicate a schematic drawing of our interpretation of the fate of the jailed struts. Panel **a** shows 2D and 3D findings directly postprocedure. 3D reconstruction shows separation of the ostium in six compartments, 2D OCT still frames show malapposition of the BVSs struts. Panel **b** shows 2D and 3D OCT findings of the same side branch at 6 months' follow-up. The malapposed struts are connected with lateral neo-intimal tissue bridges. In-between the jailed side branch struts, the formation of a neo-intimal tissue membrane was visualized (§). In addition, there was a neo-intimal tissue "bowstring" connecting the strut and the rim of the side branch ostium (white arrows). Panel **c** shows the jailed side branch at 2 years. 3D reconstruction clearly shows that the ostium is divided in only two compartments due to occlusion of the three most proximal compartments by a neo-intimal tissue membrane. From the initial three most distal compartments, two were merged into one because of breaking of a strut linking two subsequent hoops (*). Panel **d** shows complete resorption of the BVSs at 5 years, without any discernable struts at 2D-OCT. 3D-OCT reveals two compartments, separated by a tissue bridge (#).

5. Serruys PW, Onuma Y, Garcia-Garcia HM, Muramatsu T, van Geuns RJ, de Bruyne B, Dudek D et al. Dynamics of vessel wall changes following the implantation of the absorb everolimus-eluting bioresorbable vascular scaffold: A multi-imaging modality study at 6, 12, 24 and 36 months. *EuroIntervention. Journal of EuroPCR in Collaboration with the Working Group on Interventional Cardiology of the European Society of Cardiology.* 2014;9:1271–84.

6. Serruys PW, Onuma Y, Ormiston JA, de Bruyne B, Regar E, Dudek D, Thuesen L et al. Evaluation of the second generation of a bioresorbable everolimus

drug-eluting vascular scaffold for treatment of de novo coronary artery stenosis: Six-month clinical and imaging outcomes. *Circulation.* 2010;122:2301–12.

7. Serruys PW, Ormiston JA, Onuma Y, Regar E, Gonzalo N, Garcia-Garcia HM, Nieman K et al. A bioabsorbable everolimus-eluting coronary stent system (ABSORB): 2-year outcomes and results from multiple imaging methods. *Lancet.* 2009;373:897–910.

8. Nakatani S, Sotomi Y, Ishibashi Y, Grundeken MJ, Tateishi H, Tenekecioglu E, Zeng Y et al. Comparative analysis method of permanent

metallic stents (XIENCE) and bioresorbable poly-L-lactic (PLLA) scaffolds (Absorb) on optical coherence tomography at baseline and follow-up. *EuroIntervention. Journal of EuroPCR in Collaboration with the Working Group on Interventional Cardiology of the European Society of Cardiology.* 2015;11.

9. Muramatsu T, Garcia-Garcia HM, Onuma Y, Zhang YJ, Bourantas CV, Diletti R, Iqbal J et al. Intimal flaps detected by optical frequency domain imaging in the proximal segments of native coronary arteries: An innocent bystander? Insights from the TROFI Trial. *Circ J.* 2013;77:2327–33.

10. Gonzalo N, Serruys PW, Okamura T, Shen ZJ, Onuma Y, Garcia-Garcia HM, Sarno G et al. Optical coherence tomography assessment of the acute effects of stent implantation on the vessel wall: A systematic quantitative approach. *Heart.* 2009;95:1913–9.

11. Sotomi Y, Tateishi H, Suwannasom P, Dijkstra J, Eggermont J, Liu S, Tenekecioglu E et al. Quantitative assessment of the stent/scaffold strut embedment analysis by optical coherence tomography. *Int J Cardiovasc Imaging.* 2016.

12. Serruys PW, Suwannasom P, Nakatani S and Onuma Y. Snowshoe versus ice skate for scaffolding of disrupted vessel wall. *JACC Cardiovasc Interv.* 2015;8:910–3.

13. Tearney GJ, Regar E, Akasaka T, Adriaenssens T, Barlis P, Bezerra HG, Bouma B et al. Consensus standards for acquisition, measurement, and reporting of intravascular optical coherence tomography studies: A report from the International Working Group for Intravascular Optical Coherence Tomography Standardization and Validation. *J Am Coll Cardiol.* 2012;59:1058–72.

14. Onuma Y, Serruys PW, Perkins LE, Okamura T, Gonzalo N, Garcia-Garcia HM, Regar E et al. Intracoronary optical coherence tomography and histology at 1 month and 2, 3, and 4 years after implantation of everolimus-eluting bioresorbable vascular scaffolds in a porcine coronary artery model: An attempt to decipher the human optical coherence tomography images in the ABSORB trial. *Circulation.* 2010;122:2288–300.

15. Kereiakes DJ, Onuma Y, Serruys PW and Stone GW. Bioresorbable vascular scaffolds for coronary revascularization. *Circulation.* 2016;134:168–82.

16. Nakatani S, Onuma Y, Ishibashi Y, Eggermont J, Zhang YJ, Campos CM, Cho YK et al. Temporal evolution of strut light intensity after implantation of bioresorbable polymeric intracoronary scaffolds in the ABSORB cohort B trial-an application of a new quantitative method based on optical coherence tomography. *Circ J.* 2014;78:1873–81.

17. Nakatani S, Ishibashi Y, Sotomi Y, Perkins L, Eggermont J, Grundeken MJ, Dijkstra J et al. Bioresorption and vessel wall integration of a fully bioresorbable polymeric everolimus-eluting scaffold: Optical coherence tomography, intravascular ultrasound, and histological study in a porcine model with 4-year follow-up. *JACC Cardiovasc Interv.* 2016;9:838–51.

18. van Soest G, Goderie T, Regar E, Koljenovic S, van Leenders GL, Gonzalo N, van Noorden S et al. Atherosclerotic tissue characterization in vivo by optical coherence tomography attenuation imaging. *J Biomed Opt.* 2010;15:011105.

19. Ughi GJ, Adriaenssens T, Sinnaeve P, Desmet W and D'Hooge J. Automated tissue characterization of in vivo atherosclerotic plaques by intravascular optical coherence tomography images. *Biomed Opt Express.* 2013;4:1014–30.

20. Karanasos A, Tu S, van Ditzhuijzen NS, Ligthart JM, Witberg K, Van Mieghem N, van Geuns RJ et al. A novel method to assess coronary artery bifurcations by OCT: Cut-plane analysis for side-branch ostial assessment from a main-vessel pullback. *Eur Heart J Cardiovasc Imaging.* 2015;16:177–89.

# Noninvasive coronary computed tomography analysis after bioresorbable scaffold implantation

CARLOS COLLET, KOEN NIEMAN, PATRICK W.J.C. SERRUYS, AND YOSHINOBU ONUMA

## INTRODUCTION

Noninvasive coronary computed tomography angiography has shown to be an accurate method for the exclusion of significant coronary artery stenosis, with negative predictive values of 97%–99% [1,2]. However, in patients previously treated with percutaneous coronary interventions, the artifact from the metallic stent precludes appropriate luminal assessment [3]. In contrast, the bioresorbable vascular scaffold (ABSORB, Abbott Vascular, Santa Clara, CA) has a translucent polymeric backbone that allows for noninvasive coronary computed tomography angiography (CTA) [4].

In the first-in-human studies, ABSORB cohorts A and B, coronary CTA showed to be feasible at mid- and long-term follow-up. In these studies, in-scaffold luminal dimensions were quantitatively analyzed at the cross-section level. Additionally, to investigate the functional component of the treated vessel, the three-dimensional geometry was extracted and processed with computational fluid dynamics to obtain the noninvasive fractional flow reserve ($FFR_{CT}$) [5,6]. The comprehensive evaluation of the anatomy and physiology of the scaffolded region makes coronary CTA an attractive method for the follow-up of patients treated with bioresorbable vascular scaffolds.

## ACQUISITION AND RECONSTRUCTION OF CORONARY CTA IMAGES FOR SCAFFOLD EVALUATION

The recommendations for image acquisition for scaffold evaluation are similar to the recommendations for native coronary vessels [7]. Nevertheless, the required image quality is higher than for routine clinical exclusion of coronary artery disease (CAD). High-image quality and avoidance of artifacts are essential to allow quantitative assessment of the coronary arteries. The acquisition protocol should contemplate heart rate modulation with beta-blocker for heart rates ≥65/min during breath holding with the systematic use of coronary vasodilators (i.e., nitroglycerin). In addition, reconstructions aimed at improving the assessment of high-density material (radio-opaque platinum markers) should be added (i.e., thin slices and sharp reconstruction filters). The reconstruction should be optimized for the scaffolded segments, using different phases if necessary. In the ABSORB studies, tube settings depended on patient body mass index (80–140 kV), and axial scan protocols for patients with lower heart rates were recommended as radiation reduction strategies [5]. The coronary CTA were performed with CT scanners of at least 64 detectors [6].

## CORONARY CTA ANALYSIS

The selection of the best phase for analysis is an important step in the screening process. The assessment of the images should focus on the treated segment. It might be necessary to evaluate different phases to obtain the best image for analysis. Image quality is then classified as good, sufficient for analysis, or of poor quality. The presence of artifacts (e.g., motion artifacts, step artifact, and bean hardening artifact) should be described. After the selection of the best image, the automatic vessel extraction and segmentation are performed, and the treated vessel is selected for analysis.

### Qualitative analysis

Scrolling of transaxial images allows displaying the course of the treated vessel and assists identifying the radio-opaque markers located at each edge of the scaffold. Subsequently,

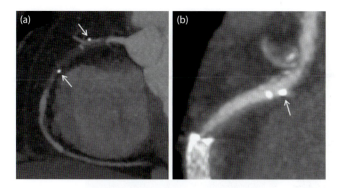

**Figure 5.4.1** Coronary CTA qualitative assessment of bioresorbable scaffold. Panel **a** shows a total occlusion at the level of a bioresorbable vascular scaffold in the proximal segment of the right coronary artery (white arrows shows the radio-opaque markers). Panel **b** shows a severe coronary stenosis in the distal part of a bioresorbable vascular scaffold in the transition to a metallic stent; note that the metal obscures the distal radio-opaque marker.

multi-planar reformation (MPR) enables rotating the vessel and the scaffolded segment on its longitudinal axis through 360 degrees. Using these maneuvers, a qualitative assessment of luminal and area stenosis of the scaffolded segment is performed. The qualitative grading of the stenosis follows the recommendations from the Society of Cardiovascular Computed Tomography (normal, minimal <25% stenosis, mild 25–49% stenosis, moderate 50–69% stenosis, severe 70–99% stenosis and occluded). In addition, the presence of other angiographic abnormalities should be described (Figure 5.4.1). Qualitative assessment of plaque composition is also performed in the scaffolded segment and proximal and distal edges. The number of cross-sections with noncalcified plaque, mixed plaque, and calcified plaque (noncalcified plaque ≤20% of total plaque area) is registered [7].

## Quantitative analysis

Luminal and vessel segmentation is visually assessed in the MPR images. To define the scaffolded region, the platinum scaffold markers are used as landmarks [8]. Automatic lumen segmentation of the vessel lumen with manual correction is performed to measure the lumen area. The cross-section analysis is performed every 1 mm, extending 5 mm beyond the device (Figures 5.4.2 and 5.4.3) [1]. The display settings are set as follows: 750 Hounsfield units; width, 250 Hounsfield units, with adjustment if necessary. The mean lumen area, minimal lumen area (MLA), and maximum lumen area are determined for each scaffold. The reference lumen area is calculated as the average between the mean vessel area proximal and distal to the scaffolded segment. The percentage of luminal area stenosis is calculated as the difference between the MLA and the reference as a percentage of the reference. A significant area of stenosis is

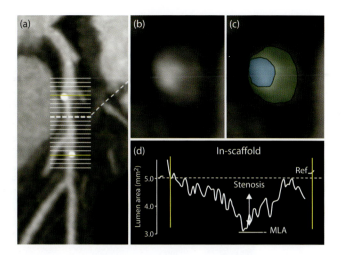

**Figure 5.4.2** Coronary CTA quantitative assessment of bioresorbable scaffold. In a multiplanar reformat image (panel **a**), the region of interest is analyzed longitudinally every 1 mm for luminal and vessel segmentation. At the level of the MLA (white dash line), contour tracing (panels **b** and **c**) quantify a luminal area of 3.22 mm$^2$. Panel **d** shows the in-scaffold lumen area curve, with the localization of the minimal lumen area (MLA).

defined as ≥75%, which approximates 50% diameter stenosis. At the level of the radio-opaque marker cross-section, the prolongation of the luminal through the center marker is recommended [5]. In a similar way, in case of calcification, a blooming artifact is assumed and luminal contour is exaggerated maintaining the circular to ellipsoid shape of the vessel lumen.

## EXPERIENCE IN THE ABSORB TRIALS

Several reports of the use of cardiac CTA for in-scaffold evaluation have been published. In the ABSORB Cohort A, the feasibility of early postimplantation cardiac CTA (72 hours) was demonstrated. A small bias was observed in CTA-derived scaffold area and length as compared to the nominal area (i.e., 7.07 mm$^2$ luminal area in 3-mm scaffold nominal diameter) and length (18 mm) [8]. In ABSORB cohort A, serial coronary CTA at 18 and 60 months was performed in 18 patients. Quantitative analysis was feasible in all patients (n = 18). All scaffold were patients with a median minimal lumen area of 3.25 mm$^2$ (interquartile range 2.20–4.30) [6]. In the ABSORB Cohort B, the new iteration of the bioresorbable vascular scaffold was evaluated with multimodality imaging. Coronary CTA was performed at 18 and 72 months. In 39 patients with serial CTA, quantitative analysis was feasible in 87% of the cases. In this series, a significant increase in mean and minimal lumen area was found. In addition, plaque composition significantly changed, with an increase in the calcified component of the plaque behind the scaffold compared to baseline [9].

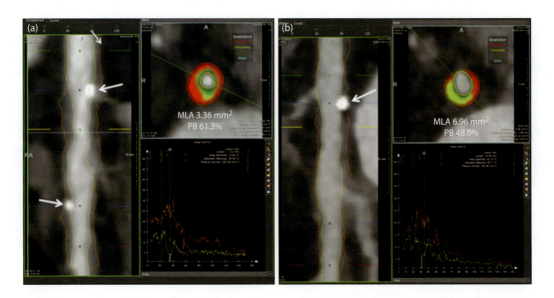

**Figure 5.4.3** Noninvasive serial evaluation with coronary CTA in a patient treated with a bioresorbable vascular scaffold (BVS). In panel **a**, at 18 months after implantation the treated region is identified by the two radio-opaque markers (white arrows). After automatic detection of the lumen (yellow line) and the vessel (orange) boundaries, the MLA is identified with an area of 3.36 mm$^2$ and a plaque burden of 61.3%. At 6-year follow-up (panel **b**), a significant increase in lumen dimension is observed with an MLA of 6.96 mm$^2$ and a 48.6% decrease in plaque burden. These images were analyzed with QAngio CT Research Edition v 3.0.14. CTA = computed tomography angiography; MLA = minimal lumen area.

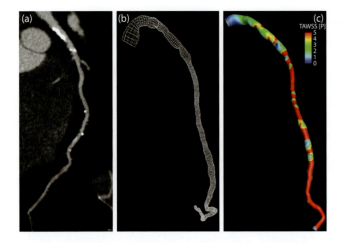

**Figure 5.4.4** Non-invasive angiographic (panel **a**) and functional assessment using FFR$_{CT}$ (panel **b**) of a patient treated with a bioresorbable vascular scaffold in the left circumflex coronary artery. A patent scaffold is observed in coronary CTA with a FFR$_{CT}$ distal to the scaffold of 0.92 with an in-scaffold gradient of 0.04. In panel **c**, the corresponding angiogram shows the patency of the scaffolded region.

In the ongoing clinical studies ABSORB II and ABSORB Japan, coronary CTA will be performed in a larger population. These studies will further increase the evidence on the ability of coronary CTA to accurately evaluate in-scaffold luminal area.

## APPLICATION OF COMPUTATIONAL FLUID DYNAMIC TO CORONARY CTA

After coronary lumen segmentation, three-dimensional (3-D) vessel reconstruction is performed. The 3-D geometry could be further processed using computational fluid dynamic and the finite element method to evaluate physiologic parameters such as fractional flow reserve and shear stress in a patient-specific model (Figure 5.4.4) [10]. In the ABSORB cohort B population with serial coronary CTA, fractional flow reserve derived from coronary CTA (i.e., FFR$_{CT}$) was performed at 18 and 72 months. The drop of pressure in-scaffold (i.e., scaffold gradient) was reported as a surrogate of the functional status of the treated region (Figure 5.4.5). The persistence of the normalization of the FFR$_{CT}$ was observed.

## VALIDATION AND REPRODUCIBILITY TESTING

For internal core lab validation of lumen area and vessel area measurements, a comparison with other imaging modalities (e.g., angiography, intravascular ultrasound [IVUS], or optical coherence tomography [OCT]) could be performed. Ideally, the correlation and level of agreement between coronary CTA-derived areas and areas derived from a higher resolution modality are quantified. Compared to angiography, a high diagnostic accuracy of coronary CTA to detect coronary stenosis ≥50% diameter stenosis has been reported (at the vessel-level sensitivity 92%, specificity 95%, positive

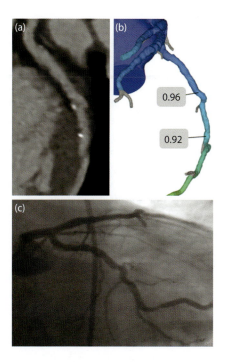

Figure 5.4.5 Coronary CTA analysis of a left anterior descending coronary artery with a bioresorbable scaffold implanted in the mid-segment (the arrows indicate the scaffold radio-opaque markers). Panel **a** shows the multiplanar reconstruction, with a patent scaffold without stenosis. Panel **b** shows the 3-D geometry extricated after vessel segmentation. Panel **c** shows the shear stress pattern at diastole with areas of high shear stress (red) and low shear stress (green and blue).

predictive value 87%, and negative predictive value 97%) [11]. Moreover, coronary CTA-derived lumen and vessel areas obtained from a tomographic cross-section could also be compared with IVUS or OCT derived areas. Previous studies comparing areas derived from coronary CTA and IVUS have reported a mean difference of +0.23 mm$^2$ (95% CI −0.04 to 0.49) for lumen area, and a mean difference of +0.13 mm$^2$ (95% CI −0.72 to 0.98) for vessel area [12]. Figure 5.4.6 shows the agreement between coronary CTA and IVUS for in-scaffold luminal and plaque measurements.

In addition, reproducibility testing is performed once a year using a standard set of three patients. The technician and the supervising cardiologist participate in the reproducibility test. The statistical department analyzes the areas and standard deviation from each analyst. If the standard deviation of the luminal area is not within the predefined range, the causes are assessed and corrective or preventive action is taken and documented.

## CONCLUSION

Coronary CTA is a clinically robust modality for bioresorbable scaffold evaluation. In the initial experience, a high feasibility for quantitative evaluation was reported. In addition to the accurate angiographic luminal evaluation, the functional assessment of the treated vessel can be obtained. Therefore, coronary CTA might emerge as the method of choice for the evaluation of patients treated with bioresorbable vascular scaffolds.

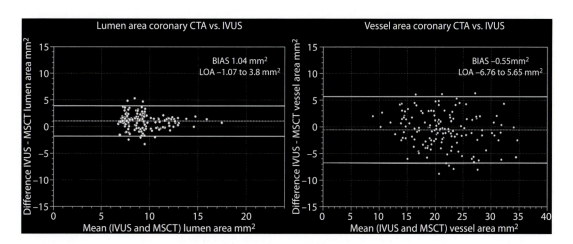

Figure 5.4.6 Bland–Altman analysis of the agreement of in-scaffold lumen and vessel area. A small bias in both parameters is observed. These data are used by the core lab for validation purposes.

# REFERENCES

1. Leber AW, Knez A, von Ziegler F, Becker A, Nikolaou K, Paul S, Wintersperger B et al. Quantification of obstructive and nonobstructive coronary lesions by 64-slice computed tomography: A comparative study with quantitative coronary angiography and intravascular ultrasound. *J Am Coll Cardiol*. 2005;46:147–54.

2. Mollet NR, Cademartiri F, van Mieghem CA, Runza G, McFadden EP, Baks T, Serruys PW et al. High-resolution spiral computed tomography coronary angiography in patients referred for diagnostic conventional coronary angiography. *Circulation*. 2005;112:2318–23.

3. Rief M, Zimmermann E, Stenzel F, Martus P, Stangl K, Greupner J, Knebel F et al. Computed tomography angiography and myocardial computed tomography perfusion in patients with coronary stents: Prospective intraindividual comparison with conventional coronary angiography. *J Am Coll Cardiol*. 2013;62:1476–85.

4. Serruys PW, Ormiston JA, Onuma Y, Regar E, Gonzalo N, Garcia-Garcia HM, Nieman K et al. A bioabsorbable everolimus-eluting coronary stent system (ABSORB): 2-year outcomes and results from multiple imaging methods. *Lancet*. 2009;373:897–910.

5. Onuma Y, Dudek D, Thuesen L, Webster M, Nieman K, Garcia-Garcia HM, Ormiston JA et al. Five-year clinical and functional multislice computed tomography angiographic results after coronary implantation of the fully resorbable polymeric everolimus-eluting scaffold in patients with de novo coronary artery disease: The ABSORB cohort A trial. *JACC Cardiovasc Interv*. 2013;6:999–1009.

6. Nieman K, Serruys PW, Onuma Y, van Geuns RJ, Garcia-Garcia HM, de Bruyne B, Thuesen L et al. Multislice computed tomography angiography for noninvasive assessment of the 18-month performance of a novel radiolucent bioresorbable vascular scaffolding device: The ABSORB trial (a clinical evaluation of the bioabsorbable everolimus eluting coronary stent system in the treatment of patients with de novo native coronary artery lesions). *J Am Coll Cardiol*. 2013;62:1813–4.

7. Leipsic J, Abbara S, Achenbach S, Cury R, Earls JP, Mancini GJ, Nieman K et al. SCCT guidelines for the interpretation and reporting of coronary CT angiography: A report of the Society of Cardiovascular Computed Tomography Guidelines Committee. *J Cardiovasc Comput Tomogr*. 2014;8:342–58.

8. Bruining N, Tanimoto S, Otsuka M, Weustink A, Ligthart J, de Winter S, van Mieghem C et al. Quantitative multi-modality imaging analysis of a bioabsorbable poly-L-lactic acid stent design in the acute phase: A comparison between 2- and 3D-QCA, QCU and QMSCT-CA. *EuroIntervention*. 2008;4:285–91.

9. Serruys PWC and Onuma, Y. Six-year follow-up of the first-in-man use of a polylactide everolimus-eluting BRS for the treatment of coronary stenosis: An assessment of FFR by multislice CT. Paper presented at: http://wwwpcronlinecom/Lectures/2016/Six-year-follow-up-of-the-first-in-man-use-of-a-polylactide-everolimus-eluting-BRS-for-the-treatment-of-coronary-stenosis-an-assessment-of-FFR-by-multislice-CT as accessed on August 3, 2016.

10. Taylor CA, Fonte TA and Min JK. Computational fluid dynamics applied to cardiac computed tomography for noninvasive quantification of fractional flow reserve: Scientific basis. *J Am Coll Cardiol*. 2013;61:2233–41.

11. Li S, Ni Q, Wu H, Peng L, Dong R, Chen L and Liu J. Diagnostic accuracy of 320-slice computed tomography angiography for detection of coronary artery stenosis: Meta-analysis. *Int J Cardiol*. 2013;168:2699–705.

12. Fischer C, Hulten E, Belur P, Smith R, Voros S and Villines TC. Coronary CT angiography versus intravascular ultrasound for estimation of coronary stenosis and atherosclerotic plaque burden: A meta-analysis. *J Cardiovasc Comput Tomogr*. 2013;7:256–66.

# Angiography is sufficient

J. RIBAMAR COSTA JR. AND ALEXANDRE ABIZAID

## INTRODUCTION

In the recent years, bioresorbable vascular scaffolds (BRSs) have been developed as an attractive alternative to metallic stents as the need for mechanical support for the healing artery is temporary, and beyond the first few months there are potential disadvantages of a permanent metallic prosthesis.

However, due to intrinsic properties related to its design and composition, the deployment of BRSs might require some caveats. One of the critical points with this technology concerns the precise vessel sizing and proper device diameter selection.

The ability of BRSs, especially the first generation ones, to be overexpanded is limited by the risk of structural fracture, which has already been described with the ABSORB, the most frequently implanted BRSs nowadays [1]. Figure 5.5.1 shows the bench behavior of ABSORB when submitted to postdilation with oversized balloon catheters.

Although other scaffolds under clinical evaluation have shown, in bench evaluations, to tolerate postdilation with bigger balloon-catheters, the safety of these procedures has not been properly addressed in the real-world clinical scenario, since the inclusion criteria in the trials evaluating these devices have been very restrictive to prevent this kind of situation. Therefore, most of the recommendations presented in this chapter are based on analysis of the ABSORB BRSs and might not be applicable to other scaffolds under development.

## SCAFFOLD SIZE SELECTION

Initially, it is important to keep in mind that currently, the ABSORB is only available in three diameters (2.5, 3.0, and 3.5 mm), and the recommended IFU (instruction for use) for this BRSs implantation is in *de novo* coronary lesions with RVD >2.5 mm and RVD <4.0 mm.

In order to obtain an adequate BVSs implantation, the five Ps rule should be carefully observed: (1) **P**roper vessel sizing; (2) **P**reparation of the lesion; (3) **P**ay attention to expansion

limits of each type of BVSs device; (4) **P**ostdilation with noncompliant balloons; and (5) **P**rescription of dual antiplatelet therapy. In this chapter we will mainly focus on the first **P** rule.

For vessel sizing, although the use of intracoronary imaging modalities (OCT, IVUS) may provide a more accurate estimation of real vessel dimension [2–4], visual estimation and online QCA still remain the most frequent tools to select a scaffold/stent, since they are usually available worldwide, require less specific training to be performed, and do not add additional cost or time to the procedure.

Two recent pools with highly experienced operators in the implantation of BRSs pointed to the routine use of intracoronary imaging in less than 20% of their cases [5,6]. Therefore, even in high volume centers, treating more complex lesions, the choice of the device is mostly based on visual estimation (>80% of the cases) or online QCA (14%) [6].

Our personal practice has also been based on visual/online QCA assessment of vessel dimensions performed after adequate lesion preparation, especially in cases of critical stenosis, when the lack of adequate coronary flow might lead to undersize of the diseased segment.

In the current stage of BVSs development, predilatation is strongly recommended in order not only to facilitate the scaffold deliverability but also to favor its adequate expansion and apposition. Predilation might also help to properly size the vessel, guiding the correct device selection. In a recent publication of Brown et al., the authors showed that BVSs expansion was significantly improved in patients where a 1:1 balloon to artery predilatation was performed [7].

## ONLINE QUANTITATIVE CORONARY ANGIOGRAPH (QCA): REFERENCE VESSEL DIAMETER (RVD) VERSUS $D_{MAX}$

In choosing to perform online QCA, the operator should use the measurement of maximum diameter ($D_{max}$) instead of interpolated reference vessel diameter (RVD) to guide the

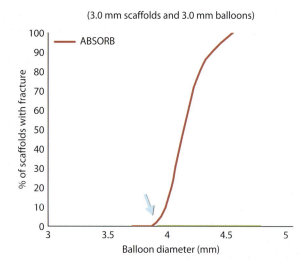

(3.0 mm scaffolds and 3.0 mm balloons)

**Figure 5.5.1** Illustrative chart on ABSORB BRSs *in vitro* expansion properties. Note that whenever this device is expanded beyond 0.8 mm of its nominal diameter, there is an exponential risk of device fracture. (Modified from Ormiston JA et al. *EuroIntervention.* 2015 May;11(1):60–7.)

BVSs size selection. While RVD represents the virtual diameter at the level of the minimum lumen diameter, representing an average of many vessel diameters between the two "normal" (healthy) segments at the lesion edges, $D_{max}$ represents the maximum lumen diameter at the level of intended implantation zone, representing the "true" landing zone in the perilesion segment within 5 mm of the segment to be scaffolded.

The interpolated RVD is influenced by the presence of side branches and tends to more often underestimate lumen size, especially in cases of tapered vessels and long/diffuse lesions. Conversely, $D_{max}$ tends to be closer to the real lumen dimensions.

Gomez-Lara et al. analyzing 52 lesions treated with $3.0 \times 18$ mm ABSORB in a cohort B substudy, showed that the use of $D_{max}$ for the BRSs selection would lead to a better scaffold deployment as later assessed by OCT [8].

Farooq et al., analyzing 202 patients treated with the ABSORB BVSs in the cohort B study and Extend Registry, concluded that the introduction of mandatory $D_{max}$ measurements of vessel size prior to ABSORB BRSs implantation significantly reduced the undersizing of the scaffold

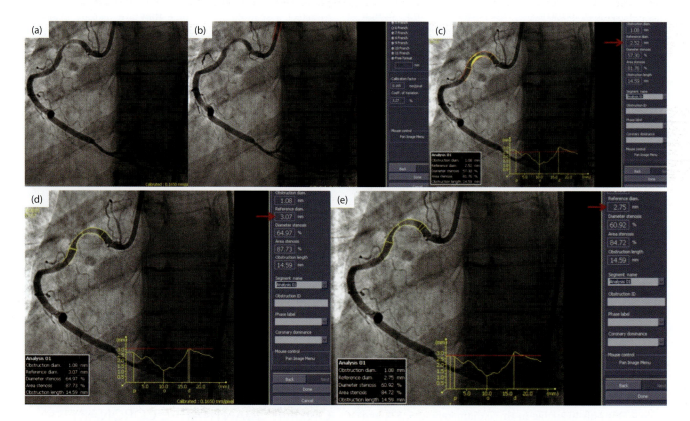

**Figure 5.5.2** Example of discrepancy between interpolated RVD and $D_{max}$ assessment. Panel **a** shows the presence of sever stenosis on a proximal segment of the RCA. Prior to QCA measurements, adequate catheter calibration should be performed (panel **b**). According to the interpolated RVD (panel **c**), the treated vessel has a diameter of 2.52 mm (red arrow). However, when $D_{max}$ is used, the distal vessel diameter within the segment to be "scaffolded" is 3.07 mm (panel **d**, red arrow) and the proximal diameter is 2.75 mm (panel **e**, red arrow). Based on $D_{max}$ measurements a $3.0 \times 18$ mm ABSORB scaffold was selected in this case. QCA = quantitative coronary angiography; RVD = reference vessel diameter; RCA = right coronary artery.

when compared to regular interpolated RVD measurement (appropriate vessel sizing with $D_{max}$ of 69.4% vs. 47.1% with RVD, p = 0.001) [9].

Therefore, at least in the beginning of the center's experience with BVSs, we recommend the regular use of $D_{max}$ to help pick the adequate scaffold size.

Overall, the choice of BRSs should be based on the largest $D_{max}$, except in those cases of extreme vessel tapering. Since ABSORB is only available at the maximum length of 28 mm, it is unlikely to have lesions with marked discrepancy between proximal and distal landing zone. In the case where multiple BRSs are required (overlapping), proximal $D_{max}$ should be obtained for each BRSs deployed. In the case where multiple BRSs are deployed, special attention should be paid to avoid excessive overlapping which has been shown, in pre-clinical evaluation, to be associated with poorer scaffold endothelializaton [10].

Figures 5.5.2 and 5.5.3 show examples of the differences in vessel diameter as assessed by $D_{max}$ and interpolated RVD.

## VISUAL VESSEL SIZE ESTIMATION

Although visual vessel size estimation remains as the most common way to select the size scaffolds/stents to be deployed in the coronary system, this is also the method with more intra observer variability.

In the previously mentioned study conducted by Farooq et al., the authors pointed to a sizing error in the choice of the BRSs in over half of the cases, which was marked improved by the use of online QCA ($D_{max}$). However, these discrepancies tend to be reduced when the operators acquire more experience with the device and its limitations.

For those who decided to select the BRSs dimension based on visual estimation, a careful review of the angiogram, comparing the vessel lumen with the known dimensions of the guiding catheter should be performed after adequate predilatation and intracoronary nitroglycerine infusion.

In case of divergence regarding vessel size, it is advisable to upsize the scaffold as recommended in the ABSORB IFU (Table 5.5.1). When deployed at low pressure (<10 atm), it is unlikely that a BRSs or a metallic stent would result in major edge dissection, even in cases of slight oversize. That is the technique we routinely use in our institution. After deploying the device at low pressure to minimize edge damages, we usually (>90% of the time) perform postdilatation with shorter, noncompliant balloons, to optimize the apposition and expansion of the device throughout its entire length. In case of an ABSORB deployment, the selection of the postdilatation balloon diameter must follow the rules previously mentioned to minimize the possibility of structural fracture.

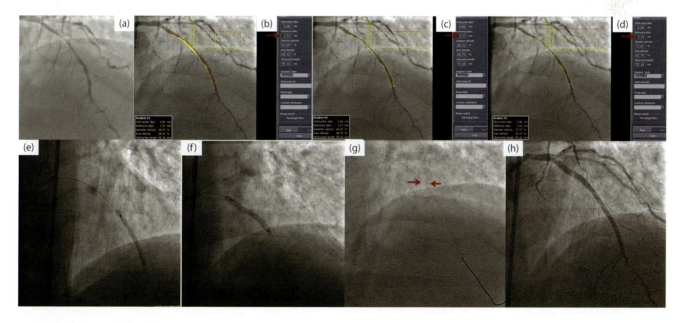

Figure 5.5.3 Example of QCA assessment of a long, diffuse LAD lesion. As noticed on panel **a**, there is a long, severe lesion at the proximal and mid segments of LAD. Also there is diffuse, nonobstructive disease on the distal segment of this vessel. On panel **b**, online QCA using interpolated RVD shows a lesion length of 55 mm and a vessel diameter of 2.53 mm (red arrow). Using $D_{max}$ assessment, one can better overcome the issue of vessel tapering, common to long lesions. Distal $D_{max}$ shows a proximal LAD of 2.57 in diameter (panel **c**, red arrow). Proximal $D_{max}$ points to a vessel of 3.19 mm (panel **d**). Based on $D_{max}$ measurements, two scaffolds with different diameters were selected. The distal BRSs was a 2.5 × 28 mm ABSORB (panel **e**) and the proximal one was a 3.0 × 28 mm (panel **f**). The scaffolds were positioned with minimal overlapping using the radio-opaque markers to guide the positioning (panel **g**, two red arrows). After postdilatation with two different noncompliant balloons (2.75 × 20 mm and 3.25 × 15 mm), the final angiography showed a satisfactory result, with minimum residual stenosis along the entire treated segment (panel **h**). QCA = quantitative coronary angiography; RVD = reference vessel diameter; LAD = left anterior descending coronary artery.

**Table 5.5.1** Scaffold selection based on vessel sizing by QCA/visual estimation (based on Abbott's ABSORB IFU)

| Target vessel diameter | ABSORB BRSs size |
|---|---|
| >2.25 mm and ≤2.5 mm | 2.5 mm |
| >2.5 mm and ≤3.3 mm | 3.0 mm |
| ≥3.3 and ≤3.8 mm | 3.5 mm |
| >3.8 mm | Do not deploy an ABSORB. Consider the use of a metallic stent |

## CONCLUSIONS

Angiography remains the most frequently used method for vessel sizing and device selection, even with the current BRSs generation and its intrinsic expansion limitations.

Careful lesion scrutiny and understanding of some "tips and tricks" might be the key for the acute success with these revolutionary devices in the daily practice. In particular, operators have to be very careful when sizing the vessels to avoid either scaffold underexpansion or the risk of fracture when trying to fix it. Especially in the beginning of the experience with BRSs, some "extra time" should be spent on proper QCA assessment.

However, there is a chance this chapter becomes soon obsolete, since for the upcoming years, a variety of novel generation BRSs [11], including a new version of the ABSORB and a few metallic BRSs, are promising to make the deployment of these devices more similar to the current practice with metallic stents, which will represent a marked step toward their broader incorporation into clinical practice.

## REFERENCES

1. Onuma Y, Serruys PW, Muramatsu T, Nakatani S, van Geuns RJ, de Bruyne B, Dudek D et al. Incidence and imaging outcomes of acute scaffold disruption and late structural discontinuity after implantation of the absorb Everolimus-Eluting fully bioresorbable vascular scaffold: Optical coherence tomography assessment in the ABSORB cohort B Trial (A Clinical Evaluation of the Bioabsorbable Everolimus Eluting Coronary Stent System in the Treatment of Patients With De Novo Native Coronary Artery Lesions). *JACC Cardiovasc Interv.* 2014;7(12):1400–11.
2. Bezerra HG, Attizzani GF, Sirbu V, Musumeci G, Lortkipanidze N, Fujino Y, Wang W et al. Optical coherence tomography versus intravascular ultrasound to evaluate coronary artery disease and percutaneous coronary intervention. *JACC Cardiovasc Interv.* 2013;6(3):228–36.
3. Kubo T, Akasaka T, Shite J, Suzuki T, Uemura S, Yu B, Kozuma K et al. OCT compared with IVUS in a coronary lesion assessment: The OPUS-CLASS study. *JACC Cardiovasc Imaging.* 2013;6(10):1095–104.
4. Tahara S, Bezerra HG, Baibars M, Kyono H, Wang W, Pokras S, Mehanna E et al. In vitro validation of new Fourier-domain optical coherence tomography. *EuroIntervention.* 2011;6(7):875–82.
5. Cortese B, Valgimigli M. Current know how on the absorb BVS technology: An experts' survey. *Int J Cardiol.* 2015;180:203–5.
6. Tamburino C, Latib A, van Geuns RJ, Sabate M, Mehilli J, Gori T, Achenbach S et al. Contemporary practice and technical aspects in coronary intervention with bioresorbable scaffolds: A European perspective. *EuroIntervention.* 2015;10(10).
7. Brown AJ, McCormick LM, Braganza DM, Bennett MR, Hoole SP, West NE. Expansion and malapposition characteristics after bioresorbable vascular scaffold implantation. *Cathet Cardiovasc Interv.* 2014;84(1):37–45.
8. Gomez-Lara J, Diletti R, Brugaletta S, Onuma Y, Farooq V, Thuesen L, McClean D et al. Angiographic maximal luminal diameter and appropriate deployment of the everolimus-eluting bioresorbable vascular scaffold as assessed by optical coherence tomography: An ABSORB cohort B trial sub-study. *EuroIntervention.* 2012;8(2):214–24.
9. Farooq V, Gomez-Lara J, Brugaletta S, Gogas BD, Garcìa-Garcìa HM, Onuma Y, van Geuns RJ et al. Proximal and distal maximal luminal diameters as a guide to appropriate deployment of the ABSORB everolimus-eluting bioresorbable vascular scaffold: A sub-study of the ABSORB Cohort B and the ongoing ABSORB EXTEND Single Arm Study. *Cathet Cardiovasc Interv.* 2012;79(6):880–8.
10. Farooq V, Serruys PW, Heo JH, Gogas BD, Onuma Y, Perkins LE, Diletti R et al. Intracoronary optical coherence tomography and histology of overlapping everolimus-eluting bioresorbable vascular scaffolds in a porcine coronary artery model: The potential implications for clinical practice. *JACC Cardiovasc Interv.* 2013 May;6(5):523–32.
11. Ormiston JA, Webber B, Ubod B, Darremont O, Webster MW. An independent bench comparison of two bioresorbable drug-eluting coronary scaffolds (Absorb and DESolve) with a durable metallic drug-eluting stent (ML8/Xpedition). *EuroIntervention.* 2015 May;11(1):60–7.

# Intravascular ultrasound is a must in bioresorbable scaffold implantation

HIROYOSHI KAWAMOTO, NEIL RUPARELIA, AND ANTONIO COLOMBO

## INTRODUCTION

Grayscale intravascular ultrasound (IVUS) is now established as an invaluable adjunctive tool in percutaneous coronary intervention (PCI) and it provides accurate and detailed anatomical information with regard to both the reference vessel and stents following implantation. This information is not only useful in aiding an operator to choose the best strategy peri-procedurally, but also has been shown to result in a lower incidence of repeat revascularization, myocardial infarction, stent thrombosis, and death [1–3].

Bioresorbable scaffolds (BRSs) are promising for the treatment of coronary artery disease and are characterized by complete scaffold absorption within 2–3 years of implantation. These properties can potentially result in the positive remodeling of the vessel wall and reduce the occurrence of late stent thrombosis [4,5]. Limited long-term data is currently available; however, outcomes appear to be favorable as assessed by several imaging modalities [6,7]. Current BRSs devices have several limitations due to scaffold fragility (poor tolerance to overexpansion) and their bulky structure (ABSORB [Abbott Vascular, Santa Clara, CA] BRSs; strut thickness 157 µm and width > 190 pm). Therefore, particular care must be taken to assess the reference vessel diameter and characterize the plaque prior to implantation to avoid complications such as strut fracture due to the limits of overexpansion with certain devices. During the course of this chapter, we discuss the indications and practical guidance for the use of IVUS when implanting a BRSs.

## ADVANTAGES OF IVUS IN BRSs IMPLANTATION

The coronary angiogram remains the "gold standard" for the assessment of coronary artery disease. However, angiographic evaluation is limited only to providing information regarding the vessel lumen as defined by contrast injection. In some cases, an angiographically "normal" coronary artery may demonstrate various degrees of atherosclerotic plaque when assessed by intravascular imaging. IVUS enables better characterization of plaque, sizing of reference vessel diameter, and optimization of stent implantation when compared to angiographic-guided PCI alone [8–10]. Current IVUS systems are in the 20–40 MHz range and produce a real-time visualization of the reference vessel with deep tissue penetration. Therefore, they enable accurate visualization not only of the vessel lumen and plaque volume (and characteristics), but also of the external elastic membrane to accurately size the reference vessel diameter.

Optical coherence tomography (OCT) is an alternative intravascular imaging modality that can also be employed in this setting [11]. The physical characteristics of both devices are summarized in Figure 5.6.1. OCT can detect scaffold struts more clearly by virtue of its high resolution (10–20 µm axially, and 20–40 µm laterally) in comparison to IVUS (100–150 pm axially, 150–300 pm laterally). However, it is limited by poor depth penetration (1–2 mm) [12] although some studies have demonstrated its efficacy in ostial lesions or large vessels such as the left main stem [13]. Additionally, OCT requires adequate clearance of blood by contrast or low-molecular-weight dextran within the vessel of interest to obtain optimal imaging, resulting in the administration of higher contrast loads. Furthermore, real-time imaging is not obtainable.

## PREPROCEDURAL EVALUATION AND DEVICE SELECTION

### Predilatation

IVUS-guided optimization after metal stent implantation has been clearly demonstrated to improve outcomes [1–3,

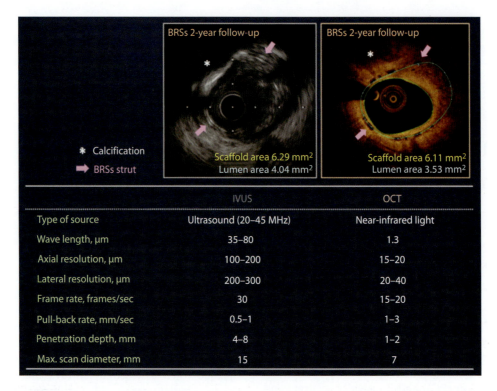

| | IVUS | OCT |
|---|---|---|
| Type of source | Ultrasound (20–45 MHz) | Near-infrared light |
| Wave length, µm | 35–80 | 1.3 |
| Axial resolution, µm | 100–200 | 15–20 |
| Lateral resolution, µm | 200–300 | 20–40 |
| Frame rate, frames/sec | 30 | 15–20 |
| Pull-back rate, mm/sec | 0.5–1 | 1–3 |
| Penetration depth, mm | 4–8 | 1–2 |
| Max. scan diameter, mm | 15 | 7 |

**\* Calcification**
**➡ BRSs strut**

BRSs 2-year follow-up — Scaffold area 6.29 mm$^2$ / Lumen area 4.04 mm$^2$

BRSs 2-year follow-up — Scaffold area 6.11 mm$^2$ / Lumen area 3.53 mm$^2$

**Figure 5.6.1** Representative images at 2-year follow-up and physical characteristics of IVUS and OCT. Both images are obtained at the same position where an ABSORB BRSs had been implanted 2 years previously. BRSs struts were visible with both modalities. OCT clearly demonstrated the homogenous pattern of the neointima and BRSs struts by virtue of its greater resolution. Vessel size was best calculated with IVUS due to the inability of OCT to visualize the elastic lamina due to poor depth penetration. BRSs = bioresorbable scaffolds; IVUS = intravascular ultrasound; OCT = optical coherence tomography.

14–16]. However, the impact of IVUS use prior to stent implantation upon clinical outcomes has not been established. With regard to BRSs implantation, predilatation of the target lesion is currently strongly recommended due to the limitations of current BRSs compared to the new generation DESs as they have less crossability and limited expandability. Thus, accurate reference vessel sizing and aggressive predilatation are essential. If calcification is detected by IVUS, then the use of a cutting balloon, scoring balloon, or rotational atherectomy to facilitate crossing and optimal expansion of BRSs is needed. It should be noted that because calcium is a strong reflector of ultrasound, IVUS can precisely identify the extent and location of vessel wall calcium. On the other hand, due to the inability of ultrasound to penetrate calcium, the resultant acoustic shadows render IVUS unable to visualize the elastic lamina [17]. In such situations, the vessel size can be evaluated by assessing the segment proximal and distal to the calcified lesion.

## BRSs selection

Due to the fragility of the BRSs (unlike metallic stents) and the risk of strut fracture, the current recommendation is that the ABSORB BRSs should only be postdilated to a maximum of 0.5 mm greater than its scaffold diameter: Other BRSs devices such as the 93.0 mm DESolve BRSs

can be expanded to 4.5 mm in diameter without strut fracture [18]. With the aid of IVUS, the correct device can be selected knowing the reference vessel diameter (Figure 5.6.2) and identifying the proximal and distal landing zone. Some studies with DESs have shown that the residual plaque burden (percentage plaque volume >50%) is associated with edge restenosis [19,20] and so the aim should be to implant proximal and distal BRSs edges at sites where the percentage plaque volume <50%. Additionally, online IVUS can precisely identify these points by correlating the IVUS findings with the angiographic image to further optimize BRSs implantation. The fact that these devices will be completely reabsorbed in time enables the strategy of full lesion coverage taking maximum advantage from the information obtained by IVUS.

## Side branch occlusion

The other concern when implanting BRSs is the occurrence of side branch occlusion and resultant periprocedural myocardial infarction [21,22]. Muramatsu et al. reported that BRSs implantation was associated with a higher incidence of postprocedural occlusion of small side branches ≤0.5 mm compared to everolimus-eluting metallic stents [22]. Some studies suggested that strut thickness/width is a potential contributing factor toward side branch occlusion

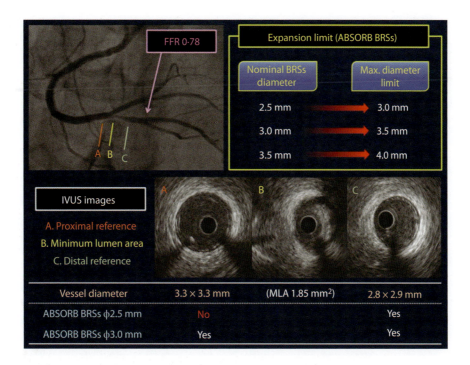

**Figure 5.6.2** Expansion limits of BRSs, and representative case. IVUS demonstrated a vessel diameter of 2.8 × 2.9 mm distally, and 3.3 × 3.3 mm proximally. Due to the limitations of expansion of the ABSORB BRSs, a ϕ2.5 mm BRSs was too small to obtain good apposition at the lesion proximal to the bifurcation (A and C). Additionally, there was only limited plaque at the ostium of side branch, suggesting that the risk of side branch occlusion was low. FFR = fractional flow reserve; BRSs = bioresorbable scaffolds; IVUS = intravascular ultrasound; MLA = minimum lumen area.

[23,24]. This observation is particularly relevant with current BRSs having struts that are thick (ABSORB 157 pm, and DESolve [Elixir Medical Corporation, Sunnyvale, CA] 150um) and wide (ABSORB; more than 190 pm). IVUS is useful in this setting and can be employed to predict the risk side branch occlusion after PCI. If no or minimal plaque is demonstrated at the ostium (Video 5.6.1), the incidence of side branch occlusion occurs in less than 10% of patients; however, the occurrence of this complication increases to 35% in the presence of significant plaque burden [25]. IVUS may therefore be particularly useful when contemplating the treatment of bifurcation lesions with BRSs to direct the selection of the best strategy such as: side branch protection, provisional approach, and two-BRSs strategy.

## OPTIMIZATION

### Is "the bigger, the better" still true in the BRSs era?

In the bare metal stent (BMSs) era, adequate stent expansion with high-pressure balloon dilatation confirmed by IVUS was found to result in a significant reduction in restenosis [14–16] and stent thrombosis [26] and this concept has been extended to newer stents. The development of new DESs, the availability of more potent antiplatelet regimens, and the attention to meticulous stent optimization have all contributed to improve outcomes with regard to the incidence of repeat revascularization, stent thrombosis, myocardial infarction, and death [1–3]. Considering these data, and taking into account that BRSs occupies more space in the vessel lumen and currently has a higher immediate recoil compared to a metal stent, it would be reasonable to assume that the concept of "the bigger, the better" would be even more valid when implanting a BRSs.

### Radial force

The radial force of a BRSs seems to be comparable to the cobalt-chromium metallic stent [27]. Brugaletta et al. reported that ABSORB BRSs tend to have less symmetrical expansion following deployment in comparison to everolimus-eluting metallic stents [28] but this was not associated with any significant differences in clinical outcomes at 6-month follow-up between the groups although the number of lesions was too small to demonstrate noninferiority. In view of the uncertain radial force and asymmetric expansion of BRSs following implantation, IVUS should be liberally employed to evaluate the expansion of BRSs even after postdilatation with a noncompliant balloon (Figure 5.6.3, Videos 5.6.2 and 5.6.3). This practice may improve the clinical outcome.

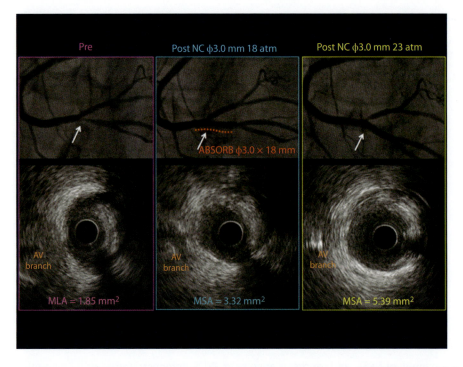

**Figure 5.6.3** Representative case of IVUS-guided postimplantation optimization. An ABSORB BRSs φ3.0 × 18 mm was deployed after pre-dilatation with a φ2.5 mm noncompliant balloon. After post-dilatation with a φ3.0 mm noncompliant balloon (18 atm), the angiographic result appeared optimal. However, the MSA was 3.32 mm² as calculated by IVUS. The MSA increased to 5.39 mm² following further high-pressure dilatation (23 atm) with the same noncompliant balloon demonstrating the importance of IVUS evaluation in optimizing BRSs strut expansion. NC = noncompliant balloon; MLA = minimum lumen area; MSA = minimum scaffold area.

## Strut thickness

The thick struts of the current BMSs had been implicated in a greater late lumen loss and neointimal atherosclerotic changes when compared to BMSs with thinner struts [29,30]. While it is not clear if this is also true for DESs, aggressive postdilatation of BRSs may also be beneficial to better embed their thick (157 m) and wide (>190 μm) struts in the vessel wall. For these reasons, we advocate optimization of the BRSs following implantation with IVUS guidance. To avoid scaffold disruption or deformation during advancement of the IVUS catheter, the operator should perform an initial postdilatation of the BRSs.

## INFLUENCE OF IVUS ON CLINICAL OUTCOMES WITH BRSs

### Short-term outcomes (within 1 year)

The ABSORB II trial, which was the first randomized study comparing BRSs with everolimus-eluting metallic stents, showed similar and favorable 1-year clinical outcomes [21]. The clinical outcomes of randomized trial and retrospective studies on BRSs are described in Table 5.6.1 [7,18,21,31–38]. Three studies reported 1-year clinical outcomes [7,21,32]. In these studies, the incidence of MACE at 1 year was 4.3–5.0%,

and that of TLR was 1.0–2.8%. However, there are no data available investigating the benefits associated with the use of IVUS in this setting.

## Scaffold thrombosis

One of the main concerns following BRSs implantation is the occurrence of scaffold thrombosis. Although ABSORB trials enrolled "simple" lesions, scaffold thrombosis occurred in almost 1% of the study population at 6 months (ABSORB EXTEND 0.8%) [7] and 12 months (ABSORB II 0.9%) [21]. In the real-world GHOST EU registry, the incidence of scaffold thrombosis increased to 2.1% at 6 months [37]. Of interest, IVUS was performed in only 14%, and postdilatation in 49% [37] and thus many cases of stent underexpansion may not have been identified accounting for these high complications rates. This hypothesis is supported by evidence demonstrating that stent underexpansion (as assessed by OCT) was a predictor of stent thrombosis [39,40]. Strut dimensions and positioning in an *in-vivo* model were found to be critical factors in modulating stent thrombogenicity [41]. This has been confirmed by real-world registries with high IVUS usage and final high-pressure postdilatation reporting low scaffold thrombosis rates [31,33,42] (Table 5.6.1). Thus, IVUS-guidance seems to be an effective strategy to reduce the rate of scaffold thrombosis.

**Table 5.6.1** Randomized trial and retrospective studies on BRSs

| | No. of patients | B2/C lesions (%) | IVUS (%) | Post-dilatation (%) | Follow-up (months) | MACE (%) | TLR (%) | Scaffold thrombosis (%) |
|---|---|---|---|---|---|---|---|---|
| **ABSORB BRSs** | | | | | | | | |
| Randomized trial | | | | | | | | |
| ABSORB II | 335 | 46.0 | 98.5 | 61.0 | 12 | 5.0 (TLF) | 1.0 | 0.9 (D/P) |
| ABSORB III | 1322 | 68.7 | 11.2 (IVUS/OCT) | 65.5 | 12 | 7.8 (TLF) | 3.0 | 1.5 (D/P) |
| ABSORB Japan | 266 | 76.0 | 68.8 (Final IVUS/OCT) | 82.2 | 12 | 4.2 (TLF) | 2.6 | 1.5 (D/P) |
| ABSORB China | 241 | 74.9 | 0.4 | 63.0 | 12 | 3.4 (TLF) | 2.9 | 0.4 (D/P) |
| EVERBIO II | 78 | 30 | N/A | 34.0 | 9 | 12.0 (DOCE) | 10.0 | 0 (D/P) |
| TROFI II (STEMI) | 95 | N/A | 0 | 50.5 | 6 | 1.1 (DOCE) | 1 patient | 1 patient (D) |
| Single- and multi-center studies | | | | | | | | |
| Costopoulos et al. 2014 | 92 | 83.9 | 82.5 | 99.3 | 6 | 3.3 | 3.3 | 0 (D/P) |
| GHOST EU registry | 1189 | 51.2 | 14.4 | 49.0 | 6 | 4.4 (TLF) | 2.5 | 2.1 (D/P) |
| Liang et al. 2013 | 35 | 75.6 | 11.4 | N/A | 2 | 0 | 0 | 0 (D/P) |
| AMC registry | 135 | 67.0 | 5.0 | 55.0 | 6 | 8.5 | 6.3 | 3 (D/P) |
| ABSORB EXTEND registry | 512 | 41.0 | N/A | N/A | 12 | 4.3 | 1.8 (ID) | 0.8 (D/P) |
| ASSURE registry | 183 | 64.6 | N/A | 12.6 | 12 | 5.0 | 2.8 | 0 (D/P) |
| RAI registry (STEMI) | 74 | N/A | 2.7 (IVUS/OCT) | N/A | 6 | N/A | 0 | 1.3 (D/P) |
| Gori et al. (ACS) | 150 | N/A | N/A | 14 | 1 | 10.7[a] | 6.6[a] | 2.7 (D/P) |
| Mattesini et al. 2014 | 73 | 100 | 100 (OCT) | 100 | 8.5 | N/A | N/A | 0 |
| **DESolve BRSs** | | | | | | | | |
| Multi-center study | | | | | | | | |
| DESolve First-in-Man | 16 | 37.5 | 100 | N/A | 12 | 0 | 0 | 0 (D/P) |

*Source:* Puricel S, Arroyo D, Corpataux N et al., *J Am Coll Cardiol* 2015;65:791–801; Gao R, Yang Y, Han Y et al., *J Am Coll Cardiol* 2015;66:2298–309; Kimura T, Kozuma K, Tanabe K et al. *Eur Heart J* 2015;36:3332–42. Ellis SG, Kereiakes DJ, Metzger DC et al., *N Engl J Med* 2015;373:1905–15; Sabate M, Windecker S, Iniguez A et al., *Eur Heart J.* 2016;37:229–40.

*Abbreviations:* BRSs = bioresorbable scaffolds; D = definite thrombosis; IVUS = intravascular ultrasound; MACE = major adverse cardiac event; P = probable thrombosis; TLR = target lesion revascularization.

[a] Including non-target/lesion revascularization.

## CONCLUSIONS

IVUS is a valuable tool when implanting a BRSs. IVUS enables operators to make precise decisions regarding the appropriate lesion preparation, device size and length prior to BRSs implantation, and to optimize results (underexpansion, residual dissection, and minimum scaffold area) following implantation. Based on the experience with BMSs and DESs, high-pressure postdilatation with IVUS-guidance following BRSs implantation would seem to be an effective strategy to reduce subsequent adverse clinical events.

Larger studies focusing on the specific impact of IVUS use on outcomes following BRSs implantation are eagerly awaited.

## VIDEOS

Video 5.6.1 Preprocedural evaluation with intravascular ultrasound.

Video 5.6.2 Intravascular ultrasound following postdilatation with noncompliant balloon (ϕ3.0 mm, 18 atm).

Video 5.6.3 Final intravascular ultrasound following additional postdilatation with noncompliant balloon (ϕ3.0 mm, 23 atm).

# REFERENCES

1. Zhang Y, Farooq V, Garcia-Garcia HM, Bourantas CV, Tian N, Dong S et al. Comparison of intravascular ultrasound versus angiography-guided drug-eluting stent implantation: A meta-analysis of one randomised trial and ten observational studies involving 19,619 patients. *EuroIntervention.* 2012;8:855–65.

2. Klersy C, Ferlini M, Raisaro A, Scotti V, Balduini A, Curti M et al. Use of IVUS guided coronary stenting with drug eluting stent: A systematic review and meta-analysis of randomized controlled clinical trials and high quality observational studies. *Int J Cardiol.* 2013;170:54–63.

3. Jang JS, Song YJ, Kang W, Jin HY, Seo JS, Yang TH et al. Intravascular ultrasound-guided implantation of drug-eluting stents to improve outcome: A meta-analysis. *JACC Cardiovasc Interv.* 2014;7:233–43.

4. Serruys PW, Ormiston JA, Onuma Y, Regar E, Gonzalo N, Garcia-Garcia HM et al. A bioabsorbable everolimus-eluting coronary stent system (ABSORB): 2-year outcomes and results from multiple imaging methods. *Lancet.* 2009;373:897–910.

5. Onuma Y, Serruys PW. Bioresorbable scaffold: The advent of a new era in percutaneous coronary and peripheral revascularization? *Circulation.* 2011;123:779–97.

6. Onuma Y, Dudek D, Thuesen L, Webster M, Nieman K, Garcia-Garcia HM et al. Five-year clinical and functional multislice computed tomography angiographic results after coronary implantation of the fully resorbable polymeric everolimus-eluting scaffold in patients with de novo coronary artery disease: The ABSORB cohort A trial. *JACC Cardiovasc Interv.* 2013;6:999–1009.

7. Abizaid A, Costa JR, Jr., Bartorelli AL, Whitbourn R, van Geuns RJ, Chevalier B et al. The ABSORB EXTEND study: Preliminary report of the twelve-month clinical outcomes in the first 512 patients enrolled. *EuroIntervention.* 2015;10(12):1396–401.

8. Russo RJ, Silva PD, Teirstein PS, Attubato MJ, Davidson CJ, DeFranco AC et al. A randomized controlled trial of angiography versus intravascular ultrasound-directed bare-metal coronary stent placement (the AVID Trial). *Circ Cardiovasc Interv.* 2009;2:113–23.

9. Jimenez-Quevedo P, Sabate M, Angiolillo DJ, Costa MA, Alfonso F, Gomez-Hospital JA et al. Vascular effects of sirolimus-eluting versus bare-metal stents in diabetic patients: Three-dimensional ultrasound results of the Diabetes and Sirolimus-Eluting Stent (DIABETES) Trial. *J Am Coll Cardiol.* 2006;47:2172–9.

10. Doi H, Maehara A, Mintz GS, Yu A, Wang H, Mandinov L et al. Impact of post-intervention minimal stent area on 9-month follow-up patency of paclitaxel-eluting stents: An integrated intravascular ultrasound analysis from the TAXUS IV, V, and VI and TAXUS ATLAS Workhorse, Long Lesion, and Direct Stent Trials. *JACC Cardiovasc Interv.* 2009;2:1269–75.

11. Prati F, Regar E, Mintz GS, Arbustini E, Di Mario C, Jang IK et al. Expert review document on methodology, terminology, and clinical applications of optical coherence tomography: Physical principles, methodology of image acquisition, and clinical application for assessment of coronary arteries and atherosclerosis. *Eur Heart J.* 2010;31:401–15.

12. Bezerra HG, Attizzani GF, Sirbu V, Musumeci G, Lortkipanidze N, Fujino Y et al. Optical coherence tomography versus intravascular ultrasound to evaluate coronary artery disease and percutaneous coronary intervention. *JACC Cardiovasc Interv.* 2013;6:228–36.

13. Fujino Y, Bezerra HG, Attizzani GF, Wang W, Yamamoto H, Chamie D et al. Frequency-domain optical coherence tomography assessment of unprotected left main coronary artery disease: A comparison with intravascular ultrasound. *Cathet Cardiovasc Interv.* 2013;82:E173–83.

14. Sbruzzi G, Quadros AS, Ribeiro RA, Abelin AP, Berwanger O, Plentz RD et al. Intracoronary ultrasound-guided stenting improves outcomes: A meta-analysis of randomized trials. *Arq Bras Cardiol.* 2012;98:35–44.

15. Parise H, Maehara A, Stone GW, Leon MB, Mintz GS. Meta-analysis of randomized studies comparing intravascular ultrasound versus angiographic guidance of percutaneous coronary intervention in pre-drug-eluting stent era. *Am J Cardiol.* 2011;107:374–82.

16. Casella G, Klauss V, Ottani F, Siebert U, Sangiorgio P, Bracchetti D. Impact of intravascular ultrasound-guided stenting on long-term clinical outcome: A meta-analysis of available studies comparing intravascular ultrasound-guided and angiographically guided stenting. *Cathet Cardiovasc Interv.* 2003;59:314–21.

17. Mintz GS, Garcia-Garcia HM, Nicholls SJ, Weissman NJ, Bruining N, Crowe T et al. Clinical expert consensus document on standards for acquisition, measurement and reporting of intravascular ultrasound regression/progression studies. *EuroIntervention.* 2011;6:1123–30, 9.

18. Verheye S, Ormiston JA, Stewart J, Webster M, Sanidas E, Costa R et al. A next-generation bioresorbable coronary scaffold system: From bench to first clinical evaluation: 6- and 12-month clinical and multimodality imaging results. *JACC Cardiovasc Interv.* 2014;7:89–99.

19. Morino Y, Tamiya S, Masuda N, Kawamura Y, Nagaoka M, Matsukage T et al. Intravascular ultrasound criteria for determination of optimal longitudinal positioning of sirolimus-eluting stents. *Circ J.* 2010;74:1609–16.

20. Sakurai R, Ako J, Morino Y, Sonoda S, Kaneda H, Terashima M et al. Predictors of edge stenosis following sirolimus-eluting stent deployment (a quantitative intravascular ultrasound analysis from the SIRIUS trial). *Am J Cardiol*. 2005;96:1251–3.

21. Serruys PW, Chevalier B, Dudek D, Cequier A, Carrié D, Iniguez A et al. A bioresorbable everolimus-eluting scaffold versus a metallic everolimus-eluting stent for ischaemic heart disease caused by de-novo native coronary artery lesions (ABSORB II): An interim 1-year analysis of clinical and procedural secondary outcomes from a randomised controlled trial. *Lancet*. 2015;385:43–54.

22. Muramatsu T, Onuma Y, Garcia-Garcia HM, Farooq V, Bourantas CV, Morel MA et al. Incidence and short-term clinical outcomes of small side branch occlusion after implantation of an everolimus-eluting bioresorbable vascular scaffold: An interim report of 435 patients in the ABSORB-EXTEND single-arm trial in comparison with an everolimus-eluting metallic stent in the SPIRIT first and II trials. *JACC Cardiovasc Interv*. 2013;6:247–57.

23. Lansky AJ, Yaqub M, Hermiller JB, Smith RS, Farhat N, Caputo R et al. Side branch occlusion with everolimus-eluting and paclitaxel-eluting stents: Three-year results from the SPIRIT III randomised trial. *EuroIntervention*. 2010;6 Suppl J:J44–52.

24. Popma JJ, Mauri L, O'Shaughnessy C, Overlie P, McLaurin B, Almonacid A et al. Frequency and clinical consequences associated with sideb-ranch occlusion during stent implantation using zotarolimus-eluting and paclitaxel-eluting coronary stents. *Circ Cardiovasc Interv*. 2009;2:133–9.

25. Furukawa E, Hibi K, Kosuge M, Nakatogawa T, Toda N, Takamura T et al. Intravascular ultrasound predictors of side branch occlusion in bifurcation lesions after percutaneous coronary intervention. *Circ J*. 2005;69:325–30.

26. Colombo A, Hall P, Nakamura S, Almagor Y, Maiello L, Martini G et al. Intracoronary stenting without anticoagulation accomplished with intravascular ultrasound guidance. *Circulation*. 1995;91:1676–88.

27. Onuma Y, Serruys PW, Gomez J, de Bruyne B, Dudek D, Thuesen L et al. Comparison of in vivo acute stent recoil between the bioresorbable everolimus-eluting coronary scaffolds (revision 1.0 and 1.1) and the metallic everolimus-eluting stent. *Cathet Cardiovasc Interv*. 2011;78:3–12.

28. Brugaletta S, Gomez-Lara J, Diletti R, Farooq V, van Geuns RJ, de Bruyne B et al. Comparison of in vivo eccentricity and symmetry indices between metallic stents and bioresorbable vascular scaffolds: Insights from the ABSORB and SPIRIT trials. *Cathet Cardiovasc Interv*. 2012;79:219–28.

29. Kitabata H, Kubo T, Komukai K, Ishibashi K, Tanimoto T, Ino Y et al. Effect of strut thickness on neointimal atherosclerotic change over an extended follow-up period (>/= 4 years) after bare-metal stent implantation: Intracoronary optical coherence tomography examination. *Am Heart J*. 2012;163:608–16.

30. Rittersma SZ, de Winter RJ, Koch KT, Bax M, Schotborgh CE, Mulder KJ et al. Impact of strut thickness on late luminal loss after coronary artery stent placement. *Am J Cardiol*. 2004;93:477–80.

31. Costopoulos C, Latib A, Naganuma T, Miyazaki T, Sato K, Figini F et al. Comparison of early clinical outcomes between ABSORB bioresorbable vascular scaffold and everolimus-eluting stent implantation in a real-world population. *Cathet Cardiovasc Interv*. 2015;85:E10–5.

32. Wohrle J, Naber C, Schmitz T, Schwencke C, Frey N, Butter C et al. Beyond the early stages: Insights from the ASSURE registry on bioresorbable vascular scaffolds. *EuroIntervention*. 2015;11(2):149–56.

33. Mattesini A, Secco GG, Dall'Ara G, Ghione M, Rama-Merchan JC, Lupi A et al. ABSORB biodegradable stents versus second-generation metal stents: A comparison study of 100 complex lesions treated under OCT guidance. *JACC Cardiovasc Interv*. 2014;7:741–50.

34. Kraak RP, Hassell ME, Grundeken MJ, Koch KT, Henriques JP, Piek JJ et al. Initial experience and clinical evaluation of the Absorb bioresorbable vascular scaffold (BVS) in real-world practice: The AMC Single Centre Real World PCI Registry. *EuroIntervention*. 2015;10(10):1160–8.

35. Ielasi A, Cortese B, Varricchio A, Tespili M, Sesana M, Pisano F et al. Immediate and midterm outcomes following primary PCI with bioresorbable vascular scaffold implantation in patients with ST-segment myocardial infarction: Insights from the multicentre "Registro ABSORB Italiano" (RAI registry). *EuroIntervention*. 2015;11(2):157–62.

36. Gori T, Schulz E, Hink U, Wenzel P, Post F, Jabs A et al. Early outcome after implantation of Absorb bioresorbable drug-eluting scaffolds in patients with acute coronary syndromes. *EuroIntervention*. 2014;9:1036–41.

37. Capodanno D, Gori T, Nef H, Latib A, Mehilli J, Lesiak M et al. Percutaneous coronary intervention with everolimus-eluting bioresorbable vascular scaffolds in routine clinical practice: Early and midterm outcomes from the European multicentre GHOST-EU registry. *EuroIntervention*. 2015;10(10):1144–53.

38. Liang M, Kajiya T, Lee CH, Chan M, Teo SG, Chan KH et al. Initial experience in the clinical use of everolimus-eluting bioresorbable vascular scaffold (BVS) in a single institution. *Int J Cardiol*. 2013;168:1536–7.

39. Parodi G, La Manna A, Di Vito L, Valgimigli M, Fineschi M, Bellandi B et al. Stent-related defects in patients presenting with stent thrombosis: Differences at optical coherence tomography between subacute and late/very late thrombosis in the Mechanism Of Stent Thrombosis (MOST) study. *EuroIntervention*. 2013;9:936–44.

40. Guagliumi G, Capodanno D, Ikejima H, Bezerra HG, Sirbu V, Musumeci G et al. Impact of different stent alloys on human vascular response to everolimus-eluting stent: An optical coherence tomography study: The OCTEVEREST. *Cathet Cardiovasc Interv*. 2013;81:510–8.

41. Kolandaivelu K, Swaminathan R, Gibson WJ, Kolachalama VB, Nguyen-Ehrenreich KL, Giddings VL et al. Stent thrombogenicity early in high-risk interventional settings is driven by stent design and deployment and protected by polymer-drug coatings. *Circulation*. 2011;123:1400–9.

42. Brown AJ, McCormick LM, Braganza DM, Bennett MR, Hoole SP, West NE. Expansion and malapposition characteristics after bioresorbable vascular scaffold implantation. *Cathet Cardiovasc Interv*. 2014;84:37–45.

# OCT is the way to go

JIANG MING FAM, NIENKE SIMONE VAN DITZHUIJZEN, JORS VAN DER SIJDE,
BU-CHUN ZHANG, ANTONIOS KARANASOS, ROBERT-JAN M. VAN GEUNS,
AND EVELYN REGAR

## INTRODUCTION—CURRENT CHALLENGES FACING BIORESORBABLE VASCULAR SCAFFOLDS IN PERCUTANEOUS CORONARY INTERVENTION

Bioresorbable vascular scaffolds (BRSs) represent a new treatment for coronary artery disease. While imaging sightings have shown a favorable healing response after scaffold implantation with complete strut resorption and recovery of vasomotor function [1] and clinical studies have demonstrated similar clinical outcomes of BRSs compared to best-in-class drug eluting metallic platform stents (MPSs) [2–4] in highly selected, simple lesions, there are still limitations facing the use of BRSs in percutaneous coronary intervention (PCI). Compared to MPSs, BRSs have a limited range of expansion, limiting their use in cases of vessel tapering. While small malapposition may be correctable by postdilatation and resolve at follow-up, large malapposition can be uncorrectable and persist at follow-up until resorption occurs. Attempts to correct large malapposition by overexpansion with a large balloon can lead to acute disruption of the scaffold (Figure 5.7.1). Therefore, exact sizing and device matching of lumen dimension is crucial. As BRSs are relatively bulky and have thicker struts (approximately 150 µm), it becomes even more important to achieve close matching of scaffold edges with minimal regions of overlap. Long regions of scaffold overlap should preferably be avoided as it increases the risk of scaffold thrombosis and also increases the risk of side branch occlusion. In addition, polymers are invisible under X-ray and thus suffer from poor visualization by coronary angiography. Most of the BRSs such as the ABSORB BVSs are equipped with radiopaque markers on both ends of the scaffold (Figure 5.7.2) or on both ends of the delivery balloon [2,5,6] whereas in the REVA bioresorbable scaffold a proprietary iodinated

material is added to the polymer that allows visualization of the entire scaffold under X-ray [7] (Figure 5.7.3). Therefore, acute placement of the scaffold can be challenging especially in regions of significant overlap or foreshortening. Finally, the paucity of visualization of the scaffold under direct angiography also makes it difficult to assess expansion of the scaffold postimplantation and the need for further scaffold optimization.

## LIMITATIONS OF ANGIOGRAPHY TO ADDRESS THESE CHALLENGES

While angiography-based imaging remains the mainstay of assessment for the vast majority of cases in PCI, it is not able to provide detailed information regarding the true anatomic extent of disease and the procedural result of the scaffold postimplantation in certain situations. Even with the use of 3D quantitative coronary analysis (QCA), angiography offers a limited longitudinal assessment particularly in vessels with eccentric luminal lesions and when there are foreshortened or overlap angiographic images [8,9]. As a result, areas of overlap segments are difficult to assess using angiography as well. If scaffold length is either too short or too long leading to inadequate lesion coverage or excessive overlap segments, these can also potentially lead to adverse clinical outcomes. Last, angiography cannot reveal the true extent of plaque composition (such as lipid core plaque and calcium distribution) affecting the diseased coronary vessel, which has been shown to be associated with clinical and procedural outcomes such as target lesion revascularization rate [10] and periprocedural myocardial infarct [11]. Thus, angiographic assessment alone provides limited information to facilitate optimal lesion coverage and the need for further lesion preparation such as the potential need for cutting balloon dilation or the use of rotational artherectomy. Failure to fully appreciate the underlying plaque composition of the

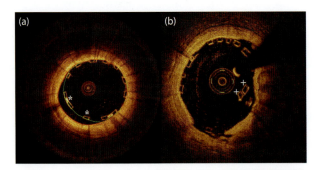

Figure 5.7.1 Panel **a** showing malapposed struts (marked *). Attempts to correct large malapposition by overexpansion with a large balloon can lead to acute disruption of the scaffold (Panel **b**: disrupted struts marked +).

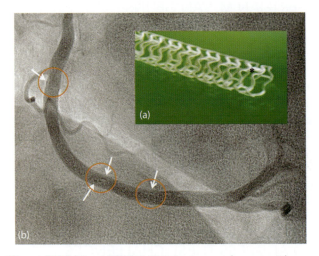

Figure 5.7.2 The ABSORB BVSs# seen on closeup with the platinum radiopaque marker (*) at one end (Panel **a**) and in the right coronary artery (RCA) after implantation (Panel **b**). The arrows indicate the radio-opaque markers of two scaffolds deployed in an overlapping manner in the RCA. (Reproduced with permission from Abbott Vascular.)

disease vessel may lead to inadequate lesion coverage or suboptimal lesion preparation thus potentially affecting scaffold expansion.

## Why preprocedural sizing on OCT is mandatory

The application of OCT, a light-based intravascular imaging technology [12], has enabled us to address the challenges facing the use of BRSs and overcome the limitations of angiography in assessing the significance of coronary stenosis and results of PCI in a clinical setting [13,14]. There are clear advantages of using OCT in the deployment of BRSs [15]. The advantages include the capability to provide accurate luminal measurements, and optimal detection of scaffold malapposition and fracture, which cannot be detected reliably on plain angiography. Last, 3-dimensional rendering and co-registration capabilities can provide additional information which can potentially improve procedural outcomes in more complex cases such as in bifurcation stenting. New OCT probes are of low profile (2.6–2.7 French), flexible, coated with a hydrophilic layer, and the acquisition speed is at least 10 times higher compared with intravascular ultrasound (IVUS). OCT catheters thus have a low delivery profile and can pass almost every lesion with few anatomical or patient exclusion criteria. The OCT imaging procedure is safe [16] and fast, providing all necessary information in just seconds. Radial access can also be used for OCT imaging, although a slight trend toward less optimal image quality and more artifacts has been observed [17]. Indeed, the latest European Society of Cardiology guidelines on myocardial revascularization has already recommended OCT as a tool in selected patients to optimize stent implantation (Class II b, level C) [18].

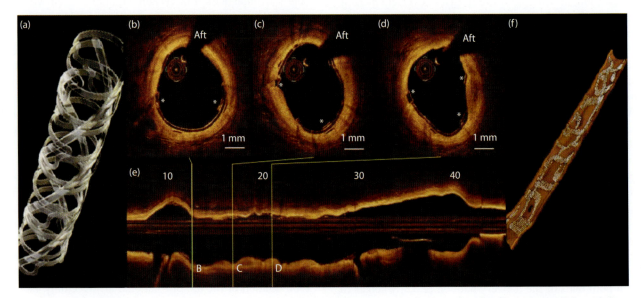

Figure 5.7.3 The REVA is designed with a unique slide-and-lock design, as can be visualized in the cartoon **(a)**, and the OCT cross-sections (* in **b, c, d**) that correspond to the letters b, c and d in the longitudinal view **(e)** of the OCT-pullback. Panel **f** shows the REVA implanted in the coronary vessel after 3-dimensional rendering. Aft: guidewire artifact.

# OCT provides accurate luminal measurements

OCT can reliably assess luminal dimensions accurately and provide quantitative indices of stent expansion in order to evaluate procedural outcomes. OCT can generate a clear and complete assessment of long coronary artery segments within a few seconds and allow for easier image interpretation compared with angiography. OCT offers a representation of the true lumen diameter over the length of the entire pullback with no projection-related error, foreshortening, or geometric distortion, which are limitations of angiographic assessment. Importantly, the information is reliable and instantaneously available making online analysis in the cath lab possible. Before the implantation of the BRSs,

luminal measurements are frequently taken to determine the severity of stenosis and the size of the "normal" reference segment. These measurements are critical as they are used to guide implantation of stent placement and sizing of the device to be implanted. OCT is especially important to make sure that the lumen diameter does not exceed the scaffold diameter by 0.5 mm to avoid incorrectable scaffold malapposition. OCT is the most accurate method in terms of comparison to phantom measurements [9] (Figure 5.7.4), has low interstudy, intraobserver, and interobserver variability, both in core lab [19] and in clinical setting [20–24], and is the best to measure scaffold length when compared with IVUS and QCA [25]. The location of minimal lumen area in relation to the diseased vessel can also be visualized clearly using the lumen profile (Figure 5.7.5), making

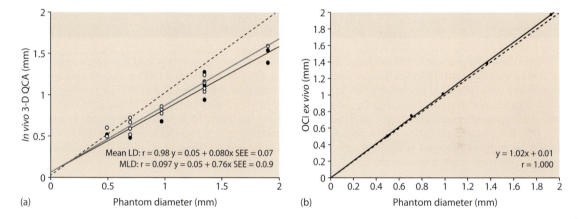

**Figure 5.7.4** Panel **a** shows 3-dimensional QCA assessment of minimum (continuous black lines) and mean luminal diameter (continuous gray lines) with catheter calibration. The dashed lines indicate the line of identity. Panel **b** shows linear regression analysis of the phantom lumen diameter versus the cross-sectional luminal diameter measured with OCT. (Reproduced with permission from Tsuchida K, van der Giessen WJ, Patterson M, Tanimoto S, García-García HM, Regar E, Ligthart JMR et al. *EuroIntervention* 2007;3:100–108.)

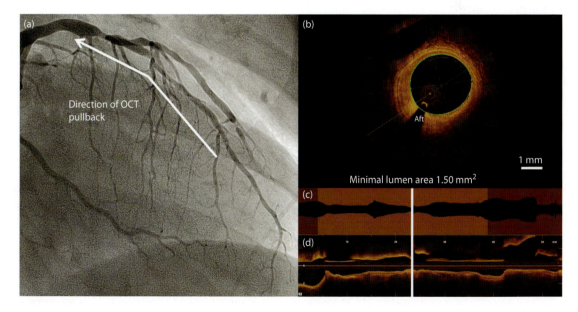

**Figure 5.7.5** Coronary angiogram (Panel **a**) and OCT pullback (Panel **b**) of the left anterior descending (LAD) artery prior to percutaneous coronary intervention (PCI). The LAD as shown with the minimal lumen area seen on the lumen (Panel **c**) and longitudinal profile (Panel **d**) in relation to the length of the diseased vessel. Aft: guidewire artifact.

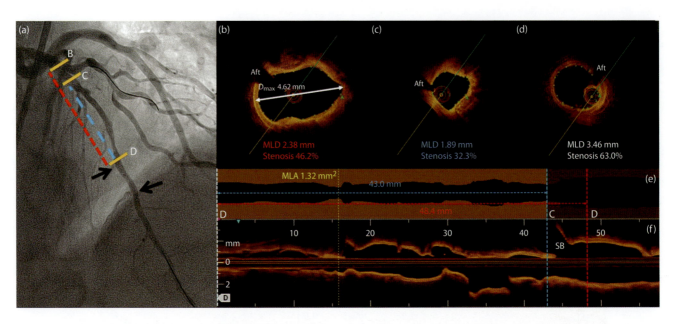

**Figure 5.7.6** Panel **a**: Angiogram of a diffusely diseased left anterior descending artery (LAD). Arrows indicating markers of a distal 2.5 × 12 mm BVSs ABSORB scaffold already implanted. OCT images of the LAD at two choice landing zones before (Panel **b**) and after (Panel **c**) the bifurcation as well as the distal landing zone (Panel **d**). The landing zone before the bifurcation was not chosen in view of its large D$_{max}$ diameter of 4.62 mm (Panel **b**). Two ABSORB BVSs (3.0 × 28 mm and 3.0 × 18 mm scaffolds) were deployed from c to d in an overlapping manner. The lumen profile (Panel **e**) and longitudinal or "L" profile (Panel **f**) show the location of the choice proximal landing zones, minimal lumen area (MLA) in relation to the distal landing zone with the required scaffold length, respectively, for optimal lesion coverage. Aft: guidewire artifact; MLD: mean lumen diameter; SB: side branch.

it possible to determine the length of lesion to be treated allowing for highly accurate assessment of scaffold length required for optimal lesion coverage. Thus by accurately determining lumen dimensions, OCT can play a potentially important role in guiding treatment strategy, in terms of the selection of an appropriate balloon and optimal scaffold diameter and length, thus avoiding unnecessary overlap segments at sidebranch ostia or inadequate lesion coverage (Figure 5.7.6).

## OCT has the ability to assess plaque morphology and characteristics

The high resolution of intracoronary OCT proffers advantages for the assessment of atherosclerotic plaque. OCT can reliably assess and quantify atherosclerotic plaque characteristics (thin fibrous cap, lipid core, and calcific plaques) (Figure 5.7.7). The implantation of struts into the necrotic cores of ruptured thin cap fibroatheromas has been associated with delayed healing in MPSs (both BMS and DESs) and increased risk of periprocedural myocardial infarct [11,26–28]. By identifying and avoiding landing sites containing lipid-rich plaque or thin cap fibroatheroma, OCT can precisely identify the optimal segment for stent deployment, the so-called "landing zone."

The BRSs has potentially less deliverability in calcified lesions where focal areas of calcification limit expansion of the BRSs more compared to MPSs [29]. Hence, adequate lesion preparation is crucial, e.g., by predilation

or lesion modification by scoring balloon angioplasty or even rotational artherectomy. OCT can provide information about the location of the calcium within the vessel wall (superficial vs. deep) and extent of involvement—calcium arc tapering, plaque type, and distribution both in the lesion and proximal to the lesion. Thus, the need for lesion preparation and postdilation may be realized upfront [30,31].

Therefore by understanding the true extent and nature of the underlying plaque in the diseased vessel wall, OCT can be used preprocedurally to guide BRSs implantation by facilitating the selection of optimal landing zones (i.e., region with largest lumen and least plaque or normal vessel segment), in so doing ensuring optimal lesion coverage and facilitate the decision making process on overall stent implantation strategy [32–36]. With online analysis in the catheterization lab, "virtual PCI planning" involving the selection of optimal landing zone (Figure 5.7.8), planning of regions of scaffold overlap (e.g., with respect to side branch ostia), and estimation of required stent length can be performed.

## OCT findings can be used to optimize scaffold expansion postdeployment

OCT demonstrated consistently high accuracy and reproducibility for the assessment of coronary stents and scaffolds, irrespective of the analysis method or software used [37]. The major concern in inadequate scaffold expansion

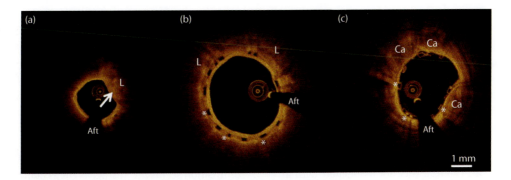

Figure 5.7.7 Different plaque characteristics that can be seen on OCT showing fibrous cap (arrow) covering a necrotic lipid core (Panel **a**) and lipid core plaque in a previously scaffolded vessel (struts marked * in Panel **b**). Panel **c** shows calcific plaques (marked Ca) in a previously scaffolded vessel (struts marked *). Aft: guidewire artifact.

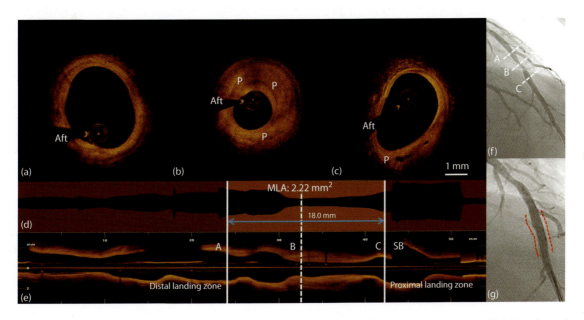

Figure 5.7.8 "Virtual PCI" planning. OCT images of the left anterior descending artery prior to scaffold implantation showing the distal landing zone (Panel **a**), minimal lumen area (Panel **b**) and proximal landing zone (Panel **c**). OCT can assess lumen dimensions accurately, assess underlying plaque composition (P), and show the location of the minimal lumen area in relation to the treated vessel on the lumen profile (Panel **d**). In this way, OCT can guide scaffold implantation strategy by assessing the scaffold length (18.0 mm in this example) required for optimal lesion coverage and avoiding side branch (SB) ostia. The side branch is seen on the longitudinal profile (Panel **e**). Panels **f** and **g** show the LAD before and after implantation of a 3.0 × 18.00 mm ABSORB BVSs scaffold (dashed line). Aft: guide wire artifact.

and incomplete strut apposition is that it can cause non-laminar and turbulent blood flow that can trigger platelet activation, thrombosis, or restenosis [38]. Intracoronary OCT also enables high-resolution, *in-vivo*, serial imaging of the scaffold and vessel microarchitecture enabling investigators and clinicians to assess the effect of vascular injury caused by the implantation procedure and mechanical integrity of the scaffold over time [14,39,40]. In complex interventional settings that involve a high risk of complications such as in scaffold thrombosis, OCT can provide critical decision making by assessing for mechanistic causes such as malapposition. In CLI-OPCI, additional post-OCT interventions were performed in 34.7% of the patients undergoing OCT assessment. Notable findings that led to

additional intervention post-OCT included edge dissection, scaffold underexpansion, and malapposition not previously detected on angiography alone [36]. In another study studying the utility of OCT in BRSs implantation, 28% of patients [41] with optimal angiographic results underwent further intervention to optimize BRSs scaffold placement following intravascular imaging. The reasons for further BRSs optimization included scaffold malapposition and scaffold underexpansion. Additional intervention in OCT-guided PCI may influence clinical outcomes as stent expansion, tissue protrusion, and dissection have been associated with early stent thrombosis [42,43] and inadequate stent expansion has been implicated in restenosis [43]. However, further prospective studies would need to be conducted.

## OCT is safe

In clinical studies [16,41,44,45], it has been shown that it is feasible to perform OCT safely during PCI. Current commercial systems use frequency domain detection (FD-OCT) that does not require vessel occlusion. As with any intracoronary instrumentation, there is a theoretical risk of intimal injury or dissection. Although particular care should be taken in patients with renal insufficiency, hemodynamic instability, and severely impaired ejection fraction contractility, the use of FD-OCT was not associated with any major complications including arterial dissection or life-threatening arrhythmias and worsening of postprocedural renal function [36].

## OCT imaging has the potential to improve outcomes

Improvement in clinical and angiographic outcomes with intracoronary imaging guided PCI was first shown in the use of IVUS in the implantation of DES [46–50]. In a meta analysis involving DES involving 19,619 patients, IVUS-guided DES deployment compared with standard angiographic guidance was associated with a reduced incidence of death (hazard ratio [HR]: 0.59, 95% confidence interval [CI]: 0.48–0.73, $p < 0.001$), major adverse cardiac events (HR: 0.87, 95% CI: 0.78–0.96, $p = 0.008$), and stent thrombosis (HR: 0.58, 95% CI: 0.44–0.77, $p < 0.001$) [48]. The incidence of myocardial infarction and target vessel revascularization was comparable between the angiography and IVUS-guided arms.

The advantages of imaging guidance observed by IVUS may also apply to OCT. This was supported by findings from an observational study in that angiographic plus OCT guidance was associated with a significantly lower risk of cardiac death or MI, even after multivariate adjustment for baseline and procedural differences between the groups (OR = 0.49 [0.25–0.96], $p = 0.037$) or propensity-score adjusted analyses [36]. Though there is limited proven prognostic value of OCT in BRSs, preliminary observations suggest a potentially beneficial role in improving outcomes [38].

## USE OF OPTICAL COHERENCE TOMOGRAPHY IN SPECIAL SITUATIONS

As the clinical indications for BRSs expand beyond simpler lesions, the need for procedural OCT to predetermine sizing becomes even more critical. The 3-dimensional rendering and co-registration capabilities of OCT facilitate the planning of PCI involving more complex anatomical subsets such as bifurcation and left main stenting. There have been positive studies that suggest that intracoronary imaging with IVUS can be of benefit in various subgroups such as small vessels [51], long lesions [50], bifurcation, and left main lesions [52,53]. Cases of BRSs use have been reported in CTOs and bifurcations as well [54,55]. Potentially, OCT can be of benefit in these subgroups.

## Bifurcation stenting

In appropriately selected patients, a BRSs potentially may be a good therapeutic option in bifurcation lesions [56]. Bifurcation lesion stenting is a potential application of OCT guidance. The unique ability of OCT to reconstruct 3-dimensional (3D) images allows better visualization of the scaffold surface and can provide additive information on luminal and lesion measurements, particularly in complex lesions such as bifurcations [57,58]. The application of 3D OCT within the coronary bifurcation seems promising, as the visualization of the complex anatomy of the bifurcation and the effects of intervention are difficult and not always reliable with 2-dimensional imaging. 3D-OCT can also produce images that indicate the relative position of the main vessel and the side-branch and help select a suitable strategy [57–59] and help identify the point of recrossing of a guidewire in a side branch through the cells of a stent implanted in the main vessel, and evaluate possible presence of struts at the ostia of the side branches following kissing balloon dilation [60]. Furthermore, in the case of BRSs, OCT could help in one-scaffold strategies by identifying change in ostium dimensions after scaffold implantation [61,62], or by assessing strut protrusion into the main vessel in side-branch ostial scaffold implantation [63].

## LIMITATIONS OF OCT

There are still limitations facing the use of OCT in certain situations. In severe cases of atherosclerosis marked by profound vessel remodeling, the extent of the disease process contributed by remodeling cannot be well assessed due to the limited penetration of OCT. OCT systems still require clearance of blood before the vessel can be imaged which is usually performed with injections of saline flushes with power injector systems limiting their use in large (>5 mm) and ostial, tortuous vessels and in patients unable to tolerate additional contrast and volume load such as patients with congestive cardiac failure or renal impairment.

## Dimensional measurements evaluated on OCT

Dimensional measurements are well defined and have been published recently [64,65]. Important and commonly used measurements are described below. Other measurements such as plaque area and strut apposition are discussed elsewhere.

The following are important measurements at the cross-sectional level that are commonly reported with OCT.

### LUMEN MEASUREMENTS

- Minimum lumen diameter: The shortest diameter through the center of mass of the lumen.
- Maximum lumen diameter: The longest diameter through the center of mass of the lumen.
- Residual area stenosis: Percentage residual area stenosis (%RAS) was calculated as: [1 − (minimal lumen area/reference lumen area] × 100.

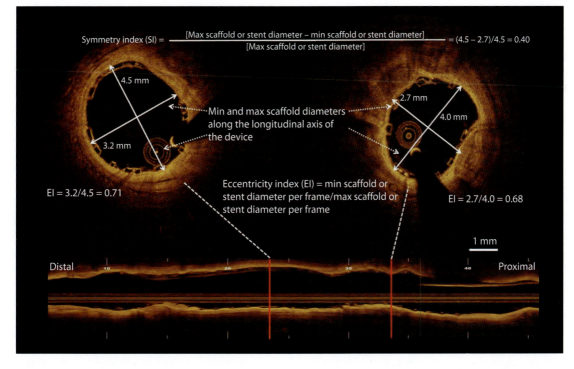

**Figure 5.7.9** OCT measurements used to assess expansion of the bioresorbable vascular scaffolds (BRSs). Both the maximum (max) and minimum (min) scaffold/stent diameters were used to calculate the eccentricity index (EI) and the symmetry index (SI) as shown. EI is defined as the ratio between min and max scaffold/stent diameter in each analyzed frame. The SI was defined as: (max stent/scaffold diameter – min stent/scaffold diameter)/(max stent/scaffold diameter).

## SCAFFOLD MEASUREMENTS

- Minimum scaffold diameter: The shortest diameter through the center of mass of the scaffold.
- Maximum scaffold diameter: The longest diameter through the center of mass of the scaffold.
- Eccentricity index: (maximum scaffold diameter – minimum stent diameter)/maximum scaffold diameter, i.e., the lower the eccentricity index the higher the difference (Figure 5.7.9).
- Symmetry index: (maximal scaffold diameter – minimal scaffold diameter)/(maximal scaffold diameter).
- Minimum scaffold area: The area bounded by the scaffold border.

## HOW TO PERFORM ONLINE OCT IN THE CATHERIZATION LAB

### Proper technique is essential

OCT analysis can be performed online using the dedicated imaging consoles. A proper technique is essential since a proper image is a prerequisite for online OCT analysis. A key challenge especially for initial users is to acquire optimal imaging of the full scaffold length especially for long and complex lesions such as CTO. Currently, commercially available systems include the Illumien™ and Illumiem Optis™ systems with the Dragonfly™ and Dragonfly Duo™ imaging catheters (LightLab/St. Jude Medical, St. Paul, MN) and the Terumo Lunawave™ with the dedicated Fastview™

imaging catheter. Both are compatible with a 6 Fr guide that can acquire frames with a pullback speed of up to 40 mm/s covering 54–150 mm within a single pullback. In contrast to IVUS, in OCT the coronary vessel needs to be cleared of blood. This is because red blood cells are opaque to light, which will lead to the light beam being scattered, resulting in severe signal attenuation. In our practice, the examined artery is cleared of blood by means of iso-osmolar X-ray or low molecular weight dextran contrast injected by power injector at rates 3–4 mL/s (total volume 10–30 mL). Multiple pullbacks or higher imaged length might be needed to cover long lesions with multiple stents.

### Online analysis

For the analysis of the images, before the performance of any measurement, calibration of the Z-offset must be performed, in order to ensure accurate sizing of vessels [66,67]. The identification of the endoluminal border and measurement of vessel diameters/area as described earlier are automatically performed by the imaging system. The whole OCT run should be replayed on the imaging console while the procedure is "live" or ongoing. Manual adjustment of the auto-detected endoluminal border is performed when required especially in regions where blood clearance is inadequate or at regions of bifurcation. Online analysis also allows the image acquired to be displaced in "L-mode" or a lumen profile view where a longitudinal restitution of the study segment where the length of interest

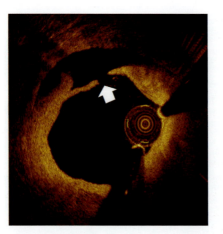

**Figure 5.7.10** Edge dissection seen after predilation prior to scaffold implantation (white arrow: dissection flap).

can be further selected to guide coronary intervention (Figure 5.7.8). Most available OCT systems record cross-sectional images in great detail, but these are not easily matched to their geographical position on the angiogram, especially when clear anatomical landmarks are missing. Important data that are acquired by OCT are therefore not always translated into clinical use. Fortunately, several systems such as Medis System, Optis I System, and Termo System Co-registration Systems have been introduced that allow for quick and easy online co-registration of angiographic and OCT images. This integration of OCT and angiographic information enables immediate utilization of such information by the operator. Optimal landing zones for optimal scaffold deployment can be chosen based on the images acquired and specific scaffold dimensions chosen. Minimum scaffold areas are calculated and further postdilation recommended if necessary. The entire pullback should also be assessed for vascular trauma such as edge dissection which sometimes is not clearly visualized angiographically (Figure 5.7.10). Such information can guide further deployment of scaffolds to treat the edge dissection in severe cases especially if there is lumen reduction, occurring over long segments or compromise of TIMI flow. If there is severe incomplete strut apposition occurring over long segments, further postdilation can be required and further pullbacks performed to check for procedural efficacy.

## CONCLUSION

The use of OCT for preprocedural guidance of BRSs implantation can provide accurate estimation of lumen dimensions and lesion length, which can help in scaffold sizing and optimal lesion coverage, which can help achieve an optimal implantation result. Moreover, use of OCT during the procedure can help identify complications and suboptimal implantation, leading to additional intervention in order to optimize scaffold expansion and apposition and achieve optimal lesion coverage. This approach shows

promise for use in more complex patient and lesion subsets and could translate to improved procedural and clinical outcomes.

## REFERENCES

1. Karanasos A, Simsek C, Gnanadesigan M, van Ditzhuijzen NS, Freire R, Dijkstra J, Tu S et al. OCT assessment of the long-term vascular healing response 5 years after everolimus-eluting bioresorbable vascular scaffold. *J Am Coll Cardiol.* 2014 Dec 9;64 (22):2343–56.
2. Ormiston JA, Serruys PW, Regar E, Dudek D, Thuesen L, Webster MW et al. A bioabsorbable everolimus-eluting coronary stent system for patients with single de-novo coronary artery lesions (ABSORB): A prospective open-label trial. *Lancet.* 2008;371(9616):899–907.
3. Serruys PW, Onuma Y, Ormiston JA, de Bruyne B, Regar E, Dudek D, Thuesen L et al. Evaluation of the second generation of a bioresorbable everolimus drug-eluting vascular scaffold for treatment of de novo coronary artery stenosis: Six-month clinical and imaging outcomes. *Circulation.* 2010 Nov 30;122(22):2301–12.
4. Serruys PW, Chevalier B, Dudek D, Cequier A, Carrié D, Iniguez A, Dominici M et al. A bioresorbable everolimus-eluting scaffold versus a metallic everolimus-eluting stent for ischaemic heart disease caused by de-novo native coronary artery lesions (ABSORB II): An interim 1-year analysis of clinical and procedural secondary outcomes from a randomised controlled trial. *Lancet.* 2015 Jan 3;385(9962):43–54.
5. Tamai H, Igaki K, Kyo E, Kosuga K, Kawashima A, Matsui S et al. Initial and 6-month results of biodegradable poly-l-lactic acid coronary stents in humans. *Circulation.* 2000;102(4):399–404.
6. Verheye S, Ormiston JA, Stewart J, Webster M, Sanidas E, Costa R et al. A next-generation bioresorbable coronary scaffold system: From bench to first clinical evaluation: 6- and 12-month clinical and multimodality imaging results. *JACC Cardiovasc Interv.* 2014;7(1):89–99.
7. Pollman MJ. Engineering a bioresorbable stent: REVA programme update. *EuroIntervention.* 2009;5 Suppl F:F54–7.
8. Tu S, Xu L, Ligthart J, Xu B, Witberg K, Sun Z, Koning G et al. In vivo comparison of arterial lumen dimensions assessed by co-registered three-dimensional (3D) quantitative coronary angiography, intravascular ultrasound and optical coherence tomography. *Int J Cardiovasc Imaging.* 2012 Aug; 28(6): 1315–1327.
9. Tsuchida K, van der Giessen WJ, Patterson M, Tanimoto S, García-García HM, Regar E et al. In vivo validation of a novel three-dimensional quantitative

coronary angiography system (CardiOp-B™): Comparison with a conventional two-dimensional system (CAAS II™) and with special reference to optical coherence tomography. *EuroIntervention*. 2007;3:100–108.

10. Onuma Y, Tanimoto S, Ruygrok P, Neuzner J, Piek JJ, Seth A, Schofer JJ et al. Efficacy of everolimus eluting stent implantation in patients with calcified coronary culprit lesions: Two-year angiographic and three-year clinical results from the SPIRIT II study. *Catheter Cardiovasc Interv*. 2010 Nov 1;76(5):634–42.

11. Lee T, Yonetsu T, Koura K, Hishikari K, Murai T, Iwai T, Takagi T et al. Impact of coronary plaque morphology assessed by optical coherence tomography on cardiac troponin elevation in patients with elective stent implantation. *Circ Cardiovasc Interv*. 2011 Aug;4(4):378–86.

12. Lowe HC, Narula J, Fujimoto JG, Jang IK. Intracoronary optical diagnostics current status, limitations, and potential. *JACC Cardiovasc Interv*. 2011;4:1257–70.

13. Prati F, Cera M, Ramazzotti V, Imola F, Giudice R, Giudice M, Propris SD et al. From bench to bedside: A novel technique of acquiring OCT images. *Circ J*. 2008;72:839–43.

14. Prati F, Regar E, Mintz GS, Arbustini E, Di Mario C, Jang IK, Akasaka T et al. Expert's OCT review document. Expert review document on methodology, terminology, and clinical applications of optical coherence tomography: Physical principles, methodology of image acquisition, and clinical application for assessment of coronary arteries and atherosclerosis. *Eur Heart J*. 2010;31:401–15.

15. Nammas W, Ligthart JM, Karanasos A, Witberg KT, Regar E. Optical coherence tomography for evaluation of coronary stents in vivo. *Expert Rev Cardiovasc Ther*. 2013 May;11(5):577–88.

16. van der Sijde J, Karanasos A, van Soest G, Van Mieghem NM, De Jaegere P, Van Geuns RJ, Diletti R et al. TCT-382 safety and feasibility of optical coherence tomography: A single center experience. *J Am Coll Cardiol*. 2014;64(11, Supplement):B112.

17. Lehtinen T, Nammas W, Airaksinen JK, Karjalainen PP. Feasibility and safety of frequency-domain optical coherence tomography for coronary artery evaluation: A single-center study. *Int J Cardiovasc Imaging*. 2013 Jun;29(5):997–1005.

18. Windecker S, Kolh P, Alfonso F, Collet JP, Cremer J, Falk V, Filippatos G et al. 2014 ESC/EACTS Guidelines on myocardial revascularization. *Eur Heart J*. 2014 Dec 7;35(46):3235-6.

19. Kubo T, Akasaka T, Shite J, Suzuki T, Uemura S, Yu B, Kozuma K et al. OCT compared with IVUS in a coronary lesion assessment: The OPUS-CLASS study. *JACC Cardiovasc Imaging*. 2013 Oct;6(10):1095–104.

20. Gonzalo N, Serruys PW, García-García HM, van Soest G, Okamura T, Ligthart J, Knaapen M et al. Quantitative ex vivo and in vivo comparison of lumen dimensions measured by optical coherence tomography and intravascular ultrasound in human coronary arteries. *Rev Esp Cardiol*. 2009 Jun;62(6):615–24.

21. Gonzalo N, Escaned J, Alfonso F, Nolte C, Rodriguez V, Jimenez-Quevedo P, Bañuelos C et al. Morphometric assessment of coronary stenosis relevance with optical coherence tomography: A comparison with fractional flow reserve and intravascular ultrasound. *J Am Coll Cardiol*. 2012 Mar 20;59(12):1080–9.

22. Ramesh S, Papayannis A, Abdel-karim AR, Banerjee S, Brilakis E. In vivo comparison of Fourier-domain optical coherence tomography and intravascular ultrasonography. *J Invasive Cardiol*. 2012 Mar;24(3):111–5.

23. Jamil Z, Tearney G, Bruining N, Sihan K, van Soest G, Ligthart J, van Domburg R et al. Interstudy reproducibility of the second generation, Fourier domain optical coherence tomography in patients with coronary artery disease and comparison with intravascular ultrasound: A study applying automated contour detection. *Int J Cardiovasc Imaging*. 2013 Jan; 29(1): 39–51. Published online 2012 May 26.

24. Tanimoto S, Rodriguez-Granillo G, Barlis P, de Winter S, Bruining N, Hamers R, Knappen M et al. A novel approach for quantitative analysis of intracoronary optical coherence tomography: High inter-observer agreement with computer-assisted contour detection. *Catheter Cardiovasc Interv*. 2008 Aug 1;72(2):228–35.

25. Gutiérrez-Chico JL, Serruys PW, Girasis C, Garg S, Onuma Y, Brugaletta S, García-García H et al. Quantitative multi-modality imaging analysis of a fully bioresorbable stent: A head-to-head comparison between QCA, IVUS and OCT. Quantitative multi-modality imaging analysis of a fully bioresorbable stent: A head-to-head comparison between QCA, IVUS and OCT. *Int J Cardiovasc Imaging*. 2012 28(3):467–78.

26. Farb A, Sangiorgi G, Carter AJ, Walley VM, Edwards WD, Schwartz RS, Virmani R. Pathology of acute and chronic coronary stenting in humans. *Circulation*. 1999 Jan 5–12;99(1):44–52.

27. Finn AV, Nakazawa G, Ladich E, Kolodgie FD, Virmani R. Does underlying plaque morphology play a role in vessel healing after drug-eluting stent implantation? *JACC Cardiovasc Imaging*. 2008 Jul;1(4):485–8.

28. Imola F, Occhipinti M, Biondi-Zoccai G, Di Vito L, Ramazzotti V, Manzoli A, Pappalardo A et al. Association between proximal stent edge positioning on atherosclerotic plaques containing lipid pools and postprocedural myocardial infarction (from the CLI-POOL Study). *Am J Cardiol*. 2013 Feb 15;111(4):526–31.

29. Tanimoto S, Serruys PW, Thuesen L, Dudek D, de Bruyne B, Chevalier B, Ormiston JA. Comparison of in vivo acute stent recoil between the bioabsorbable everolimus-eluting coronary stent and the everolimus-eluting cobalt chromium coronary stent: Insights from the absorb and spirit trials. *Catheter Cardiovasc Interv.* 2007;70:515–523.

30. Shaw E, Allahwala UK, Cockburn JA, Hansen TCE, Mazhar J, Figtree GA, Hansen PS et al. The effect of coronary artery plaque composition, morphology and burden on Absorb bioresorbable vascular scaffold expansion and eccentricity—A detailed analysis with optical coherence tomography. *Int J Cardiol.* 184 (2015) 230–236.

31. Gonzalo N, Serruys PW, Okamura T, Shen ZJ, Garcia-Garcia HM, Onuma Y et al. Relation between plaque type and dissections at the edges after stent implantation: An optical coherence tomography study. *Int J Cardiol.* 2011;150(2):151–5.

32. Reiber JH, Serruys PW, Kooijman CJ, Wijns W, Slager CJ, Gerbrands JJ, Schuurbiers JC et al. Assessment of short-, medium-, and long-term variations in arterial dimensions from computer-assisted quantitation of coronary cineangiograms. *Circulation.* 1985;71:1–8.

33. Di Mario C, Haase J, den Boer A, Reiber JH, Serruys PW. Edge detection versus densitometry in the quantitative assessment of stenosis phantoms: An in vivo comparison in porcine coronary arteries. *Am Heart J.* 1992;124:1181–9.

34. Serruys PW, Booman F, Troost GJ, Reiber JHC, Gerbrands JJ, van de Brand M, Cherrier F et al. Computerized Quantitative coronary angiography applied to percutaneous transluminal coronary angioplasty: Advantages and limitations. In: Kaltenbach M, Gruentzig A, Rentrop K, Bussman WD, Eds. *Transluminal Coronary Angioplasty and Intracoronary Thrombolysis.* Berlin: Springer-Verlag; 1982:110–124.

35. Dvir D, Marom H, Guetta V, Kornowski R. Three-dimensional coronary reconstruction from routine single-plane coronary Angiograms: In vivo quantitative validation. *Int J Cardiovasc Interv.* 2005;7:141–5.

36. Prati F, Di Vito L, Biondi-Zocca G, Occhipinti M, Alessio La Manna, Tamburino C, Burzotta F et al. Angiography alone versus angiography plus optical coherence tomography to guide decision-making during percutaneous coronary intervention: The Centro per la Lotta contro l'Infarto-Optimisation of Percutaneous Coronary Intervention (CLI-OPCI) study. *EuroIntervention.* 2012:823–829.

37. Okamura T, Onuma Y, Garcia-Garcia HM, van Geuns RJ, Wykrzykowska JJ, Schultz C, van der Giessen WJ et al. First-in-man evaluation of intravascular optical frequency domain imaging (OFDI) of Terumo: A comparison with intravascular ultrasound and quantitative coronary angiography. *EuroIntervention.* 2011 Apr;6(9):1037–45.

38. Karanasos A, Van Mieghem NM, van Ditzhuijzen N, Felix C, Daemen J, Autar A, Onuma Y et al. Angiographic and optical coherence tomography insights into bioresorbable scaffold thrombosis. A single-center experience. *Circ Intv* (in press).

39. Takarada S, Imanishi T, Liu Y, Ikejima H, Tsujioka H, Kuroi A, Ishibashi K et al. Advantage of next-generation frequency-domain optical coherence tomography compared with conventional time-domain system in the assessment of coronary lesion. *Catheter Cardiovasc Interv.* 2010;75:202–6.

40. Fujino Y, Bezerra HG, Attizzani GF, Wang W, Yamamoto H, Chamie D, Kanaya T et al. Frequency-domain optical coherence tomography assessment of unprotected left main coronary artery disease—A comparison with intravascular ultrasound. *Catheter Cardiovasc Interv.* 2013;82:E173–83.

41. Allahwala UK, Cockburn JA, Shaw E, Figtree GA, Hansen PS, Bhindi R. Clinical utility of optical coherence tomography (OCT) in the optimisation of Absorb bioresorbable vascular scaffold deployment during percutaneous coronary intervention. *EuroIntervention.* 2015 Feb;10(10):1154–9.

42. Choi SY, Witzenbichler B, Maehara A, Lansky AJ, Guagliumi G, Brodie B, Kellett MA Jr et al. Intravascular ultrasound findings of early stent thrombosis after primary percutaneous intervention in acute myocardial infarction: A harmonizing outcomes with revascularization and stents in acute myocardial infarction (HORIZONS-AMI) substudy. *Circ Cardiovasc Interv.* 2011 Jun;4(3):239–47.

43. Liu X, Doi H, Maehara A, Mintz GS, de Ribamar Costa Jr J, Sano K et al. Avolumetric intravascular ultrasound comparison of early drug-eluting stent thrombosis versus restenosis. *JACC Cardiovasc Interv.* 2009;2(5):428–34.

44. Imola F, Mallus MT, Ramazzotti V, Manzoli A, Pappalardo A, Di Giorgio A, Albertucci M et al. Safety and feasibility of frequency domain optical coherence tomography to guide decision making in percutaneous coronary intervention. *EuroIntervention.* 2010;6:575–81.

45. Vicecone N, Chan PH, Alegria-Barrero E, Ghilencea L, Lindsay A, Foin N, Di Mario C. Frequency domain optical coherence tomography for guidance of coronary stenting. *Int J Cardiol.* 2011 Dec 30.

46. Parise H, Maehara A, Stone GW et al. Metanalysis of randomized studies comparing intravascular ultrasound versus angiographic guidance of percutaneous coronary intervention in pre drug eluting era. *Am J Cardiol.* 2011; 107 (3): 374–382.

47. Keane D, Haase J, Slager CJ, Montauban van Swijndregt E, Lehmann KG, Ozaki Y, di Mario C et al. Comparative validation of quantitative coronary

angiography systems. Results and implications from a multicenter study using a standardized approach. *Circulation*. 1995;91:2174–83.

48. Zhang Y, Farooq V, Garcia-Garcia HM, Bourantas CV, Tian N, Dong S, Li M et al. Comparison of intravascular ultrasound versus angiography-guided drug-eluting stent implantation: A meta-analysis of one randomised trial and ten observational studies involving 19,619 patients. *EuroIntervention*. 2012;8:855–865.

49. Fitzgerald PJ, Oshima A, Hayase M, Metz JA, Bailey SR, Baim DS, Cleman MW et al. Final results of the can routine ultrasound influence stent expansion (cruise) study. *Circulation*. 2000;102:523–530.

50. Oemrawsingh PV, Mintz GS, Schalij MJ, Zwinderman AH, Jukema JW, and van der Wall EE. Intravascular ultrasound guidance improves angiographic and clinical outcome of stent implantation for long coronary artery stenoses: Final results of a randomized comparison with angiographic guidance (TULIP study). *Circulation*. 2003;107:62– 67.

51. Park SW, Lee CW, Hong MK et al. Randomized comparison of coronary stenting with optimal balloon angioplasty for treatment of lesions in small coronary arteries. *Eur Heart J*. 2000;21:1785–1789.

52. Kim JS, Hong MK, Ko YG et al. Impact of intravascular ultrasound guidance on long term clinical outcomes in patients treated with drug eluting stent for bifurcational lesions: Data from a Korean multicentre bifurcation registry. *Am Heart J*. 2011; 161 (1): 180–187.

53. Park SJ, Kim YH, Park DW et al. Impact of ultrasound guidance on long term mortality in stenting for unprotected left main coronary artery stenosis. *Circ Cardiovasc Interv*. 2009;2: 167–177.

54. Vaquerizo B, Barros A, Pujadas S, Bajo E, Estrada D, Miranda-Guardiola F, Rigla J et al. Bioresorbable everolimus-eluting vascular scaffold for the treatment of chronic total occlusions: CTO-ABSORB pilot study. *EuroIntervention*. 2015 11(5):555–563.

55. Jaguszewski M, Ghadri JR, Zipponi M, Bataiosu DR, Diekmann J, Geyer V, Neumann CA et al. Feasibility of second-generation bioresorbable vascular scaffold implantation in complex anatomical and clinical scenarios. *Clin Res Cardiol*. 2015 Feb;104(2):124-35.

56. Everaert B, Felix C, Koolen J, den Heijer P, Henriques J, Wykrzykowska JJ, van der Schaaf R et al. Appropriate use of bioresorbable vascular scaffolds in percutaneous coronary interventions: A recommendation from experienced users: A position statement on the use of bioresorbable vascular scaffolds in the Netherlands. *Neth Heart J*. 2015 Mar;23(3):161–5.

57. Farooq V, Serruys PW, Heo JH, Gogas BD, Okamura T, Gomez-Lara J et al. New insights into the coronary artery bifurcation hypothesisgenerating concepts utilizing 3-dimensional optical frequency domain imaging. *JACC Cardiovasc Interv*. 2011;4(8):921–31.

58. Di Mario C, Iakovou I, van der Giessen WJ, Foin N, Adrianssens T, Tyczynski P, Ghilencea L et al. Optical coherence tomography for guidance in bifurcation lesion treatment. *EuroIntervention*. 2010;6:J99–106.

59. Okamura T, Serruys PW, and Regar E. The fate of bioresorbable struts located at a side branch ostium: Serial three-dimensional optical coherence tomography assessment. *Eur Heart J*. May 2010: 2179.

60. Okamura T, Yamada J, Nao T, Suetomi T, Maeda T, Shiraishi K et al. Three-dimensional optical coherence tomography assessment of coronary wire re-crossing position during bifurcation stenting. *EuroIntervention*. 2011;7 (7):886–7.

61. Karanasos A, Tu S, van der Heide E, Reiber JH, and Regar E. Carina shift as a mechanism for side-branch compromise following main vessel intervention: Insights from three-dimensional optical coherence tomography. *Cardiovasc Diagn Ther*. 2012 Jun;2(2):173–7.

62. Karanasos A, Tu S, van Ditzhuijzen NS, Ligthart JM, Witberg K, Van Mieghem N, van Geuns RJ et al. A novel method to assess coronary artery bifurcations by OCT: Cut-plane analysis for side-branch ostial assessment from a main-vessel pullback. *Eur Heart J Cardiovasc Imaging*. 2015 Feb;16(2):177-89.

63. Karanasos A, Li Y, Tu S, Wentzel JJ, Reiber JH, van Geuns RJ, Regar E. Is it safe to implant bioresorbable scaffolds in ostial side-branch lesions? Impact of "neo-carina" formation on main-branch flow pattern. Longitudinal clinical observations. *Atherosclerosis*. 2015 Jan;238(1):22–5.

64. Tearney GJ, Regar E, Akasaka T et al. Consensus standards for acquisition, measurement, and reporting of intravascular optical coherence tomography studies: A report from the International Working Group for Intravascular Optical Coherence Tomography Standardization and Validation. *J Am Coll Cardiol*. 2012;59:1058–72.

65. Garcia-Garcia HM, Serruys PW, Stone GW et al. Assessing bioresorbable coronary devices: Methods and parameters. *JACC Cardiovasc Imaging*. 2014 Nov;7(11):1130–48.

66. Bezerra HG et al Intracoronary optical coherence tomography: A comprehensive review clinical and research applications. *JACC Cardiovasc Interv*. 2009;2(11):1035–1046.

67. Mehanna EA, Attizzani GF, Kyono H, Hake M, and Bezerra HG. Assessment of coronary stent by optical coherence tomography, methodology and definitions. *Int J Cardiovasc Imaging*. 2011 Feb;27(2):259–69.

# Imaging to evaluate the bioresorbable scaffold—Clinicians' perspective: I need both (IVUS and OCT)

JOSEP GOMEZ-LARA AND ANTONIO SERRA

## INTRODUCTION

Bioresorbable vascular scaffolds (BVSs) have been shown as effective as metallic drug-eluting stents in patients with coronary artery disease at 1 year of follow-up [1]. However, the temporal scaffolding of the vessel with complete or partial restoration of the vessel vasomotion, restoration of the coronary anatomy, healing of culprit plaques with thick neointima cap, and avoidance of pathologic plaque remodeling have emerged as the key targets with this technology at mid-long-term follow-up [2–4]. In addition, the use of concomitant medical treatments capable of decreasing the plaque burden and the "systemic vulnerability" of high-risk patients, such as statins, HDL-raising therapies, or PCSK9 inhibitors, may be the cornerstone of future treatments for coronary artery disease.

Intravascular imaging techniques, such as intravascular ultrasound (IVUS) and optical coherence tomography (OCT), allow assessing the vessel wall dynamic changes and showing complementary observations such as: composition and dimensions of the culprit lesion, preparation of the lesion prior to scaffold implantation, optimization of the BVSs deployment, healing process of the scaffold during the temporary scaffolding, and the surveillance of the bioresorption [4]. In a series of 53 event-free highly selected stable patients included in the ABSORB Cohort B study, IVUS and OCT were performed at baseline, 6 or 12 months, 24 or 36 months, and 5 years [4]. In this study, polymeric scaffolds were no longer visible by IVUS nor OCT at 5 years. The analysis of the vessel changes from postprocedure to 5 years showed mild decrease in mean lumen area (as assessed by OCT), mild decrease in plaque area (as assessed by IVUS), and no modification of the vessel volume (as assessed by IVUS). Moreover, the angiographic analysis of

the "in-scaffold" segment showed vasodilatation after intracoronary dose of nitroglycerin in most of the cases.

Although intravascular imaging techniques are usually not necessary in noncomplex lesions, its use in complex lesions, such as coronary chronic total occlusions (CTO) or bifurcated lesions, may help operators to optimize scaffold implantation and may have clinical impact. Coronary CTO successfully treated with stent implantation has been associated with dynamic changes of the occluded vessel, such as lumen enlargement, that can predispose to late-acquired malapposition [5,6]. Bifurcation lesions with side-branch jailing are also associated with persistent nonapposed struts. Due to its temporary presence in the vessel, the use of bioresorbable vascular scaffolds (BVSs) in coronary CTO and bifurcation lesions can overcome late adverse events related to stent malappostion.

## IVUS AND OCT ASSESSMENT OF CULPRIT LESIONS PRIOR TO BVS IMPLANTATION

Assessment of plaque and vessel characteristics prior to BVSs implantation is of interest due to different causes. First, suboptimal scaffold implantation, such as scaffold underexpansion, has been related with higher risk of thrombosis [7]. Although severe calcified lesions are rarely observed, patients with angiographic calcium or suboptimal balloon expansion may merit intravascular imaging before BVSs implantation. In patients with coronary CTO, 30% of lesions have severe calcification [8]. IVUS imaging allows assessment of calcium rings and is able to ensure the proper rupture of the calcium ring before scaffold implantation.

On the other hand, the placement of the coronary wire in the medial space in patients undergoing CTO interventions has been associated with intramural hematomas. A total of 34% of successfully recanalized CTO have intramural hematomas [8]. IVUS imaging is capable of assessing intramural hematomas and visualizing the medial location of the coronary wire. In a series of 38 cases with coronary CTO treated with a BVSs, IVUS imaging was performed immediately after lesion recanalization (wire crossing and mild predilatation) [9]. The IVUS images obtained immediately after CTO recanalization were used to decide the balloon size (with a balloon-to-artery ratio of 0.7–1:1) and the balloon type (noncompliant or cutting balloons) [9]. In this study, only one patient (2.6%) with subintimal wiring (wire located in the media layer) presented with coronary perforation after predilatation with a noncompliant balloon and needed to be treated with a graft stent [9].

Finally, polymeric BVSs have limited expansion of the device with risk of scaffold rupture in cases of device overexpansion. Therefore, accurate sizing of the vessel is of interest in order to prevent size mismatch between the scaffold size and vessel dimension [10]. Intravascular imaging techniques allow assessing the reference lumen diameter (in segments with no or minimal plaque burden located proximal and/or distal to the culprit lesion) and assessing the "to be scaffolded segment length" prior to BVSs implantation. The lumen area of the reference segment is usually overestimated with IVUS and is measured precisely with OCT due to the technical differences of each technique. Similarly, fast OCT pullbacks allow more accurate segment length measurements as compared to slow IVUS pullbacks. However, coregistration systems between angiography and intravascular imaging techniques also allow accurate segment length measurements. Table 5.8.1 shows the potential utility of IVUS and OCT in complex percutaneous coronary interventions.

**Table 5.8.1** Potential utility of intravascular imaging techniques in percutaneous coronary interventions

| | OCT | IVUS |
|---|---|---|
| Assessment of the proximal stump and proper entrance of the wire in the case of blunt stump | Difficult<br>Only in cases with >2 mm lateral branches at the proximal stump. | Easy<br>Short tip catheters allow imaging in case of absent lateral branches at the proximal stump. |
| Assessment of intimal wiring into the chronic total occlusion | Difficult<br>Blood needs to be completely removed from the lumen to achieve good quality images. OCT catheters (long tip) require to cross >25 mm the CTO and to perform aggressive predilatation prior to imaging. | Easy<br>Imaging can be performed without the need of crossing the CTO and there is no need of aggressive predilatation with short tip catheters. |
| Assessment of subintimal hematoma prior to stenting | Feasible<br>In case of large plaques subintimal hematomas can be ignored. | Easy<br>In case of severe calcified plaques it can be difficult. |
| Assessment of plaque characteristics and proper preparation in the case of calcified plaques | Feasible<br>In the case of large plaques deep calcium can be ignored. | Feasible<br>In the case of severe calcified plaques, rupture of calcium rings can be difficult. |
| Assessment of the vessel size (media diameter) | Feasible<br>In the case of large plaques the OCT signal does not visualize the media layer. | Easy<br>In the case of severe calcified plaques, it can be difficult due to the echo shadow. |
| Assessment of optimal BVSs implantation: | | |
|   Strut malapposition | Easy | Feasible |
|   Strut fracture | Easy | Difficult |
|   Scaffold underexpansion | Easy | Feasible |
|   Thrombus | Easy | Difficult |
|   Plaque protrusion | Easy | Difficult |
|   Subintimal location | Easy | Feasible |
|   In-scaffold dissections | Easy | Difficult |
|   Edge dissections | Easy | Feasible |
|   Geographical miss | Easy | Feasible |

*Abbreviations:* BVSs = bioresorbable vascular scaffolds; CTO = chronic total occlusion; IVUS = intravascular ultrasound; OCT = optical coherence tomography.

## OPTIMIZATION OF BVS IMPLANTATION

IVUS renders the polymeric struts as hyper-refractive boxes with an important echogenic blooming effect that confers a double strut appearance. Assessment of lumen perimeter is usually hampered by the blooming effect of the polymeric struts. Moreover, polymeric struts are usually unseen in calcified lesions because of the similar echogenicity between polymer and calcium. On the contrary, OCT renders polymeric struts as a black central core surrounded by a light-scattering frame. The four sides of the polymeric struts are clearly visible and there is no

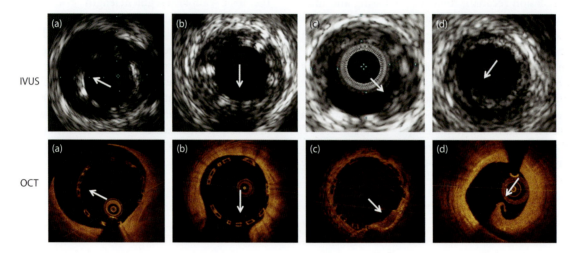

Figure 5.8.1 Qualitative findings after scaffold implantation between IVUS and OCT. Matched images between IVUS and OCT of incomplete strut/scaffold apposition (a), side-branch struts (b), tissue protrusion (c), and edge dissection (d).

Table 5.8.2 Optical coherence tomography criteria of optimal scaffold deployment

| OCT findings (definitions) | When to perform further interventions | When to not perform further interventions |
|---|---|---|
| Edge dissections (Linear rim of tissue with a width >200 μm and a clear separation from the vessel wall) | Flow limitation and/or >5 consecutive cross-sections with dissection >180 degrees of the lumen perimeter. | <180 degrees of the lumen perimeter. |
| Malapposition (Separation of the abluminal side of the strut to the vessel wall) | >200 μm of malapposition length in 5 consecutive cross-sections. | In the case of side branches or in the case of large malappositions with risk of scaffold fracture by overstretching. |
| Underexpansion (In-stent MLA <70% of the average reference lumen area outside the scaffolded segment) | Signs of angiographic balloon underexpansion or scaffold recoil after implantation. The MLA cross-section usually has eccentric scaffold perimeter. | Long scaffolded segments with vessel tapering and no evidence of balloon underexpansion or scaffold recoil. |
| Minimal lumen area <4.5 mm² (Lumen perimeter measured behind the abluminal side of the struts) | Usually associated with some degree of underexpansion. | No signs of underexpansion. |
| Scaffold fracture (Overhanging struts with or without malapposition or isolated struts at the luminal center without obvious connection to other surrounding struts) | Minor scaffold disruptions (<5 cross-sections). | In the case of follow-up imaging strut disruptions may be part of the bioresorption process. |
| Intrastent plaque/thrombus protrusion (Tissue or thrombus prolapsing between stent struts or located in the lumen >500 μm thick) | Diffuse protrusion extending >5 cross-sections. | In the case of clear thrombus upgrade of anticoagulant and antiplatelet treatment may be considered. |

*Source:* Modified from Prati F, Romagnoli E, Burzotta F, Limbruno U, Gatto L, La Manna A, Versaci F et al. *JACC Cardiovasc Imaging.* 2015;8:1297–305.

shadow behind the struts. Therefore, scaffold/strut apposition and expansion are easily assessed with OCT [11]. Figure 5.8.1 shows the IVUS and OCT characteristics of bioresorbable scaffolds.

Nonoptimal scaffold/strut apposition and expansion with BVSs have been associated with higher risk of scaffold thrombosis [7]. The thicker strut size of the scaffolds, as compared with current metallic stents, causes larger flow alterations surrounding the struts and this can predispose the patient to platelet aggregation and thrombosis [12]. There is limited information on the optimal deployment criteria after scaffold implantation. The CLI-OPCI II study recommended five OCT criteria for metallic stent implantation. These criteria included: edge dissections, malapposition, underexpansion, small minimal lumen area, and tissue/thrombus protrusion [13]. Table 5.8.2 shows the modification of those OCT criteria for scaffold implantation according to our criteria that also includes scaffold fracture.

## SERIAL IMAGING OF BVS WITH IVUS AND OCT

The healing process of the different metallic drug-eluting stents (DESs) is extremely heterogeneous. However, it is well known that >75% of malapposed struts immediately after stent implantation are apposed and covered at 6–12 months of follow-up [14]. Small malappositions (<200 μm distance from malapposed strut to the vessel wall and <2 mm length of longitudinal malappositon) are usually healed at follow-up [14]. Similar results have been reported with BVSs, as assessed by OCT, at 6–12 months of follow-up [15].

However, cases of late-acquired malapposition with metallic and bioresorbable DES at mid-term of follow-up have also been described [6,7]. Late-acquired malapposition can occur due to several causes: (1) pathologic vessel remodeling because polymer/drug hypersensibility; (2) stent/scaffold fractures; and finally (3) cases of lumen and vessel enlargement a few hours/days after scaffold

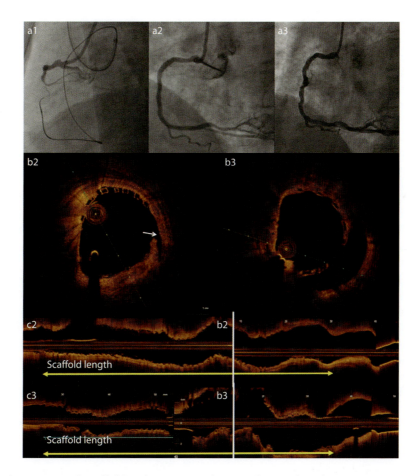

**Figure 5.8.2**  One-year late-acquired scaffold malapposition due to subintimal implantation. Patient with chronic total occlusion of the right coronary artery (RCA) treated with two BVSs by retrograde approach. **(a1)** Angiograms of the lesion with the retrograde wire; **(a2)** angiogram of the final result after two scaffold implantation; **(a3)** angiogram of the RCA at 1 year of follow-up (the patient remained asymptomatic); **(b2)** OCT cross-section immediately after scaffold implantation (arrow shows rupture of the media and scaffold in subintimal location); **(b3)** same OCT cross-section at 1 year (several struts with late-acquired malapposition); **(c2)** longitudinal OCT cross-section immediately after scaffold implantation; **(c3)** longitudinal OCT cross-section showing large segments with scaffold malapposition at 1 year follow-up.

implantation. The former mechanism has been described in patients treated with first-generation DES. It has been also described in patients with subintimal stent/scaffold implantation in patients with CTO [6]. The second mechanism has been described in patients treated with BVSs due to polymer bioresorption and loss of the radial force [15]. Finally, lumen and vessel enlargement have been described in patients with ST-elevation myocardial infarction (due to vessel spasm) and in patients undergoing to CTO procedures [5]. Figure 5.8.2 shows an illustrative case of BVSs implantation in coronary-CTO imaged with serial OCT imaging.

Serial intravascular imaging of noncomplex lesions in stable patients treated with BVSs showed 11% of patients with scaffold malappositon and 8% with late-acquired malapposition at 6 months [15]. Serial intravascular imaging of coronary CTO treated with BVSs showed 29% of patients with scaffold malapposition and 12% of patients with late-acquired malapposition at 1 year [6]. In all cases, BVSs can overcome most of the risks of late malapposition due to its temporary presence into the lumen. At 5 years of the scaffold implantation, scaffolds are no longer visible and there are no traces in human coronary arteries, as assessed by intravascular imaging techniques [4].

On the other hand, lack of strut coverage has been also described as an important predictor of stent thrombosis. Lesion complexity is an important predictor of strut coverage. Noncomplex lesions in stable patients treated with BVSs presented with >5% of uncovered struts in <10% of cases; but 42% of CTO lesions treated with BVSs presented with >5% of uncovered struts at 1 year [6]. As stated previously, the use of BVSs in complex lesions can overcome the risks of thrombosis when the scaffold will eventually disappear.

## CONCLUSION

BVSs have been shown effective in the treatment of patients with coronary artery disease. The use of intravascular imaging techniques is not necessary in noncomplex cases in the hands of experienced operators. However, both IVUS and OCT are advisable in the initial experiences with this device and in complex cases. IVUS allows the assessment of the vessel wall dynamics and the bioresorption process and OCT provides an accurate assessment of the scaffold characteristics and bioresorption.

## REFERENCES

1. Stone GW, Gao R, Kimura T, Kereiakes DJ, Ellis SG, Onuma Y, Cheong WF et al. 1-year outcomes with the Absorb bioresorbable scaffold in patients with coronary artery disease: A patient-level, pooled meta-analysis. *Lancet*. 2016.
2. Gomez-Lara J, Brugaletta S, Farooq V, van Geuns RJ, De Bruyne B, Windecker S, McClean D et al. Angiographic geometric changes of the lumen arterial wall after bioresorbable vascular scaffolds and metallic platform stents at 1-year follow-up. *JACC Cardiovasc Interv*. 2011;4:789–99.
3. Brugaletta S, Heo JH, Garcia-Garcia HM, Farooq V, van Geuns RJ, de Bruyne B, Dudek D et al. Endothelial-dependent vasomotion in a coronary segment treated by ABSORB everolimus-eluting bioresorbable vascular scaffold system is related to plaque composition at the time of bioresorption of the polymer: Indirect finding of vascular reparative therapy? *Eur Heart J*. 2012;33:1325–33.
4. Serruys PW, Ormiston J, van Geuns RJ, de Bruyne B, Dudek D, Christiansen E, Chevalier B et al. A polylactide bioresorbable scaffold eluting everolimus for treatment of coronary stenosis: 5-year follow-up. *J Am Coll Cardiol*. 2016;67:766–76.
5. Gomez-Lara J, Teruel L, Homs S, Ferreiro JL, Romaguera R, Roura G, Sanchez-Elvira G et al. Lumen enlargement of the coronary segments located distal to chronic total occlusions successfully treated with drug-eluting stents at follow-up. *EuroIntervention*. 2014;9:1181–8.
6. Vaquerizo B, Barros A, Pujadas S, Bajo E, Jimenez M, Gomez-Lara J, Jacobi F et al. One-year results of bioresorbable vascular scaffolds for coronary chronic total occlusions. *Am J Cardiol*. 2016;117:906–17.
7. Cuculi F, Puricel S, Jamshidi P, Valentin J, Kallinikou Z, Toggweiler S, Weissner M et al. Optical coherence tomography findings in bioresorbable vascular scaffolds thrombosis. *Circ Cardiovasc Interv*. 2015;8:e002518.
8. Fujii K, Ochiai M, Mintz GS, Kan Y, Awano K, Masutani M, Ashida K et al. Procedural implications of intravascular ultrasound morphologic features of chronic total coronary occlusions. *Am J Cardiol*. 2006;97:1455–62.
9. Vaquerizo B, Barros A, Pujadas S, Bajo E, Estrada D, Miranda-Guardiola F, Rigla J et al. Bioresorbable everolimus-eluting vascular scaffold for the treatment of chronic total occlusions: CTO-ABSORB pilot study. *EuroIntervention*. 2015;11:555–63.
10. Gomez-Lara J, Diletti R, Brugaletta S, Onuma Y, Farooq V, Thuesen L, McClean D et al. Angiographic maximal luminal diameter and appropriate deployment of the everolimus-eluting bioresorbable vascular scaffold as assessed by optical coherence tomography: An ABSORB cohort B trial sub-study. *EuroIntervention*. 2012;8:214–24.
11. Gomez-Lara J, Brugaletta S, Diletti R, Gogas BD, Farooq V, Onuma Y, Gobbens P et al. Agreement and reproducibility of gray-scale intravascular ultrasound and optical coherence tomography for the analysis of the bioresorbable vascular scaffold. *Cathet Cardiovasc Interv*. 2011;79:890–902.
12. Kolandaivelu K, Swaminathan R, Gibson WJ, Kolachalama VB, Nguyen-Ehrenreich KL, Giddings VL, Coleman L et al. Stent thrombogenicity early

in high-risk interventional settings is driven by stent design and deployment and protected by polymer-drug coatings. *Circulation*. 2011;123:1400–9.

13. Prati F, Romagnoli E, Burzotta F, Limbruno U, Gatto L, La Manna A, Versaci F et al. Clinical Impact of OCT Findings During PCI: The CLI-OPCI II Study. *JACC Cardiovasc Imaging*. 2015;8:1297–305.

14. Gutierrez-Chico JL, Wykrzykowska JJ, Nuesch E, van Geuns RJ, Koch KT, Koolen JJ, di Mario C et al. Vascular tissue reaction to acute malapposition in human coronary arteries: Sequential assessment with optical coherence tomography. *Circ Cardiovasc Interv*. 2012;5:20–9, S1–8.

15. Gomez-Lara J, Radu M, Brugaletta S, Farooq V, Diletti R, Onuma Y, Windecker S et al. Serial analysis of the malapposed and uncovered struts of the new generation of everolimus-eluting bioresorbable scaffold with optical coherence tomography. *JACC Cardiovasc Interv*. 2011;4:992–1001.

<br>

# 5.9

# Multislice computed tomography as a modality of follow-up

ANTONIO L. BARTORELLI, DANIELE ANDREINI, SIMONA ESPEJO, AND MANUEL PAN

## INTRODUCTION

Fully bioresorbable vascular scaffolds (BVSs) have several advantages over current metallic drug-eluting stents (DESs). Indeed, they do not only provide transient scaffolding properties with drug-delivery capabilities and reestablish normal flow in diseased coronary segments but may also restore vascular integrity and function introducing a novel therapeutic potential. By avoiding a permanent metallic cage, the coronary vessel may recover pulsatility, vasomotion, and responsiveness to shear stress and physiological cyclic strain [1–3]. Moreover, full scaffold bioresorption eliminates the risk that foreign materials, such as nonendothelialized stent struts and drug polymers, can persist long-term creating a potential trigger for late coronary thrombosis. Thus, this novel technology has the potential to overcome many of the safety concerns regarding metallic DESs and possibly convey additional clinical benefits [4]. However, the clinical advantages of BVSs technology over the currently available metallic DESs need to be investigated further. Thus, large studies with specific end points and long-term follow-up may be necessary to confirm that these new devices may obtain better outcome after percutaneous treatment of coronary artery disease (CAD) patients. Non-invasive coronary imaging with coronary computed tomography angiography (CCTA) will play a major research and clinical role in the follow-up of patients treated with BVSs for evaluating neointimal growth and arterial remodeling of the scaffolded segment. Currently, the BVSs technology is still in an early phase and only a few studies are available on CCTA follow-up in patients treated with these devices. Therefore, this chapter will focus on the ABSORB BVSs (Abbott Laboratories, Abbott Park, IL) that was the first bioresorbable device to undergo noninvasive assessment with CCTA and to date has accumulated the largest amount of data.

## CORONARY COMPUTED TOMOGRAPHY ANGIOGRAPHY

For decades, new percutaneous coronary therapies have required invasive coronary angiography (ICA) for follow-up assessment. Considering the good diagnostic accuracy of CCTA in the absence of metal stents and the advantages in safety, patient convenience, and cost, CCTA offers a noninvasive alternative to ICA for both clinical care and research. At the present time, CCTA is considered a reliable diagnostic method for the evaluation of patients with known or suspected CAD. This imaging tool demonstrated high diagnostic performance for the detection of significant coronary stenosis [5], particularly in specific clinical subsets [6–8], and the ability to correctly rule out the presence of CAD. Starting from 2006, the European and American Society of Cardiology and Radiology have identified the appropriate clinical indications for CCTA clinical use including: (1) exclusion of significant coronary narrowing in patients with chest pain and intermediate pretest probability of CAD, those with acute chest pain and new-onset heart failure, or in those who are candidates for valve surgery, (2) diagnosis of coronary artery anomalies, and (3) assessment of coronary artery bypass grafts [5,9]. A strong diagnostic value of CCTA has been already demonstrated by a large amount of data in patients with stable chest pain, leading the European Society of Cardiology to include CCTA in the guidelines on the management of stable CAD as the first-line imaging technique in patients with low-to-intermediate pretest likelihood of CAD [10]. However, even though CCTA is gaining widespread acceptance for noninvasive evaluation of coronary arteries, the associated radiation exposure is still causing concern. Nowadays, according to the principle of optimization as pointed out by the International Commission of Radiological Protection, the number of individuals exposed and the magnitude of the radiation dose they receive should be kept as low as reasonably achievable (ALARA concept). Accordingly, several strategies for reducing radiation exposure with multi-slice computed tomography (MSCT) have been developed: modification of x-ray output such as low tube voltage and tube current set-up [11,12], tube current modulation-ECG triggered [11–13], prospective ECG triggering [14–16], adaptive iterative reconstruction algorithm rather than filtered back projection algorithm [17–19], reduction of the extent or duration of x-ray exposure such as optimization of scan length, dual source CT [20] or high pitch CT [21,22], and reduction of z-over-beaming and/or z-over-scanning such as large detector (256-slices and 320-slices) scanners [23,24]. Indeed, using a combination of multiple effective dose reduction strategies a sub-millisievert CCTA is a realistic achievement.

## EVALUATION OF CORONARY STENTS WITH CCTA

A correct evaluation of stent patency by CCTA may be particularly difficult. The main hurdles are blooming artifacts caused by metallic stent struts that may impair stent lumen visualization and quantification of lumen narrowing by neointimal hyperplasia (Figure 5.9.1). Previous studies showed that CCTA has a very high negative predictive value (NPV), ranging from 78% to 100%, for excluding in-stent restenosis (ISR), while the positive predictive value (PPV) is markedly worse (25–100%). However, CCTA performance has been improved by recent scanner generation, including dual-source CT, which decreased the number of stented segments excluded from analysis. To date, four meta-analyses have been published on the value of CCTA for coronary stent evaluation [25–28]. The overall sensitivity, specificity, PPV, and NPV for assessable stents, as reported by Kumbhani et al., were 91%, 91%, 68%, and 98%, respectively [26]. Two meta-analyses were based on the identical set of clinical studies, but reached controversial conclusions. While Sun and Almutairi stated that CCTA is a reliable alternative to ICA [27], Kumbhani et al. reached the conclusion that stress imaging remains the most acceptable noninvasive technique for diagnosing ISR [26]. The latest and largest meta-analysis, including 24 studies, 1300 patients, and more than 200 stents showed an overall CCTA stent evaluability of 90%, with sensitivity, specificity,

PPV, NPV, and diagnostic accuracy of 90%, 92%, 73%, 97%, and 92%, respectively [28]. Aside from blooming and motion artifacts, stent-related factors such as stent diameter, strut thickness, stent design, and stent deployment technique may influence CCTA visualization of the stented vessel lumen. There is consensus that stents with a diameter <3 mm are less likely to be accessible than stents with a diameter ≥3 mm [29–31]. The role of strut thickness is still controversial, with studies in which this parameter affected stent lumen assessment and other studies that found no impact. However, it is important to note that in the latter studies the cut-off for distinguishing thin from thick strut stents was higher (110 μm vs. 120 μm or <140 μm vs. >140 μm) [32,33]. The role of stent material has been demonstrated by *in vitro* studies and confirmed in patients by Oncel et al. and Andreini et al. studies [34–36]. Indeed, Andreini et al. showed higher diagnostic accuracy for the cobalt-chromium alloy stents as compared to stainless steel stents. In addition, they demonstrated that long and bifurcation lesions requiring elaborate procedures and involving multiple and overlapping stents are other factors limiting stent lumen visualization [35,36] (Figure 5.9.2). This is likely due to a larger amount of metal owing to multiple strut layers at the ostium of side branches and at overlapping sites resulting from these complex procedures [28]. Finally, the effect of stent design (open vs. closed cell) remains unclear [30]. Recently, a new generation high-definition scanner with improved in-plane spatial resolution (230 μm) demonstrated to allow a more accurate detection and quantification of ISR [37] (Figure 5.9.3).

## NONINVASIVE ASSESSMENT OF BVS WITH CCTA

In contrast to radio-opaque metallic stents, which hinder in-stent luminal assessment with CCTA because of blooming artifacts, the polymeric BVSs is radio-lucent except for two

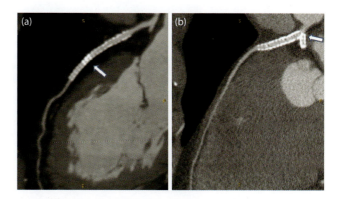

Figure 5.9.2 Examples of CCTA focal beam-hardening artifacts due to drug-eluting stent overlap in the left anterior descending coronary artery (**a**, arrow) and at the site of a bifurcation lesion between the proximal left anterior descending and left circumflex coronary arteries treated with the T-stenting technique (**b**, arrow). The large amount of metal due to a double strut layer impedes evaluation of stent patency.

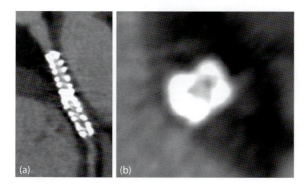

Figure 5.9.1 Long axis (**a**) and short axis (**b**) CCTA curved reconstruction of a right coronary artery treated with a drug-eluting stent. Note the severe and diffuse beam-hardening artifacts due to metallic struts that hinder evaluation of the stent lumen.

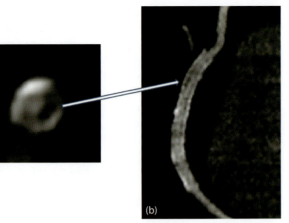

Figure 5.9.3 Moderate neointimal hyperplasia of a drug-eluting stent implanted in a right coronary artery can be detected with CCTA in short axis **(a)** and long axis **(b)** reconstructions using a high-definition scanner with improved in-plane spatial resolution.

metallic markers located at both extremities. Thus, CCTA delineates easily the contours of the scaffolded vessel and noninvasive imaging follow-up has provided reliable angiographic assessment up to 3 to 5 years after implantation and may therefore become an alternative to ICA [35]. Moreover, when compared to angiographic follow-up, CCTA might be a more cost-effective follow-up modality and surely avoids the potential complications of ICA.

## Platinum radio-opaque markers

The BVSs is radiolucent and completely dissolves in a few years after implantation except for two pairs of very small (244 μm) cylindrical platinum radio-opaque markers separated by a distance of 147 μm at both proximal and distal scaffold edges that remain embedded in the neointimal tissue growing over time on the scaffold (Figure 5.9.4). The presence of these markers enables to locate where the BVSs was implanted in the coronary vessel after all polymeric struts have bioresorbed, therefore facilitating visualization by CCTA of coronary segments treated with this innovative device and allowing a better assessment of the index vessel lumen. Indeed, knowing where a BVSs has been placed in the artery is important for routine follow-up after PCI and in the event of future revascularization procedures. However, calcium deposits may interfere with the identification of radio-opaque markers due to overlapping attenuation measured by Hounsfield units and distinction between calcified spots and metallic markers may be difficult. Nevertheless, as compared to calcium deposits, metallic markers usually have higher blooming artifacts and peak intensity and this may help their detection. Of note, the radio-opaque markers positioned at the BVSs extremities appear much larger than they really are and as a single marker because of the blooming effect due to partial volume averaging that is typical of highly radio-opaque objects imaged by MSCT.

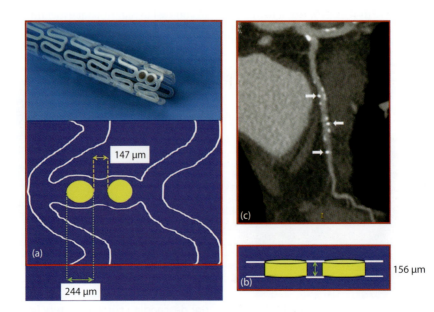

Figure 5.9.4 The Abosorb BVSs has two pairs of cylindrical platinum radio-opaque markers at both proximal and distal edges (244 μm in diameter and 156 μm thick) separated by a distance of 147 μm **(a)**. Three-year CCTA follow-up of patients enrolled in the ABSORB Extend trial and treated with two 3.0-mm × 18-mm BVSs **(b)**. Note the good patency of the scaffolded segment and the BVSs radio-opaque markers (arrows) that can be differentiated from the adjacent calcific nodules by higher peak intensity.

## ABSORB studies

In 71 out of 101 patients who were treated with an ABSORB BVSs and enrolled in the nonrandomized, multicenter, single-arm ABSORB (A Clinical Evaluation of the Bioabsorbable Everolimus Eluting Coronary Stent System in the Treatment of Patients With de Novo Native Coronary Artery Lesions) Cohort B trial [3], CCTA follow-up was performed mainly with 64-slice CT technology [38]. Vessel cross-sections were reconstructed at approximately 1-mm longitudinal increments, extending 5 mm beyond the BVSs, using the scaffold radio-opaque markers as landmark indicators. Four CCTA (6%) scans were noninterpretable, while six (8%) scans were qualitatively evaluable only. In the 61 quantitatively assessable arteries, the average mean in-scaffold lumen area was 5.1 ± 1.4 mm² (2.6–8.2 mm²), the proximal and distal reference areas were 5.3 ± 2.0 mm² and 4.3 ± 1.5 mm², respectively, the minimal lumen area was 3.5 ± 1.0 mm² (1.6–5.6 mm²), and the maximum lumen area was 7.0 ± 2.1 mm² (3.1–13.3 mm²). The average area stenosis was 22.7 ± 22.4% (−64.2% to +72.0%). The minimal lumen area was <25% of nominal in one case of a small posterolateral branch (minimal lumen area 1.6 mm², reference 2.1 mm²).

At 5-year follow-up, 18 patients enrolled in the first-in-human ABSORB cohort A trial and treated with the BVSs underwent CCTA [39]. Quantitative analysis of the scaffolded segments was feasible in all patients. All scaffolds were patent, with a median minimal lumen area of 3.25 mm² (interquartile range [IQR]: 2.20–4.33 mm²) and a median area stenosis of 33.3% (IQR: 12.8–43.8%). These studies demonstrate that CCTA could be an alternative to ICA for the noninvasive follow-up of BVSs allowing quantitative analysis of the treated coronary arteries.

## Evaluation of ABSORB BVS with CCTA in the real world

For practical clinical purposes, CCTA can be used to detect restenosis after successful BVSs implantation (Figure 5.9.5). Additionally, this technique provides information about the patterns of restenosis (focal, diffuse, or at BVSs edges). Other interesting information provided by CCTA assessment are the follow-up findings after BVSs treatment of complex coronary disease such as bifurcation lesions, chronic total occlusions (CTO), and long or diffuse lesions.

### BIFURCATION LESIONS

Once treatment of bifurcation lesions is planned with a BVSs, the provisional stenting technique seems to be an appropriate approach [40]. When the one-stent technique is chosen, two very simple strategies may be considered: (1) one BVSs across the bifurcation and nothing else (preferred by most

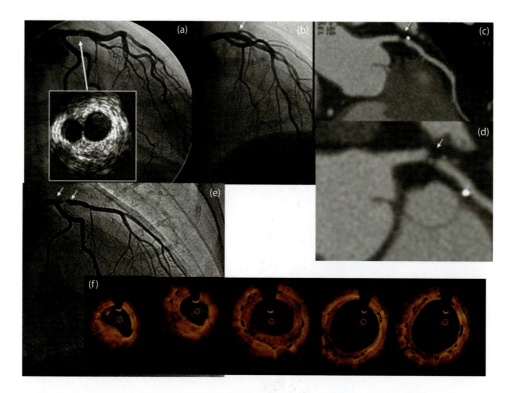

Figure 5.9.5 Example of a BVSs restenosis detected by CCTA. A severe stenosis of the proximal left anterior descending coronary artery is visible at baseline angiography and IVUS (**a**). Acute angiographic result after BVSs implantation (**b**). Six-month CCTA follow-up revealed severe restenosis at BVSs proximal edge (**c, d**). Invasive coronary angiography showed close correlation with the CCTA image (**e**). Optical coherence tomography at the time of invasive evaluation showed neointimal proliferation at the BVSs proximal edge causing severe luminal stenosis (**f**, left panels).

interventional cardiologists), and (2) side branch predilation followed by one BVSs deployed across the bifurcation. These strategies have the advantage of avoiding scaffold deformation, but they cannot be used in all cases and lateral dilation of side branch through the BVSs struts may be needed. Limited information is available regarding the fate of side branches covered by a BVSs [41]. Moreover, it is not clear if the BVSs struts jailing the side branch ostium undergo a resorption process similar to that occurring when the struts are fully apposed to the vessel wall. Valuable information

may be obtained with CCTA to resolve these questions giving insight into the fate of side branches covered by BVSs (Figures 5.9.6 and 5.9.7). If lateral dilation of the SB through the BVSs struts is performed, deformation of the scaffold or even strut fractures may occur. Again, CCTA may be a valuable follow-up tool to evaluate these patients (Figure 5.9.8).

## CHRONIC TOTAL OCCLUSIONS (CTO)

These lesions are the most challenging to be treated with a percutaneous coronary approach. Although technology

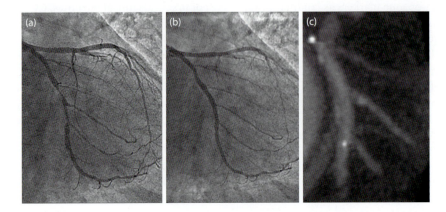

Figure 5.9.6 Tandem lesions of the left circumflex coronary artery involving two side branches (a) were successfully treated with one 3.5-mm × 28-mm BVSs across the side branches and nothing else (b). Note that both side branches remained patent without significant ostium compromise after BVSs deployment. Six-month CCTA follow-up showed a good result in the scaffolded segment and at the side branch ostia (c). Note that the radio-opaque markers enable to locate where the BVSs was implanted.

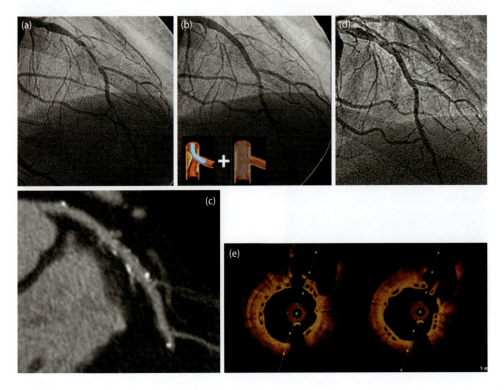

Figure 5.9.7 A bifurcation lesion (Medina 1,1,1) of the left anterior descending coronary artery (a) was treated with diagonal branch predilation followed by implantation of a 3.0-mm × 28-mm BVSs (b). At 1-year follow-up, CCTA demonstrated a good result at the bifurcation site (c) that was confirmed by invasive angiography (d) and optical coherence tomography (e).

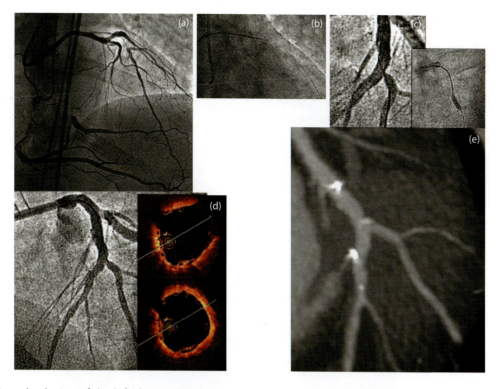

Figure 5.9.8  Complex lesion of the left descending coronary artery (chronic total occlusion plus bifurcation lesion) **(a)**. After antegrade CTO recanalization **(b)**, a 3.5-mm × 18-mm BVSs was implanted and dilation of the diagonal branch through the BVSs struts was performed with a 2.5-mm balloon at 8 atm **(c)** with good acute result confirmed by optical coherence tomography assessment **(d)**. At 6-month follow-up, CCTA showed an excellent result **(e)**. Note the blooming effect of the two BVSs radio-opaque markers.

improvements and development of specific skills by the operators have considerably increased the success rate, failures continue to be higher than in non-CTO procedures. In addition, after recanalization, a long coronary segment is usually treated with implantation of long and frequently multiple DESs. Indeed, deployment of multiple BVSs in this type of lesion may be an attractive alternative. The scaffold reabsorption could provide theoretical long-term advantages compared with metallic DESs than can be assessed with CCTA [4]. When an occluded artery is reopened, it may be difficult to know the true size of the distal vessel. Moreover, significant lumen and vessel enlargement has been shown at follow-up distally to a successfully opened CTO [42]. Both facts can lead to underestimation of the real vessel diameter and stent undersizing with the resulting risk of late stent malapposition and thrombosis [43]. Disappearance of the scaffold struts implies vessel uncaging and, therefore, the long-term consequences of this problem can be avoided. A recent study demonstrated that CCTA is able to show the recovery of distal vessel size over time [44] (Figure 5.9.9). Indeed, CCTA can provide follow-up information about vessel patency, positive remodeling of the scaffolded and distal segments, and late outcome of CTO treated with BVSs using complex techniques (Figure 5.9.10).

### LONG AND DIFFUSE LESIONS

It is known that the length of the stented vessel is a strong predictor of adverse events at follow-up such as stent thrombosis and the need for repeat revascularization [45,46]. Additionally, permanent caging of the artery inhibits the recovery of the physiological propriety of the vessel. Use of BVSs may avoid the issues associated with permanent implantation of long and multiple metallic DESs. As in the previous complex coronary lesions, CCTA is a valuable tool to perform a noninvasive follow-up of these patients assessing the patency of the entire scaffolded segment. Of note, the metallic radio-opaque markers of the BVSs may allow the detection of overlapped segments or gaps between scaffolds when a long vessel reconstruction is performed (Figure 5.9.11).

## NONINVASIVE FRACTIONAL FLOW RESERVE ASSESSMENT FOR BVS FOLLOW-UP

On the basis of physiological modeling and with the input of clinical and CCTA data, coronary blood flow and pressure during hyperemia can be simulated for functional coronary artery disease assessment. This analysis, defined CCTA-based fractional flow reserve ($FFR_{CT}$), was developed by HeartFlow, Inc. (Redwood City, CA) and has been recently introduced to evaluate the hemodynamic significance of coronary lesions in a more accurate fashion [47]. This approach is based on computational fluid dynamics, simulates maximal hyperemia in the coronary tree reconstructed from CCTA, and is able to compute FFR across the coronaries and to detect flow-limiting

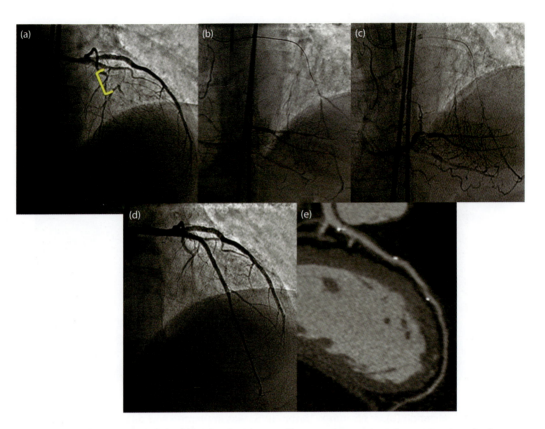

Figure 5.9.9 A chronic total occlusion of the left anterior descending coronary artery (**a**, square bracket) was successfully treated with antegrade recanalization (**b, c**) and implantation of two BVSs achieving an excellent acute result (**d**). At 6-month CCTA follow-up, a significant increase of the distal vessel size was observed (**e**).

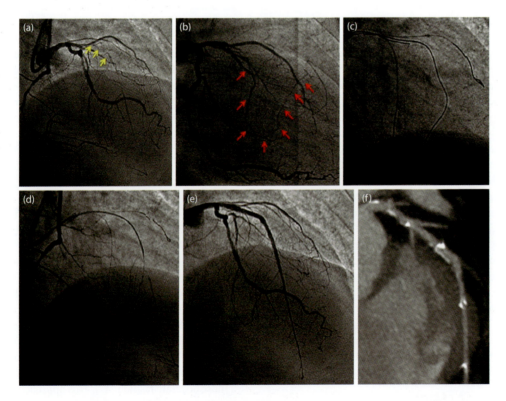

Figure 5.9.10 A long chronic total occlusion of the left anterior descending coronary artery (**a**, yellow arrows) was successfully treated with retrograde recanalization through a septal-septal collateral (**b**, red arrows, **c, d**) and implantation of three BVSs (**e**). At 6-month's follow-up, CCTA demonstrated vessel patency without restenosis of the long scaffolded segment (**f**).

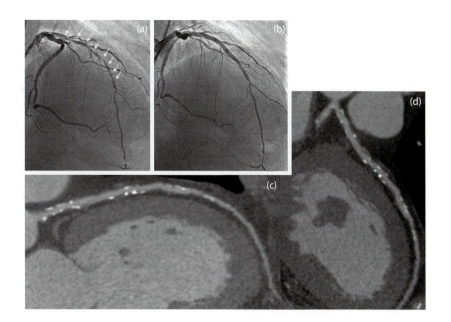

Figure 5.9.11  A long lesion of a diffusely diseased left anterior descending coronary artery (**a**, arrows) was successfully treated with implantation of two long BVSs, a 3.0-mm × 28-mm scaffold distally and a 3.5-mm × 28-mm scaffold proximally (**b**). At 6 months, CCTA showed full patency of the long scaffolded segment (**c, d**). Note that the metal-free BVSs struts allow unrestricted evaluation of the treated segment.

lesions. Although this technique cannot overcome the intrinsic limitations of CCTA, it may improve the sensitivity and specificity of the noninvasive evaluation of patients with CAD and of those already treated with stenting. The $FFR_{CT}$ higher accuracy is likely due to the fact that it takes into account not only the vessel stenosis but also the lesion length, the impact of serial narrowing on FFR as well as the myocardial area supplied by the stenotic artery. As a rule, the $FFR_{CT}$ gradient is calculated as the $FFR_{CT}$ distal-$FFR_{CT}$ proximal difference across the stenotic site. A $FFR_{CT}$ numeric value <0.80, defined as the ratio between coronary and aortic computed mean pressure, is considered significant. The feasibility of

$FFR_{CT}$ for the follow-up of patients treated with the BVSs was assessed in the ABSORB cohort B study [39]. Among patients undergoing CCTA at follow-up, $FFR_{CT}$ could be performed in 38 (57%) and measured 0.92 ± 0.06 (0.77–0.99) proximal and 0.89 ± 0.06 (0.74–0.97) distal to the scaffolded segment (Figure 5.9.12). The average gradient was −0.03 ± 0.04 (+0.01 to −0.23). There was no significant correlation between area stenosis and minimal lumen area or $FFR_{CT}$ gradient. The largest $FFR_{CT}$ gradient (−0.23) was associated with 9.4% area stenosis only, a minimal lumen area of 3.2 mm², and low $FFR_{CT}$ values in all distal branches, suggesting systematic underestimation. The $FFR_{CT}$ gradient ranged between −0.02 and −0.09 in patients

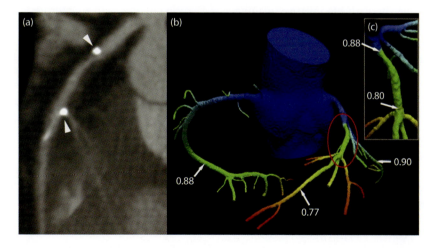

Figure 5.9.12  Follow-up CCTA performed 18 months after BVSs deployment in patients enrolled in the ABSORB trial. The two platinum radio-opaque markers indicating the location of the scaffold are clearly visible (**a**, arrowheads). CCTA-based fractional flow reserve ($FFR_{CT}$) is calculated throughout the coronary arteries and displayed as yellow to red for low $FFR_{CT}$ and from blue to green for $FFR_{CT}$ within the normal range (**b**). In this case, $FFR_{CT}$ decreases from 0.88 to 0.80 from the proximal to the distal edge of the scaffolded coronary segment (**c**).

with an area stenosis ≥50%. Noninvasive FFR$_{CT}$ was also feasible in 13 out of 18 patients undergoing 5-year CCTA follow-up in the ABSORB cohort A trial [38]. Image artifacts impeded FFR$_{CT}$ in four patients, whereas in one case FFR$_{CT}$ could not be calculated because of incomplete documentation of the entire coronary tree. Indeed, high quality of CCTA images of all coronary arteries is crucial for FFR$_{CT}$ because three-dimensional modeling of the entire coronary tree is indispensable for flow simulation. More recently, assessment of FFR by MSCT at 6-year follow-up in patients enrolled in the ABSORB cohort B MSCT substudy has been reported at the euroPCR 2016 meeting [48]. The study demonstrated that long-term serial noninvasive CCTA with functional assessment (FFR$_{CT}$) is feasible, allowing qualitative diagnosis of patency in the vast majority of patients (51/54, 94%). Moreover, it confirmed that late lumen enlargement is related to decrease of plaque/media which is associated with adaptive remodeling. Finally, FFR$_{CT}$ correlated with minimal lumen area (R = 0.56) and trans-scaffold FFR$_{CT}$ gradient was able to assess noninvasively the long-term performance of BRSs. It is likely that the unceasing advancements of MSCT technology and the consequent optimization of the acquired coronary images will improve further FFR$_{CT}$ feasibility in the near future.

## CONCLUSIONS

Rapid progress of MSCT technology has permitted more accurate coronary images with improved spatial and temporal resolution and has resulted in the recognition of CCTA as a dependable noninvasive diagnostic modality for the evaluation of CAD. However, visualization and evaluation of the stent lumen by CCTA is still challenging due to blooming artifacts caused by metallic stent struts. The polymeric BVSs is radio-lucent and allows delineating easily the contours of the scaffolded vessel by CCTA. Considering the good diagnostic accuracy for scaffolded vessel assessment and the advantages in safety, patient convenience, and cost, CCTA offers a reliable alternative to invasive imaging and will play an increasing clinical and research role in the future for the follow-up of patients treated with the BVSs and other polymeric and bioresorbable vascular devices.

## REFERENCES

1. Serruys PW, Ormiston JA, Onuma Y, Regar E, Gonzalo N, Garcia-Garcia HM, Nieman K et al. A bioabsorbable everolimus-eluting coronary stent system (ABSORB): 2-year outcomes and results from multiple imaging modalities. *Lancet.* 2009; 373:897–910.
2. Brugaletta S, Cogas BD, García-García HM, Farooq V, Girasis C, Heo JH, van Geuns RJ et al. Vascular compliance changes of the coronary vessel wall after bioresorbable vascular scaffold implantation in the treated and adjacent segments. *Circ J.* 2012; 767:1616–23.
3. Serruys PW, Onuma Y, Dudek D, Smits PC, Koolen J, Chevalier B, de Bruyne B et al. Evaluation of the second generation of a bioresorbable everolimus-eluting vascular scaffold for the treatment of de novo coronary artery stenosis. *J Am Coll Cardiol.* 2011; 58:1578–88.
4. Onuma Y, Serruys PW. Bioresorbable Scaffold. The advent of a new era in percutaneous coronary and peripheral revascularization? *Circulation.* 2011; 123:779–97.
5. Taylor AJ, Cerqueira M, Hodgson JM, Mark D, Min J, O'Gara P, Rubin GD et al. ACCF/SCCT/ACR/AHA/ASE/ASNC/NASCI/SCAI/SCMR 2010 appropriate use criteria for cardiac computed tomography. A report of the American College of Cardiology Foundation Appropriate Use Criteria Task Force, the Society of Cardiovascular Computed Tomography, the American College of Radiology, the American Heart Association, the American Society of Echocardiography, the American Society of Nuclear Cardiology, the North American Society for Cardiovascular Imaging, the Society for Cardiovascular Angiography and Interventions, and the Society for Cardiovascular Magnetic Resonance. *J Am Coll Cardiol.* 2010; 56:1864–94.
6. Andreini D, Pontone G, Pepi M, Ballerini G, Bartorelli AL, Magini A, Quaglia C et al. Diagnostic accuracy of multidetector computed tomography coronary angiography in patients with dilated cardiomyopathy. *J Am Coll Cardiol.* 2007; 49:2044–50.
7. Pontone G, Andreini D, Bertella E, Cortinovis S, Mushtaq S, Foti C, Annoni A et al. Pre-operative CT coronary angiography in patients with mitral valve prolapse referred for surgical repair: Comparison of accuracy, radiation dose and cost versus invasive coronary angiography. *Int J Cardiol.* 2013; 167:2889–94.
8. Leber AW, Johnson T, Becker A, von Ziegler F, Tittus J, Nikolaou K, Reiser M et al. Diagnostic accuracy of dual-source multi-slice CT-coronary angiography in patients with an intermediate pretest likelihood for coronary artery disease. *Eur Heart J.* 2007; 28:2354–60.
9. Abbara S, Arbab-Zadeh A, Callister TQ, Desai MY, Mamuya W, Thomson L, Weigold WG. SCCT guidelines for performance of coronary computed tomographic angiography: A report of the Society of Cardiovascular Computed Tomography Guidelines Committee. *J Cardiovasc Comput Tomogr.* 2009; 3:190–204.
10. Task Force Members, Montalescot G, Sechtem U, Achenbach S, Andreotti F, Arden C, Budaj A et al. 2013 ESC guidelines on the management of stable coronary artery disease: The Task Force on the management of stable coronary artery disease of the European Society of Cardiology. *Eur Heart J.* 2013; 34:2949–3003.
11. Pontone G, Andreini D, Bartorelli AL, Bertella E, Mushtaq S, Annoni A, Formenti A et al. Radiation dose and diagnostic accuracy of multidetector

computed tomography for the detection of significant coronary artery stenoses A meta-analysis. *Int J Cardiol.* 2012; 160:155–64.

12. Hausleiter J, Meyer T, Hadamitzky M, Huber E, Zankl M, Martinoff S, Kastrati A et al. Radiation dose estimates from cardiac multislice computed tomography in daily practice: Impact of different scanning protocols on effective dose estimates. *Circulation.* 2006; 113:1305–10.

13. Paul JF, Abada HT. Strategies for reduction of radiation dose in cardiac multislice CT. *Eur Radiol.* 2007; 17:2028–37.

14. Husmann L, Valenta I, Gaemperli O, Adda O, Treyer V, Wyss CA, Veit-Haibach P et al. Feasibility of low-dose coronary CT angiography: First experience with prospective ECG-gating. *Eur Heart J.* 2008; 29:191–7.

15. Maruyama T, Takada M, Hasuike T, Yoshikawa A, Namimatsu E, Yoshizumi T. Radiation dose reduction and coronary assessability of prospective electrocardiogram-gated computed tomography coronary angiography: Comparison with retrospective electrocardiogram-gated helical scan. *J Am Coll Cardiol.* 2008; 52:1450–5.

16. Pontone G, Andreini D, Bartorelli AL, Cortinovis S, Mushtaq S, Bertella E, Annoni A et al. Diagnostic accuracy of coronary computed tomography angiography: A comparison between prospective and retrospective electrocardiogram triggering. *J Am Coll Cardiol.* 2009; 54:346–55.

17. Hara AK, Paden RG, Silva AC, Kujak JL, Lawder HJ, Pavlicek W. Iterative reconstruction technique for reducing body radiation dose at CT: Feasibility study. *Am J Roentgenol.* 2009; 193:764–71

18. Leipsic J, Nguyen G, Brown J, Sin D, Mayo JR. A prospective evaluation of dose reduction and image quality in chest CT using adaptive statistical iterative reconstruction. *Am J Roentgenol.* 2010; 195:1095–9.

19. Pontone G, Andreini D, Bartorelli AL, Bertella E, Mushtaq S, Foti C, Formenti A et al. Feasibility and diagnostic accuracy of a low radiation exposure protocol for prospective ECG-triggering coronary MDCT angiography. *Clin Radiol.* 2012; 67:207–15.

20. Achenbach S, Ropers U, Kuettner A, Anders K, Pflederer T, Komatsu S, Bautz W et al. Randomized comparison of 64-slice single- and dual-source computed tomography coronary angiography for the detection of coronary artery disease. *JACC Cardiovasc Imaging.* 2008; 1:177–86.

21. McCollough CH, Primak AN, Saba O, Bruder H, Stierstorfer K, Raupach R, Suess C et al. Dose performance of a 64-channel dual-source CT scanner. *Radiology.* 2007; 243:775–84.

22. Achenbach S, Marwan M, Schepis T, Pflederer T, Bruder H, Allmendinger T, Petersilka M et al. High-pitch spiral acquisition: A new scan mode for coronary CT angiography. *J Cardiovasc Comput Tomogr.* 2009; 3:117–21.

23. Mori S, Nishizawa K, Kondo C, Ohno M, Akahane K, Endo M. Effective doses in subjects undergoing computed tomography cardiac imaging with the 256-multislice CT scanner. *Eur J Radiol.* 2008; 65:442–8.

24. Rybicki FJ, Otero HJ, Steigner ML, Vorobiof G, Nallamshetty L, Mitsouras D, Ersoy H et al. Initial evaluation of coronary images from 320-detector row computed tomography. *Int J Cardiovasc Imaging.* 2008; 24:535–46.

25. Carrabba N, Schuijf JD, De Graaf FR, Parodi G, Maffei E, Valenti R, Palumbo A et al. Diagnostic accuracy of 64-slice computed tomography coronary angiography for the detection of in-stent restenosis: A meta-analysis. *J Nucl Cardiol.* 2010; 17:470–8.

26. Kumbhani DJ, Ingelmo CP, Schoenhagen P, Curtin RJ, Flamm SD, and Desai MY. Meta-analysis of diagnostic efficacy of 64-slice computed tomography in the evaluation of coronary in-stent restenosis, *Am J Cardiol.* 2009; 12:1675–81.

27. Sun Z and Almutairi AMD. Diagnostic accuracy of 64 multislice CT angiography in the assessment of coronary in-stent restenosis: A meta-analysis, *Eur J Radiol.* 2010; 73:266–73.

28. Andreini D, Pontone G, Mushtaq S, Pepi M, Bartorelli AL. Multidetector computed tomography coronary angiography for the assessment of coronary in-stent restenosis. *Am J Cardiol.* 2010; 105:645–55.

29. Cademartiri F, Schuijf JD, Pugliese F, Mollet NR, Jukema JW, Maffei E, Kroft LJ et al. Usefulness of 64-slice multislice computed tomography coronary angiography to assess in-stent restenosis. *J Am Coll Cardiol.* 2007; 49:2204–10.

30. Ehara M, Kawai M, Surmely JF, Matsubara T, Terashima M, Tsuchikane E, Kinoshita Y et al. Diagnostic accuracy of coronary in-stent restenosis using 64-slice computed tomography: Comparison with invasive coronary angiography. *J Am Coll Cardiol.* 2007; 49:951–9.

31. Carrabba N, Bamoshmoosh M, Carusi LM, Parodi G, Valenti R, Migliorini A, Fanfani F et al. Usefulness of 64-slice multidetector computed tomography for detecting drug eluting in-stent restenosis. *Am J Cardiol.* 2007; 100:1754–8.

32. Schuijf JD, Pundziute G, Jukema JW, Lamb HJ, Tuinenburg JC, van der Hoeven BL, de Roos A et al. Evaluation of patients with previous coronary stent implantation with 64-section CT. *Radiology.* 2007; 245:416–23.

33. Pflederer T, Marwan M, Renz A, Bachmann S, Ropers D, Kuettner A, Anders K et al. Noninvasive assessment of coronary in-stent restenosis by dual-source computed tomography. *Am J Cardiol.* 2009; 103:812–7.

34. Oncel D, Oncel G, Tastan A, Tamci B. Evaluation of coronary stent patency and in-stent restenosis with dual-source CT coronary angiography without heart rate control. *Am J Roentgenol.* 2008; 191:56–63.

35. Andreini D, Pontone G, Bartorelli AL, Trabattoni D, Mushtaq S, Bertella E, Annoni A et al. Comparison of feasibility and diagnostic accuracy of 64-slice multidetector computed tomography coronary angiography versus invasive coronary angiography versus intravascular ultrasound for evaluation of in-stent restenosis. *Am J Cardiol.* 2009; 103:1349–58.

36. Andreini D, Pontone G, Bartorelli AL, Mushtaq S, Trabattoni D, Bertella E, Cortinovis S et al. High diagnostic accuracy of prospective ECG-gating 64-slice computed tomography coronary angiography for the detection of in-stent restenosis: In-stent restenosis assessment by low-dose MDCT. *Eur Radiol.* 2011; 21:1430–8.

37. Andreini D, Pontone G, Mushtaq S, Bartorelli AL, Bertella E, Trabattoni D, Montorsi P et al. Coronary in-stent restenosis: Assessment with CT coronary angiography. *Radiology.* 2012; 265:410–7.

38. Onuma Y, Dudek, D, Thuesen L, Webster M, Nieman K, Garcia-Garcia HM, Ormiston JA et al. Five-year clinical and functional multislice computed tomography angiographic results after coronary implantation of the fully resorbable polymeric everolimus-eluting scaffold in patients with de novo coronary artery disease: The ABSORB cohort A trial. *JACC Cardiovasc Interv.* 2013; 6:999–1009.

39. Nieman K, Serruys PW, Onuma Y, van Geuns RJ, Garcia-Garcia HM, de Bruyne B, Thuesen L et al. Multislice computed tomography angiography for noninvasive assessment of the 18-month performance of a novel radiolucent bioresobable vascular scaffolding device. The ABSORB trial. *J Am Coll Cardiol.* 2013; 62:1813–4.

40. Tamburino C, Latib A, van Geuns RJ, Sabate M, Mehilli J, Gori T, Achenbach S et al. Contemporary practice and technical aspects in coronary intervention with bioresorbable scaffolds: A European perspective. *EuroIntervention.* 2015; 11(1):45–52.

41. Muramatsu T, Onuma Y, García-García HM, Farooq, Bourantas CV, Morel MA, Li X et al. Incidence and short-term clinical outcomes of small side branch occlusion after implantation of an everolimus-eluting bioresorbable vascular scaffold. An interim report of 435 patients in the ABSORB-EXTEND single-arm trial in comparison with an everolimus-eluting metallic stent in the SPIRIT first and II trials. *JACC Cardiovasc Interv.* 2013; 6:247–257.

42. Gomez-Lara J, Teruel L, Homs S, Ferreiro JL, Romaguera R, Roura G, Sánchez-Elvira G et al. Lumen enlargement of the coronary segments located distal to chronic total occlusions successfully treated with drug-eluting stents at follow-up. *EuroIntervention.* 2014; 9:1181–8.

43. Valenti R, Vergara R, Migliorini A, Parodi G, Carrabba N, Cerisano G, Dovellini EV et al. Predictors of reocclusion after successful drug-eluting stent supported percutaneous coronary intervention of chronic total occlusion. *J Am Coll Cardiol.* 2013; 61:545–50.

44. Ojeda S, Pan M, Romero M, Suárez de Lezo J, Mazuelos F, Segura J, Espejo S et al. Outcomes and computed tomography scan follow-up of bioresorbable vascular scaffold for the percutaneous treatment of chronic total coronary artery occlusion. *Am J Cardiol.* 2015 Jun 1; 115(11):1487–93.

45. Shirai S, Kimura T, Nobuyoshi M, Morimoto T, Ando K, Soga Y, Yamaji K et al. Impact of multiple and long sirolimus-eluting stent implantation on 3-year clinical outcomes in the j-Cypher registry. *JACC Cardiovasc Interv.* 2010; 3:180–8.

46. Naidu SS, Krucoff MW, Rutledge DR, Mao VW, Zhao W, Zheng Q, Wilburn O et al. Contemporary incidence and predictors of stent thrombosis and other major adverse cardiac events in the year after XIENCE V implantation. Results from the 8,061-patient XIENCE V United States study. *JACC Cardiovasc Interv.* 2012; 5:626–35.

47. Taylor CA, Fonte TA, Min JK. Computational fluid dynamics applied to cardiac CT for noninvasive quantification of fractional flow reserve: Scientific basis. *J Am Coll Cardiol.* 2013; 61:2233–41.

48. Serruys PW, Collet C, Onuma Y on behalf of the ABSORB Investigators. Follow-up of the first-in-man use of a polylactide everolimus-eluting BRS for the treatment of coronary stenosis: An assessment of FFR by multislice CT. http://www.pcronline.com /Lectures/2016/Six-year.

# PART 6

# Clinical evidence of randomized and nonrandomized trials: Personal perspective

# What are appropriate clinical endpoints? From device failure assessment to angina evaluation

MAIK J. GRUNDEKEN, YOSHINOBU ONUMA, AND PATRICK W.J.C. SERRUYS

## INTRODUCTION: THE HISTORICAL FOCUS ON TREATMENT FAILURE INSTEAD OF TREATMENT SUCCESS

Angina pectoris is chest pain caused by ischemia of the myocardium secondary to a supply/demand mismatch [1]. In most cases, myocardial ischemia is caused by one or more flow-limiting stenoses in one or more of the epicardial coronary arteries, while in a minority it is caused by coronary vasospasms (Prinzmetal's angina) or microvascular dysfunction [2–5]. In the elective setting, PCI is performed to alleviate patients from their angina by treating flow-limiting coronary stenoses. However, ever since the introduction of coronary interventions by balloon angioplasty, clinical research evaluating PCI treatment is mostly focused on the quantification of the failure of the different techniques and devices, including the number of deaths, peri-procedural myocardial infarctions (MIs), spontaneous (recurrent) MIs, repeat (target vessel/lesion) revascularizations, and stent thrombosis (ST). In this perspective, it is quite remarkable that there has been much less focus on the success of the device in terms of quantifying the reduction of angina burden. This development was most likely driven by the difficulties to objectively assess angina in clinical trials. As the Academic Research Consortium (ARC) committee discussed in their consensus document on endpoint definitions, angina "does not lend itself as readily to objective assessment as the other proposed end points and is better measured as a stand-alone end point with the use of formal, validated health status instruments" [6]. The general thought is that it is easier to objectively assess the conventional clinical endpoints.

For the all-cause mortality endpoint this seems indeed to be true. However, for other clinical endpoints there are some challenges as well, such as to objectify the clinical indication of target lesion revascularizations (TLR) [7] or the ongoing debate on the appropriate definitions of periprocedural

MI [8,9]. With the introduction of bioresorbable scaffolds (BRSs), new challenges in defining clinical endpoints arose. For instance, how to call a thrombosis at the site of the implanted BRSs after its complete resorption? You still may call it ST, arguing that the BRSs resorption resulted in local inflammation with unfavorable vessel wall healing causing the ST, but you may argue against that this should be considered a spontaneous recurrent MI, assuming the BRSs "did its job" and left the vessel uncaged. Alternatively, you may want to call it "intra-marker thrombosis," although this definition will be problematic since not all BRSs currently under development have proximal and distal markers so that the exact initial position of the implanted device cannot be identified once the BRSs is completely resolved. The same dilemmas account for revascularizations of the treated segments. How should you call a repeat percutaneous coronary intervention (PCI) of a segment with "intra-marker (neo-)atherosclerosis" after complete resorption of the BRSs? The ARC committee is currently working on adaptation of the current definitions to uniform and standardize the nomenclature in the BRSs literature. This is important because we need objective tools to compare the safety of new BRSs with current generation drug-eluting stents (DESs) and with other BRSs.

However, developments in the field of PCI might shift the focus from these "hard clinical endpoints," quantifying the failure, toward the success of the treatment (i.e., a sustained reduction of angina burden), including clear definitions and guidance on how to assess angina by the new ARC definitions, for the following reasons:

1. The incidence of the conventional endpoints becomes very low in contemporary clinical stent trials. In some all-comers trials the event rates are even as low as ~6% for the composite endpoint of cardiac death, MI, and CI-TLR at 1 year [10], so that it will be more and more challenging to design appropriate trials to demonstrate noninferiority of new devices.

2. The incidence of angina has consistently been reported to be 20% or higher at 1-year post-PCI [11–15]. There is an unmet need to better understand the etiology of angina, including other reasons than fixed epicardial stenosis alone.

3. After the full biodegradation of BRSs, restoration of pulsatility, cyclical strain, physiological shear stress, and mechanotransduction might result in less angina in the long-term when compared to metallic stents.

Angina can be assessed in two distinctive ways. The first is to obtain angina complaints directly from the patient, without any interference from a physician/investigator, via a so-called "patient-reported outcome" (PRO) instrument. Alternatively, angina can be reported by the physician/investigator who interpreted the patient's complaints, with or without additional information (recent coronary angiograms, results from ischemia testing, etc.), as being of ischemic origin, and thus angina, or not (the so-called "site-reported" angina). We will discuss both methodologies in extent below.

## ASSESSMENT OF ANGINA: PATIENT-REPORTED OUTCOMES VERSUS SITE-REPORTED OUTCOMES

### Patient-reported outcomes

A PRO instrument quantifies the status of a patient's health condition in which the information comes directly from the patient. The main advantage is that there is no interpretation by the treating physician and/or investigator, avoiding any bias from the outcome assessor. The U.S. Food and Drug Administration (FDA) supports the use of PROs, and even allows the use of PRO instruments to support claims in approved medical product labeling, as discussed in the FDA document *Guidance for Industry—Patient-Reported Outcome Measures: Use in Medical Product Development to Support Labeling Claims* [16]. A PRO instrument should fit in an appropriate "conceptual framework." This conceptual framework defines the concepts measured by the PRO instrument and a description of, and relationship between, items, domain, and concept(s) measured.

A very simple example of a PRO instrument that we will use to illustrate the conceptual framework is the visual analogue scale (VAS) for pain (Figure 6.1.1). In the VAS for pain, patients indicate on a straight line how much pain they experience, with both ends of the line indicating "no pain" and "worst possible pain imaginable," respectively (Figure 6.1.1). In this PRO instrument, there is only one item (pain scale from 0 to 10), representing one domain ("pain"), supporting the general concept ("perception of pain"). Such PRO instruments can be easily used in daily clinical practice, for instance after administration of pain medication to assess whether it relieved the patient's discomfort. However, most patients' health statuses are not so easy to assess and would require a more thorough PRO instrument with a more complex conceptual framework.

The most widely used PRO to assess angina is the Seattle Angina Questionnaire (SAQ), developed and validated by John Spertus in the mid-1990s [17]. As shown in Figure 6.1.2, the SAQ has five domains, including "physical limitation," "angina stability," "angina frequency," "treatment satisfaction," and "disease perception." For each domain, the patient is questioned by a different number of "items." For each domain, a score can be calculated from 0 (worst possible health status) to 100 (best possible health status; no angina). All five domains contribute to the general concept ("angina"). The SAQ is well-validated [17], widely used in cardiovascular trials [18–22], and SAQ scores are strongly associated with both hard clinical endpoints and resource

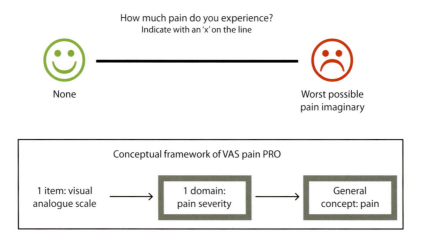

**Figure 6.1.1** The visual analogue scale (VAS) for pain. The VAS for pain is an example of a simple patient-reported outcome (PRO) instrument. The upper panel shows an example of a VAS for a pain PRO instrument on which the patient is asked to indicate on the straight line how much pain he or she is experiencing, with both ends of the line indicating "no pain" and "worst possible pain imaginable," respectively. The lower panel shows the conceptual framework of this PRO: There is only one item (pain scale from 0 to 10), representing one domain ("pain"), supporting the general concept ("patient's perception of his or her pain"). Such PRO instruments can be easily used in daily clinical practice, for instance after administration of pain medication to assess whether it relieved patient's discomfort.

utilization [23,24]. An example of how the SAQ scores are presented is shown in Figure 6.1.3.

Although PRO instruments have a major strength in the sense that the information is coming directly from the patient, avoiding any bias from the physician, there are also precautions that have to be taken into consideration when using PRO instruments and interpreting the obtained data:

1. The PRO instrument should be tested on reliability (including test-retests, internal consistency tests, and inter-reviewer reproducibility if applicable), should be validated (both on content validity [the evidence from

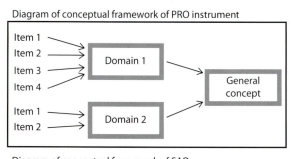

Diagram of conceptual framework of PRO instrument

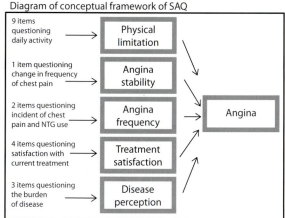

Diagram of conceptual framework of SAQ

**Figure 6.1.2** Conceptual framework of the Seattle Angina Questionnaire (SAQ). The upper panel illustrates the concept of a more complex conceptual framework, as described by the U.S. Food and Drug Administration (FDA). There are multiple items for each domain and multiple domains supporting a certain general concept. The lower panel shows the conceptual framework of the SAQ. The SAQ has five domains, including "physical limitation," "angina stability," "angina frequency," "treatment satisfaction," and "disease perception." For each domain, the patient is questioned by a different number of "items." For each domain, a score can be calculated from 0 (worst possible health status) to 100 (best possible health status; no angina). All 5 domains contribute to the general concept ("angina"). (From U.S. Department of Health and Human Services Food and Drug Administration Center for Drug Evaluation and Research [CDER] Center for Biologics Evaluation and Research [CBER] Center for Devices and Radiological Health [CDRH]. Guidance for Industry Patient-Reported Outcome Measures: Use in Medical Product Development to Support Labeling Claims. December 2009.)

qualitative studies that item and domains are appropriate and comprehensive relative to its intended measurement concept, population, and use] and construct validity [the evidence of proven existing logical relationships between items, domains, and concepts]), and should be tested on its ability to detect changes [16,17].

2. The PRO instrument should be applied on the appropriate target population. This seems logical, but you cannot use a single-item VAS pain score to assess a patient's general well-being, and you cannot use the SAQ to assess pain other than ischemic chest pain.

3. It is essential to maintain the patient's blinding. Since a PRO instrument evaluates the patient's perspective on his or her health status, it is absolutely essential that the patient is blinded for his or her treatment if a (change) in health status is attributed to a certain treatment. Otherwise, placebo and/or Hawthorne effects might influence the results.

4. The so-called "recall period" of the PRO should be respected. Every PRO instrument is validated with a certain recall period. If patients must recall over a long period, this might undermine the content validity of the instrument (i.e., they cannot remember correctly). In general, a short recall period, or even the assessment of the current health status ("how do you feel today?" rather than "how did you feel the last past months?"), is preferable. The recall period of the SAQ is 4 weeks. This means that the patient is questioned about his angina complaints occurring 4 weeks prior to the assessment. In other words, when the angina complaints are resolved >4 weeks before the SAQ (due to successful repeat revascularization, for instance), the SAQ will not reflect the patient's health status at the time the patient had the angina complaint, but rather at the time of the SAQ assessment and the 4 weeks before. This implies that when there is a considerable amount of time in-between the PRO assessments, changes in health status might not be captured if they evolve after the last PRO assessment and are resolved before the recall period of the new PRO assessment. To resolve this issue, a daily (digital) angina diary can be applied as was done in the TERISA trial [25].

5. If the number of items is too extensive, there is the risk of noncompliance. The PRO should be constructed in such way that the items cover all aspects of the concept, avoiding too much overlap. The point of "saturation" is reached when additional items no longer add relevant information on the investigated concept of interest. Interestingly, recently a short 7-item version of the SAQ has been introduced which proved to preserve the high test-retest reliability, responsiveness, and prognostic ability compared to the original 19-item SAQ with the benefit it is more practical and less time-consuming to complete [26].

## Site-reported outcomes

In contrast with PRO assessment, health status is not obtained directly from the patient when using a site-reported approach. Site-reported outcomes are outcomes that are

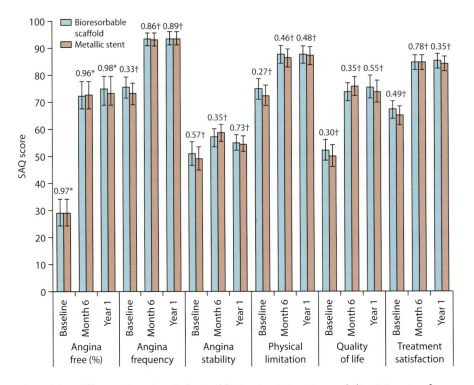

**Figure 6.1.3** The results of the different domains ("physical limitation," "angina stability," "angina frequency," "treatment satisfaction," and "disease perception") of the Seattle Angina Questionnaire (SAQ) as assessed at three different follow-up time points (1 month, 6 months, and 1 year) in the ABSORB II trial. (With permission from Serruys PW, Chevalier B, Dudek D, Cequier A, Carrie D, Iniguez A, Dominici M et al. *Lancet.* 2015;385:43–54.)

reported by the treating physician/investigator in the (electronic) case report form ([e]CRF). In most trials, angina status is simply scored in the (e)CRF during each (unscheduled) study visit by stating whether the patient experiences angina at the time of the study visits. In most (e)CRFs, the investigator is able to choose between mutually exclusive options: "no angina," "stable angina," "unstable angina," or "silent ischemia." In some trials, there are additional options such as "angina-equivalent" or "indeterminate." In case the patient is scored as having "stable angina," the Canadian Cardiology Society (CCS) angina classification is widely used to report on the angina severity and is defined as follows [27]:

- *CCS Grade I:* Ordinary physical activity does not cause angina, such as walking and climbing stairs. Angina with strenuous or rapid or prolonged exertion at work or recreation.
- *CCS Grade II:* Slight limitation of ordinary activity. Walking or climbing stairs rapidly, walking uphill, walking or stair climbing after meals, or in cold, or in wind, or under emotional stress, or only during the few hours after awakening. Walking more than two blocks on the level and climbing more than one flight of ordinary stairs at a normal pace and in normal conditions.
- *CCS Grade III:* Marked limitation of ordinary physical activity. Walking one or two blocks on the level and climbing one flight of stairs in normal conditions and at normal pace.
- *CCS Grade IV:* Inability to carry on any physical activity without discomfort, angina syndrome may be present at rest.

Historically, the presence or absence of angina (either as dichotomous variable or in mutually exclusive categories as described above) and the CCS classification (in case of stable angina) have been reported as rates during the baseline and the follow-up study visits, and might be considered to be a "cross-sectional" analytic approach.

More recently, in the ABSORB II trial, an exploratory post-hoc analysis was performed using the cardiac adverse event (AE) forms from the eCRF [28]. In this trial, the study sites needed to fill out dedicated cardiac AE forms for every cardiac-related adverse event patients experienced during the trial. On these cardiac AE forms, the angina status had to be indicated by the investigator. Because these forms also needed to be filled out for cardiac events occurring in-between visits, a "cumulative incidence" of site-reported angina episodes could be assessed. This analysis showed a difference in cumulative incidence of angina episodes in favor of the ABSORB everolimus-eluting bioresorbable vascular scaffold (BVSs; Abbott Vascular, Santa Clara, CA) compared to the XIENCE everolimus-eluting stent (Abbott Vascular, Santa Clara, CA) (Figure 6.1.4). A potential advantage of such analytic approach is that also angina episodes that are resolved before the next study visit are taken into account. As shown by a recent 2-year follow-up study of the DUTCH-PEERS trial (randomizing between zotarolimus-eluting stents [ZESs] and EES), around 20% of patients had a change (increase or decrease) in angina complaints between the 1-year and 2-year follow-up study visit. These findings indicate the dynamic nature of angina: angina may recur post-PCI but may also be resolved again during the follow-up of the trial due to (changes in) treatment.

However, the post-hoc cumulative angina analysis in the ABSORB II trial had some major limitations, which also have to be taken into account in general when interpreting site-reported data. First, the trial was single-blinded and the non-blinded study site personnel assessed the angina status when filling out the cardiac AE forms. Therefore, a reporting bias may have occurred in favor of the ABSORB BVSs. Reporting of angina might differ from site-to-site, introducing inaccuracies. No clear definitions were provided on the different angina categories and especially in the "angina-equivalent" category there were some inconsistencies observed, with study sites filling out the accompanying free text field with "atypical chest pain," suggesting the patient did not experience angina complaints. There was no independent adjudication by a clinical event committee. Finally, there has been no pathophysiological explanation for a favorable effect of a BRSs on angina complaints <6 months, while in the ABSORB II trial a difference in cumulative angina incidence between ABSORB BVSs and the XIENCE EES was already observed within this period (Figure 6.1.4). Importantly, the more recent ABSORB III trial, randomizing 2008 patients between treatment with ABSORB BVSs (1322 patients) or XIENCE EES (686 patients), using a similar methodology to evaluate site reported angina

as in ABSORB II, did not show a difference at 12 months follow-up (18.3% vs. 18.4%, $p = 0.93$) [29].

The ongoing ABSORB IV randomized trial will probably shed more light on this issue. This trial, randomizing 3000 patients in a 1:1 fashion to treatment with the ABSORB BVSs or XIENCE EES, has a primary endpoint on 1-year angina, powered for superiority. The assessment of angina is done in a rigorous way. PROs (SAQ, Rose Dyspnea Scale [RDS], and EuroQoL 5D [EQ5D]) are assessed frequently at 1, 3, 6, 9, 12, 24, and 36 months. Site-reported outcomes (at 1, 3, 6, 9, 12, 24, and 36 months) are reported via a detailed 5-page CRF including standard questions on angina, including severity, localization, accompanying complaints, triggers, etc. An independent clinical event committee will review these 5 eCRF pages of each study visit to adjudicate whether the patient has angina. Although the trial is single blinded, study site personnel who conduct the clinical follow-up are blinded and not present at the index procedure. To reduce the possibilities of patient unblinding, the patients wear headphones playing music throughout the index procedure. Interestingly, a "perception analysis" will be performed as well. This analysis investigates how the patients' belief which device they have received does affect PRO assessment. A perception assessment questionnaire will be administered ≥4 hours to ≤7 days post-index procedure: the patients will be asked whether they think they know which treatment

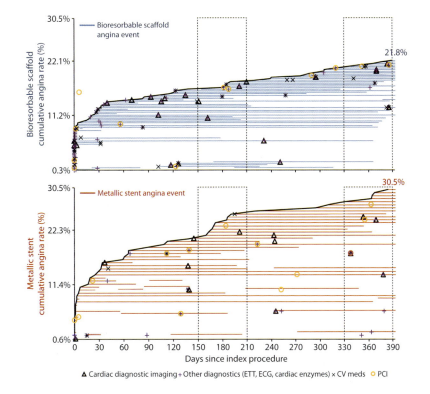

**Figure 6.1.4** Time to first occurrence and duration of angina. Figure shows the time to first occurrence (black curves) and duration (blue horizontal bars for the ABSORB group, red horizontal bars for the XIENCE group) of angina in the ABSORB II trial. The rectangulars indicate the timing of the two cross-sectional time windows of 4 weeks during which the Seattle Angina Questionnaire (SAQ) had to be completed by the patients. ETT = exercise tolerance testing; ECG = electrocardiogram; PCI = percutaneous coronary intervention. (With permission from Serruys PW, Chevalier B, Dudek D, Cequier A, Carrie D, Iniguez A, Dominici M et al. *Lancet.* 2015;385:43–54.)

they have received. If they think they know, they will be asked which device they have received, how certain they are, and how they knew which device they have received. Angina outcomes will subsequently not only be analyzed according to treatment arm, but also according to perception of treatment received. This analysis will provide us insights whether the device itself or the perception of the patient on the received treatment is the most important determinant to develop angina complaints during follow-up. The results from the ABSORB IV trial will provide us important information whether the ABSORB BVSs indeed reduces the angina burden compared to the metallic XIENCE EES within the first year of follow-up.

## ANGINA REDUCTION WITH BRSs: POSSIBLE EXPLANATIONS

Even if the ABSORB IV trial will also find a different angina incidence within the first year of follow-up, its pathophysiological mechanism is thus far not understood. Besides placebo and/or Hawthorne effects, there are some mechanistic hypotheses. For the ABSORB BVSs, it has been shown that within scaffold, vasomotion of any kind was not observed at 6 months [30], while at 1-year follow-up 8 out 19 patients showed a vasodilatory response and 10 out of 19 patients had vasoconstriction within the scaffolded segment after the maximum dosage of acetylcholine [31]. A natural physiological response of vasodilatation following acethylcholine administration requires complete anatomical and functional integrity of coalescent endothelial cells (see Chapter 5.1). These results therefore suggested that mechanical integrity of the BVSs was still intact at 6 months (i.e., the BVSs was still a "rigid tube" without any motion). At 1 year, however, the BVSs lost some of its mechanical integrity due to the bioresorption process, resulting in the return of vasomotion within the scaffolded segment, although complete anatomical and functional integrity of coalescent endothelial cells was not yet restored in the majority of patients. Biodegradation with return of vasomotion can therefore not explain any differences in angina between the BRSs and metallic stents within the first 6 months, and can only partly explain a potential difference from 6 months to 1 year.

Myocardial ischemia is not only caused by "fixed" flow-limiting stenosis of the epicardial coronary arteries, but can also be caused by "dynamic" flow-limiting lesions (i.e., vasospasms) and/or by microvascular dysfunction. Since there were no differences in acute luminal dimensions between the ABSORB BVSs and the XIENCE EES, as assessed with quantitative coronary angiography and intravascular ultrasound, within the ABSORB II trial, some hypothesized that the BVSs might influence the endothelial and microvascular function differently than metallic drug-eluting stents (DESs). Endothelial dysfunction in coronary segments distal to implanted DESs have been described and this endothelial dysfunction seems to be DESs-type specific; related to polymer and drug eluted [32–34]. This might be different

with BVSs. The better conformability of the BVSs over the metallic EES, as shown as less difference in curvature and angle between pre- and post-implantation [18,35], which does influence local shear stresses at the stent edges [36], also shows that BRSs are different devices, mechanically speaking, than metallic DESs. Furthermore, it has been thought that the large surface area of the BVSs struts are embedded less easily than thinner metallic struts (i.e., "ice-skate vs. snow shoe" effect) [37]. Whether these differences in endothelial (dys)function, conformability, and the issue of tissue penetration may lead to differences in endothelial or microvascular response needs further investigation.

Unpublished non-randomized data in human and porcine models have shown differences in post-procedural microvascular resistance (as determined with thermodilution) between the ABSORB BVSs and the metallic DESs: The microvasculature resistance decreases after BVSs implantation and increases after implantation of metallic DESs acute post-procedural [personal communication Nick West and Alec Sheehy] and this will further be evaluated in the randomized EMPIRE-BVSs study (see Chapter 6.3). The longer-term effect of ABSORB BVSs on myocardial flow and microvascular function compared with XIENCE EES will be assessed in the randomized VANISH trial (ClinicalTrials.gov Identifier: NCT01876589) and the ABSORB II physiology substudy (see Chapter 6.3). VANISH (Impact of vascular reparative therapy on vasomotor function and myocardial perfusion: a randomized $H_{215}O$ PET/CT study) investigates the impact of ABSORB BVSs (compared to XIENCE EES) on the endothelium-dependent vasodilation and subsequent maximum hyperemic perfusion of the total myocardium using $H_{215}O$ PET/CT. Patients will undergo these PET/CT assessment at 30 days, 1 year, and 3 years to assess the myocardial blood flow over time. The ABSORB II physiology substudy will assess intracoronary pressure and flow (using Doppler technique) in 41 patients being randomized in the ABSORB II trial and who return for their scheduled 3-year repeat angiogram. Outcomes will include coronary flow reserve (CFR), hyperemic microvascular resistance (HMR), and instantaneous hyperemic diastolic velocity-pressure slope (IHDVPS). IHDVPS proved to be very sensitive to detect structural microcirculatory changes, is considered to be the equivalent to hyperemic diastolic conductance, and is defined as the slope of the pressure–flow velocity relationship between the mid- and end-diastole under maximal hyperemia [38]. A higher IHDVPS value (i.e., a steeper slope) indicates better hyperemic diastolic conductance, and thus less microvascular impairment (see Chapter 6.3). These ongoing studies will investigate the potential influence of ABSORB BVSs on the coronary and microvascular hemodynamics and will provide us further insights in possible explanations on the potential benefit of BRSs in terms of angina reduction.

## CONCLUSIONS

Historically, clinical research evaluating PCI treatment is mostly focused on the quantification of the failure of the treatment including (cardiac) death, MI, repeat revascularizations, and ST. However, even in all-comers trials including patients with ACS, contemporary devices show 1-year event rates as low as 6%, while the incidence of angina is still reported to be around 20% or higher at 1 year. Fully bioresorbable scaffolds have different properties than metallic DESs, which might result in improvement in angina complaints during follow-up. Therefore, there is the need to shift our focus to assessing the burden of angina after PCI. Angina can be assessed using patient-reported outcomes (PRO) or site-reported outcomes, both with their own strengths and weaknesses. More future studies are needed to investigate potential pathophysiological mechanisms to understand the potential differences in angina incidence between BRSs and metallic stents. Currently ongoing studies are investigating the relation between bioresorbable scaffolds and intracoronary pressure/flow, microvascular function, and total myocardial flow.

# REFERENCES

1. Task Force Members, Montalescot G, Sechtem U, Achenbach S, Andreotti F, Arden C, Budaj A et al. 2013 ESC guidelines on the management of stable coronary artery disease: The Task Force on the management of stable coronary artery disease of the European Society of Cardiology. *Eur Heart J*. 2013;34:2949–3003.

2. Zaya M, Mehta PK and Merz CN. Provocative testing for coronary reactivity and spasm. *J Am Coll Cardiol*. 2014;63:103–9.

3. Oliva PB, Potts DE and Pluss RG. Coronary arterial spasm in Prinzmetal angina. Documentation by coronary arteriography. *N Eng J Med*. 1973;288:745–51.

4. Crea F, Camici PG and Bairey Merz CN. Coronary microvascular dysfunction: An update. *Eur Heart J*. 2014;35:1101–11.

5. Takahashi J, Nihei T, Takagi Y, Miyata S, Odaka Y, Tsunoda R, Seki A et al. Prognostic impact of chronic nitrate therapy in patients with vasospastic angina: Multicentre registry study of the Japanese coronary spasm association. *Eur Heart J*. 2015;36:228–37.

6. Cutlip DE, Windecker S, Mehran R, Boam A, Cohen DJ, van Es GA, Steg PG et al. Clinical end points in coronary stent trials: A case for standardized definitions. *Circulation*. 2007;115:2344–51.

7. Topol EJ and Nissen SE. Our preoccupation with coronary luminology. The dissociation between clinical and angiographic findings in ischemic heart disease. *Circulation*. 1995;92:2333–42.

8. Woudstra P, Grundeken MJ, van de Hoef TP, Wallentin L, Fox KA, de Winter RJ and Damman P. Prognostic relevance of PCI-related myocardial infarction. *Nat Rev Cardiol*. 2013;10:231–6.

9. Moussa ID, Klein LW, Shah B, Mehran R, Mack MJ, Brilakis ES, Reilly JP et al. Consideration of a new definition of clinically relevant myocardial infarction after coronary revascularization: An expert consensus document from the Society for Cardiovascular Angiography and Interventions (SCAI). *J Am Coll Cardiol*. 2013;62:1563–70.

10. Pilgrim T, Heg D, Roffi M, Tuller D, Muller O, Vuilliomenet A, Cook S et al. Ultrathin strut biodegradable polymer sirolimus-eluting stent versus durable polymer everolimus-eluting stent for percutaneous coronary revascularisation (BIOSCIENCE): A randomised, single-blind, non-inferiority trial. *Lancet*. 2014;384:2111–22.

11. Boden WE, O'Rourke RA, Teo KK, Hartigan PM, Maron DJ, Kostuk WJ, Knudtson M et al. Optimal medical therapy with or without PCI for stable coronary disease. *N Engl J Med*. 2007;356:1503–16.

12. Serruys PW, Ormiston JA, Onuma Y, Regar E, Gonzalo N, Garcia-Garcia HM, Nieman K et al. A bioabsorbable everolimus-eluting coronary stent system (ABSORB): 2-year outcomes and results from multiple imaging methods. *Lancet*. 2009;373:897–910.

13. Abdallah MS, Wang K, Magnuson EA, Spertus JA, Farkouh ME, Fuster V and Cohen DJ. Quality of life after PCI vs CABG among patients with diabetes and multivessel coronary artery disease: A randomized clinical trial. *JAMA*. 2013;310:1581–1590.

14. Hlatky MA, Boothroyd DB, Bravata DM, Boersma E, Booth J, Brooks MM, Carrie D et al. Coronary artery bypass surgery compared with percutaneous coronary interventions for multivessel disease: A collaborative analysis of individual patient data from ten randomised trials. *Lancet*. 2009;373:1190–7.

15. Sen H, Lam MK, Lowik MM, Danse PW, Jessurun GA, van Houwelingen KG, Anthonio RL et al. Clinical events and patient-reported chest pain in all-comers treated with resolute integrity and promus element stents: 2-year follow-up of the DUTCH PEERS (DUrable Polymer-Based STent CHallenge of Promus ElemEnt Versus ReSolute Integrity) randomized trial (TWENTE II). *JACC Cardiovasc Interv*. 2015.

16. U.S. Department of Health and Human Services Food and Drug Administration Center for Drug Evaluation and Research (CDER) Center for Biologics Evaluation and Research (CBER) Center for Devices and Radiological Health (CDRH). Guidance for Industry Patient-Reported Outcome Measures: Use in Medical Product Development to Support Labeling Claims. December 2009.

17. Spertus JA, Winder JA, Dewhurst TA, Deyo RA, Prodzinski J, McDonell M and Fihn SD. Development and evaluation of the Seattle Angina Questionnaire: A new functional status measure for coronary artery disease. *J Am Coll Cardiol*. 1995;25:333–41.

18. Serruys PW, Chevalier B, Dudek D, Cequier A, Carrie D, Iniguez A, Dominici M et al. A bioresorbable everolimus-eluting scaffold versus a metallic everolimus-eluting stent for ischaemic heart disease caused by de-novo native coronary artery lesions (ABSORB II): An interim 1-year analysis of clinical and procedural secondary outcomes from a randomised controlled trial. *Lancet*. 2015;385:43–54.

19. Abdallah MS, Wang K, Magnuson EA, Spertus JA, Farkouh ME, Fuster V, Cohen DJ and FREEDOM Trial Investigators. Quality of life after PCI vs CABG among patients with diabetes and multivessel coronary artery disease: A randomized clinical trial. *JAMA*. 2013;310:1581–90.

20. Arnold SV, Magnuson EA, Wang K, Serruys PW, Kappetein AP, Mohr FW, Cohen DJ and Investigators. Do differences in repeat revascularization explain the antianginal benefits of bypass surgery versus percutaneous coronary intervention?: Implications for future treatment comparisons. *Circ Cardiovasc Qual Outcomes*. 2012;5:267–75.

21. Weintraub WS, Spertus JA, Kolm P, Maron DJ, Zhang Z, Jurkovitz C, Zhang W et al. Effect of PCI on quality of life in patients with stable coronary disease. *N Engl J Med*. 2008;359:677–87.

22. Cohen DJ, Van Hout B, Serruys PW, Mohr FW, Macaya C, den Heijer P, Vrakking MM et al. Quality of life after PCI with drug-eluting stents or coronary-artery bypass surgery. *N Engl J Med*. 2011;364:1016–26.

23. Arnold SV, Morrow DA, Lei Y, Cohen DJ, Mahoney EM, Braunwald E and Chan PS. Economic impact of angina after an acute coronary syndrome: Insights from the MERLIN-TIMI 36 trial. *Circ Cardiovasc Qual Outcomes*. 2009;2:344–53.

24. Spertus JA, Jones P, McDonell M, Fan V and Fihn SD. Health status predicts long-term outcome in outpatients with coronary disease. *Circulation*. 2002;106:43–9.

25. Arnold SV, Kosiborod M, Li Y, Jones PG, Yue P, Belardinelli L and Spertus JA. Comparison of the Seattle Angina Questionnaire With Daily Angina Diary in the TERISA Clinical Trial. *Circ Cardiovasc Qual Outcomes*. 2014;7:844–50.

26. Chan PS, Jones PG, Arnold SA and Spertus JA. Development and validation of a short version of the Seattle angina questionnaire. *Circ Cardiovasc Qual Outcomes*. 2014;7:640–7.

27. Campeau L. Letter: Grading of angina pectoris. *Circulation*. 1976;54:522–3.

28. Grundeken MJ, White RM, Hernandez JB, Wykrzykowska JJ, Ishibashi Y, Staehr P, Veldhof S et al. The incidence and relevance of site-reported versus patient reported angina: Insights from the ABSORB II randomized trial comparing ABSORB everolimus eluting bioresorbable scaffold with XIENCE everolimus eluting metallic stent. *Eur Heart J Qual Care Clin Outcomes*. 2016;2:108–16.

29. Ellis SG, Kereiakes DJ, Metzger DC, Caputo RP, Rizik DG, Teirstein PS, Litt MR et al. Everolimus-eluting bioresorbable scaffolds for coronary artery disease. *N Engl J Med*. 2015;373:1905–15.

30. Brugaletta S, Heo JH, Garcia-Garcia HM, Farooq V, van Geuns RJ, de Bruyne B, Dudek D et al. Endothelial-dependent vasomotion in a coronary segment treated by ABSORB everolimus-eluting bioresorbable vascular scaffold system is related to plaque composition at the time of bioresorption of the polymer: Indirect finding of vascular reparative therapy? *Eur Heart J*. 2012;33:1325–33.

31. Serruys PW, Onuma Y, Dudek D, Smits PC, Koolen J, Chevalier B, de Bruyne B et al. Evaluation of the second generation of a bioresorbable everolimus-eluting vascular scaffold for the treatment of de novo coronary artery stenosis: 12-month clinical and imaging outcomes. *J Am Coll Cardiol*. 2011;58:1578–88.

32. Hamilos M, Ribichini F, Ostojic MC, Ferrero V, Orlic D, Vassanelli C, Karanovic N et al. Coronary vasomotion one year after drug-eluting stent implantation: Comparison of everolimus-eluting and paclitaxel-eluting coronary stents. *J Cardiovasc Transl Res*. 2014;7:406–12.

33. Hamilos M, Sarma J, Ostojic M, Cuisset T, Sarno G, Melikian N, Ntalianis A et al. Interference of drug-eluting stents with endothelium-dependent coronary vasomotion: Evidence for device-specific responses. *Circ Cardiovasc Interv*. 2008;1:193–200.

34. Hamilos MI, Ostojic M, Beleslin B, Sagic D, Mangovski L, Stojkovic S, Nedeljkovic M et al. Differential effects of drug-eluting stents on local endothelium-dependent coronary vasomotion. *J Am Coll Cardiol*. 2008;51:2123–9.

35. Gomez-Lara J, Garcia-Garcia HM, Onuma Y, Garg S, Regar E, De Bruyne B, Windecker S et al. A comparison of the conformability of everolimus-eluting bioresorbable vascular scaffolds to metal platform coronary stents. *JACC Cardiovasc Interv*. 2010;3:1190–8.

36. Wentzel JJ, Whelan DM, van der Giessen WJ, van Beusekom HM, Andhyiswara I, Serruys PW, Slager CJ et al. Coronary stent implantation changes 3-D vessel geometry and 3-D shear stress distribution. *J Biomech*. 2000;33:1287–95.

37. Serruys P, Suwannasom P, Nakatani S and Onuma Y. Snowshoe versus ice skate for scaffolding of disrupted vessel wall. *JACC Cardiovasc Interv*. 2015;8:910–913.

38. Escaned J, Colmenarez H, Ferrer MC, Gutierrez M, Jimenez-Quevedo P, Hernandez R, Alfonso F et al. Diastolic dysfunction in diabetic patients assessed with Doppler echocardiography: Relationship with coronary atherosclerotic burden and microcirculatory impairment. *Rev Esp Cardiol*. 2009;62:1395–403.

# Angina reduction after BRSs implantation: Correlation with changes in coronary hemodynamics

NICK E.J. WEST, ADAM J. BROWN, AND STEPHEN P. HOOLE

## INTRODUCTION: ANGINA REDUCTION AFTER PCI: NEED FOR IMPROVEMENT?

Despite huge advances in interventional cardiology, as a specialty we remain rooted in the immediate: most novel devices are assessed at short-term time points with low-frequency clinical endpoints that have to be combined into composites in order to provide a reasonable chance of demonstrating either noninferiority or superiority [1,2]. As far as longer-term patient prognosis goes, percutaneous coronary intervention (PCI) provides at best a modest impact, with benefits largely confined to patients with substantial ischemic burden [3] or acute ST-elevation myocardial infarction [4].

What then, is the role of PCI? Originally, this novel intervention was designed as a treatment adjunct to medical therapy to reduce the frequency of anginal; the treatment itself, in the words of Andreas Grüntzig, would need "a prospective randomized trial...to evaluate its usefulness in comparison with surgical and medical management" [5]. Such trials have come and gone, with PCI proving efficacious in low-complexity multivessel disease compared with coronary artery bypass graft surgery in the short-term [6], but showing little benefit in prognosis or angina reduction when compared with optimal guideline-driven medical therapy [7].

Disappointingly, most clinical trials still demonstrate persistent/recurrent angina in between 20% and 30% of patients 1 year after metallic drug-eluting stent (DES) implantation [8–10], with important healthcare-economic consequences in terms of requirement for ongoing medications, further hospital appointments, admissions, and investigation [11]. Furthermore, deteriorating anginal status is strongly associated with increased mortality [12,13].

If angina reduction and longer-term patient-oriented outcomes are the primary role of PCI in stable patients, there is certainly room for improvement, and it is highly likely that if this were achieved, prognostic benefits may follow. Whether such improvements will be through improved targeting of ischemia-inducing lesions, addition of enhanced procedural/postprocedural pharmacotherapy, or utilization of new devices/techniques remains to be seen.

## ANGINA REDUCTION AFTER BIORESORBABLE VASCULAR SCAFFOLD IMPLANTATION: FACT OR FANTASY?

Bioresorbable vascular scaffolds (BRSs) are an emerging and novel treatment for coronary artery disease [14]: similar to but essentially differing from conventional metallic stents, they provide the short-term scaffolding required to prevent acute vessel closure during PCI, deliver antiproliferative drug in the same way as DES but subsequently resorb in a benign fashion over varying timeframes to leave nothing behind. Of currently available devices in this class, only the ABSORB bioresorbable vascular scaffold (BVS; Abbott Vascular, Santa Clara, CA) has a substantial body of supporting data. At present, randomized controlled trials of BVSs against best-in-class DESs have confirmed comparable (noninferior) clinical outcomes at 1 year with longer-term clinical benefits yet to be determined [15,16].

Interestingly, the first report of the pivotal ABSORB II randomized trial also hinted at patient benefits outside of conventional hard clinical outcome measures—a significant observed reduction in the rate of recurrent or worsening angina occurring as early as 1 year of follow-up (Figure 6.2.1) [15]. A similar, hypothesis-generating 1-year (short-term) difference had previously been observed in

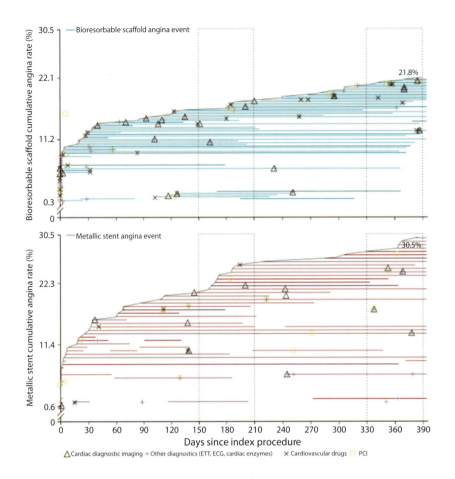

**Figure 6.2.1** Anginal episodes collected from adverse event reports in the ABSORB II randomized trial [15]. Recurrent or worsening anginal episodes picked up by adverse event reporting showed a significant reduction in patients treated with BVSs (top panel, blue graph), compared with DES (bottom panel, red graph). Symbols on graph represent culminated hospital episodes resulting from angina. (Reprinted from *Lancet*, Vol. 385, Serruys PW et al. A bioresorbable everolimus-eluting scaffold versus a metallic everolimus-eluting stent for ischemic heart disease caused by de-novo native coronary artery lesions (ABSORB II): An interim 1-year analysis of clinical and procedural secondary outcomes from a randomised controlled trial, pp. 43–54, Copyright 2015, with permission from Elsevier.)

a post-hoc comparison of patients from the real-world ABSORB-EXTEND registry [17] with a propensity-matched population of patients receiving a single 3.0 × 18 mm everolimus-eluting DES in the SPIRIT IV study [18]. In ABSORB II, anginal status assessed by the standardized 5-domain Seattle Angina Questionnaire was similar in the two treatment groups, but angina episodes assessed through protocol-driven adverse event reporting overcomes the issue of patient recall and takes into account earlier episodes that may have occurred. Furthermore, supporting this finding were significant reductions in the use of nitrates and premature ischemia-driven termination of protocol-driven exercise tread-mill testing at 6 months in patients receiving BVSs, and a subsequent directionally consistent but nonsignificant trend toward less use of nitrates and all revascularizations at 1 year. However, it should be emphasized that, while exciting and thought-provoking, this finding was not a powered primary endpoint and thus the findings should be viewed as exploratory.

Subsequent randomized controlled trials have been designed to investigate these findings further, with ABSORB III having a prespecified post-PCI angina endpoint [19] and the larger ABSORB IV study dedicated directly to addressing angina status with a co-primary endpoint and a raft of healthcare-economic and quality-of-life as well as perceptual analyses [20]. Disappointingly, ABSORB III failed to replicate the preliminary observations from the ABSORB-EXTEND/SPIRIT IV analysis and ABSORB II (Figure 6.2.2), demonstrating no difference in patient-reported angina at 1 year of follow-up [16], although lack of central adjudication of this endpoint and issues with vessel sizing below protocol stipulation (and hence likely reduced area of distribution) may have contributed. The influence of patient perception may have also been important as patients were blinded to their treatment group allocation, and it was the DES group that overperformed compared with histori-cal data. Whether angina reduction proves to be a reality or a statistical vagary will be determined both by the results of ABSORB IV and the planned combined angina data

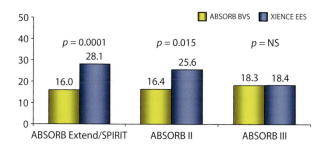

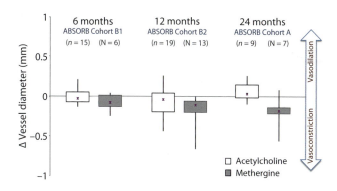

**Figure 6.2.2** Frequency of reported angina in the retrospective, propensity-matched ABSORB-EXTEND/SPIRIT IV population (data on file, Abbott Vascular) and the ABSORB II and III randomized controlled trials [15,16]. In both the ABSORB-EXTEND/SPIRIT IV analysis and in ABSORB II, a similar magnitude of benefit in terms of angina episodes was seen in BVSs-treated patients (gold bars) compared with metallic DES counterparts (blue bars). In ABSORB III, no difference was observed, with metallic DES-treated patients overperforming in terms of angina reporting when compared with historical data.

**Figure 6.2.3** Epicardial coronary vasomotor responses in human patients treated with BVSs. Changes in vessel diameter (vertical axis) to physiological stimulation with acetylcholine (endothelium-dependent relaxation, open boxes) and methergine (constriction, greyed boxes) show little meaningful biological difference before 12 months (left and center datasets, ABSORB cohorts B1 and B2), with more significant changes at 2 years post-implant. Later data from ABSORB cohort 5 demonstrated that the majority of BVSs-treated vessels exhibited endothelium-independent relaxation to intracoronary nitrates. (From Serruys PW. First report of the 5-year cohort B multimodality imaging results. Presented at TCT 2015.)

from ABSORB III and IV, but such a finding, if proved true, would represent a definite advantage for this therapy over conventional DES.

## Possible mechanisms underlying angina reduction after BRSs implantation

A reduction in angina emerging as early as 6 months after PCI (in ABSORB II) and being apparent at 12 months (in both the ABSORB EXTEND/SPIRIT IV analysis and ABSORB II) may be explained by a variety of possible mechanisms: early return of vasomotion, improved conformability compared with metallic DES and compliance mismatch have all been proposed, but given the non-blinded nature of both ABSORB-EXTEND and ABSORB II, the placebo and "Hawthorne" effects cannot be discounted (the latter referring to altered behaviors when individuals are aware they are being studied).

Clearly, although late improvements in angina could be mediated via the preserved or even increased luminal geometry documented on serial intravascular imaging at late follow-up after full BVSs resorption [21], alternative mechanisms must be sought to account for such an observation so early after implantation.

Epicardial vessel reactivity to physiological stimuli has recently been reported in previously scaffolded vessels at 5-year follow-up [21,22], although the earliest time point studied to date where biologically relevant changes in vasomotion in human arteries was evident was at 2 years [23] (Figure 6.2.3).

The structural integrity of the BVSs persists beyond 6 months, the first follow-up point where angina reduction was clinically observed [15]. By this time the device has already begun to resorb, but changes in vascular function below the level that might be measured by conventional techniques cannot be ruled out, with loss of mechanical

"caging" of the vessel possibly important in allowing vessel accommodation in response to increased demand for flow. Interestingly, the primary endpoints of the ABSORB II study [24] failed to demonstrate any difference in epicardial vasomotor function between BVSs and metallic DES at 3 years, although shortcomings in methodology (resolution of QCA 200 μm vs. magnitude of observed vessel diameter change approximately 60 μm) may be in part responsible for this.

The improved conformability of the BVSs to coronary anatomy [25,26] may limit deep medial penetration and vessel injury seen with metallic DESs (Figure 6.2.4), and this may thereby reduce vessel stretch and improve compliance mismatch compared with metallic DESs. This in turn may reduce pain triggered by local neurogenic pathways or cellular signaling consequent on mechanotransduction related to wall strain [27].

Despite a lack of overt vasomotor function at six months, compliance at the scaffolded site is significantly increased by this time point, with concurrent disappearance of compliance mismatch between the scaffolded and adjacent segments [26], theoretically leading to a more laminar flow pattern, homogeneous and even endothelial/wall stresses, and an atheroprotective environment [28,29], providing a solid scientific rationale that such mechanisms could be linked to angina reduction at an early time point.

Any or all of such potential underlying mechanisms could and should have demonstrable hemodynamic changes underpinning them; if macrovascular testing methods cannot detect such changes, what of methods designed to detect changes in coronary microvascular function?

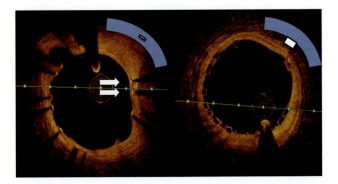

**Figure 6.2.4** Possible mechanism for increased vessel injury with metallic DES over BVSs. Metallic stent struts (left panel) may penetrate deep into the media (diagram, inset) resulting in more profound vascular responses and mechanotransduction resulting from stretch injury, compared with BVSs struts (right panel), often sitting on or penetrating in more shallow fashion the vessel wall (diagram, inset). The relatively large "footprint" and strut thickness (156 µM) of the BVSs precludes its use as a surrogate "scoring" device compared with the thinner-struts of contemporary metallic DES ($\approx$80 µM) and limits deep medial injury.

## CORONARY VASCULAR FUNCTION

A full discussion of coronary physiology and testing methods is outside the scope of this chapter, but a brief overview and relevant methodologies are summarized; comprehensive contemporary reviews of regulation of coronary vascular tone/remodeling and of microvascular function testing techniques provide the rationale for such mechanisms being important in the mediation of angina both in the presence and absence of coronary artery disease, and after PCI [30–32].

The coronary vascular tree, in simplistic terms, can be considered to be composed of two principal elements (Figure 6.2.4): the epicardial coronary arteries and the microcirculation (further subdivided into prearterioles and arterioles); while gross changes in epicardial vessel function can be judged by a variety of testing techniques with direct angiographic visualization, the microcirculation cannot be detected by conventional means and must be tested indirectly. Furthermore, the function of the different parts of the vascular bed may be assessed by different, sometimes overlapping techniques.

### Coronary vasomotor function and testing

Epicardial coronary arteries are essentially conduit vessels with little resistance and therefore contribute minimally to overall coronary flow reserve (CFR). However, the ability of a vessel to dilate and constrict to physiological stimuli is an essential part of vascular homeostasis, with pulsatile flow and concomitant increased shear stresses increasing endothelial bioavailability of antiatherogenic,

antiproliferative, and antiaggregatory substances including nitric oxide, prostaglandin I2, and transforming growth factor-ß [33,34], and a functional epicardial vessel endothelium may exert effects on the coronary microcirculation (Figure 6.2.5).

Testing for epicardial vasomotor function may be achieved through direct infusion of vasoactive agents into the coronary artery during selective coronary angiography [35] with concomitant quantitative coronary angiographic assessment of vessel diameter changes. Although noninvasive surrogates for coronary endothelial function do exist, their correlation with acetylcholine-derived coronary responses is poor [36]. Endothelium-dependent relaxation characterized by a dilatory response to acetylcholine is perhaps the most useful and physiologically relevant parameter, as such a response implies a restored, intact, functional endothelial layer [37,38]. Rapid atrial pacing to cause flow-mediated dilatation or administration of direct nitric oxide donors such as intracoronary nitrates may also be used, but neither of these techniques rely on the presence of functional endothelium although they do demonstrate vasoactive ability, something entirely lacking from "caged" and immobile metallic DES-treated vessels.

Provocative testing with ergonovine is now rarely performed, but methergine may be administered to induce a muscular constrictive response, although this is a somewhat less specific test for physiological vessel function.

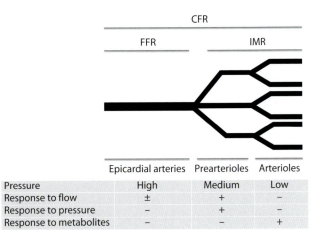

| | CFR | | |
| --- | --- | --- | --- |
| | FFR | IMR | |
| | Epicardial arteries | Prearterioles | Arterioles |
| Pressure | High | Medium | Low |
| Response to flow | ± | + | − |
| Response to pressure | − | + | − |
| Response to metabolites | − | − | + |

**Figure 6.2.5** Features of the coronary microcirculation and tests to interrogate microvascular function. Principal pathways of vascular responsiveness for the different segments of the coronary circulation are summarized in the table (lower panel); investigations and the respective parts of the coronary tree that they address are shown (top panel, above schematic)—while fractional flow reserve (FFR) may be used to interrogate the severity and functional significance of an epicardial arterial stenosis, the index of microcirculatory resistance (IMR) provides an accurate estimation of the microvasculature's function, independent of upstream epicardial stenosis. The coronary flow reserve (CFR) addresses the ability of the entire coronary circulation to increase myocardial blood flow.

## Vasomotor function after BRSs implantation

As previously described, vasomotion has been documented to return as the BVSs begins its resorption process, with vascular responses and pulsatile flow evident in a porcine model as early as 12–18 months after implantation [39], associated with a far less disordered intimal response compared with DES and a differentiated, mature and contractile smooth muscle cell phenotype seen histologically. In humans (with existing coronary disease in contrast to the disease-free animal model), vascular responses do not become definitively obvious until two years after PCI with a BVSs [24] (Figure 6.2.3), but nevertheless, despite such findings not directly improving patient symptoms or hard outcomes, the physiological implications of a functional endothelial layer are important as they betoken improved vascular homeostasis that may yield longer-term benefits and are a stark discriminant compared with vessels "caged" with conventional metallic DES.

## Coronary microvascular dysfunction and assessment methods

Coronary microvascular dysfunction has been identified as a mechanism of myocardial ischemia that may operate both in and without the presence of conventional obstructive coronary artery disease [31]. Further, not only does the function of the microvasculature alter with disease, but chronic changes may manifest as structural changes and adverse vascular remodeling at the arteriolar level which, dependent on pathophysiology, may be reversible with appropriate treatments [40]. Impaired coronary microvascular function (coronary flow reserve [CFR] and index of microcirculatory resistance [IMR]) is associated with increased risk of adverse outcomes including future cardiac events and periprocedural myocardial infarction after PCI [41–44].

In contrast to epicardial responses, visualized angiographically, coronary microcirculatory function is tested indirectly, and may be assessed invasively or noninvasively [31,32]. Validated noninvasive methods of assessing CFR include echocardiography (Doppler and myocardial contrast), cardiac magnetic resonance imaging, positron emission tomography (PET), and computed tomography-derived CFR, while invasive methods utilized in the cardiac catheter lab center on pressure or Doppler wire assessments to derive indices such as CFR, IMR, and coronary blood flow velocity [31]. Each method has its own particular advantages and disadvantages, including the need for specialized equipment (e.g., PET) or local expertise (e.g., Doppler wire) to produce reliable and reproducible results.

## Coronary microcirculatory changes after BRSs implantation

Interest in microcirculatory responses after BVSs implantation were driven by the observations of improved epicardial vasoreactivity and reduced angina rates in BVSs-treated patients in ABSORB II, findings that would suggest some alteration or improvement in coronary hemodynamics especially given the relatively reduced acute lumen gain and increased late loss at 6 months with BVSs [15].

The single-center VANISH trial [45] randomized patients undergoing PCI to receive either a DES or a BVSs and used PET imaging and cold pressor and adenosine-mediated maximal hyperemia to assess myocardial blood flow and CFR. Although the study is designed to complete after three years, an interim report of hemodynamic changes at 1 month were recently presented and published [45]. The authors found that myocardial blood flow to the treated vascular territory assessed by PET was similar between treatment groups, but that CFR of the treated territory was statistically lower in BVSs patients, despite mean values all being above the "normal" cutoff value (Figure 6.2.6). There were some differences in implantation technique between groups and incidence of periprocedural myocardial infarction (which itself may alter coronary hemodynamic indices) was not recorded, but overall the results cannot be viewed as surprising: at 1 month, the BVSs retains structural integrity and is unlikely to exhibit epicardial reactivity, and the timeframe is too short to realistically allow microvascular remodeling to have occurred. Clearly, future follow-up will be interesting to determine whether reported reduced angina rates at 1 year are manifest as evolutionary hemodynamic improvements.

Although CFR effectively interrogates the ability of the whole coronary tree to increase flow as an integrated measure of blood flow through both epicardial vessels and microcirculation, function of the microvasculature itself can be isolated by measurement of IMR using intracoronary thermodilution and the temperature-sensor on an intracoronary pressure wire (St. Jude Medical, St. Paul, MN). Although mathematical corrections are required for contribution of collateral vessels and changes due to central venous pressure, this index provides a validated and reproducible clinically useful index [31,46]. In a small single-center observational study (EMPIRE-BVSs pilot study [46]), IMR values measured immediately after PCI was performed with either a DESs or a BVSs demonstrated a directionally opposite and statistically significant reduction in the BVSs compared with the DES, with all individuals within-group showing uniform responses in terms of direction of change in IMR measurements (Figure 6.2.7). In this study, there was no change in the incidence of periprocedural myonecrosis to account for such difference, and some differences in baseline characteristics again make these findings exploratory. However, only metabolic or autonomic changes (including preconditioning or neurohormonal change) rather than structural adaptation can explain this result, given the immediacy of such findings. Such findings, although ostensibly at odds with those from VANISH, are not mutually exclusive: immediate changes in microcirculatory function (therefore not related to microcirculatory remodeling) may

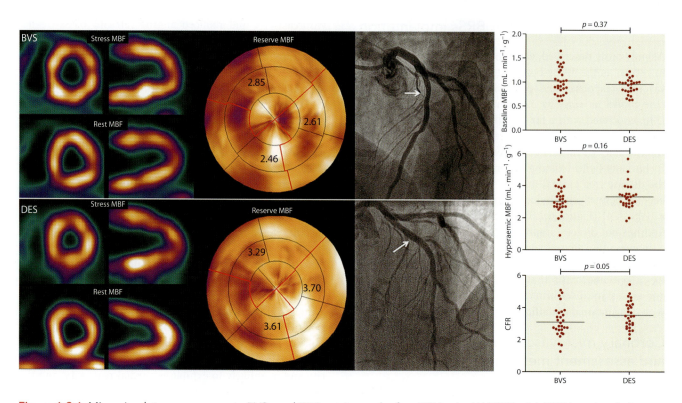

**Figure 6.2.6** Microcirculatory responses to BVSs and DESs at 1 month after PCI in the VANISH trial. PET imaging (left panel) with accompanying coronary angiograms of patients receiving BVSs (top panel) and DESs (bottom panel) in the VANISH trial. Mean baseline/hyperemic MBF and CFR were above normal cutoff values for both groups, but despite no differences in MBF measurements, there was a statistically significant reduction in CFR in the BVSs-treated group (right panel). (Reprinted from *EuroIntervention*, Vol. 12, Stuijfzand WJ et al. Evaluation of myocardial blood flow and coronary flow reserve after implantation of a bioresorbable vascular scaffold versus metal drug-eluting stent: an interim one-month analysis of the VANISH trial, pp. e584–594, Copyright 2016, with permission from Europa Digital & Publishing.)

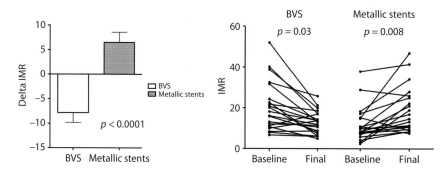

**Figure 6.2.7** Microcirculatory responses to BVSs and DESs immediately after PCI in the EMPIRE-BVSs pilot study. Measurement of IMR immediately before and after PCI showed a directionally opposite and statistically significant change for BVSs compared with DESs, with hyperemic corrected IMR falling in patients receiving BVSs (left panel). Individuals within the group showed uniform responses in terms of direction of change in IMR measurements (right panel).

occur and subsequently alter qualitatively by 1 month (as studied in VANISH). Given that changes in angina frequency were not evident until later in ABSORB II, these hemodynamic/physiological changes may represent a continuum of developing change in vascular/microvascular structure and function. A larger randomized controlled trial to investigate these preliminary findings further is underway (EMPIRE-BVSs [NCT03076476]) and will address in particular implant technique and its possible

effect on preconditioning and deployment characteristics as confounders.

Finally, a physiological substudy of the ABSORB II population [15] has been designed to provide a detailed intracoronary physiological assessment at 3 years' invasive follow-up; in this population, patients that have received BVSs and DESs will undergo intracoronary measurements of pressure and flow velocity to derive intracoronary pressure-flow velocity loops, CFR, and IMR [48]. This study will yield the most comprehensive assessment at a time point remote enough from the index procedure to definitively determine whether functional alterations in the microcirculatory function might differ between treatment groups at a time point when the BVSs-treated cohort will have experienced complete resorption at the scaffolded site.

## CONCLUSIONS AND FUTURE DIRECTIONS

Although interest in the phenomenon of angina reduction with BVSs/BRSs rather waned with the negative findings of ABSORB III, the potential impact of such benefits should not be underestimated. Notwithstanding the huge healthcare-economic and quality of life costs associated with ongoing post-PCI angina that might be ameliorated, there is the issue of mortality: should angina reduction with BRSs prove reality, this might provide a stepping stone to the holy grail of improved prognosis in carefully selected elective patients undergoing PCI. Results of the large-scale ABSORB IV study, dedicated to investigating this phenomenon in detail, and the potentially large (5000 patients) dataset that will result from combination of ABSORB II and IV are therefore awaited with interest.

In the meantime, detailed but, by necessity, smaller-scale physiological investigations also hint at differences in vascular function between BVSs- and DESs-treated vessels, apparently at early time points when neither vascular remodeling nor BVSs degradation/resorption have had the opportunity to occur. Longer-term planned follow-up of VANISH, the forthcoming EMPIRE-BVSs study, and the ABSORB II physiological substudy will yield further important mechanistic insights into the hypothesis-generating observations of reduced angina frequency and its microcirculatory correlates. Without doubt, the enticing prospect of a novel therapy that may definitively reduce post-PCI angina through changes in coronary physiology makes this an area of novel scientific research of potentially enormous impact.

## REFERENCES

1. Serruys PW. Assessing percutaneous intervention: Re-appraising the significance of residual angina. *EuroIntervention.* 2015; 10: 1253.
2. Lim E, Brown A, Helmy A, Mussa S, Altman D. Composite outcomes in cardiovascular research: A survey of randomized trials. *Ann Intern Med.* 2008; 149: 612–617.
3. Shaw LJ, Berman DS, Maron DJ et al. Optimal medical therapy with or without percutaneous coronary intervention to reduce ischemic burden: Results from the Clinical Outcomes Utilizing Revascularization and Aggressive Drug Evaluation (COURAGE) trial nuclear substudy. *Circulation.* 2008; 117: 1283–1291.
4. Keeley EC, Boura JA, Grines CL. Primary angioplasty versus intravenous thrombolytic therapy for acute myocardial infarction: A quantitative review of 23 randomised trials. *Lancet.* 2003; 361: 13–20.
5. Gruntzig AR, Senning A, Siegenthaler WE. Nonoperative dilatation of coronary-artery stenosis—Percutaneous transluminal coronary angioplasty. *N Engl J Med.* 1979; 301: 61–68.
6. Mohr FW, Morice MC, Kappetein AP et al. Coronary artery bypass graft surgery versus percutaneous coronary intervention in patients with three-vessel disease and left main coronary disease: 5-year follow-up of the randomized, clinical SYNTAX trial. *Lancet.* 2013; 381: 629–638.
7. Boden WE, O'Rourke RA, Teo KT et al. Optimal medical therapy with or without PCI for stable coronary disease. *N Engl J Med.* 2007; 356: 1503–1516.
8. Tonino PA, De Bruyne B, Pijls NH et al. Fractional flow reserve versus angiography for guiding percutaneous coronary intervention. *N Engl J Med.* 2009; 360: 213–224.
9. Cohen DJ, Van Hout B, Serruys PW et al. Quality of life after PCI with drug-eluting stents or coronary-artery bypass surgery. *N Engl J Med.* 2011; 364: 1016–1026.
10. Abdallah MS, Wang K, Magnuson EA et al. Quality of life after PCI vs CABG among patients with diabetes and multivessel coronary artery disease: A randomized clinical trial. *JAMA.* 2013; 310: 1581–1590.
11. Ben-Yehuda O, Kazi DS, Bonafede M et al. Angina and associated healthcare costs following percutaneous coronary intervention: A real-world analysis from a multi-payer database. *Catheter Cardiovasc Interv.* 2016; Jan 17 (epub ahead of print).
12. Spertus JA, Jones P, McDonnell M, Fan V, Fihn SD. Health status predicts long-term outcome in outpatients with coronary disease. *Circulation.* 2002; 106: 43–49.
13. Mozaffarian D, Bryson CL, Spertus JA, McDonnell MB, Fihn SD. Anginal symptoms consistently predict total mortality among outpatients with coronary artery disease. *Am Heart J.* 2003; 146: 1015–1022.
14. Wiebe J, Nef HM, Hamm CW. Current status of bioresorbable scaffolds in the treatment of coronary artery disease. *J Am Coll Cardiol.* 2014; 64: 2541–2551.
15. Serruys PW, Chevalier B, Dudek D et al. A bioresorbable everolimus-eluting scaffold versus a metallic everolimus-eluting stent for ischaemic heart disease caused by de-novo native coronary lesions (ABSORB II): An interim 1-year analysis of clinical and procedural secondary outcomes from a randomized controlled trial. *Lancet.* 2015; 385: 43–54.
16. Ellis SG, Kereiakes DJ, Metzger DC et al. Everolimus-eluting bioresorbable scaffolds for coronary artery disease. *N Engl J Med.* 2015; 170: 641–651.

17. Abizaid A, Ribamar Costa J Jr, Bartorelli A et al. The ABSORB EXTEND study: Preliminary report of the twelve-month clinical outcomes in the first 512 patients enrolled. *EuroIntervention.* 2015; 10: 1396–1401.

18. Brener SJ, Kereiakes DJ, Simonton CA et al. Everolimus-eluting stents in patients undergoing percutaneous coronary intervention: Final 3-year results of the clinical evaluation of the XIENCE V everolimus eluting coronary stent system in the treatment of subjects with de novo native coronary artery lesions trial. *Am Heart J.* 2013; 166: 1035–1042.

19. Kereiakes DJ, Ellis SG, Popma JJ et al. Evaluation of a fully bioresorbable in patients with coronary artery disease: Design of and rationale for the ABSORB III randomized trial. *Am Heart J.* 2015; 170: 641–651.

20. Stone GW. Assessing whether superiority exists: Design, rationale and status of ABSORB IV. Presented at TCT 2015.

21. Simsek C, Karanasos A, Magro M et al. Long-term invasive follow-up of the everolimus-eluting bioresorbable vascular scaffold: Five-year results of multiple invasive imaging modalities. *EuroIntervention.* 2016; 11: 996–1003.

22. Serruys PW. First report of the 5-year cohort B multimodality imaging results. Presented at TCT 2015.

23. Serruys PW, Ormiston JA, Onuma Y et al. A bioabsorbable everolimus-eluting coronary stent system (ABSORB): 2-year outcomes and results from multiple imaging methods. *Lancet.* 2009; 373: 897–910.

24. Serruys PW, Chevalier B, Sotomi Y et al. Comparison of an everolimus-eluting bioresorbable scaffold with an everolimus-eluting metallic stent for the treatment of coronary artery stenosis (ABSORB II): A 3 year, randomised, controlled, single-blind, multicentre clinical trial. *Lancet.* 2016; 388: 2479–2491.

25. Gomez-Lara J, Brugaletta S, Farooq V et al. Angiographic geometric changes of the lumen arterial wall after bioresorbable vascular scaffolds and metallic platform stents at 1-year follow-up. *JACC Cardiovasc Interv.* 2011; 4: 789–799.

26. Gomez-Lara J, Garcia-Garcia HM, Onuma Y et al. A comparison of the conformability of everolimus-eluting bioresorbable vascular scaffolds to metal platform coronary stents. *JACC Cardiovasc Interv.* 2010; 3: 1190–1198.

27. Brugaletta S, Gogas BD, Garcia-Garcia HM et al. Vascular compliance changes of the coronary vessel wall after bioresorbable vascular scaffold implantation in the treated and adjacent segments. *Circ J.* 2012; 76: 1616–1623.

28. Schwarzacher SP, Tsao PS, Ward M et al. Effects of stenting on adjacent vascular distensibility and neointima formation: Role of nitric oxide. *Vasc Med.* 2001; 6: 139–144.

29. Ward MR, Hibi K, Shaw JA et al. Effects of stent implantation on upstream coronary artery compliance—A cause of late plaque rupture? *Am J Cardiol.* 2005; 96: 673–675.

30. Pries AR, Badimon L, Bugiardini R et al. Coronary vascular regulation, remodeling, and collateralization: Mechanisms and clinical implications on behalf of the working group on coronary pathophysiology and microcirculation. *Eur Heart J.* 2015; 36: 3134–3146.

31. Camici PG, d'Amati G, Rimoldi O. Coronary microvascular dysfunction: Mechanisms and functional assessment. *Nat Rev Cardiol.* 2015; 12: 48–62.

32. Hirata K, Amudha K, Elina R et al. Measurement of coronary vasomotor function: Getting to the heart of the matter in cardiovascular research. *Clin Sci.* 2004; 107: 449–460.

33. Chien S. Mechanotransduction and endothelial cell homeostasis: The wisdom of the cell. *Am J Physiol Heart Circ Physiol.* 2007; 292: H1209–1224.

34. Traub O, Berk BC. Laminar shear stress: Mechanisms by which endothelial cells transduce an atheroprotective force. *Arterioscler Thromb Vasc Biol.* 1998; 18: 677–685.

35. Raitakari OT, Celermajer DS. Testing for endothelial dysfunction. *Ann Med.* 2009; 32: 293–304.

36. Monnink SHJ, Tio RA, van Boven AJ, van Gilst WH, van Veldhuisen. The role of coronary endothelial function testing in patients suspected for angina pectoris. *Int J Cardiol.* 2004; 96: 123–129.

37. Hofma SH, van der Giessen WJ, van Dalen BM et al. Indication of long-term endothelial dysfunction after sirolimus-eluting stent implantation. *Eur Heart J.* 2006; 27: 166–170.

38. Sabate M, Kay IP, van der Giessen et al. Preserved endothelial-dependent vasodilatation in coronary segments previously treated with balloon angioplasty and intracoronary irradiation. *Circulation.* 1999; 100: 1623–1629.

39. Lane JP, Perkins LE, Sheehy AJ et al. Lumen gain and restoration of pulsatility after implantation of a bioresorbable vascular scaffold in porcine coronary arteries. *JACC Cardiovasc Interv.* 2014; 7: 668–695.

40. Neglia D, Fommei E, Varela-Carver A et al. Perindopril and indapamide reverse coronary microvascular remodeling and improve flow in arterial hypertension. *J Hypertens.* 2011; 29: 364–372.

41. Murthy VL, Naya M, Taqueti VR et al. Effects of sex on coronary microvascular dysfunction and cardiac outcomes. *Circulation.* 2014; 129: 2518–2527.

42. Layland JJ, Whitbourn RJ, Burns AT et al. The index of microcirculatory resistance identifies patients with periprocedural myocardial infarction in elective percutaneous coronary intervention. *Heart.* 2012; 98: 1492–1497.

43. van de Hoef TP, Bax M, Damman P et al. Impaired coronary autoregulation is associated with long-term fatal events in patients with stable coronary artery disease. *Circ Cardiovasc Interv.* 2013; 6: 329–335.

44. van de Hoef TP, Bax M, Meuwiseen M et al. Impact of coronary microvascular function on long-term cardiac mortality in patients with acute ST-segment-elevation myocardial infarction. *Circ Cardiovasc Interv.* 2013; 6: 207–215.

45. Stuijfzand WJ, Raijmakers PG, Driessen RS et al. Evaluation of myocardial blood flow and coronary flow reserve after implantation of a bioresorbable vascular scaffold versus metal drug-eluting stent: An interim one-month analysis of the VANISH trial. *EuroIntervention.* 2016; 12: e584–594.

46. Lee JM, Layland J, Jung J et al. Integrated physi-ologic assessment of ischemic heart disease in real-world practice using index of microcirculatory resistance and fractional flow reserve. Insights from the international index of microcirculatory resistance registry. *Circ Cardiovasc Interv.* 2015; 8: e002857.

47. Hoole SP, Brown AJ, McCormick LM, West NEJ. Implantation of bioresorbable vascular scaffolds improves the index of microvascular resistance. *J Am Coll Cardiol.* 2014; 63 (12_S) (Abstract].

48. Escaned J. Post-PCI angina after ABSORB implanta-tion: Overview on the available data. Presented at EuroPCR 2015.

6.3

# Comparison of everolimus-eluting bioresorbable scaffolds with everolimus-eluting metallic stents for treatment of coronary artery stenosis: Three-year follow-up of the ABSORB II randomized trial

CARLOS COLLET, YOHEI SOTOMI, BERNARD CHEVALIER, ANGEL RAMÓN CEQUIER FILLAT,
DIDIER CARRIÉ, JAN PIEK, A.J. VAN BOVEN, MARCELLO DOMINICI,
DARIUSZ DUDEK, DOUGAL MCCLEAN, STEFFEN HELQVIST, MICHAEL HAUDE,
SEBASTIAN REITH, MANUEL DE SOUSA ALMEIDA, GIANLUCA CAMPO,
ANDRÉS IÑIGUEZ, ROBERT-JAN M. VAN GEUNS, PIETER SMITS, MANEL SABATÉ,
STEPHAN WINDECKER, YOSHINOBU ONUMA, AND PATRICK W.J.C. SERRUYS

## INTRODUCTION

At the time of the ABSORB II study design in July 2011, commercialization of the ABSORB scaffold (Abbott Vascular, Santa Clara, CA) was just starting, following approval with CE mark in December 2010. At that time, clinical evidence of the everolimus-eluting ABSORB scaffold had been attained without the use of a comparator. There was a need to conduct a trial with the metallic comparator that was at that time the best-in-class drug-eluting stent. The aims of the trial were to assess the additional value of the technology in order to generate evidence-based data that would support the introduction of this novel device in clinical practice and to guide interventional cardiologists in its early use.

The ABSORB II trial is a prospective, randomized, active-controlled, single-blind, parallel 2-arm, multicenter clinical trial. A total of 501 subjects were randomized either to treatment with the everolimus-eluting bioresorbable scaffold (ABSORB) or treatment with the everolimus-eluting metallic stent (XIENCE, Abbott Vascular) in 2:1 ratio at 46 sites in Europe and New Zealand. The trial protocol allowed the treatment of up to two *de novo* native coronary artery lesions. The protocol describing the inclusion criteria, exclusion criteria, the methods of quantitative

coronary angiography, and quantitative intravascular ultrasound has been published elsewhere [1–3]. All patients and treating physicians were asked to adhere to the published guidelines in terms of tobacco usage, exercise, healthy food intake, maintaining an adequate weight (body mass index) and waist circumference, achieving target blood lipid levels, and blood pressure control [4]. Subjects were blinded to the treatment arm for the duration of the trial. Study staff were instructed not to reveal the treatment to the patients or the referring physicians. A data safety monitoring board reviewed the cumulative safety data from the trial at given intervals for the purpose of safeguarding the interests of the participants. All patients provided informed consent before being included in the trial and all participating sites received medical ethics committee approval for the study. Subjects had clinical follow-up at 30 and 180 days and at 1, 2, and 3 years.

Repeat invasive imaging was scheduled at 3 years, with angiography and intravascular ultrasound for assessment of co-primary endpoints. In case of repeat treatment of the target lesion, the luminal dimensions prior to the treatment were carried forward to the 3-year follow-up for statistical purposes. Angiography was documented prior to and after intracoronary administration of nitrate to assess vasomotion. Multiple matched angiographic views were used for the assessment of vasomotion and long-term luminal dimensions [5–7]. Seattle Angina Questionnaires were collected at preimplantation, at 180-days, and at 1-, 2-, and 3-year follow-up [8]. Exercise testing including ECG recording was performed at 180 days, 1, 2, and 3 years [9]. ST-T depression of 0.1 mV at maximal exercise or chest pain during exercise was considered as indicative of ischemia [9,10].

The co-primary endpoints at 3 years were vasomotion assessed by change in mean lumen diameter assessed by quantitative coronary angiography (QCA) pre- and postintracoronary nitrate administration, as well as angiographic late luminal loss (minimum lumen diameter [MLD] at follow-up postnitrate—MLD postprocedure postnitrate). The co-primary endpoints were analyzed for the Intent-to-Treat (ITT) population, on a lesion basis. For the endpoint of vasomotion, the comparison was tested using a two-sided t-test. For the endpoint of late luminal loss, noninferiority was tested using a one-sided asymptotic test, against a noninferiority margin of 0.14 mm. If noninferiority was met with higher value in the ABSORB arm, then superiority would be tested using a two-sided t-test. The p-value <0.05 was considered statistically significant.

Intravascular ultrasound secondary endpoints were quantitative analysis of lumen area, plaque area, and vessel area. Outcomes measured for composite clinical secondary endpoints were death (cardiac vs. vascular vs. noncardiovascular), myocardial infarction (Q-wave vs. non-Q-wave; attributable vs. nonattributable to target vessel), target-lesion revascularization, target-vessel revascularization, nontarget-vessel revascularization, and all coronary revascularizations (all revascularizations clinically indicated vs. nonclinically indicated). Composite clinical secondary endpoints were death plus all myocardial infarction, cardiac death plus myocardial infarction attributable to target vessel plus clinically indicated target-lesion revascularization (device-oriented composite endpoint [DOCE]); and death plus all myocardial infarction plus all revascularization (patient-oriented composite endpoint [POCE]). Myocardial infarction per protocol was defined as the development of new pathological Q-wave or creatine kinase rise of two or more times upper limit of normal accompanied by creatine kinase-MB rise [2,11,12]. The sample size for the trial was calculated on the basis of the first co-primary endpoint (superiority for vasomotion). Assuming a two-tailed superiority t-test, a 2:1 randomization ratio, an α of 0.05, and true changes in mean lumen diameter of 0.07 mm for the bioresorbable scaffold and 0 mm for the metallic stent (standard deviation 0.20 mm for both) [13,14], we estimated that 260 lesions in the bioresorbable scaffold arm and 130 lesions in the metallic stent arm would be needed for 90% power. Allowing for a 29% attrition rate and 10% of patients with dual lesions, we estimated that 334 patients in the bioresorbable scaffold arm and 167 patients in the metallic stent arm would be needed.

Considering the 390 lesions available for quantitative coronary angiography assessments, the study has 89% power to detect noninferiority in the second co-primary endpoint of late luminal loss (assuming the true means are equal in both arms with a standard deviation of 0.45 mm and a noninferiority margin [δ] of 0.14 mm). The endpoint analyses presented in this report were performed on an intent-to-treat basis. For binary variables, counts, percentages, and exact 95% confidence intervals using the Clopper–Pearson method were calculated. For continuous variables, means, standard deviations, and 95% confidence intervals for the mean using the Gaussian approximation were calculated. Chi-square or Fisher's exact test was used to compare binary variables, and the Student's t-test or the Wilcoxon signed rank test was used to compare continuous variables. For time-to-event variables, survival curves were constructed using Kaplan–Meier estimates, and log rank test results are for hypothesis-generating purposes only. Analyses were performed using SAS software version 9.3 (SAS Institute, Cary, NC).

## BASELINE DEMOGRAPHIC, LESIONS AND PROCEDURAL CHARACTERISTICS OF THE ABSORB II POPULATION

Table 6.3.1 shows patient demographics and risk factors at baseline. The prevalence of diabetes was 24%, with 6.6 and 8.4% being insulin dependent. Twenty-one percent of patients presented with unstable angina. More than 80% of patients had single-vessel disease. The complexity of the treated lesions is described according to the AHA/ACC classification. Device success and procedural success as well as technique of implantation have been previously reported [15]. All lesions were predilated with the exception of two lesions in the metallic stent group. For quantitative coronary angiography, preprocedural measurements did not differ between the two groups, whereas for quantitative intravascular ultrasound, both preprocedural vessel area and plaque area were larger in the metallic stent group than in the bioresorbable scaffold group. Rates of clinical device success and clinical procedural success were similar in the two treatment groups. The nominal size of devices used and the acute recoil after device implantation were also similar between treatment groups. Balloon dilatation after device implantation was in 61% in the ABSORB group compared to 59% in the XIENCE group (p = 0.67). However, dilatation pressure was significantly higher and balloon diameter at the highest pressure during implantation or postdilatation of the device was significantly larger in the metallic stent group. Therefore, the acute gain in minimum lumen diameter (by quantitative coronary angiography) and minimum lumen area (by quantitative intravascular ultrasound), and the final minimum lumen diameter and minimum lumen area, were significantly larger in the metallic stent group than in the bioresorbable scaffold group. The incidence of side branch occlusion and any anatomic complications assessed by angiography was similar between the two treatment arms (side branch occlusion: ABSORB:

Table 6.3.1 Characteristics of patients and lesions at baseline

| | ABSORB (N = 335, L = 364) | XIENCE (N = 166, L = 182) | Difference [95% CI] |
|---|---|---|---|
| Age (year) | 61.5 (10.0) | 60.9 (10.0) | 0.6 [−1.2, 2.5] |
| Male, n (%) | 253 (75.5) | 132 (79.5) | −4.00% [−11.30, 4.03] |
| Body mass index, kg/m² | 27.9 (4.1) | 28.1 (3.7) | −0.2 [−0.9, 0.5] |
| Current tobacco use, n (%) | 79 (23.6) | 36 (21.7) | 1.90% [−6.17, 9.28] |
| Hypertension, n (%) (history and/or requiring medication) | 231 (69.0) | 119 (71.7) | −2.73% [−10.87, 5.95] |
| Dyslipidemia, n (%) (history and/or requiring medication) | 252 (75.2) | 133 (80.1) | −4.90% [−12.15, 3.09] |
| LDL Cholesterol <2 mmol/L (80 mg/dL), n (%) | 113 (34.9) | 51 (31.9) | 3.00% [−6.06, 11.59] |
| All diabetes, n (%) | 80 (23.9) | 40 (24.1) | −0.22% [−8.44, 7.40] |
| Diabetes mellitus treated with insulin, n (%) | 22 (6.6) | 14 (8.4) | −1.87% [−7.53%, 2.74] |
| Family history of premature CAD, n (%) | 112 (36.6) | 64 (41.3) | −4.69% [−14.12, 4.59] |
| Prior cardiac intervention in target vessel, n (%) | 14 (11.7) | 5 (8.9) | 2.74% [−8.56, 11.35] |
| Prior MI, n (%) | 93 (28) | 48 (28.9) | −0.90% [−9.52, 7.22] |
| Recent myocardial infarction with normalized enzyme, n (%) | 11 (3.3) | 3 (1.8) | 1.48% [−2.19, 4.25] |
| Stable angina, n (%) | 214 (63.9) | 107 (64.5) | −0.58% [−9.25, 8.44] |
| Stable angina CCS III or IV, n (%) | 47 (22) | 24 (22.4) | −0.47% [−10.58, 8.66] |
| Unstable angina, n (%) | 68 (20.3) | 37 (22.3) | −1.99% [−9.96, 5.33] |
| Unstable angina Braunwald Class III, n (%) | 16 (23.5) | 10 (27.0) | −3.50% [−21.57, 12.74] |
| Silent ischemia, n (%) | 42 (12.5) | 19 (11.4) | 1.09% [−5.44, 6.73] |
| Single vessel disease, n (%) | 278 (83) | 141 (84.9) | −1.95% [−8.35, 5.26] |
| Target vessel | n = 364 lesions | n = 182 lesions | |
| Left anterior descending artery, n (%) | 163 (44.8) | 84 (46.2) | −1.37% [−10.19, 7.38] |
| Left circumflex artery, n (%) | 106 (29.1) | 42 (23.1) | 6.04% [−1.94, 13.41] |
| Right coronary artery, n (%) | 95 (26.1) | 56 (30.8) | −4.67% [−12.90, 3.18] |
| Two or more lesion treated, n (%) | 29/335 (8.7) | 16/166 (9.6) | −0.69% [−6.86, 4.52] |
| Calcification (moderate or severe), n (%) | 46 (12.7) | 28 (15.5) | −2.80% [−9.50, 3.14] |
| ACC/AHA Lesion Class, n (%) | | | |
| A | 5 (1.4) | 1 (0.6) | 0·82% [−1.82, 2.68] |
| B1 | 193 (53.2) | 90 (50) | 3.17% [−5.70, 12.00] |
| B2 | 159 (43.8) | 87 (48.3) | 4.53% [−13.35, 4.31] |
| C | 6 (1.7) | 2 (1.1) | 0.54% [−2.44, 2.61] |

Note: Data are n (%) or mean (SD) unless otherwise stated.

5.3% vs. XIENCE: 7.6%, $p = 0.07$; any anatomic complication: ABSORB: 16.4% vs. EES: 19.9%, $p = 0.39$). There were no differences in the incidence of cardiac biomarkers rise and periprocedural myocardial infarction between ABSORB and XIENCE [16].

By means of intravascular ultrasound, the preprocedural minimum lumen area (MLA) was comparable between the two arms. However, preprocedural vessel area (XIENCE 11.61 mm² vs. ABSORB 10.71 mm², respectively; $p = 0.014$) and plaque area (XIENCE 9.47 mm² vs. ABSORB 8.63 mm², respectively; $p = 0.016$) at the site of MLA were significantly larger in the XIENCE arm than in the ABSORB arm. The postprocedural lumen area at the site of preprocedural MLA was significantly smaller in the ABSORB arm (5.55 mm² vs. 6.40 mm², respectively; $p < 0.001$). The increase of vessel

area tended to be smaller in the ABSORB arm (2.34 mm² vs. 2.66 mm², respectively; $p = 0.066$). As a result, there were significant differences in acute gain for the minimal lumen areas (3.46 mm² vs. 4.27 mm², respectively; $p < 0.001$). In addition, device expansion defined as the ratio of postprocedural lumen area at the site of preprocedural MLA to the expected inner device area calculated from the largest balloon used during procedure was 62 ± 12% of the predicted lumen area with the ABSORB, whereas the XIENCE stent achieved 71 ± 15% ($p < 0.001$). Lower acute gain (lowest tertile) occurred more frequently in the ABSORB arm than in the XIENCE arm (risk ratio: 3.04; 95% confidence interval [CI]: 1.94–4.76). ABSORB use, maximal inner device or balloon diameter throughout procedure, vessel, and plaque areas at the MLA site, and negative remodeling were significantly associated with lower acute gain in the multivariate model [17]. Also, the implantation of the ABSORB scaffold was more frequently associated with postprocedural asymmetric and eccentric morphology compared to the XIENCE stent. Postprocedural device asymmetry was independently associated with device-oriented cardiac events 1-year follow-up [18].

## CO-PRIMARY ANGIOGRAPHIC ENDPOINTS

The vasomotor reactivity test was analyzable for 388 lesions. At 3-year follow-up angiography, the increase in mean lumen diameter postintracoronary injection of nitrate was comparable in both arms (ABSORB 258 paired lesions 0.047 ± 0.109 mm vs. XIENCE 130 paired lesions 0.056 ± 0.117 mm, $p_{superiority}$ = 0.49). In both arms, the vasodilation of the proximal and distal edge was larger than the scaffolded or stented segment themselves (Figure 6.3.1) [10].

Follow-up angiographic analysis was available in 298 lesions in ABSORB and 151 lesions in XIENCE. Angiographic results are tabulated in Table 6.3.2.

In device, the in-stent/scaffold late luminal loss was 0.371 ± 0.449 mm vs. 0.250 ± 0.250 mm ($p_{noninferiority}$ = 0.78) in ABSORB and XIENCE, respectively. The criteria for noninferiority were not met. Minimum lumen diameter at follow-up was 1.86 ± 0.54 mm versus 2.25 ± 0.37 mm in ABSORB and XIENCE, respectively ($p < 0.001$). The percentage diameter stenosis at follow-up was 26 ± 17% vs. 16 ± 8% in ABSORB and XIENCE ($p < 0.001$), respectively. Binary restenosis was 7.0% (21/298) versus 0.7% (1/151) for the ABSORB and XIENCE, respectively ($p = 0.003$).

In segment, binary restenosis was 8.4% (25/296) versus 3.3% (5/151) for the ABSORB and XIENCE, respectively ($p = 0.04$) [10].

## INTRAVASCULAR ULTRASOUND

At 3-year follow-up, intravascular ultrasound was available in 247 lesions in ABSORB and 136 lesions in XIENCE (Table 6.3.2). Out of 32 patients who underwent repeat target lesion revascularization, 19 underwent intravascular imaging prior to repeat treatment of target lesions, whereas the remaining 13 were not assessed. Acute gain in minimum lumen area postprocedure was significantly different

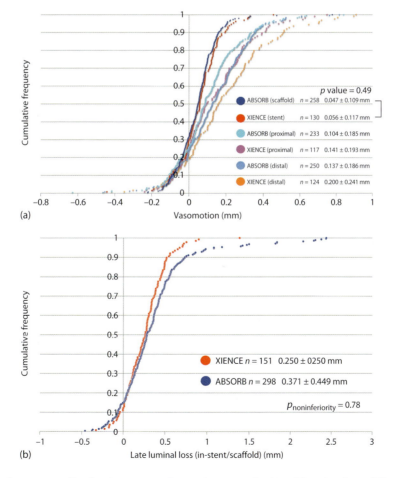

**Figure 6.3.1** Cumulative frequency distribution curve of co-primary endpoints. The absolute differences in mean lumen diameter (mm) pre- and postintracoronary nitrate injection **(a)** and late luminal loss **(b)** for the ABSORB and the XIENCE. (Reproduced with permission of Serruys PW et al. *Lancet.* 2016 Nov 19;388(10059):2479–2491.)

Table 6.3.2 Angiographic and intravascular ultrasound analyses preprocedure, postprocedure and at follow-up (3 years)

| | ABSORB | XIENCE | Difference [95% confidence interval] | p value |
|---|---|---|---|---|
| **Angiographic analysis** | **298 lesions** | **151 lesions** | | |
| Lesion length obstruction (mm) | 13.94 (6.65) | 13.40(6.01) | 0.54 [–0.69, 1.77] | 0.39 |
| Total scaffolded or stented length (mm) | 21.06 (9.07) | 20.71 (6.96) | 0.35 [–1.18, 1.88] | 0.66 |
| **In-scaffold/stent assessment** | | | | |
| **Reference vessel diameter** | | | | |
| Preprocedure diameter (mm) | 2.59 (0.39) | 2.61 (0.40) | –0.0152 [–0.0932, 0.0628] | 0.7 |
| Postprocedure diameter (mm) | 2.64 (0.36) | 2.79 (0.34) | –0.15 [–0.21, –0.08] | <0.001 |
| Follow-up diameter (mm) | 2.50 (0.40) | 2.67 (0.34) | –0.17 [–0.24, –0.10] | <0.001 |
| **Minimum lumen diameter** | | | | |
| Preprocedure diameter (mm) | 1.06 (0.33) | 1.06 (0.30) | 0.00 [–0.06, 0.06] | 0.99 |
| Postprocedure diameter (mm) | 2.22 (0.33) | 2.50 (0.33) | –0.28 [–0.34, –0.21] | <0.001 |
| Acute gain (mm) | 1.16 (0.38) | 1.45 (0.37) | –0.29 [–0.36, –0.21] | <.0001 |
| Follow-up diameter (mm) | 1.86 (0.54) | 2.25 (0.37) | –0.39 [–0.48, –0.31] | <0.001 |
| **Percent diameter stenosis** | | | | |
| Preprocedure percent diameter stenosis (%) | 58.90 (11.31) | 59.15 (11.42) | –0.25 [–2.49, 1.99] | 0.83 |
| Postprocedure percent diameter stenosis (%) | 15.61 (6.63) | 10.06 (4.85) | 5.55 [4.47, 6.64] | <0.001 |
| Follow-up percent diameter stenosis (%) | 25.84 (17.26) | 15.72 (8.33) | 10.12 [7.75, 12.50] | <0.001 |
| Binary restenosis (%) | 7.0% [4.41%, 10.57%] | 0.7% [0.02%, 3.63%] | 6.38% [2.55%, 9.91%] | 0.003 |
| Net gain (mm) | 0.80 (0.61) | 1.20 (0.44) | –0.41 [–0.51, –0.31] | <0.0001 |
| **In-segment assessment** | | | | |
| Binary restenosis (%) | 8.4% [5.50%, 12.14%] | 3.3% [1.08%, 7.56%] | 5.08% [0.11%, 9.23%] | 0.042 |
| **Co-primary endpoints** | | | | |
| Vasomotion (mm) | 0.047 (0.109) | 0.056 (0.117) | –0.0084 [–0.0326, 0.0157] | 0.492* |
| Late loss (mm) | 0.37 (0.45) | 0.25 (0.25) | 0.12 [0.06, 0.19] | 0.78** 0.0003 |
| **Grayscale intravascular ultrasonographic analysis in scaffolded/stented segment** | | | | |
| | **247 lesions** | **136 lesions** | | |
| **Mean vessel area** | | | | |
| Preprocedure area (mm²) | 11.42 (3.43) | 12.35 (3.22) | –0.93 [–1.64, –0.22] | 0.0101 |
| Postprocedure area (mm²) | 13.04 (3.51) | 14.25 (3.35) | –1.21 [–1.93, –0.50] | 0.001 |
| Follow-up area (mm²) | 13.79 (3.66) | 14.56 (3.33) | –0.77 [–1.50, –0.05] | 0.037 |
| **Mean total plaque area** | | | | |
| Preprocedure plaque area/media (mm²) | 6.61 (2.49) | 7.32 (2.41) | –0.71 [–1.23, –0.18] | 0.0084 |
| Postprocedure plaque area/media (mm²) | 6.99 (2.40) | 7.44 (2.23) | –0.45 [–0.93, 0.03] | 0.066 |
| Follow-up plaque area/media (mm²) | 7.66 (2.27) | 7.90 (2.15) | –0.24 [–0.70, 0.22] | 0.31 |
| **Mean lumen area** | | | | |
| Preprocedure mean lumen area (mm²) | 4.81 (1.41) | 5.02 (1.38) | –0·22 [–0.52, 0.08] | 0.1568 |
| Postprocedure mean lumen area (mm²) | 6.05 (1.45) | 6.81 (1.52) | –0.76 [–1.08, –0.45] | <0.001 |
| Follow-up mean lumen area (mm²) | 6.12 (1.88) | 6.66 (1.53) | –0.54 [–0.89, –0.19] | 0.003 |

(Continued)

Table 6.3.2 (Continued) Angiographic and intravascular ultrasound analyses preprocedure, postprocedure and at follow-up (3 years)

| | ABSORB | XIENCE | Difference [95% confidence interval] | p value |
|---|---|---|---|---|
| **Minimal lumen area** | | | | |
| Preprocedure minimal lumen area (mm$^2$) | 2.01 (0.71) | 2.11 (0.79) | −0.09 [−0.26, 0.07] | 0.2714 |
| Postprocedure minimal lumen area (mm$^2$) | 4.88 (1.39) | 5.72 (1.46) | −0.84 [−1.14, −0.53] | <0.001 |
| Acute gain in minimal lumen area (mm$^2$) | 2.89 (1.28) | 3.64 (1.28) | −7.54 [−1.03, −0.48] | <0.001 |
| Follow-up minimal lumen area (mm$^2$) | 4.32 (1.48) | 5.38 (1.51) | −1.06 [−1.38, −0.75] | <0.001 |
| Mean change in minimal lumen area from postprocedure to 3 years (mm$^2$) | −0.56 (1.11) | −0.33 (0.97) | −0.23 [−0.44, −0.01] | 0.04 |
| Incomplete malapposition area (mm$^2$)+ | 2.18 (n = 1) | 1.50 ± 1.17 (n = 14) | 0.6786 [−1.9560, 3.3133] | 0.5873 |
| **Major secondary endpoint** | | | | |
| Mean change in mean lumen area from postprocedure to 3 years (mm$^2$) | 0.07 (1.20) | −0.15 (0.70) | 0.23 [0.04, 0.42] | 0.02 |
| **Virtual histology analysis in scaffolded/stented segment** | | | | |
| | 212 lesions | 114 lesions | | |
| Preprocedural dense calcium (%) | 4.92 (4.94) | 4.22 (3.60) | 0.70 [−0.26, 1.67] | 0.15 |
| Preprocedural necrotic core (%) | 16.17 (6.99) | 15.51 (6.18) | 0.66 [−0.86, 2.18] | 0.39 |
| Postprocedural dense calcium (%) | 6.28 (3.54) | 8.79 (3.46) | −2.50 [−3.30, −1.70] | <0.001 |
| Postprocedural necrotic core (%) | 14.32 (4.70) | 15.71 (4.03) | −1.40 [−2.37, −0.42] | 0.005 |
| 3-year dense calcium (%) | 5.47 (3.49) | 11.22 (4.72) | −5.76 [−6.75, −4.76] | <0.001 |
| 3-year necrotic core (%) | 11.60 (4.11) | 15.91 (3.86) | −4.30 [−5.20, −3.40] | <0.001 |

Note: Data are n (%) or mean (SD) unless otherwise stated. * p for superiority, ** p for noninferiority, + The values were calculated as a mean within the lesions with malapposition.

(ABSORB 244 paired lesions 2.85 ± 1.24 mm$^2$ vs. XIENCE 135 paired lesions 3.59 ± 1.34 mm$^2$, $p < 0.001$) and late luminal loss in minimum lumen area was also significantly different (ABSORB 0.56 ± 1.11 mm$^2$ vs. XIENCE 0.33 ± 0.97 mm$^2$, $p = 0.04$) between the two arms. Minimum lumen area at 3-year follow-up was 4.32 ± 1.48 mm$^2$ for ABSORB and 5.38 ± 1.51 mm$^2$ for XIENCE ($p < 0.001$).

Postprocedure, the mean lumen area of the XIENCE arm was significantly larger than the ABSORB arm (6.05 ± 1.45 mm$^2$ vs. 6.81 ± 1.52 mm$^2$, $p < 0.001$). At follow-up, there were no changes in the mean lumen area of the ABSORB (+0.07 ± 1.20 mm$^2$, $p = 0.54$), while there was a significant decrease of the mean lumen area of the XIENCE (−0.15 ± 0.70 mm$^2$, $p = 0.01$).

## EXERCISE TESTING

An analysis of exercise testing was prespecified in the protocol. Three hundred fifty-seven (71%) patients received an exercise test at 3 years (Table 6.3.3). All the electrocardiographic signs and symptoms among the subjects without prior repeat revascularization ($n = 307, 61\%$) were comparable between both arms (≥0.1 mV ST depression or chest pain, ABSORB: 17.3% vs. XIENCE: 11.8%, $p = 0.23$) [10].

## SEATTLE ANGINA QUESTIONNAIRE

Figure 6.3.2 shows the five domains of the Seattle Angina Questionnaire related to angina stability, frequency, physical limitation, disease perception, and treatment satisfaction. Substantial improvement in every domain at 3 years was documented with respect to the preprocedural assessment without significant difference between the two treatment arms. Before the procedure, 94 (29%) and 48 (29%) patients subsequently assigned to the ABSORB arm and the XIENCE arm, respectively, were free from angina, whereas at 3 years, 230 (74%) patients in the ABSORB arm and 113 (73%) patients in the XIENCE arm were angina-free [10].

## CLINICAL EVENTS

Clinical follow-up was available in 321 cases (96%) in ABSORB and 161 cases (97%) in XIENCE. Sixteen patients

Table 6.3.3 Exercise test (intent-to-treat population, excluding tests subsequent to any revascularization)

| | Bioresorbable scaffold group | Metallic stent group | Difference [95% confidence interval] | p value |
|---|---|---|---|---|
| Participated in exercise test | 71.3% (239/335) | 72.3% (120/166) | −0.95% [−8.99%, 7.63%] | 0.825 |
| Participated in exercise test: Subjects with exercise test and no prior repeat revascularization | 60.6% (203/335) | 56.0% (93/166) | 4.57% [−4.49%, 13.72%] | 0.3272 |
| Treadmill | 54.2% (110/203) | 52.7% (48/91) | 1.44% [−10.64%, 13.62%] | 0.8189 |
| Cycling | 45.8% (93/203) | 47.3% (43/91) | −1.44% [−13.62%, 10.64%] | 0.8189 |
| Maximum heart rate (beats per min) | 131.0 (21.3) | 136.2 (21.0) | −5.2 [−10.4, 0.1] | 0.0541 |
| Diastolic blood pressure at peak exercise (mmHg) | 79.5 (14.7) | 83.9 (20.2) | −4.4 [−9.1, 0.3] | 0.0654 |
| Systolic blood pressure at peak exercise (mmHg) | 178.1 (29.8) | 181.9 (28.5) | −3.8 [−11.1, 3.5] | 0.302 |
| Maximum workload (watts) | 133.85 ± 44.49 (80) | 145.05 ± 39.16 (39) | −11.21 [−27.12, 4.71] | 0.17 |
| Maximum workload (METS) | 8.92 ± 2.82 (121) | 9.85 ± 2.74 (53) | −0.92 [−1.83, −0.02] | 0.045 |
| Terminated by physician due to >0.2 mV ST depression | 4.0% (2/50) | 0.0% (0/20) | 4.00% [−12.37%, 13.46%] | 1 |
| Test terminated by patient (dyspnea) | 15.9% (22/138) | 10.4% (7/67) | 5.49% [−5.40%, 14.28%] | 0.2897 |
| Test terminated by patient (angina) | 1.4% (2/138) | 4.5% (3/67) | −3.03% [−10.98%, 1.68%] | 0.3328 |
| Exercise duration (min) | 8.57 (3.36) | 9.23 (3.27) | −0.66 [−1.48, 0.16] | 0.1136 |
| ≥0.1 mV ST depression | 13.9% (28/201) | 7.5% (7/93) | 6.40% [−1.89%, 13.08%] | 0.11 |
| Chest pain during exercise | 4.5% (9/202) | 4.3% (4/93) | 0.15% [−6.43%, 4.76%] | 1.0 |
| ≥0.1 mV ST depression or chest pain | 17.3% (35/202) | 11.8% (11/93) | 5.50% [−3.83%, 13.23%] | 0.23 |
| **Antianginal medication** | | | | |
| β blocker | 69.5% | 65.9% | 3.52% [−8.09, 15.14] | 0.548 |
| Calcium channel blocker | 23.6% | 24.2% | −0.53% [−11.09, 10.03] | 0.921 |
| Nitrate | 18.7% | 26.4% | −7.65% [−18.18, 2.87] | 0.137 |

*Note:* Data are n (%) or mean (SD) unless otherwise stated.

withdrew their consent, 1 patient was withdrawn by physician, 2 patients were lost to follow-up, and 14 patients died (Figure 6.3.3). Table 6.3.4 and Figure 6.3.4 report the POCE and DOCE. The DOCE showed significant difference in rates of events (10.4% vs. 5.0%, $p = 0.043$, Figure 6.3.4a), driven by target vessel myocardial infarction (TVMI) in the ABSORB arm (7.1% vs. 1.2%, $p = 0.006$), 52% of which were periprocedural, based on the per-protocol and historical definition of the World Health Organization. In the XIENCE arm, all TVMI were periprocedural. In contrast, the POCE did not differ between ABSORB and XIENCE (20.9% vs. 24.2%, $p = 0.40$, Figure 6.3.4b) with a higher rate of nonclinically indicated revascularizations (5.5% vs. 11.2%, $p = 0.03$) in the XIENCE arm that counterbalances the higher rate of TVMI in the ABSORB arm. Figures 6.3.4c and d also provide the landmark analysis of DOCE and POCE at 30 days and demonstrate the impact of the 3-year protocol mandated imaging that triggered subsequent revascularizations, clinically indicated or not.

Over the period of 3 years, there were 8 definite scaffold thrombosis (1 acute, 1 subacute, 6 very late) and 1 late probable scaffold thrombosis in the ABSORB arm (2.8%), and no definite or probable stent thrombosis in the XIENCE arm (0%) ($p = 0.0335$). These 9 scaffold thromboses were associated with ST elevation myocardial infarction, and 1 patient died 13 days postscaffold thrombosis [10].

## DISCUSSION

The main findings of the present study can be summarized as follows: (1) At 3 years, the trial did not meet its co-primary endpoints of superior vasomotor reactivity and noninferior late luminal loss with respect to XIENCE; (2) a higher rate of device oriented composite endpoint mainly due to myocardial infarction in the vascular territory of the scaffolded vessel was observed in the ABSORB arm; and (3) the patient oriented composite endpoint, anginal status, and exercise testing were comparable for both devices at 3 years.

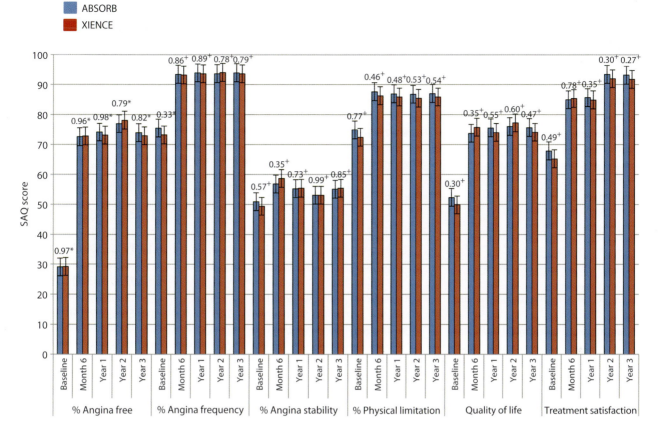

Figure 6.3.2  Seattle Angina Questionnaire responses. Figure shows five domains of the Seattle Angina Questionnaire related to angina stability, frequency, physical limitation, disease perception, and treatment satisfaction in addition to the number of patients with no angina. The bars show 95% CIs. SAQ = Seattle Angina Questionnaire. *p value from posthoc test. †p value from χ² test. (From Serruys PW et al. *Lancet*. 2016 Nov 19;388(10059):2479–2491.)

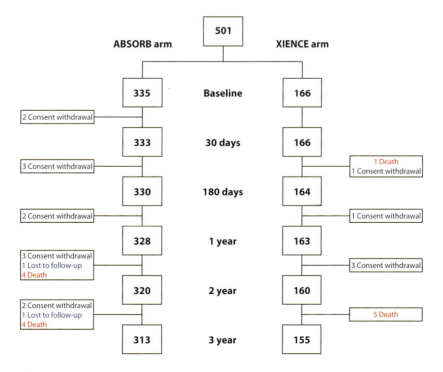

Figure 6.3.3  Study flowchart.

Table 6.3.4 Secondary clinical outcomes at 3-year follow-up

| | ABSORB | XIENCE | Relative risk | Difference [95% CI] | p value |
|---|---|---|---|---|---|
| All deaths | 2.5% (8/326) | 3.7% (6/161) | 0.66 [0.23, 1.87] | −1.27% [−5.61%, 1.79%] | 0.56 |
| Cardiac deaths | 0.9% (3/326) | 1.9% (3/161) | 0.49 [0.10, 2.42] | −0.94% [−4.47%, 1.19%] | 0.4 |
| Myocardial infarction per protocol | 8.3% (27/326) | 3.1% (5/161) | 2.67 [1.05, 6.80] | 5.18% [0.48%, 9.10%] | 0.03 |
| Q-wave | 3.1% (10/326) | 1.2% (2/161) | 2.47 [0.55, 11.14] | 1.83% [−1.64%, 4.47%] | 0.35 |
| Non-Q-wave | 5.2% (17/326) | 1.9% (3/161) | 2.80 [0.83, 9.41] | 3.35% [−0.62%, 6.57%] | 0.08 |
| Target vessel myocardial infarction | 7.1% (23/326) | 1.2% (2/161) | 5.68 [1.36, 23.79] | 5.81% [1.89%, 9.24%] | 0.006 |
| Q-wave myocardial infarction | 2.8% (9/326) | 0.0% (0/161) | NA [NA] | 2.76% [0.09%, 5.16%] | 0.03 |
| Non-Q-wave myocardial infarction | 4.3% (14/326) | 1.2% (2/161) | 3.46 [0.80, 15.03] | 3.05% [−0.56%, 5.98%] | 0.08 |
| Nontarget vessel myocardial infarction | 1.2% (4/326) | 1.9% (3/161) | 0.66 [0.15, 2.91] | −0.64% [−4.19%, 1.61%] | 0.69 |
| Q-wave myocardial infarction | 0.3% (1/326) | 1.2% (2/161) | 0.25 [0.02, 2.70] | −0.94% [−4.12%, 0.74%] | 0.26 |
| Non-Q-wave myocardial infarction | 0.9% (3/326) | 0.6% (1/161) | 1.48 [0.16, 14.13] | 0.30% [−2.58%, 2.12%] | 1 |
| All target-lesion revascularization | 7.4% (24/326) | 5.0% (8/161) | 1.48 [0.68, 3.22] | 2.39% [−2.72%, 6.54%] | 0.32 |
| Clinically indicated target-lesion revascularization | 6.1% (20/326) | 1.9% (3/161) | 3.29 [0.99, 10.92] | 4.27% [0.20%, 7.65%] | 0.04 |
| Nonclinically indicated target-lesion revascularization | 1.2% (4/326) | 3.1% (5/161) | 0.40 [0.11, 1.45] | −1.88% [−5.91%, 0.71%] | 0.16 |
| All target-vessel revascularization | 10.1% (33/326) | 11.8% (19/161) | 0.86 [0.50, 1.46] | −1.68% [−8.21%, 3.89%] | 0.57 |
| Clinically indicated target-vessel revascularization | 7.1% (23/326) | 7.5% (12/161) | 0.95 [0.48, 1.85] | −0.40% [−6.02%, 4.16%] | 0.87 |
| Nonclinically indicated target-vessel revascularization | 3.4% (11/326) | 6.8% (11/161) | 0.49 [0.22, 1.11] | −3.46% [−8.66%, 0.47%] | 0.08 |
| Nontarget-vessel revascularization | 6.7% (22/326) | 11.8% (19/161) | 0.57 [0.32, 1.03] | −5.05% [−11.36%, 0.20%] | 0.06 |
| Clinically indicated nontarget-vessel revascularization | 5.2% (17/326) | 9.3% (15/161) | 0.56 [0.29, 1.09] | −4.10% [−9.92%, 0.56%] | 0.09 |
| Nonclinically indicated nontarget-vessel revascularization | 2.5% (8/326) | 4.3% (7/161) | 0.56 [0.21, 1.53] | −1.89% [−6.41%, 1.32%] | 0.27 |
| All revascularization | 15.0% (49/326) | 20.5% (33/161) | 0.73 [0.49, 1.09] | −5.47% [−13.18%, 1.52%] | 0.13 |
| Clinically indicated revascularization | 11.0% (36/326) | 15.5% (25/161) | 0.71 [0.44, 1.14] | −4.49% [−11.53%, 1.67%] | 0.16 |
| Nonclinically indicated revascularization | 5.5% (18/326) | 11.2% (18/161) | 0.49 [0.26, 0.92] | −5.66% [−11.79%, −0.64%] | 0.02 |

(Continued)

Table 6.3.4 (Continued) Secondary clinical outcomes at 3-year follow-up

| | ABSORB | XIENCE | Relative risk | Difference [95% CI] | p value |
|---|---|---|---|---|---|
| Composite secondary endpoints | | | | | |
| Cardiac death, target-vessel myocardial infarction, and clinically indicated target-lesion revascularization (target-lesion failure; device-oriented composite endpoint) | 10.4% (34/326) | 5.0% (8/161) | 2.10 [0.99, 4.43] | 5.46% [0.10%, 9.96%] | 0.04 |
| Cardiac deaths* | 0.9% (3/326) | 1.9% (3/161) | 0.49 [0.10, 2.42] | −0.94% [−4.47%, 1.19%] | 0.4 |
| Target vessel myocardial infarction* | 6.4% (21/326) | 1.2% (2/161) | 5.19 [1.23, 21.84] | 5.20% [1.34%, 8.53%] | 0.01 |
| Clinically indicated target-lesion revascularization* | 3.1% (10/326) | 1.9% (3/161) | 1.65 [0.46, 5.90] | 1.20% [−2.54%, 3.98%] | 0.56 |
| All death, all myocardial infarction, and all revascularization (patient-oriented composite endpoint) | 20.9% (68/326) | 24.2% (39/161) | 0.86 [0.61, 1.22] | −3.36% [−11.60%, 4.25%] | 0.4 |
| All deaths* | 2.5% (8/326) | 3.7% (6/161) | 0.66 [0.23, 1.87] | −1.27% [−5.61%, 1.79%] | 0.56 |
| All myocardial infarction* | 7.7% (25/326) | 3.1% (5/161) | 2.47 [0.96, 6.33] | 4.56% [−0.08%, 8.40%] | 0.049 |
| All revascularization* | 10.7% (35/326) | 17.4% (28/161) | 0.62 [0.39, 0.98] | −6.66% [−13.87%, −0.30%] | 0.04 |
| Thrombosis endpoints | | | | | |
| Definite scaffold or stent thrombosis | 2.5% (8/321) | 0.0% (0/158) | NA | 2.49% [−0.18%, 4.84%] | 0.06 |
| Acute (0–1 day) | 0.3% (1/335) | 0.0% (0/166) | NA | 0.30% [−1.98%, 1.67%] | 1 |
| Sub-acute (2–30 days) | 0.3% (1/334) | 0.0% (0/166) | NA | 0.30% [−1.98%, 1.68%] | 1 |
| Late (31–365 days) | 0.0% (0/329) | 0.0% (0/164) | NA | 0.00% [−2.29%, 1.15%] | 1 |
| Very late (>365 days) | 1.8% (6/329) | 0.0% (0/164) | NA | 1.82% [−0.67%, 3.92%] | 0.19 |
| Definite or probable scaffold or stent thrombosis | 2.8% (9/321) | 0.0% (0/158) | NA | 2.80% [0.09%, 5.24%] | 0.03 |
| Acute (0–1 day) | 0.3% (1/335) | 0.0% (0/166) | NA | 0.30% [−1.98%, 1.67%] | 1 |
| Sub-acute (2–30 days) | 0.3% (1/334) | 0.0% (0/166) | NA | 0.30% [−1.98%, 1.68%] | 1 |
| Late (31–365 days) | 0.3% (1/329) | 0.0% (0/164) | NA | 0.30% [−2.00%, 1.70%] | 1 |
| Very late (>365 days) | 1.8% (6/329) | 0.0% (0/164) | NA | 1.82% [−0.67%, 3.92%] | 0.19 |
| Patients on dual antiplatelet therapy at day 1095 | 30.5% (102/334) | 29.5% (49/166) | NA | 1.02% [−7.69%, 9.24%] | 0.81 |
| Duration (day) of dual antiplatelet therapy within 1095 days | 565.5 ± 324.2 (334) | 561.0 ± 319.1 (166) | NA | 4.5 [−55.5, 64.4] | 0.88 |

Note: The denominator excludes patients who were lost to follow-up or who withdrew the consent, except for those who died or experienced the corresponding endpoint before their withdrawal of consent. * The numbers are hierarchical counts in the composite endpoints.

Abbreviation: NA = not available.

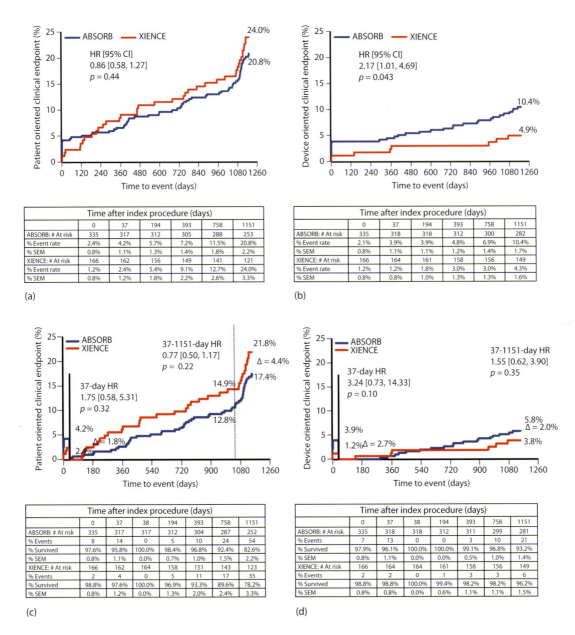

**Figure 6.3.4** Kaplan-Meier curves for the patient and device oriented composite clinical endpoints (**a** and **b**). Panels **c** and **d** present landmark analyses at 30 days.

## Vasomotion

In designing the present randomized trial, the assumption was made that the metallic stent would not be affected by vasomotion as previously reported in the literature [7,19,20]. The overall vasodilation of the scaffold observed in the present study (0.047 ± 0.109 mm) is very similar to the vasodilation observed in the first-in-man study at 3 years (0.054 ± 0.12 mm) [21] and in the ABSORB Japan randomized trial at 2 years (0.06 ± 0.14 mm) [22].

Past publications performed vasomotion studies in metallic stent segments 6–9 months after implantation in an early phase of vessel wall healing [23]. It might be hypothesized that the myogenic components of the wall structure at

36 months in response to nitrate billows between the tether points of the metallic stent ring structures that are separated by 1600 micron. Although this billowing might not be individually visible on angiography due to its limited imaging resolution (200 micron), it may effect changes in boundary by detection algorithm that results in a statistical difference between the populations. Future studies with higher resolution intravascular imaging could elucidate these findings.

## Angiographic late luminal loss

The angiographic in-device late luminal loss in the present study (0.39 ± 0.48 mm) is larger than the late luminal loss

(0.29 ± 0.43 mm) observed in the first-in-man trial [21], but comparable to the 2-year late luminal loss (0.36 ± 0.38 mm) observed in the ABSORB Japan trial [22]. Comparative measurement of luminal dimension obtained by angiography immediately postimplantation of ABSORB and XIENCE has been flawed by methodological bias in quantification, with systematic underestimation of the scaffolded lumen dimension due to thick polymeric struts when compared to the stented lumen with thin metallic struts [24]. Nevertheless, at follow-up in both cases the comparative method is again reliable since the endoluminal lining consists of a continuous layer of neointimal tissue covering the polymeric and metallic struts. Therefore, the minimum lumen diameter on angiography and minimum lumen area on intravascular ultrasound at follow-up must be considered objective assessments of the respective performance of the two devices.

## Intravascular ultrasound

Difference in device volume and backscattering between the polymeric scaffolds and metallic stents are known to affect the intravascular ultrasound assessment of the immediate change in plaque media and lumen volume postprocedure differently, and may together with the difference in balloon diameter and inflation pressure partially explain the significant difference in mean and minimum lumen area immediately postprocedure [3,21]. However, at 3-year follow-up, this methodological bias should no longer interfere with the intravascular ultrasound assessment of luminal dimension for the same above-mentioned reasons. Therefore, the minimum lumen area in the ABSORB arm is objectively smaller than in the XIENCE arm, corresponding to a larger late luminal loss in minimum lumen area in the ABSORB arm when compared to the XIENCE arm. As previously demonstrated in the first-in-man trial, the mean lumen area of the ABSORB arm enlarges with time, whereas in the XIENCE arm it decreases significantly. The sequential intravascular ultrasound measurements in the first-in-man trial indicated that substantial change in vessel area, plaque media, and lumen area still occurred between 3 and 5 years. In other words, the complete wall dynamic change resulting from bioresorption of the scaffold can only be fully assessed at 5 years [7].

## Clinical events

From a patient perspective, overall clinical performance of the two arms is comparable, in terms of the POCE, exercise test, and patient reported outcomes as assessed by the Seattle Angina Questionnaire. In the POCE, the rate of non-clinically indicated revascularization was doubled in the XIENCE arm than in the ABSORB arm. In the ABSORB arm, there were 23 (7.1%) adjudicated target vessel myocardial infarctions of which 12 were periprocedural, which was adjudicated according to the WHO definition. Using these criteria, the periprocedural myocardial infarction rate in the current trial was 3.9% versus 1.2% in the ABSORB and the XIENCE arm, respectively, whereas it was 0.6% in both arms when the more contemporary SCAI definition was applied [25]. For this reason, landmark analyses were performed at 30 days to more objectively assess the performance of the devices without artificial differences of periprocedural events (Figure 6.3.4c and d). Further evolution of comparative device performances after 3 years should be investigated in large-scale long-term randomized trials.

There were 6 definite very late scaffold thromboses reported between 1 and 3 years. In the present study, no systematic optical coherence tomography or ultrasound imaging was performed at the time of the event in an attempt to elucidate the mechanistic aetiology of the very late scaffold thromboses. One single case investigated with OCT showed at the site of thrombosis a marked eccentricity of the lumen that was not present postprocedure (Figure 6.3.5). The use of dual antiplatelet therapy at 3 years was 34.4% and 32.5% in the ABSORB and XIENCE arm ($p = 0.672$), respectively. Of note, the patients with late or very late scaffold thrombosis were not on dual antiplatelet therapy. Conversely, no late and very late scaffold thrombosis occurred in 63 patients who never interrupt dual antiplatelet therapy up to 3 years. The benefit and need for prolonged dual antiplatelet therapy after bioresorbable scaffold implantation is at the present time entirely speculative and the present results cannot be extrapolated to the other bioresorbable technology. Changes in polymer resorption time, strut thickness, and design of scaffolding platform warrant further investigation.

There are some limitations to be addressed. This was the first randomized trial of the ABSORB scaffold. The operators therefore were not experienced with the use of a scaffold device as compared to the long experience with a metallic stent. The implantation techniques used for a scaffold device at the time of enrolment were different from the currently recommended optimal implantation techniques [26]. The co-primary endpoint of superior vasomotion was not met due to the fact that the metallic stents exhibited an unexpected change in diameter thus far not reported in the literature. The analysis of clinical events such as device-oriented and patient-oriented endpoints was underpowered from a statistical point of view.

In conclusion, the trial did not meet its co-primary endpoints of superior vasomotor reactivity and noninferior late luminal loss with respect to the XIENCE. The mechanistic part of the trial failed to demonstrate that the late luminal loss was comparable for the bioresorbable scaffold when compared to the metallic stents. A higher rate of device-oriented cardiovascular events was observed with the ABSORB mainly driven by a higher rate of target vessel myocardial infarction. In addition, the incidence of very late scaffold thrombosis is a worrisome signal that warrants further careful monitoring of the patient having a clinical follow-up of longer than 2 years.

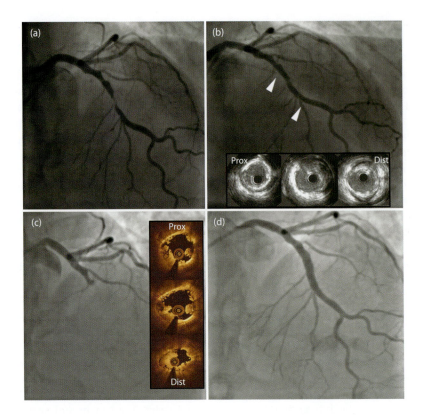

Figure 6.3.5 Very late scaffold thrombosis case. 58-year-old male with a history of dyslipidemia and hypertension. Underwent PCI in the mid-segment of the LAD guided by quantitative coronary angiography with $D_{max}$ (prox) of 3.25 mm and $D_{max}$ (dist) of 2.57 mm; 85% DS; lesion length of 14 mm (a). After predilatation with a noncompliant 3.0 × 155 mm balloon catheter, one ABSORB BVSs 3.0 × 18 mm was successfully deployed at 11 atm following postdilatation with a 3.25 balloon at 12 atm. Residual stenosis was 24% with a good angiographic result and final intravascular ultrasound evaluation revealed a well-apposed scaffold, minimum lumen area of 5.01 mm², and an eccentricity index of 0.87 (b). At 967 days, the patient presented with acute myocardial infarction due to an occlusion of the treated segment. Optical coherence tomography evaluation showed no malapposition, no fracture, and the presence of uncovered struts and an eccentricity index of 0.57 (c). The patient was on aspirin alone at the time of the event. He was treated with two drug-eluting stents (4.0 × 24 mm and 3.5 × 8 mm) and restarted dual-antiplatelet therapy with ticagrelor.

# REFERENCES

1. Onuma Y, Serruys PW, Gomez J et al. Comparison of in vivo acute stent recoil between the bioresorbable everolimus-eluting coronary scaffolds (revision 1.0 and 1.1) and the metallic everolimus-eluting stent. *Catheter Cardiovasc Interv. Official Journal of the Society for Cardiac Angiography & Interventions.* 2011;78(1):3–12.

2. Diletti R, Serruys PW, Farooq V et al. ABSORB II randomized controlled trial: A clinical evaluation to compare the safety, efficacy, and performance of the Absorb everolimus-eluting bioresorbable vascular scaffold system against the XIENCE everolimus-eluting coronary stent system in the treatment of subjects with ischemic heart disease caused by de novo native coronary artery lesions: Rationale and study design. *Am Heart J.* 2012;164(5):654–63.

3. Sotomi Y, Tateishi H, Suwannasom P et al. Quantitative assessment of the stent/scaffold strut embedment analysis by optical coherence tomography. *Int J Cardiovasc Imaging.* 2016;32(6):871–83.

4. Montalescot G, Sechtem U, Achenbach S et al. 2013 ESC guidelines on the management of stable coronary artery disease: The Task Force on the management of stable coronary artery disease of the European Society of Cardiology. *Eur Heart J.* 2013; 34(38):2949–3003.

5. Suryapranata H, Serruys PW, De Feyter PJ, Verdouw PD, Hugenholtz PG. Coronary vasodilatory action after a single dose of nicorandil. *Am J Cardiol.* 1988; 61(4):292–7.

6. Suryapranata H, Maas A, MacLeod DC, de Feyter PJ, Verdouw PD, Serruys PW. Coronary vasodilatory action of elgodipine in coronary artery disease. *Am J Cardiol.* 1992;69(14):1171–7.

7. Serruys PW, Ormiston J, van Geuns RJ et al. A polylactide bioresorbable scaffold eluting everolimus for treatment of coronary stenosis: 5-year follow-up. *J Am Coll Cardiol.* 2016;67(7):766–76.

8. Spertus JA, Winder JA, Dewhurst TA et al. Development and evaluation of the Seattle Angina Questionnaire: A new functional status measure for coronary artery disease. *J Am Coll Cardiol.* 1995; 25(2):333–41.

9. Gibbons RJ, Balady GJ, Bricker JT et al. ACC/AHA 2002 guideline update for exercise testing: Summary article: A report of the American College of Cardiology/American Heart Association Task Force on Practice Guidelines (Committee to Update the 1997 Exercise Testing Guidelines). *Circulation.* 2002; 106(14):1883–92.

10. Serruys PW, Chevalier B, Sotomi Y et al. Comparison of an everolimus-eluting bioresorbable scaffold with an everolimus-eluting metallic stent for the treatment of coronary artery stenosis (ABSORB II): A 3 year, randomised, controlled, single-blind, multicentre clinical trial. *Lancet.* 2016;388(10059):2479–2491.

11. Serruys PW, Onuma Y, Ormiston JA et al. Evaluation of the second generation of a bioresorbable everolimus drug-eluting vascular scaffold for treatment of de novo coronary artery stenosis: Six-month clinical and imaging outcomes. *Circulation.* 2010;122(22): 2301–12.

12. Ormiston JA, Serruys PW, Regar E et al. A bioabsorbable everolimus-eluting coronary stent system for patients with single de-novo coronary artery lesions (ABSORB): A prospective open-label trial. *Lancet.* 2008;371(9616):899–907.

13. Gomez-Lara J, Brugaletta S, Diletti R et al. A comparative assessment by optical coherence tomography of the performance of the first and second generation of the everolimus-eluting bioresorbable vascular scaffolds. *Eur Heart J.* 2011;32(3):294–304.

14. Serruys PW, Ormiston JA, Onuma Y et al. A bioabsorbable everolimus-eluting coronary stent system (ABSORB): 2-year outcomes and results from multiple imaging methods. *Lancet.* 2009;373(9667): 897–910.

15. Serruys PW, Chevalier B, Dudek D et al. A bioresorbable everolimus-eluting scaffold versus a metallic everolimus-eluting stent for ischaemic heart disease caused by de-novo native coronary artery lesions (ABSORB II): An interim 1-year analysis of clinical and procedural secondary outcomes from a randomised controlled trial. *Lancet.* 2015;385(9962):43–54.

16. Ishibashi Y, Nakatani S, Sotomi Y et al. Relation between bioresorbable scaffold sizing using QCA-$D_{max}$ and clinical outcomes at 1 year in 1,232 patients from 3 study cohorts (ABSORB cohort B, ABSORB EXTEND, and ABSORB II). *JACC Cardiovasc Interv.* 2015;8(13):1715–26.

17. Sotomi Y, Ishibashi Y, Suwannasom P et al. Acute gain in minimal lumen area following implantation of everolimus-eluting ABSORB biodegradable vascular scaffolds or XIENCE metallic stents:

18. Suwannasom P, Sotomi Y, Ishibashi Y et al. The impact of post-procedural asymmetry, expansion, and eccentricity of bioresorbable everolimus-eluting scaffold and metallic everolimus-eluting stent on clinical outcomes in the ABSORB II trial. *JACC Cardiovasc Interv.* 2016;9(12):1231–42.

19. Hamilos MI, Ostojic M, Beleslin B et al. Differential effects of drug-eluting stents on local endothelium-dependent coronary vasomotion. *J Am Coll Cardiol.* 2008;51(22):2123–9.

20. Maier W, Windecker S, Kung A et al. Exercise-induced coronary artery vasodilation is not impaired by stent placement. *Circulation.* 2002;105(20): 2373–7.

21. Serruys PW, Onuma Y, Garcia-Garcia HM et al. Dynamics of vessel wall changes following the implantation of the absorb everolimus-eluting bioresorbable vascular scaffold: A multi-imaging modality study at 6, 12, 24 and 36 months. *EuroIntervention.* 2014;9(11):1271–84.

22. Onuma Y, Sotomi Y, Shiomi H et al. Two-year clinical, angiographic, and serial optical coherence tomographic follow-up after implantation of everolimus-eluting bioresorbable scaffold and everolimus-eluting metallic stent: Insights from the randomized ABSORB Japan trial. *EuroIntervention. Journal of EuroPCR in Collaboration with the Working Group on Interventional Cardiology of the European Society of Cardiology* 2016: in press.

23. Otsuka F, Pacheco E, Perkins LE et al. Long-term safety of an everolimus-eluting bioresorbable vascular scaffold and the cobalt-chromium XIENCE V stent in a porcine coronary artery model. *Circ Cardiovasc Interv.* 2014;7(3):330–42.

24. Sotomi Y, Onuma Y, Suwannasom P et al. Is quantitative coronary angiography reliable in assessing the lumen gain after treatment with the everolimus eluting bioresorbable polylactide scaffold? *EuroIntervention. Journal of EuroPCR in Collaboration with the Working Group on Interventional Cardiology of the European Society of Cardiology* 2016; in press.

25. Ishibashi Y, Muramatsu T, Nakatani S et al. Incidence and potential mechanism(s) of post-procedural rise of cardiac biomarker in patients with coronary artery narrowing after implantation of an everolimus-eluting bioresorbable vascular scaffold or everolimus-eluting metallic stent. *JACC Cardiovasc Interv.* 2015; 8(8):1053–63.

26. Puricel S, Cuculi F, Weissner M et al. Bioresorbable coronary scaffold thrombosis: Multicenter comprehensive analysis of clinical presentation, mechanisms, and predictors. *J Am Coll Cardiol.* 2016;67(8):921–31.

# The ABSORB China trial

RUNLIN GAO ON BEHALF OF THE ABSORB CHINA INVESTIGATORS

## INTRODUCTION

The everolimus-eluting bioresorbable vascular scaffolds (BVSs) (ABSORB, Abbott Vascular, Santa Clara, CA) is designed to provide comparable radial strength and antirestenotic efficacy to metallic DESs in the first year after implantation, and superior long-term benefits after the scaffold bioresorbs. Over the past year, three prospective pivotal randomized controlled trials have demonstrated the noninferiority of the BVSs to cobalt-chromium everolimus-eluting stents (CoCr-EES; XIENCE V, Abbott Vascular) in either 1-year target lesion failure (ABSORB III [1] and ABSORB Japan [2]) or 12–13 months angiographic in-segment late loss (ABSORB China [3] and ABSORB Japan [2]). BVSs is thus as safe and effective as the best-in-class CoCr-EES at 1 year of implant, a critical finding as more than 125,000 BVSs scaffolds have been implanted worldwide to date.

ABSORB China [3] is the first BVSs randomized trial with a powered primary endpoint of angiographic in-segment late loss at 1 year designed for regulatory approval of BVSs in China. The 1-year results were presented as a late-breaking trial at TCT 2015 and simultaneously published online in the *Journal of American College of Cardiology* [3].

## METHODS

### Study design, patient population, and randomization

ABSORB China is a prospective, randomized, active-controlled, open-label, multicenter trial designed to evaluate the safety and efficacy of BVSs compared with CoCr-EES. The study was approved by institutional ethic committees. All patients signed written informed consent prior to randomization. Eligible patients were ≥18 years with evidence of myocardial ischemia, and suitable for elective (nonemergent) PCI, with a maximum of two de novo coronary artery lesions with reference vessel diameter 2.5–3.75 mm and length ≤24 mm as assessed by online quantitative coronary angiography (QCA) or visual estimation. Only one non-target lesion in a non-target vessel was allowed, which had to be successfully treated without complications prior to patient randomization. Patients with recent myocardial infarction (MI) whose biomarker had not returned to normal, unstable cardiac arrhythmias, and left ventricular ejection fraction <30% were ineligible. Other exclusions included patients who had prior PCI in the target vessel within the past 12 months, in a nontarget vessel within 30 days prior, or in whom future staged PCI either in a target vessel or nontarget vessel was planned. Left main stenoses, bifurcation lesions with a side branch ≥2.0 mm diameter or ≥50% diameter stenosis (DS) or requiring guidewire protection, ostial lesions, lesions with moderate or heavy calcification, myocardial bridges, and thrombus were also disallowed.

A total of 480 eligible patients who provided written informed consent were randomized in a 1:1 ratio to receive BVSs or CoCr-EES at 24 sites in China. Randomization was performed after successful treatment of the nontarget lesion (if present) and successful predilation of the target lesion, and via an interactive voice/web response system.

### Treatment strategy, medications, and follow-up

Predilatation was required, with postdilatation per investigator discretion. Each target lesion had to be covered by a single study stent, although use of a second device as randomized was allowed for bailing out edge dissection or other procedural issues. A loading dose of aspirin (≥300 mg) and either clopidogrel (≥300 mg) or ticagrelor (180 mg) 6–24 hours before the index procedure was required. Following PCI, aspirin 100 mg daily for at least 5 years was prescribed, with clopidogrel (75 mg daily) or ticagrelor (90 mg twice a day) for a minimum of 12 months. Clinical follow-up was planned at 30 days, 6 months, 9 months, and at 1, 2, 3, 4, and 5 years postprocedure. Routine follow-up angiography was planned in all patients at 1 year (±28 days) for their primary endpoint.

## Endpoints

The primary endpoint of ABSORB China was to determine if BVSs was non-inferior to CoCr-EES in angiographic in-segment late loss (LL) at 1 year in the per-treatment-evaluable (PTE) population. Patients in the PTE population were assigned into their arms based on the treatment received and were disqualified if they had prespecified major protocol deviations. Secondary endpoints included acute device and procedural success; stent/scaffold thrombosis (ST) based on ARC definition; the device-oriented composite endpoint (DoCE, TLF; the composite of cardiac death, target vessel [TV-MI], or ischemia-driven target lesion revascularization [ID-TLR]); the patient-oriented composite endpoint (PoCE, the composite of all-cause death, all MI, or all revascularization); and various clinical components of the composite endpoints. Angiographic secondary endpoints included in-device LL, in-device and in-segment minimal lumen diameter (MLD), in-device and in-segment % diameter stenosis (DS), and in-device and in-segment binary restenosis (ABR).

## Trial management

Clinical endpoint events were adjudicated by an independent clinical events committee that was blinded to device assignment. QCA data was assessed by an independent angiographic core laboratory. A data safety and monitoring board reviewed the cumulative safety data from the trial at prespecified intervals throughout the trial. On-site monitoring was performed on 100% of data.

## Sample size calculation

A non-inferiority margin of 0.15 mm for the primary endpoint was agreed on with the China regulatory authorities. By assuming no difference in the mean in-segment LL and standard deviation of 0.47 mm for both devices, and an anticipated 70% angiographic follow-up rate, randomizing 480 patients would provide 80% power to demonstrate non-inferiority of BVSs to CoCr-EES with a one-sided alpha of 2.5%.

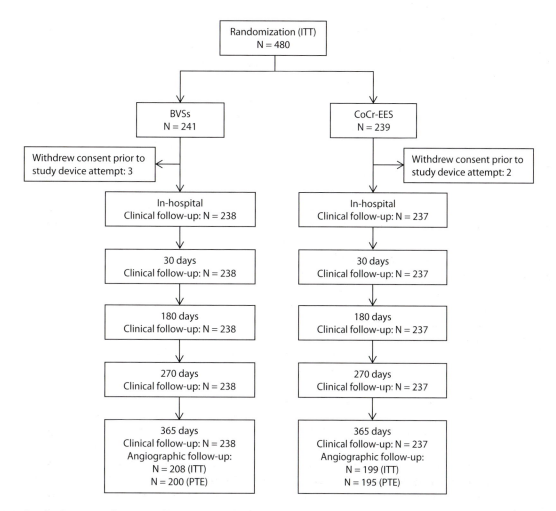

**Figure 6.4.1** Study design and patient disposition. BVSs = bioresorbable vascular scaffolds, CoCr-EES = cobalt-chromium everolimus-eluting stent, PTE = per-treatment-evaluable, ITT = intention-to-treat. (Adopted from Gao R, Yang Y, Han Y, Huo Y, Chen J, Yu B, Su X et al., on behalf of the ABSORB China Investigators. *J Am Coll Cardiol* 2015;66:2298–2309.)

## RESULTS

Between July 2013 and March 2014, 480 patients were randomized at 24 sites in China (241 to BVSs and 239 to CoCr-EES). Subject disposition is shown in Figure 6.4.1. Five patients withdrew consent before the use of any study device. Four crossovers occurred, two in each group. Among the 480 patients in the ITT population, the PTE population consisted of 460 patients (228 BVSs and 232 CoCr-EES). The results presented here will be for the ITT population unless explicitly stated. Patient demographics, risk factors, and lesion characteristics at baseline were well-balanced between the two arms. Single target lesion treatment dominated in BVSs and CoCr-EES patients (94.5% and 93.7%, respectively), and 8.4% and 6.8%, respectively, had a single non-target lesion treated. Mean device diameters were identical (3.1 mm) and device length was also similar (22.8 mm vs. 22.3 mm, $p = 0.80$) between the BVSs and CoCr-EES groups. Use of intravascular imaging was infrequent. Device postdilatation was performed in a greater proportion in the BVSs cases than in CoCr-EES (63.0% vs. 54.4%,

$p = 0.05$). Acute clinical device success (98.0% vs. 99.6%, $p = 0.22$) and procedural success (97.0% and 98.3%, $p = 0.37$) were comparable in BVSs and CoCr-EES treated patients, respectively. The discharge medication use was similar. The baseline lesion length, reference vessel diameter, MLD and % DS were balanced between groups (Table 6.4.1). The postprocedure in-segment MLD, acute gain and % DS were similar with both devices. However, within the device the postprocedural MLD and acute gain were less with the BVSs compared to CoCr-EES, and the % DS was greater with the BVSs compared to CoCr-EES (Table 6.4.1).

One-year angiographic follow-up data were available in 86.3% (208/241) BVSs patients and in 83.3% (199/239) CoCr-EES patients per ITT, and 87.7% (200 of 228) and 84.1% (195 of 232) per PTE. The primary endpoint of 1 year in-segment LL in the PTE population based on per subject analysis was $0.19 \pm 0.38$ mm for BVSs versus $0.13 \pm 0.38$ mm for CoCr-EES; the one-side 97.5% upper confidence limit of the difference was 0.14 mm, which is lower than the noninferiority margin of 0.15 mm, thus achieving noninferiority of BVSs compared to CoCr-EES ($p_{noninferiority} = 0.01$). A sensitivity

**Table 6.4.1** Angiographic results (core laboratory), intention-to-treat population

| | BVSs (N = 238) (L = 251) | CoCr-EES (N = 237) (L = 252) | Difference [95% CI] | p-value |
|---|---|---|---|---|
| Preprocedure | | | | |
| Lesion length, mm | 14.1 ± 0.32 | 13.9 ± 0.30 | 0.2 (–0.7, 1.1) | 0.66 |
| RVD, mm | 2.81 ± 0.03 | 2.82 ± 0.03 | –0.01 (–0.09, 0.07) | 0.83 |
| MLD, mm | 0.98 ± 0.03 | 1.01 ± 0.03 | –0.03 (–0.10, 0.05) | 0.48 |
| % DS | 65.3 ± 0.82 | 64.5 ± 0.82 | 0.8 (–1.4, 3.1) | 0.48 |
| Postprocedure | | | | |
| RVD, mm | 2.84 ± 0.03 | 2.85 ± 0.03 | –0.01 (–0.09, 0.06) | 0.73 |
| In-segment MLD, mm | 2.30 ± 0.03 | 2.29 ± 0.03 | 0.01 (–0.07, 0.08) | 0.86 |
| In-device MLD, mm | 2.48 ± 0.02 | 2.59 ± 0.03 | –0.11 (–0.18, –0.04) | 0.002 |
| In-segment % DS | 19.0 ± 0.43 | 19.7 ± 0.52 | –0.7 (–2.0, 0.6) | 0.32 |
| In-device % DS | 12.2 ± 0.47 | 8.7 ± 0.46 | 3.5 (2.2, 4.8) | <0.0001 |
| In-segment acute gain, mm | 1.32 ± 0.03 | 1.28 ± 0.03 | 0.04 (–0.05, 0.12) | 0.40 |
| In-device acute gain, mm | 1.51 ± 0.03 | 1.59 ± 0.03 | –0.09 (–0.17, 0.00) | 0.04 |
| Total stent/scaffold length, mm | 20.6 ± 0.39 | 20.7 ± 0.35 | –0.1 (–1.2, 0.9) | 0.78 |
| One-year follow-up | | | | |
| RVD, mm | 2.80 ± 0.03 | 2.82 ± 0.03 | –0.02 (–0.10, 0.06) | 0.64 |
| In-segment MLD, mm | 2.13 ± 0.03 | 2.17 ± 0.03 | –0.03 (–0.12, 0.06) | 0.46 |
| In-device MLD, mm | 2.27 ± 0.03 | 2.50 ± 0.03 | –0.23 (–0.31, –0.14) | <0.0001 |
| In-segment % DS | 23.5 ± 0.84 | 23.0 ± 0.92 | 0.5 (–1.9, 3.0) | 0.66 |
| In-device % DS | 18.5 ± 0.92 | 11.3 ± 0.76 | 7.3 (5.0, 9.6) | <0.0001 |
| In-segment LL, mm | 0.18 ± 0.03 | 0.13 ± 0.03 | 0.05 (–0.02, 0.13) | 0.15 |
| In-device LL, mm | 0.23 ± 0.03 | 0.10 ± 0.02 | 0.13 (0.06, 0.20) | 0.0001 |
| In-segment ABR (%) | 3.9 ± 1.34 | 2.8 ± 1.13 | 1.1 (–2.3, 4.5) | 0.5.3 |
| In-device ABR (%) | 2.9 ± 1.16 | 0.75 ± 0.56 | 2.1 (–0.4, 4.7) | 0.10 |

*Source:* Adapted from Gao R, Yang Y, Han Y, Huo Y, Chen J, Yu B, Su X et al., on behalf of the ABSORB China Investigators. *J Am Coll Cardiol* 2015;66:2298–2309.

*Note:* Results of all analyses are adjusted using generalized estimating equations (GEE) for cases in which two lesions were present in a single patient. Data are presented as least square mean ± standard error. N = number of patients; L = number of target lesions; CI = confidence interval; RVD = reference vessel diameter; MLD = minimum lumen diameter; % DS = percent diameter stenosis; ABR = angiographic binary restenosis.

**Table 6.4.2** One-year in-segment late loss in the per-treatment-evaluable and intention-to-treat populations

|  | BVSs | CoCr-EES | Difference (upper one-sided 97.5% CL) | Non-inferiority p-value |
|---|---|---|---|---|
| Per-treatment-evaluable population | N = 200 | N = 195 |  |  |
| In-segment LL (mm) (per subject)* | 0.19 ± 0.38 | 0.13 ± 0.38 | 0.06 (0.14) | 0.01 |
| Intention-to-treat population | N = 208 | N = 199 |  |  |
| In-segment LL (mm) (per subject) | 0.18 ± 0.39 | 0.13 ± 0.38 | 0.05 (0.13) | 0.01 |

*Source:* Adapted from Gao R, Yang Y, Han Y, Huo Y, Chen J, Yu B, Su X et al., on behalf of the ABSORB China Investigators. *J Am Coll Cardiol* 2015;66:2298–2309.
* Study primary endpoint. † Least square mean ± standard error. LL = late loss; CL = confidence limit.

analysis based on per subject in the ITT population similarly showed noninferiority of BVSs to CoCr-EES for 1-year in-segment LL (Table 6.4.2). The late loss cumulative frequency distribution curves are shown in Figure 6.4.2. Other ITT-based angiographic in-segment measures were also similar between the two devices at 1-year follow-up. BVSs

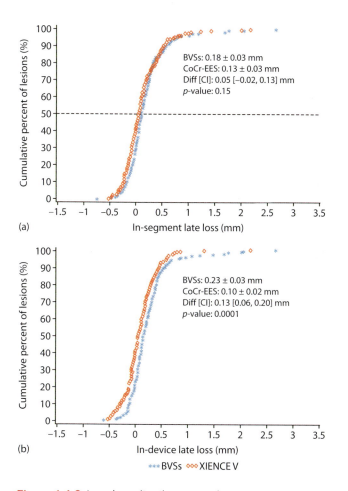

(a)

(b)

*** BVSs  ◇◇◇ XIENCE V

**Figure 6.4.2** Late loss distribution in the intention-to-treat population. Cumulative frequency distribution for 1-year in-segment (panel **a**) and in-device (panel **b**) late loss. Summary data based on GEE analysis, and presented as least square mean ± standard error. (Adopted from Gao R, Yang Y, Han Y, Huo Y, Chen J, Yu B, Su X et al., on behalf of the ABSORB China Investigators. *J Am Coll Cardiol* 2015;66:2298–2309.)

had a slightly smaller MLD and larger % DS compared to CoCr-EES within the device at 1 year. The in-device LL at 1 year was greater with the BVSs compared to CoCr-EES. Angiographic binary restenosis (ABR) rates at 1 year were low and comparable between the BVSs and CoCr-EES, whether measured in-device or in-segment (Table 6.4.1).

One-year clinical follow-up was completed in 98.8% (238/241) BVSs patients and in 237/239 (99.2%) CoCr-EES patients. BVSs and CoCr-EES also had similar 1-year rates of TLF (3.4% vs. 4.2%, respectively, p = 0.62) and PoCE (8.0% vs. 9.7%, p = 0.51). Likewise, the component measures of these endpoints were similar between both devices, other than lower 1-year all-cause mortality with the BVSs (0% vs. 2.1%, p = 0.03). The periprocedural MI rates were low and similar between the BVSs and CoCr-EES by the protocol definition (CK-MB >5x URL; 1.3% vs. 0.4%, respectively, p = 0.62).

There were no definite scaffold or stent thromboses during the 1-year follow-up period. One BVSs patient developed an MI within the distribution of the target vessel 15 days postprocedure which was initially treated medically. Angiography performed 6 days later demonstrated 20.7% and 21.6% in-device and in-segment diameter stenoses, respectively, at the target lesion site, without thrombus evident. Nonetheless this event was adjudicated as a probable scaffold thrombosis. There were no other thrombosis events. Thus, the 1-year rate of definite/probable scaffold/stent thrombosis was 0.4% with BVSs and 0% with CoCr-EES (p = 1.0).

## DISCUSSION

In-segment LL is a robust measure of clinical effectiveness as it accounts for restenosis both within the device as well as the peri-device margins. In the ABSORB China randomized trial, the BVSs was non-inferior to CoCr-EES for the primary endpoint of angiographic in-segment LL at 1 year. The mean 1-year in-segment LL for the BVSs in the present trial (0.19 mm) is less than the 0.30 mm mean in-segment LL with BVSs at 9 months in EVERBIO II, which enrolled an all-comers population [4]; however, it is slightly greater than the 0.13 mm at 13 months in the ABSORB Japan trial [2]. Other angiographic in-segment measures were similar between the two devices postprocedure and at follow-up. In-device acute gain was lower and 1-year in-device LL was greater with the BVSs compared to CoCr-EES; however, the small differences in 1-year in-device LL in the present study (and the non-significant differences in in-segment LL) between BVSs and CoCr-EES are not likely to be clinically meaningful. The rates of in-device and in-segment ABR (2.9% and 3.9%, respectively) and 1-year ID-TLR (2.5%) are comparable to the rates of in-device and in-segment ABR (0.8% and 2.8%, respectively) and ID-TLR (2.1%) observed with CoCr-EES, indicating that the BVSs is an effective PCI device.

The BVSs and CoCr-EES also demonstrated comparable rates of acute device and procedural success, with similar 1-year rates of the PoCE, the DoCE, MI, TLR, and scaffold/ stent thrombosis. The results were similar with reports from the ABSORB II [5], ABSORB Japan [2], and ABSORB III [1]. Stent and scaffold thrombosis rates were very low in our trial. Only one patient with the BVSs experienced a probable scaffold thrombosis, and no definite thromboses occurred.

BVSs, the first generation of a novel bioresorbable scaffolds (BRSs), have thicker struts and a larger crossing profile than contemporary metallic DESs. Aggressive predilatation was recommended, and postdilatation was performed at a higher rate with the BVSs than CoCr-EES, which may have helped achieve high rates of acute procedural success with only a 2.0% bailout rate. Nonetheless, improvements in implantation technique (e.g., routine postdilatation or more frequent use of intravascular imaging guidance, which was rarely used in the present study) and device iterations (thinner struts with reduced recoil) may further improve deliverability and angiographic and clinical outcomes, especially in complex lesions.

In conclusion, in the present multicenter randomized trial, the BVSs was noninferior to CoCr-EES for the primary endpoint of in-segment LL at 1 year. The BVSs had comparable rates of 1-year angiographic restenosis and clinical outcomes compared to CoCr-EES, with low rates of death, MI, and scaffold thrombosis, demonstrating the safety and effectiveness of the BVSs in treating *de novo* coronary lesions in a Chinese population.

# REFERENCES

1. Ellis SG, Kereiakes DJ, Metzger C, Caputo RP, Rizik DG, Teirstein PS, Litt MR et al. ABSORB III Investigators. Everolimus-eluting bioresorbable vascular scaffolds in patients with coronary artery disease: The ABSORB III trial. *N Engl J Med.* 2015; 373: 1905–15.
2. Kimura T, Kozuma K, Tanabe K, Nakamura S, Yamane M, Muramatsu T, Saito S et al. ABSORB Japan Investigators. A randomized trial evaluating everolimus-eluting Absorb bioresorbable scaffolds vs. everolimus-eluting metallic stents in patients with coronary artery disease: ABSORB Japan. *Eur Heart J.* 2015;36:3332–42.
3. Gao R, Yang Y, Han Y, Huo Y, Chen J, Yu B, Su X et al. ABSORB China Investigators. Bioresorbable vascular scaffolds versus metallic stents in patients with coronary artery disease: ABSORB China trial. *J Am Coll Cardiol.* 2015;66:2298–2309.
4. Puricel S, Arroyo D, Copataux N, Baeriswyl G, Lehmann S, Kallinikou Z, Muller O et al. Comparison of everolimus- and biolimus-eluting coronary stents with everolimus-eluting bioresorbable vascular scaffolds. *J Am Coll Cardiol.* 2015;65:791–801.
5. Serruys PW, Chevalier B, Dudek D, Cequier A, Carrié D, Iniguez A, Dominici M et al. A bioresorbable everolimus-eluting scaffold versus a metallic everolimus-eluting stent for ischaemic heart disease caused by de-novo native coronary artery lesions (ABSORB II): An interim 1-year analysis of clinical and procedural secondary outcomes from a randomized controlled trial. *Lancet.* 2015;385:43–54.

# ABSORB Japan

TAKESHI KIMURA

## DESIGN OF THE ABSORB JAPAN

By providing antiproliferative drug-eluting capability without the chronic limitations of permanent metallic implants, bioresorbable vascular scaffolds (BVSs) may provide long-term benefits over metallic stents [1]. Imaging studies for up to 5 years after ABSORB BVS implantation have suggested favorable vascular responses, including restoration of vasomotion and endothelium dependent vasodilation, late lumen enlargement with plaque regression and vessel remodeling, and formation of a stable-appearing neointima [1–3]. Studies are ongoing to determine whether these long-term changes after BVS implantation might mitigate the risk of very late (>1 year) adverse events reported after metallic drug-eluting stents (DESs) implantation, namely very late stent thrombosis and restenosis (for example, due to neo-atherosclerosis) [4]. However, even if the BVS demonstrates long-term advantages compared to the metallic DESs, it is important to ensure at least comparable (noninferior) short- and mid-term (i.e., 1 year) safety and efficacy profiles. To examine the clinical and angiographic outcomes of the ABSORB BVS relative to cobalt-chromium everolimus-eluting stents (CoCr-EESs), the ABSORB Japan, a randomized, controlled trial comparing the ABSORB BVS with CoCr-EES was designed to support regulatory approval of the ABSORB BVS in Japan [5].

ABSORB Japan was a prospective, multicenter, randomized, single-blind, active-controlled clinical trial in which 400 patients undergoing coronary stent implantation from 38 investigational sites in Japan were randomized in a 2:1 ratio to treatment with the ABSORB everolimus-eluting BVS or the XIENCE Prime/Xpedition CoCr-EES (both Abbott Vascular, Santa Clara, CA). Patients were eligible if they were ≥20 years of age and had evidence of myocardial ischemia (stable angina, unstable angina, or silent ischemia). We excluded patients with left ventricular ejection fraction <30%, estimated glomerular filtration rate <30 mL/min/1.73 m², recent myocardial infarction, and those at high bleeding risk. The study allowed treatment of up to two *de novo* native lesions in separate epicardial coronary arteries.

Key angiographic inclusion criteria included reference vessel diameter ≥2.5 to ≤3.75 mm, lesion length ≤24 mm and percent diameter stenosis (DS) ≥50% to <100%. Key angiographic exclusion criteria included left main or ostial location; excessive vessel tortuosity or extreme lesion angulation; heavy calcification proximal to or within the target-lesion; myocardial bridge; restenotic lesion; target vessel containing thrombus; and bifurcation lesion with side branch ≥2 mm in diameter, requiring protection guidewire or dilatation (Figure 6.5.1a).

Patients were randomized in a 2:1 ratio to BVSs versus CoCr-EESs using a central randomization service (Figure 6.5.1a). Randomization was stratified by the presence of diabetes mellitus and the number of lesions to be treated. Patients were also allocated randomly to one of three intravascular imaging subgroups; intravascular ultrasound (IVUS) group (150 patients), optical coherence tomography (OCT)-1 group (125 patients), or OCT-2 group (125 patients), based on the schedules of intravascular imaging. Patients were blinded to their treatment assignment through the completion of 5-year follow-up, while study investigators doing the procedure were not blinded.

The study allowed treatment of up to two *de novo* native coronary artery lesions. If a patient had two lesions in separate vessels and only one lesion was eligible for randomization, the second lesion could be treated as a non-study lesion. The nonstudy lesion had to be treated successfully prior to treatment of the study target lesion. Successful predilatation of the target lesion was mandatory. Sizes of the BVS available in the study were: 2.5, 3.0, and 3.5 mm in diameter, and 8, 12, 18, and 28 mm in length. Treatment with the same size matrix was required for patients assigned to the CoCr-EES arm. The target lesion had to be treated with a single study device, and planned overlapping was not allowed. Postdilatation of the BVS was not mandatory but was allowed, using a low profile, high-pressure, noncompliant balloon with diameter ≤0.5 mm larger than the nominal BVS size. Postdilatation of the CoCr-EES was per standard of care. Postprocedural intravascular imaging with the assigned modality was to

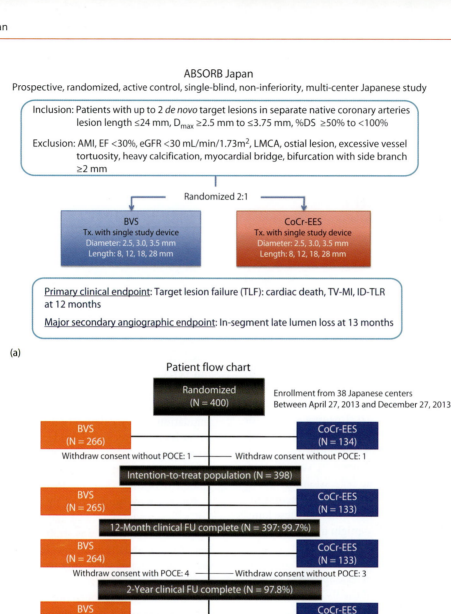

**ABSORB Japan**
Prospective, randomized, active control, single-blind, non-inferiority, multi-center Japanese study

Inclusion: Patients with up to 2 *de novo* target lesions in separate native coronary arteries lesion length ≤24 mm, $D_{max}$ ≥2.5 mm to ≤3.75 mm, %DS ≥50% to <100%

Exclusion: AMI, EF <30%, eGFR <30 mL/min/1.73m², LMCA, ostial lesion, excessive vessel tortuosity, heavy calcification, myocardial bridge, bifurcation with side branch ≥2 mm

Randomized 2:1

**BVS**
Tx. with single study device
Diameter: 2.5, 3.0, 3.5 mm
Length: 8, 12, 18, 28 mm

**CoCr-EES**
Tx. with single study device
Diameter: 2.5, 3.0, 3.5 mm
Length: 8, 12, 18, 28 mm

Primary clinical endpoint: Target lesion failure (TLF): cardiac death, TV-MI, ID-TLR at 12 months

Major secondary angiographic endpoint: In-segment late lumen loss at 13 months

(a)

**Patient flow chart**

Randomized
(N = 400)

Enrollment from 38 Japanese centers
Between April 27, 2013 and December 27, 2013

BVS (N = 266) — CoCr-EES (N = 134)

Withdraw consent without POCE: 1 — Withdraw consent without POCE: 1

Intention-to-treat population (N = 398)

BVS (N = 265) — CoCr-EES (N = 133)

12-Month clinical FU complete (N = 397: 99.7%)

BVS (N = 264) — CoCr-EES (N = 133)

Withdraw consent with POCE: 4 — Withdraw consent without POCE: 3

2-Year clinical FU complete (N = 97.8%)

BVS (N = 261) — CoCr-EES (N = 130)

(b)

**Figure 6.5.1** Study design of ABSORB Japan Trial. **(a)** Inclusion/exclusion criteria and primary/secondary endpoints. **(b)** Patient flow during 2-year follow-up.

be performed in the IVUS and OCT-1 groups, while it was not allowed in the OCT-2 group.

All patients were maintained on a thienopyridine for at least 12 months, and aspirin indefinitely. Clinical follow-up was scheduled up to 5 years. Follow-up angiography was planned in all patients at 13 months.

The primary endpoint of the study was target lesion failure (TLF: a composite of cardiac death, myocardial infarction attributable to target vessel [TV-MI], or ischemia-driven target lesion revascularization [ID-TLR]) at 1 year, powered for noninferiority of BVS versus CoCr-EES. The major secondary endpoint was angiographic in-segment late lumen loss (LLL) at 13 months. Clinical endpoint definitions, including stent/scaffold thrombosis (ST), were based on the Academic Research Consortium definitions, except for peri-procedural non-Q wave MI, which was defined as a postprocedural CK-MB >5x URL, similar to the definition used in the ABSORB III US trial

and the ABSORB China trial [6]. Device success is defined as successful deployment of the assigned device with attainment of final in-device DS <30% by quantitative coronary angiography (QCA). Procedure success is defined as successful deployment of the assigned device with attainment of final in-device DS <30% by QCA without the occurrence of TLF during the hospital stay (maximum of 7 days).

The primary endpoint of 12-month TLF was evaluated using the difference in the event rates (BVS–CoCr-EES) in the intention-to-treat (ITT) population. The hypothesis test was designed to evaluate noninferiority of BVS to CoCr-EES (margin of 8.6% for a 9.0% assumed event rate in both groups that was agreed on with the Pharmaceutical and Medical Device Agency in Japan) using the likelihood score method by Farrington and Manning [7]. Randomizing 400 patients 2:1 to BVSs versus CoCr-EESs, with an anticipated 1-year follow-up rate of 97%, provided

90% power to demonstrate noninferiority of BVSs for TLF at a one-sided significance level of 0.05. The major secondary endpoint of in-segment LLL was tested for noninferiority (margin of 0.195 mm and SD of 0.5 mm for both arms) using an asymptotic Z test statistic at a one-sided significance level of 0.05. Randomizing 400 patients 2:1 to BVSs versus CoCr-EESs (assuming 15% of patients would have two target lesions), with an anticipated angiographic follow-up rate at 13 months of 90%, provided 98% power to demonstrate noninferiority of BVS for LLL.

## PATIENT POPULATION

Between April 27, 2013 and December 27, 2013, 400 patients were enrolled and randomly assigned to BVS (266 patients) or CoCr-EES (134 patients). Clinical follow-up at 12 months

was available in 264 (99.2%) patients in the BVS arm and 133 (98.8%) patients in the CoCr-EES arm (Figure 6.5.1b).

Baseline demographic variables, risk factors, and lesion characteristics were comparable between the treatment arms (Table 6.5.1). The mean age was 67.2 years and 36.0% of patients had diabetes. Stable coronary artery disease was present in 88.0% of patients. Ninety-seven percent of patients had treatment of one study target lesion only.

## RESULTS FROM THE ABSORB JAPAN TRIAL

### Procedural results

Predilatation was performed using slightly undersized balloons with moderate inflation pressures. The rates of

Table 6.5.1 Baseline characteristics of the study population (intention-to-treat population)

| | BVS | CoCr-EES |
|---|---|---|
| **Patients** | | |
| Number of patients | 266 | 134 |
| Age (years) | 67.1 ± 9.4 | 67.3 ± 9.6 |
| Male | 210 (78.9%) | 99 (73.9%) |
| Body mass index (kg/m$^2$) | 24.0 ± 3.0 | 24.3 ± 3.0 |
| Current smoker | 53 (19.9%) | 29 (21.6%) |
| Hypertension | 208 (78.2%) | 107 (79.9%) |
| Dyslipidemia | 218 (82.0%) | 110 (82.1%) |
| Diabetes mellitus | 96 (36.1%) | 48 (35.8%) |
| – Treated with insulin | 24 (9.0%) | 11 (8.2%) |
| HbA1c (%) | 6.2 ± 1.1 | 6.2 ± 0.8 |
| Prior intervention to target vessel | 9 (3.4%) | 7 (5.2%) |
| Prior myocardial infarction | 42/262 (16.0%) | 32 (23.9%) |
| Family history of premature CAD | 16/246 (6.5%) | 10/124 (8.1%) |
| Current evidence of ischemia | | |
| – Stable angina | 170 (63.9%) | 88 (65.7%) |
| – Unstable angina | 26 (9.8%) | 22 (16.4%) |
| – Silent ischemia | 70 (26.3%) | 24 (17.9%) |
| Number of target lesions | | |
| – One | 257 (96.6%) | 131 (97.8%) |
| – Two | 9 (3.4%) | 3 (2.2%) |
| Non-study lesion treated | 20 (7.5%) | 10 (7.5%) |
| **Target Lesions*** | | |
| Total number of target lesions | 275 | 137 |
| Left anterior descending | 127 (46.2%) | 58 (42.3%) |
| Left circumflex/ramus | 63 (22.9%) | 36 (26.3%) |
| Right coronary artery | 85 (30.9%) | 43 (31.4%) |
| Calcification (moderate/severe) | 76/274 (27.7%) | 45 (32.8%) |
| Calcification (severe) | 19/274 (6.9%) | 15 (10.9%) |
| Tortuosity (moderate/severe) | 23/274 (8.5%) | 11 (8.0%) |
| Eccentric lesion | 223/273 (81.7%) | 113 (82.5%) |

*Note:* There were no significant differences between groups.
*Abbreviations:* BVS = bioresorbable vascular scaffold; CAD = coronary artery disease; CoCr-EES = cobalt-chromium everolimus-eluting stent.
* Core laboratory assessed.

clinical device and procedural success were similar in both groups, with slightly longer procedure duration in the BVS arm (Table 6.5.2). Of three acute device failures in the BVS arm, two were deployment failures (lesions subsequently treated with CoCr-EES), and one lesion had in-device DS of ≥30% after BVSs implantation. Nominal device diameter and expected final balloon diameter were similar between the two arms, with postdilatation performed in a similar proportion of patients but at slightly lower inflation pressure with BVSs. In-device acute gain and minimal luminal

diameter (MLD) were significantly smaller in the BVS arm than in the CoCr-EES arm. However, in-segment MLD and DS were similar between the two arms (Table 6.5.3).

## One year clinical follow-up results

Within 12 months, the primary endpoint of TLF occurred in 11/265 BVS patients (4.2%) and in 5/133 CoCr-EES patients (3.8%) (relative risk 1.10, 95% confidence interval 0.39–3.11) (Figure 6.5.2a). The upper one-sided 95% confidence limit

Table 6.5.2 Procedural results

| | BVS (P = 266) (L = 275) (D = 280) | CoCr-EES (P = 134) (L = 137) (D = 138) | p-value |
|---|---|---|---|
| Post OCT/IVUS assigned | 183 (68.8%) | 92 (68.7%) | 1.00 |
| Procedure duration (min) | 49.8 ± 24.8 | 44.9 ± 21.7 | 0.04 |
| **Procedural Information (per lesion)** | | | |
| Assigned device implanted | 272 (98.9%) | 137 (100%) | 0.55 |
| Bailout device used | 5 (1.8%) | 1 (0.7%) | 0.67 |
| Total device length per lesion (mm) | 20.2 ± 5.8 | 19.5 ± 5.8 | 0.22 |
| **Predilatation (per lesion)** | | | |
| Predilatation performed | 275 (100%) | 137 (100%) | 1.00 |
| – Semicompliant balloon | 143 (52.0%) | 64 (46.7%) | 0.31 |
| – Noncompliant balloon | 97 (35.3%) | 54 (39.4%) | 0.41 |
| – Scoring or cutting balloon | 54 (19.6%) | 26 (19.0%) | 1.00 |
| Nominal balloon diameter (mm) | 2.80 ± 0.37 | 2.86 ± 0.36 | 0.15 |
| Predilatation balloon pressure (atm) | 11.6 ± 3.8 | 11.9 ± 3.7 | 0.52 |
| **Device Deployment (per device)** | | | |
| Nominal device diameter (mm) | 3.09 ± 0.37 | 3.13 ± 0.38 | 0.30 |
| Deployment pressure (atm) | 10.4 ± 3.0 | 11.2 ± 2.7 | 0.003 |
| Expected device diameter at deployment (mm) | 3.30 ± 0.43 | 3.19 ± 0.42 | 0.01 |
| **Postdilatation (per lesion)** | | | |
| Postdilatation performed | 226 (82.2%) | 106 (77.4%) | 0.25 |
| Nominal balloon diameter (mm) | 3.18 ± 0.44 | 3.29 ± 0.51 | 0.0495 |
| Balloon pressure (atm) | 15.5 ± 4.2 | 16.0 ± 3.9 | 0.24 |
| Expected postdilatation balloon diameter (mm) | 3.32 ± 0.44 | 3.45 ± 0.49 | 0.02 |
| >0.5 mm larger than the BVS diameter | 9 (4.0%) | – | – |
| **Final Balloon (per lesion)** | | | |
| Balloon pressure (atm) | 14.7 ± 4.1 | 15.1 ± 4.1 | 0.36 |
| Expected final balloon diameter (mm) | 3.34 ± 0.45 | 3.41 ± 0.48 | 0.15 |
| **Acute Success** | | | |
| Device success (per lesion) | 271 (98.9%)* | 136 (99.3%) | 1.00 |
| Procedural success (per patient) | 259 (97.7%)** | 132 (98.5%) | 0.72 |

*Note:* One patient in the BVS arm had CoCr-EES implantation without attempt of assigned BVSs due to lack of BVS inventory, and was excluded from the acute success analysis.

Expected balloon/device diameter was determined from the compliance chart according to the maximum inflation pressure.

*Abbreviations:* BVS = bioresorbable vascular scaffold; CoCr-EES = cobalt-chromium everolimus-eluting stent; D = device number; DS = diameter stenosis; ITT = intention-to-treat; IVUS = intravascular ultrasound; L = lesion number; OCT = optical coherence tomography; P = patient number; QCA = quantitative coronary angiography; TLF = target lesion failure.

* N = 274 and ** N = 265.

**Table 6.5.3** Quantitative coronary angiographic results (full-analysis-set)

| | BVS | CoCr-EES | *p*-value |
|---|---|---|---|
| **Baseline** | | | |
| Number of lesions | 272 | 137 | |
| Lesion length (mm) | 13.5 ± 5.28 | 13.3 ± 5.52 | 0.78 |
| Reference vessel diameter (mm) | 2.72 ± 0.44 | 2.79 ± 0.46 | 0.11 |
| MLD (mm) | 0.96 ± 0.33 | 0.99 ± 0.36 | 0.42 |
| DS (%) | 64.6 ± 11.2 | 64.7 ± 10.9 | 0.93 |
| **Postprocedure** | | | |
| Number of lesions | 272 | 137 | |
| Reference vessel diameter (mm) | 2.76 ± 0.42 | 2.85 ± 0.43 | 0.04 |
| In-segment MLD (mm) | 2.21 ± 0.39 | 2.26 ± 0.43 | 0.19 |
| In-device MLD (mm) | 2.42 ± 0.38 | 2.64 ± 0.40 | <0.0001 |
| In-segment DS (%) | 19.9 ± 6.7 | 20.6 ± 8.7 | 0.44 |
| In-segment acute gain (mm) | 1.25 ± 0.41 | 1.28 ± 0.45 | 0.56 |
| In-device acute gain (mm) | 1.46 ± 0.40 | 1.65 ± 0.40 | <0.0001 |
| **Follow-up at 13 months** | | | |
| Number of lesions | 260 | 129 | |
| Reference vessel diameter (mm) | 2.70 ± 0.42 | 2.80 ± 0.44 | 0.046 |
| In-segment MLD (mm) | 2.08 ± 0.45 | 2.15 ± 0.50 | 0.18 |
| In-device MLD (mm) | 2.23 ± 0.47 | 2.48 ± 0.53 | <0.0001 |
| In-segment DS (%) | 23.4 ± 11.3 | 23.7 ± 12.3 | 0.87 |
| In-segment binary restenosis | 5 (1.9%) | 5 (3.9%) | 0.31 |
| In-device late lumen loss (mm) | 0.19 ± 0.31 | 0.16 ± 0.33 | 0.35 |
| In-segment net gain (mm) | 1.12 ± 0.47 | 1.15 ± 0.47 | 0.56 |
| In-device net gain (mm) | 1.28 ± 0.49 | 1.48 ± 0.48 | 0.0001 |

*Abbreviations:* BVS = bioresorbable vascular scaffold; CoCr-EES = cobalt-chromium everolimus-eluting stent; DS = diameter stenosis; MLD = minimal lumen diameter.

\* N = 128.

of the 0.4% difference in the rate of TLF (BVS – CoCr-EES) was 3.95%, less than the predefined noninferiority margin of 8.6%, demonstrating noninferiority of BVS to CoCr-EES ($p_{noninferiority} < 0.0001$). Peri-procedural MI rates were similar with the two devices (1.1% and 1.5%), as were the rates of definite/probable ST (1.5% in each group) (Figure 6.5.2b). Definite ST occurred in 4 patients (1.5%) in the BVS arm, and in 1 patient (0.8%) in the CoCr-EES arm. At 12 months, 97.0% and 93.3% of patients in the BVS and CoCr-EES arms, respectively, were taking dual antiplatelet therapy ($p = 0.08$).

## Thirteen month angiographic follow-up result

Angiographic follow-up at 13 months was performed in 262/270 (95.6%) target-lesions in the BVS arm and in 129/137 (94.2%) target lesions in the CoCr-EES arm at 395 ± 28 days after device implantation. The major secondary endpoint of 13-month angiographic in-segment LLL was 0.13 ± 0.30 mm in the BVS arm, and 0.12 ± 0.32 mm in the CoCr-EES arm (Table 6.5.3). The upper one-sided 95% confidence limit of the difference in in-segment LLL was 0.07 mm, less than

the predefined noninferiority margin of 0.195 mm, demonstrating noninferiority of BVS to CoCr-EES ($p_{noninferiority} < 0.0001$). In-device LLL was also not significantly different between the two arms, although in-device MLD and DS at 13 months were slightly smaller in the BVS arm. However, in-segment MLD, DS, and binary restenosis were similar in the two arms (Table 6.5.3). There were no significant differences in clinical or angiographic outcomes according to the performance of postprocedural intravascular imaging.

## Two year clinical follow-up results

At 2 years, 391 patients (98%, BVS: 261 patients, and CoCr-EES: 130 patients) had clinical follow-up [7]. At 2 years, almost half of the patients were on dual antiplatelet regimen (BVS: 52.3%, CoCr-EES: 50.7%, $p = 0.78$) (Figure 6.5.2a). The 2-year TLF rate was not significantly different between the BVS and CoCr-EES arms (7.3% and 3.8%, relative risk 1.89, 95% confidence interval 0.72–4.96, $p = 0.18$). The numerically higher rate of TLF in the BVS arm was mainly driven by ID-TLR (5.4% and 2.3%, $p = 0.16$) as well as TV-MI (5.0% and 3.1%, $p = 0.38$). However, the rate of all

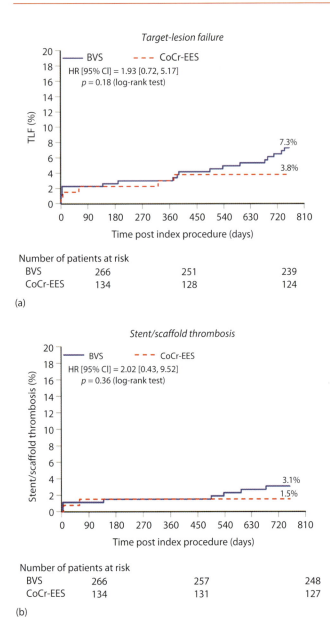

(a)

(b)

**Figure 6.5.2** ABSORB Japan 2-year follow-up. **(a)** TLF. **(b)** Definite/probable ST.

TLR was similar in both arms (5.7% and 5.4%, *p* = 0.38). The definite/probable ST rates were 3.1% and 1.5% (*p* = 0.51), respectively (Figure 6.5.2b).

From 1 to 2 years, there were 4 MI cases (1.6%, 2 non-Q-wave MI and 2 Q-wave MI) in the BVS arm related to very late scaffold thrombosis (VLST) occurring at various time points ranging from 494 to 679 days after the index procedure. All the 4 VLST cases did not belong to the OCT-1 subgroup and, therefore, did not undergo OCT imaging at postprocedure. These 4 VLST cases had relatively large angiographic reference vessel diameter, and the scaffolds were widely patent at 1-year follow-up angiography in all cases. One case was not on any antiplatelet therapy at the time of VLST. On OCT performed post-VLST in 3 cases, malapposition and late strut discontinuities protruding into the lumen (intraluminal dismantling) were observed in all cases (Figure 6.5.3a).

## Serial OCT follow-up at baseline and at 2 years

As an imaging substudy, 125 patients were allocated randomly to the OCT-1 subgroup to undergo serial OCT follow-up at postprocedure and at 2 and 3 years. In the

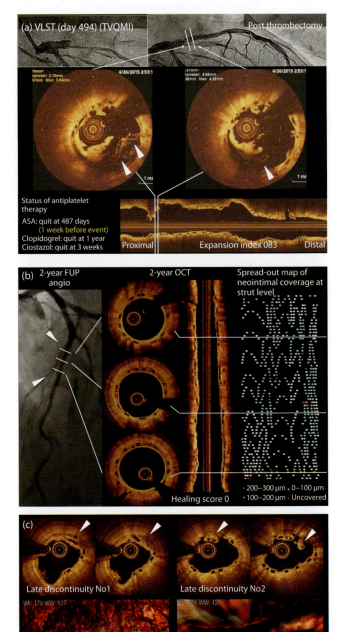

**Figure 6.5.3** OCT images from ABSORB Japan. **(a)** Very late scaffold thrombosis. **(b)** Good healing response. **(c)** Strut discontinuities without clinical events.

OCT-1 group, postprocedural OCT was performed using a frequency domain imaging system (C7/C8 system, LightLab Imaging, Westford, MA, or Lunawave system, Terumo Corporation, Tokyo, Japan). When significant incomplete strut apposition was observed on OCT, it was allowed to perform additional postdilatation. Whenever additional postdilatation was performed, coronary angiography and OCT were to be repeated. At the 2-year follow-up, coronary angiography was repeated in the same projections as at postprocedure. OCT was performed in target lesion including 5 mm distal and 5 mm proximal to the stent/scaffold. The imaging data was analyzed in the independent core laboratories (Quantitative Coronary Angiography [QCA]: Beth Israel Deaconess Medical Centre, Boston, MA, and OCT: Cardialysis, Rotterdam, the Netherlands).

OCT assessment of the stented/scaffolded coronary segment was performed using the final OCT recordings sent to an independent Core Laboratory for off-line analysis using QIVUS software (ver 3.0, MEDIS, Leiden, the Netherlands). It was not possible to blind the analysts to the device type based on the characteristic appearance of BVS and CoCr-EES struts by OCT. Taking into account the difference in optical properties of cobalt chromium and polylactide, OCT analysis was performed using comparative methods [8]. For the OCT endpoint analysis, stent area and derived measures are based on the abluminal stent contour [8]. Definitions of OCT imaging endpoints were reported previously [9].

Among the 125 patients in the OCT-1 subgroup, postprocedure OCT was evaluated in 77 patients (81 lesions) in the BVS arm, and in 42 patients (43 lesions) in the CoCr-EES arm, while 2-year OCT was evaluated in 73 patients (77 lesions) in the BVS arm, and in 37 patients (38 lesions) in the CoCr-EES arm.

Quantitative measurements of device and flow area at postprocedure were comparable between the BVS and CoCr-EES arms (Table 6.5.4). The BVS scaffold area was more eccentric than the CoCr-EES. Malapposed struts were less frequently seen with BVS than with CoCr-EES, although ISA area was small and not different between the two arms. The BVS struts had less embedment than CoCr-EES struts (Table 6.5.4). In qualitative analysis, there was no acute disruption of polymeric struts.

OCT at 2 years demonstrated a uniform tissue coverage in most of the lesions in both the BVS and CoCr-EES arms (Figure 6.5.3b). The dimension of stent and scaffold was stable over 2 years after implantation (Tables 6.5.4 and 6.5.5), while there was a trend toward greater neointimal growth with BVS than with CoCr-EES (Table 6.5.5). As a result, the mean and minimum flow area was smaller in the BVS arm than in the CoCr-EES arm, which was consistent with the smaller in-device minimum lumen diameter by QCA ($2.08 \pm 0.56$ mm and $2.37 \pm 0.5$ 8 mm, $p = 0.01$). However, the vessel healing on OCT was complete and similar in both the BVS and CoCr-EES arms. The tissue characteristics at the site of minimal scaffold/stent area were similar in both the arms, with most of the characterized tissues being homogeneous. Coverage of the struts was nearly complete in both arms, while the ISA areas were minimal, resulting in minimal healing scores in both arms (Table 6.5.5).

The serial OCT of the scaffold segment allowed the assessment of strut discontinuities, whether they were persistent or late acquired. The overhang or stacked struts were found at

**Table 6.5.4** Baseline OCT findings in the OCT-1 subgroup

|  | BVS | CoCr-EES | *p*-value |
|---|---|---|---|
| Number of lesions evaluated | N = 81 | N = 43 | |
| Mean flow area (mm²) | 6.84 ± 1.98 | 7.29 ± 2.41 | 0.26 |
| Minimum flow area (mm²) | 5.60 ± 1.81 | 5.95 ± 2.23 | 0.35 |
| Mean abluminal scaffold/stent area (mm²) | 7.74 ± 2.10 | 8.05 ± 2.49 | 0.46 |
| Minimum abluminal scaffold/stent area (mm²) | 6.55 ± 1.99 | 6.90 ± 2.44 | 0.40 |
| Mean scaffold/stent eccentricity | 0.86 ± 0.04 | 0.88 ± 0.03 | <0.001 |
| Minimum scaffold/stent eccentricity | 0.79 ± 0.08 | 0.84 ± 0.06 | <0.001 |
| Asymmetry index of scaffold/stent | 0.28 ± 0.09 | 0.23 ± 0.07 | 0.006 |
| Mean lumen diameter (mm) | 3.03 ± 0.42 | 3.02 ± 0.52 | 0.94 |
| % Malapposed strut | 2.00 (0.68, 6.37) | 6.35 (3.61, 14.94) | 0.005 |
| Mean ISA area, overall (mm²) | 0.03 (0.00, 0.09) | 0.06 (0.01, 0.12) | 0.34 |
| Lesion with ≥1 malapposed struts | 67 [82.7] | 40 [93.0] | 0.17 |
| Lesion with acute disruption | 0% | – | |
| Median embedment depth per lesion (µm) | 50 (42, 59) | 84 (67, 98) | <0.001 |
| Strut level analysis | | | |
| Number of struts analyzed | N = 14633 | N = 9048 | |
| Malapposed struts | 715 [4.9] | 849 [9.4] | <0.001 |

*Note:* Data area expressed as mean ± SD, median (interquartile range), or number [percentage].
*Abbreviations:* BVS = bioresorbable vascular scaffold; CoCr-EES = cobalt-chromium everolimus-eluting stent; ISA = incomplete strut apposition; OCT = optical coherence tomography.

**Table 6.5.5** Two-year follow-up OCT findings in the OCT-1 subgroup

| | BVS | CoCr-EES | p-value |
|---|---|---|---|
| Number of lesions evaluated | N = 77 | N = 38 | |
| Mean flow area (mm²) | 5.55 ± 1.98 | 6.60 ± 2.41 | 0.01 |
| Minimum flow area (mm²) | 4.10 ± 1.79 | 5.05 ± 1.97 | 0.01 |
| Mean strut area (mm²) | 0.28 ± 0.06 | 0.08 ± 0.01 | <0.0001 |
| Minimum strut area (mm²) | 0.12 ± 0.06 | 0.03 ± 0.01 | <0.0001 |
| Mean abluminal scaffold/stent area (mm²) | 7.91 ± 2.24 | 8.40 ± 2.61 | 0.31 |
| Minimum abluminal scaffold/stent area (mm²) | 6.31 ± 2.05 | 7.11 ± 2.42 | 0.07 |
| Neointimal area (mm²) (including on top and in-between struts) | 2.08 ± 0.66 | 1.82 ± 0.67 | 0.051 |
| Neointimal area (mm²) (on top of struts) | 1.10 ± 0.52 | 1.03 ± 0.59 | 0.52 |
| Qualitative analysis of neointima | | | 0.3 |
| Homogeneous | 73 (95%) | 34 (90%) | |
| Heterogeneous | 1 (1.3%) | 0 (0%) | |
| Layered | 3 (3.9%) | 4 (10.5%) | |
| Mean scaffold/stent eccentricity (abluminal) | 0.87 ± 0.05 | 0.92 ± 0.03 | <0.001 |
| Minimum scaffold/stent eccentricity (abluminal) | 0.75 ± 0.09 | 0.84 ± 0.05 | <0.001 |
| Asymmetry index of scaffold/stent (abluminal) | 0.34 ± 0.09 | 0.24 ± 0.08 | <0.001 |
| Flow lumen volume (mm³) | 111.10 ± 48.83 | 131.30 ± 62.59 | 0.06 |
| Strut volume (mm³) | 5.59 ± 1.98 | 1.64 ± 0.46 | <0.001 |
| Stent/scaffold volume (mm³) (abluminal) | 158.32 ± 58.95 | 167.37 ± 71.92 | 0.47 |
| Neointimal volume (on top and in-between struts) (mm³) | 41.74 ± 15.37 | 36.22 ± 17.03 | 0.08 |
| Neointimal volume (on top of struts) (mm³) | 22.00 ± 11.05 | 20.22 ± 13.54 | 0.45 |
| ISA volume (mm³) (abluminal) | 0.00 (0.00, 0.00) | 0.00 (0.00, 0.00) | 0.83 |
| Late strut discontinuities | 19/77 (25%) | NA | |
| **Healing score** | 0.00 (0.00, 1.35) | 0.00 (0.00, 1.04) | 0.66 |
| % Strut with ISA | 0.10 ± 0.45 | 0.24 ± 0.65 | 0.19 |
| Mean ISA area, overall (mm²) | 0.00 (0.00, 0.00) | 0.00 (0.00, 0.00) | 0.24 |
| Mean ISA area, ISA location (mm²) | 0.85 ± 0.75* | 0.74 ± 0.74** | 0.81 |
| Lesion with ISA | 6 (7.8%) | 6 (15.8%) | 0.19 |
| Lesion with persistent ISA | 3 (3.9%)*** | 4 (10.5%) | 0.17 |
| Lesion with late acquired ISA | 2 (2.6%)*** | 2 (5.3%) | 0.47 |
| Covered struts (%) | 100.00 (99.42, 100.00) | 100.00 (99.69, 100.00) | 0.44 |
| Lesion with ≥1 uncovered struts | 26 (33.8%) | 10 (26.3%) | 0.42 |
| Lesion with ≥1 covered and malapposed struts | 6 (7.8%) | 6 (15.8%) | 0.19 |
| Lesion with ≥1 uncovered and malapposed struts | 1 (1.3%) | 0 (0.0%) | 0.48 |
| **Strut level analysis** | (N = 13469) | (N = 8264) | |
| ISA strut | 17 (0.12%) | 16 (0.19%) | 0.22 |
| Persistent ISA | 7 (0.05%) | 10 (0.12%) | 0.077 |
| Late acquired ISA | 9 (0.07%) | 6 (0.07%) | 0.88 |
| Uncovered struts | 77 (0.6%) | 33 (0.4%) | 0.08 |
| Covered and malapposed struts | 16 (0.1%) | 16 (0.2%) | 0.16 |
| Uncovered and malapposed struts | 1 (0.0%) | 0 (0.0%) | 0.43 |

*Note:* Data area expressed as mean ± SD, median (interquartile range), or number [percentage].

*Abbreviations:* BVS = bioresorbable vascular scaffold; CoCr-EES = cobalt-chromium everolimus-eluting stent; ISA = incomplete strut apposition; OCT = optical coherence tomography.

* N = 66; ** N = 39; *** N = 76.

2 years in approximately a quarter of the BVS arm, although there was no acute strut disruption at postprocedure OCT. However, the majority of such struts was well covered and apposed (Table 6.5.5). In only three cases, such struts were uncovered and malapposed (Figure 6.5.3c). There were no adverse events associated with these findings.

## DISCUSSION

In the ABSORB Japan randomized trial, the ABSORB BVS was comparable to the CoCr-EES for the primary clinical endpoint of 12-month TLF. The BVS was also demonstrated to be comparable for the major secondary angiographic endpoint of in-segment LLL at 13 months. Other important findings included the low incidence of ID-TLR at 12 months and angiographic in-segment DS and binary restenosis at 13 months with the BVS, similar to that with the CoCr-EES, despite smaller in-device MLD and DS immediately after the BVS procedure. Safety measures with BVS, including the rates of death, MI (all and peri-procedural), and ST, occurred with similar frequency as with CoCr-EES, a DESs with an excellent safety record [10].

In the ABSORB Japan, the 12-month rate of definite/probable ST was 1.5% with both the BVS and CoCr-EES. The observed ST rate in the BVS arm in this study is consistent with recently published BVS studies, while the ST rate in the CoCr-EES arm was somewhat higher than expected, given enrolment of mostly noncomplex lesions [11–13]. This observation was likely due to chance given the low rates of ST with wide confidence intervals (0.4%–3.9% for the BVS and 0.2%–5.3% for the CoCr-EES). However, pooled analysis of the four ABSORB trials (ABSORB II, ABSORB Japan, ABSORB 3, and ABSORB China) suggested higher 1-year ST risk of the BVS relative to the CoCr-EES [14]. Patients with scaffold thrombosis tended to have device implants in small vessels (<2.5 mm in diameter), and had small postprocedure in-device MLDs (all <2.5 mm). Although the BVSs did not have a greater rate of ST than the CoCr-EESs in small vessels in the present study, smaller final in-device MLD in concert with the larger strut thickness of BVSs compared with newer generation metallic DESs might contribute to a greater propensity for ST. Therefore, improving BVS implantation strategy and technique to ensure a 1:1 ratio of BVS to artery diameter, and optimizing BVS expansion with aggressive predilatation and postdilatation to achieve optimal scaffold expansion may improve outcomes [15,16]. Furthermore, due to early concerns of strut fracture, investigators conservatively chose postdilatation balloon diameters [17]. It has since been learned that strut fracture will not occur if the postdilatation balloon is not sized >0.5 mm larger than the BVS scaffold diameter, regardless of pressure [18]. Use of intravascular imaging guidance to ensure optimal scaffold expansion, freedom from edge dissections, and residual disease may also improve device safety. Finally, development of a next generation BVS with thinner struts is underway, and is expected to further improve outcomes [19].

At 2-year follow-up, there was no significant difference in TLF rates between the BVS and CoCr-EES arms. However, there was a numerical excess of VLST between 1 year and 2 years in the BVS arm as compared with the CoCr-EES arm (4 patients [1.6%] and 0 patients [0%]). There is a scarcity of data on VLST stemming from the randomized trials, except for the ABSORB II trial that showed 2-year definite VLST rates of 0.6% in the BVS arm and 0% in the CoCr-EES arm. Among the BVS registries reporting outcomes beyond 1 year, the reported VLST rate was ranging 0.6%–0.8% [16,20], which might be slightly higher than those for CoCr-EES (approximately 0.2%) [21,22]. The results from the future pooled analyses of the randomized trials are warranted to provide further insights on the VLST risk of BVSs relative to metallic DESs.

In the four VLST cases, the scaffolds were widely patent at 1-year angiographic follow-up, suggesting that the occurrence of VLST could relate to the structural abnormalities undetectable on angiography. In three cases, OCT at the time of or shortly after VLST demonstrated strut discontinuities, malapposition, and/or uncovered struts (intraluminal dismantling). These findings are in line with the previous reports by Karanosos et al. and Räber et al. demonstrating that incomplete lesion coverage, malapposition, strut discontinuities, and underexpansion of the scaffold were frequently observed by OCT in patients presenting with definite BVS VLST [16,23]. The causal relationship of such OCT abnormalities and VLST, however, still remains undetermined. First, after the mechanical integrity of the scaffold disappears at 6 months after implantation, the scaffold structure becomes malleable so that wiring, thrombus aspiration, ballooning, or imaging procedure could induce strut discontinuities or malapposition [24]. Second, single OCT imaging only at the time of event could not differentiate the persistent acute disruption/malapposition and late acquired discontinuities. In general, late discontinuities occur frequently as part of a programmed process of bioresorption [24]. The question remains whether the late discontinuities are bystander findings or the cause of the late event, and if so, what is the trigger to induce VLST. Of note, VLST did not occur in the OCT-1 subgroup where postimplantation OCT was performed. Healing responses at 2 years was excellent with very rare uncovered and malapposed strut discontinuities in the OCT-1 group. The role of postprocedure OCT in preventing VLST should be evaluated in the future investigation. Recently, Mangiameli et al. reported a case of OCT-defined neoatherosclerosis observed in the BVS scaffold [25]. However, the healing responses in the OCT-1 subgroup were good and similar in both the BVS and CoCr-EES arms with almost complete strut coverage, minimal ISA, and homogenous in-device tissue growth, suggesting that VLST may not be due to ubiquitous adverse responses including neoatherosclerosis in the advanced bioresorption process of the scaffolds. Further studies are mandatory to investigate the VLST risk of BVS relative to metallic DESs, and the underlying mechanisms of BVS VLST.

# REFERENCES

1. Ormiston JA, Serruys PW, Regar E, Dudek D, Thuesen L, Webster MW, Onuma Y et al. A bioabsorbable everolimus-eluting coronary stent system for patients with single de-novo coronary artery lesions (ABSORB): A prospective open-label trial. *Lancet.* 2008;371:899–907.

2. Serruys PW, Onuma Y, Garcia-Garcia HM, Muramatsu T, van Geuns RJ, de Bruyne B, Dudek D et al. Dynamics of vessel wall changes following the implantation of the absorb everolimus eluting bioresorbable vascular scaffold: A multi-imaging modality study at 6, 12, 24 and 36 months. *EuroIntervention.* 2014;9:1271–1284.

3. Simsek C, Karanasos A, Magro M, Garcia-Garcia HM, Onuma Y, Regar E, Boersma E et al. Long-term invasive follow-up of the everolimus-eluting bioresorbable vascular scaffold: Five-year results of multiple invasive imaging modalities. *EuroIntervention.* 2016;11:996–1003.

4. Kimura T, Morimoto T, Nakagawa Y, Kawai K, Miyazaki S, Muramatsu T, Shiode N et al. Very late stent thrombosis and late target lesion revascularization after sirolimus-eluting stent implantation: Five-year outcome of the j-cypher registry. *Circulation.* 2012;125:584–591.

5. Kimura T, Kozuma K, Tanabe K, Nakamura S, Yamane M, Muramatsu T, Saito S et al. A randomized trial evaluating everolimus-eluting Absorb bioresorbable scaffolds vs. everolimus-eluting metallic stents in patients with coronary artery disease: ABSORB Japan. *Eur Heart J.* 2015;36:3332–3342.

6. Onuma Y, Kimura T, *EuroIntervention* 2016 planned for publication simultaneously with ESC presentation.

7. Farrington CP, Manning G. Test statistics and sample size formulae for comparative binomial trials with null hypothesis of non-zero risk difference or non-unity relative risk. *Stat Med.* 1990;9:1447–1454.

8. Nakatani S, Sotomi Y, Ishibashi Y, Grundeken M, Tateishi H, Tenekecioglu E, Zeng Y et al. Comparative analysis method of permanent metallic stents (XIENCE) and bioresorbable poly-L-lactide (PLLA) scaffolds (Absorb) on optical coherence tomography at baseline and follow-up. *EuroIntervention.* 2015;11.

9. Raber L, Onuma Y, Brugaletta S, Garcia-Garcia HM, Backx B, Iniguez A, Jensen LO et al. Arterial healing following primary PCI using the Absorb everolimus-eluting bioresorbable vascular scaffold (Absorb BVS) versus the durable polymer everolimus-eluting metallic stent (XIENCE) in patients with acute ST-elevation myocardial infarction: Rationale and design of the randomised TROFI II study. *EuroIntervention.* 2015;11.

10. Palmerini T, Biondi-Zoccai G, Della Riva D, Stettler C, Sangiorgi D, D'Ascenzo F, Kimura T et al. Stent thrombosis with drug-eluting and bare-metal stents: Evidence from a comprehensive network meta-analysis. *Lancet.* 2012;379:1393–1402.

11. Kimura T, Morimoto T, Natsuaki M, Shiomi H, Igarashi K, Kadota K, Tanabe K et al. Comparison of everolimus-eluting and sirolimus-eluting coronary stents: 1-year outcomes from the randomized evaluation of sirolimus-eluting versus everolimus-eluting stent trial (RESET). *Circulation.* 2012;126:1225–1236.

12. Capodanno D, Gori T, Nef H, Latib A, Mehilli J, Lesiak M, Caramanno G et al. Percutaneous coronary intervention with everolimus-eluting bioresorbable vascular scaffolds in routine clinical practice: Early and midterm outcomes from the European multicentre GHOST-EU registry. *EuroIntervention.* 2015;10:1144–1153.

13. Brugaletta S, Gori T, Low AF, Tousek P, Pinar E, Gomez-Lara J, Scalone G et al. Absorb bioresorbable vascular scaffold versus everolimus-eluting metallic stent in ST-segment elevation myocardial infarction: 1-year results of a propensity score matching comparison: The BVS-EXAMINATION Study (bioresorbable vascular scaffold-a clinical evaluation of everolimus eluting coronary stents in the treatment of patients with ST-segment elevation myocardial infarction). *J Am Coll Cardiol Intv.* 2015;8:189–197.

14. Stone GW, Gao R, Kimura T, Kereiakes DJ, Ellis SG, Onuma Y, Cheong WF et al. 1-year outcomes with the Absorb bioresorbable scaffold in patients with coronary artery disease: A patient-level, pooled meta-analysis. *Lancet.* 2016;387:1277–1289.

15. Tamburino C, Latib A, van Geuns RJ, Sabate M, Mehilli J, Gori T, Achenbach S et al. Contemporary practice and technical aspects in coronary intervention with bioresorbable scaffolds: A European perspective. *EuroIntervention.* 2015;11:45–52.

16. Puricel S, Cuculi F, Weissner M, Schmermund A, Jamshidi P, Nyffenegger T, Binder H et al. Bioresorbable coronary scaffold thrombosis: Multicenter comprehensive analysis of clinical presentation, mechanisms, and predictors. *J Am Coll Cardiol.* 2016;67:921–931.

17. Gomez-Lara J, Radu M, Brugaletta S, Farooq V, Diletti R, Onuma Y, Windecker S et al. Serial analysis of the malapposed and uncovered struts of the new generation of everolimus-eluting bioresorbable scaffold with optical coherence tomography. *JACC Cardiovasc Interv.* 2011;4:992–1001.

18. Ormiston JA, Webber B, Ubod B, Darremont O, Webster MW. An independent bench comparison of two bioresorbable drug-eluting coronary scaffolds (Absorb and DESolve) with a durable metallic drug-eluting stent (ML8/Xpedition). *EuroIntervention.* 2015;11:60–67.

19. Wiebe J, Bauer T, Dorr O, Mollmann H, Ham CW, Nef HM. Implantation of a novolimus-eluting bioresorbable scaffold with a strut thickness of 100 µm showing evidence of self-correction. *EuroIntervention*. 2015;11:204.

20. Karanasos A, Van Mieghem N, van Ditzhuijzen N, Felix C, Daemen J, Autar A, Onuma Y et al. Angiographic and optical coherence tomography insights into bioresorbable scaffold thrombosis: Single-center experience. *Circ Cardiovasc Interv*. 2015;8.

21. de la Torre Hernandez JM, Alfonso F, Gimeno F, Diarte JA, Lopez-Palop R, Perez de Prado A, Rivero F et al. Thrombosis of second-generation drug-eluting stents in real practice results from the multicenter Spanish registry ESTROFA-2 (Estudio Espanol Sobre Trombosis de Stents Farmacoactivos de Segunda Generacion-2). *JACC Cardiovasc Interv*. 2010;3:911–919.

22. Raber L, Magro M, Stefanini GG, Kalesan B, van Domburg RT, Onuma Y, Wenaweser P et al. Very late coronary stent thrombosis of a newer-generation everolimus-eluting stent compared with early-generation drug-eluting stents: A prospective cohort study. *Circulation*. 2012;125:1110–1121.

23. Raber L, Brugaletta S, Yamaji K, O'Sullivan CJ, Otsuki S, Koppara T, Taniwaki M et al. Very Late Scaffold Thrombosis: Intracoronary Imaging and Histopathological and Spectroscopic Findings. *J Am Coll Cardiol*. 2015;66:1901–1914.

24. Onuma Y, Serruys PW, Muramatsu T, Nakatani S, van Geuns RJ, de Bruyne B, Dudek D et al. Incidence and imaging outcomes of acute scaffold disruption and late structural discontinuity after implantation of the absorb Everolimus-eluting fully bioresorbable vascular scaffold: Optical coherence tomography assessment in the ABSORB cohort B Trial (A Clinical Evaluation of the Bioabsorbable Everolimus Eluting Coronary Stent System in the Treatment of Patients With De Novo Native Coronary Artery Lesions). *JACC Cardiovasc Interv*. 2014;7:1400–1411.

25. Mangiameli A, Ohno Y, Attizzani GF, Capodanno D, Tamburino C. Neoatherosclerosis as the cause of late failure of a bioresorbable vascular scaffold. *JACC Cardiovasc Interv*. 2015;8:633–634.

# What have we learned from meta-analysis of 1-year outcomes with the ABSORB bioresorbable scaffold in patients with coronary artery disease?

YOHEI SOTOMI, CARLOS COLLET, TAKESHI KIMURA, RUNLIN GAO, DEAN J. KEREIAKES,
GREGG W. STONE, STEPHEN G. ELLIS, YOSHINOBU ONUMA, AND PATRICK W.J.C. SERRUYS

## INTRODUCTION

The ABSORB BVSs (Abbott Vascular, Santa Clara, CA; hereafter referred to as BVSs) is a 150 μm thick bioresorbable poly(l-lactide) scaffold with a conformal bioresorbable poly(d,l-lactide) coating (total thickness 7 μm) that elutes everolimus. Randomized trials comparing this device to the XIENCE cobalt-chromium everolimus-eluting stent (CoCr-EESs; Abbott Vascular) were done to support regulatory approval in Europe, Asia, and the United States, and have only recently been reported. These studies were designed to show the noninferiority of the BVSs compared with the CoCr-EESs for 1-year clinical and angiographic outcomes, since improved results with the BVSs compared with drug-eluting stents are not expected to become evident until 3–5 years after implantation. However, none of these trials were powered to exclude small differences in composite adverse event rates between devices, or to detect differences in rarely occurring safety endpoints, and their outcomes according to specific patient and lesion characteristics. Currently, several meta-analyses have been published [1–7]. In this chapter, we present the summary of what we have learned from these meta-analyses.

## DIFFERENT META-ANALYTIC APPROACH

As of August 2016, seven meta-analyses comparing BVSs with drug eluting stents (DESs), mainly CoCr-EESs, are available. A summary of these seven meta-analyses is depicted in Table 6.6.1. All meta-analyses except for the ones by Stone et al. and by Kang et al. are standard study-level meta-analyses. The meta-analysis by Stone et al. is patient level, while the meta-analysis by Kang et al. is study level but with the Bayesian design. Three meta-analyses included both randomized controlled trials and observational studies [3,6,7], whereas the other four meta-analyses included only randomized controlled trials [1,2,4,5]. The results of these meta-analyses need to be interpreted with great caution for the following reasons [8]. First, the results of each meta-analysis have not been uniformly reported for all the potential endpoints of interest. Target vessel myocardial infarction was significantly increased in the BVSs arm compared to the CoCr-EESs arm, although this endpoint was reported only in the meta-analyses from Stone et al. and Lipinski et al. Second, the available follow-up was shorter in the meta-analysis of Lipinski et al., and last in some cases there was a variation in endpoint definitions (i.e., myocardial infarction as opposed to target-vessel myocardial infarction; target lesion revascularization as opposed to ischemia-driven target lesion revascularization). Consistent findings across all meta-analyses were comparable all-cause death and patient oriented composite endpoint, and the approximately twofold increase in definite or probable device thrombosis with the BVSs, which was significant in four out of seven studies.

In contrast to the study level analyses, a patient-level, pooled meta-analysis from Stone et al. offers three important advantages: time-to-event curves (and landmark analysis)

Table 6.6.1 Summary of currently available meta-analyses

| Meta-analysis | Type | Patient number | Included trials | Risk estimates of clinical endpoints: BVSs vs. others | | | | | | | | |
| | | | | Odd ratio [95% confidence interval] | | | | | | | | |
| | | | | All cause death | Cardiac death | PoCE | DoCE | All MI | TVMI | TVR | TLR | Definite or probable ScT |
| --- | --- | --- | --- | --- | --- | --- | --- | --- | --- | --- | --- | --- |
| Stone et al. [1] | Patient level analysis | BVSs 2164 pts vs. CoCr-EESs 1225 pts | ABSORB China, ABSORB II, ABSORB III, ABSORB Japan | 1.12 [0.47-2.69] | 1.26 [0.33-4.82] | 1.09 [0.89-1.34] | 1.22 [0.91-1.64] | 1.34 [0.97-1.85] | 1.45 [1.02-2.07] | 1.14 [0.80-1.62] | 1.14 [0.73-1.79] | 2.09 [0.92-4.75] |
| Cassese et al. [2] | Study level analysis | BVSs 2337 pts vs. CoCr-EESs 1401 pts | ABSORB China, ABSORB II, ABSORB III, ABSORB Japan, EVERBIO II, TROFI II | 0.95 [0.45-2.00] | NA | NA | 1.20 [0.90-1.60] | 1.36 [0.98-1.89] | NA | NA | 0.97 [0.66-1.43] | 1.99 [1.00-3.98] |
| Banach et al. [3] | Study level analysis | BVSs 3000 pts vs. DESs 2483 pts vs. BMSs 290 pts | BVSs-RAI, Costopoulos et al., EVERBIO II, ABSORB II, Gori et al., BVSs-EXAMINATION, ABSORB Japan, Muramatsu et al. ABSORB III, ABSORB China | 0.71 [0.39-1.29] | 1.00 [0.52-1.94] | 0.91 [0.68-1.22] | 1.12 [0.87-1.46] | 1.36 [1.00-1.85] | 1.44 [1.02-2.04] | 0.99 [0.74-1.33] | 0.92 [0.66-1.28] | NA |
| Bangalore et al. [4] | Study level analysis | BVSs 2337 pts vs. CoCr-EESs 1401 pts | ABSORB China, ABSORB II, ABSORB III, ABSORB Japan, EVERBIO II, TROFI II | 1.11 [0.53-2.33] | 1.39 (0.43-4.43) | NA | NA | 1.35 [0.98-1.86] | NA | 1.00 [0.74-1.35] | 1.06 [0.73-1.54] | 2.11 [0.99-4.47] |
| Kang et al. [5] | Bayesian network meta-analysis | BVSs 2332 pts vs. CoCr-EESs 29649 pts vs. other DESs 82548 vs. BMSs 11986 | 147 Randomized clinical trials | 1.13 [0.52-2.73] | 1.39 [0.43-5.46] | NA | NA | 1.44 [0.99-2.13] | NA | 1.03 [0.71-1.49] | 1.08 [0.63-1.84] | 2.28 [1.07-6.29] |
| Lipinski et al. [6] | Study level analysis | BVSs 1948 pts vs. DESs 2150 pts | ABSORB II, EVERBIO II, ABSORB EXTEND, BVSs EXAMINATION, BVSs-RAI, Costopoulos et al., Gori et al., Mattesini et al., PRAGUE-19 | 0.40 [0.15-1.06] | 0.80 [0.40-1.59] | 0.87 [0.66-1.16] | NA | 2.06 [1.31-3.22] | NA | 0.77 [0.48-1.25] | 0.87 [0.59-1.28] | 2.06 [1.07-3.98] |
| Mukete et al. [7] | Study level analysis | BVSs 3263 pts vs. CoCr-EESs 2325 pts | ABSORB China, ABSORB II, ABSORB III, ABSORB Japan, BVSs EXAMINATION, ABSORB Extend | NA | 1.14 [0.54-2.39] | NA | 1.19 [0.94-1.52] | 1.63 [1.18-2.25] | NA | NA | 0.98 [0.69-1.40] | 2.10 [1.13-3.87] |

Abbreviations: BMSs = bare metal stents; BVSs = ABSORB bioresorbable vascular scaffolds; CoCr-EESs = XIENCE cobalt-chromium everolimus-eluting stents; DESs = drug eluting stents; NA = not available; ScT = scaffold thrombosis.

can be generated to elucidate the temporal sequence of events; multivariable analyses can be done to ascertain the individual predictors of outcomes; and the consistency of treatment effects can be analyzed in clinically relevant subgroups. In this chapter, we focus on the insights from the patient-level pooled meta-analysis from Stone et al. [1].

## RESULTS FROM THE PATIENT-LEVEL POOLED META-ANALYSIS

In the four prospective randomized controlled trials, ABSORB China, ABSORB II, ABSORB III, and ABSORB Japan, a total of 3389 patients were enrolled at 301 centers from North America, Europe, and the Asia-Pacific region, of whom 2164 were randomly assigned to the BVSs and 1225 to the CoCr-EESs. One-year follow-up was complete in 3355 (99%) of 3389 patients. It is important to note that the lesion complexity evaluated in these four trials was limited, which is typical for the pivotal trials of coronary stents/scaffolds. Although this patient level meta-analysis did not include the EVERBIO II and TROFI II trials, this fact is less relevant due to their small numbers and the confirmation of findings by a sensitivity analysis [1]. Aspirin (BVSs 98.3% [2084/2119] vs. CoCr-EESs 97.5% [1173/1203], $p = 0.09$), adenosine diphosphate antagonist (BVSs 95.4% [2022/2120] vs. CoCr-EESs 95.6% [1147/1200], $p = 0.78$), and combined dual anti-platelet therapy use (BVSs 94.0% [1990/2116] vs. CoCr-EESs 93.8% [1126/1200], $p = 0.81$) were similar between the groups, although the more potent agents ticagrelor and prasugrel were used more frequently with BVSs than with CoCr-EESs (BVSs 18.8% [398/2120] vs. CoCr-EESs 14.8% [178/1200], $p = 0.004$). The number of events in the pooled device groups and the summary meta-analysis statistics for 21 ischemic endpoints are shown in Table 6.6.2. Figure 6.6.1 shows selected time-to-event Kaplan–Meier curves. The summary treatment effect for the 1-year relative rates of the patient-oriented composite endpoint of death, myocardial infarction, or revascularization did not differ significantly between BVSs and CoCr-EESs (Relative Risk [RR] 1.09 [95% CI 0.89–1.34], $p = 0.38$). Similarly, the 1-year relative rates of the device-oriented composite endpoint (target lesion failure) did not differ between the two devices (RR 1.22 [95% CI 0.91–1.64], $p = 0.17$). However, target lesion failure tended to be higher with BVSs than with CoCr-EESs within 30 days, whereas target lesion failure rates were similar between the two devices between 30 days and 1 year. The relative rates of cardiac and all-cause mortality and all myocardial infarction (including periprocedural or nonperiprocedural myocardial infarction, and nontarget vessel-related myocardial infarction) did not differ significantly between the two devices, although target vessel-related myocardial infarction was greater with the BVSs than with the CoCr-EESs. Definite or probable device thrombosis at 1 year was slightly more common with the BVSs than with the CoCr-EE, although this difference was not statistically significant. Effectiveness measures, including ischemia-driven target lesion revascularization, ischemia-driven target vessel

revascularization, and all revascularization, occurred at similar frequency in the BVSs and CoCr-EESs groups. No significant heterogeneity between the four studies was present for any of the assessed endpoints. The main study-level treatment effects were similar in a sensitivity analysis in which the TROFI II and EVERBIO II trials were added to the four ABSORB trials [1].

Subgroup analysis for the 1-year relative rates of the patient-oriented composite endpoint demonstrated no significant interactions between treatment effects and most subgroups, except for diabetes (CoCr-EESs tended to perform better in nondiabetic patients, but not in diabetic patients) and reference vessel diameter (CoCr-EESs tended to perform better in larger vessels but not in smaller vessels; Figure 6.6.2). Subgroup analysis for the 1-year relative rates of the device-oriented composite endpoint of target lesion failure demonstrated no significant interactions between treatment effects and most subgroups, except for American College of Cardiology–American Heart Association lesion class (CoCr-EESs tended to perform better in noncomplex A/B1 lesions but not in more complex B2/C lesions; Figure 6.6.3). Since the subgroup analysis was inherently underpowered, and interaction testing was not adjusted for multiple comparisons, all subgroup findings should be regarded as hypothesis-generating. However, the subgroup analysis implicated a disparity of efficacy of BVSs in some specific populations. Several subgroups with significant interactions should be evaluated in further clinical studies.

The most important finding of the patient-level pooled meta-analysis is that the 1-year rates of the patient-oriented composite endpoint of death, myocardial infarction, or revascularization were similar with BVSs and CoCr-EESs. The 1-year rates of the device-oriented composite endpoint of cardiac death, target vessel-related myocardial infarction, or ischemia-driven target lesion revascularization also did not differ significantly with BVSs and CoCr-EESs. These outcomes were similar after multivariable adjustment for small differences in baseline variables, and when the TROFI II and EVERBIO II trials were included. Patient-related and device-related treatment effects were consistent across most clinically relevant subgroups analyzed. These findings therefore provide reassurance that overall patient-related and device-related outcomes within the first year are not substantially compromised with use of BVSs. These results are especially noteworthy because the comparator device in the four trials was the CoCr-EESs, which is the metallic drug-eluting stent associated with the lowest rate of stent thrombosis and greatest freedom from adverse events [9]. Additionally, the BVSs was used for the first time by most of the investigators in these studies, and historically interventional device-related outcomes have improved over time with increasing experience.

Nonetheless, some differences between devices were evident that warrant discussion. In particular, although overall rates of myocardial infarction were not significantly increased with BVSs, target vessel-related myocardial infarction occurred more frequently with the BVSs than

Table 6.6.2 Summary for all ischemic endpoints from patient-level pooled meta-analysis

| | BVSs (n = 2164) | CoCr-EESs (n = 1225) | Fixed-effects RR (95% CI) | p value | I² | p value for heterogeneity |
|---|---|---|---|---|---|---|
| Patient-oriented composite endpoint (mortality, myocardial infarction, or revascularization) | 255/2147 (11.9%) | 129/1212 (10.6%) | 1.09 (0.89–1.34) | 0.38 | 5.1% | 0.37 |
| Device-oriented composite endpoint (target lesion failure) | 141/2147 (6.6%) | 63/1212 (5.2%) | 1.22 (0.91–1.64) | 0.17 | 0% | 0.78 |
| Early (0–30 days) | 89/2154 (4.1%) | 32/1222 (2.6%) | 1.49 (1.00–2.22) | 0.051 | 0% | 0.91 |
| Late (30 days–1 year; landmark) | 53/2140 (2.5%) | 31/1211 (2.6%) | 0.97 (0.62–1.51) | 0.9 | 0% | 0.84 |
| All-cause mortality | 17/2147 (0.8%) | 9/1212 (0.7%) | 1.12 (0.47–2.69) | 0.8 | NA | NA |
| Cardiac | 8/2147 (0.4%) | 4/1212 (0.3%) | 1.26 (0.33–4.82) | 0.74 | NA | NA |
| Non-cardiac | 9/2147 (0.4%) | 5/1212 (0.4%) | 1.02 (0.32–3.25) | 0.97 | NA | NA |
| All myocardial infarction | 123/2147 (5.7%) | 49/1212 (4.0%) | 1.34 (0.97–1.85) | 0.08 | 0% | 0.71 |
| Peri-procedural (ABSORB III definition) | 62/2126 (2.9%) | 26/1196 (2.2%) | 1.29 (0.82–2.03) | 0.27 | 0% | 0.75 |
| Peri-procedural (SCAI definition) | 16/2126 (0.8%) | 9/1196 (0.8%) | 0.97 (0.44–2.14) | 0.94 | 0% | 0.63 |
| Non-peri-procedural (ABSORB III definition) | 61/2144 (2.8%) | 22/1211 (1.8%) | 1.48 (0.91–2.40) | 0.11 | 0% | 0.93 |
| Target vessel-related myocardial infarction | 110/2147 (5.1%) | 40/1212 (3.3%) | 1.45 (1.02–2.07) | 0.04 | 0% | 0.8 |
| Non-target vessel-related myocardial infarction | 15/2147 (0.7%) | 11/1212 (0.9%) | 0.75 (0.34–1.66) | 0.48 | 0% | 0.94 |
| All revascularization | 169/2147 (7.9%) | 93/1212 (7.7%) | 1.02 (0.80–1.30) | 0.89 | 21.9% | 0.28 |
| Ischaemia-driven target lesion revascularization | 57/2147 (2.7%) | 28/1212 (2.3%) | 1.14 (0.73–1.79) | 0.56 | 0% | 0.91 |
| Ischaemia-driven target vessel revascularization | 92/2147 (4.3%) | 45/1212 (3.7%) | 1.14 (0.80–1.62) | 0.47 | 11.2% | 0.34 |
| Device thrombosis (definite or probable) | 28/2130 (1.3%) | 7/1204 (0.6%) | 2.09 (0.92–4.75) | 0.08 | 0% | 0.4 |
| Definite | 24/2130 (1.1%) | 6/1204 (0.5%) | 2.06 (0.85–5.03) | 0.11 | 0% | 0.84 |
| Probable | 4/2130 (0.2%) | 1/1204 (0.1%) | 2.28 (0.28–18.51) | 0.44 | NA | NA |
| Early (0–30 days) | 20/2152 (0.9%) | 6/1221 (0.5%) | 1.76 (0.72–4.34) | 0.22 | 0% | 0.7 |
| Late (30 days–1 year; landmark) | 8/2128 (0.4%) | 1/1204 (0.1%) | 4.10 (0.52–32.56) | 0.18 | NA | NA |

Note: Data are n/N (%); the denominator in each cell is the number of eligible patients (1-year follow-up or earlier event).
Abbreviations: BVSs = ABSORB bioresorbable vascular scaffolds; CoCr-EESs = XIENCE cobalt-chromium everolimus-eluting stents; NA = not applicable (cannot test for heterogeneity because no events were present in one cell in three of the four trials); RR = risk ratio; SCAI = Society of Cardiovascular Angiography and Interventions.

with the CoCr-EESs, due in part to nonsignificant increases in periprocedural myocardial infarction and device thrombosis with the BVSs. However, most periprocedural myocardial infarctions are not prognostically important [10], and clinically relevant large periprocedural myocardial infarction according to the Society of Cardiac Angiography and Interventions criteria occurred in only 0.8% of patients with each device. Although not significant, a 0.6% absolute increase in definite device thrombosis contributed to the 1.0% absolute difference in non-periprocedural target

vessel-related myocardial infarctions with the BVSs compared with the CoCr-EESs, with the remainder attributed to target vessel-related myocardial infarctions not related to device thrombosis. Device and procedure success rates were also somewhat lower with the BVSs than with the CoCr-EESs. Both greater strut thickness and postprocedural in-device diameter stenosis following BVSs versus CoCr-EESs might have contributed to these target vessel myocardial infarction-related events. Improved procedural technique with the BVSs (more aggressive plaque modification before BVSs

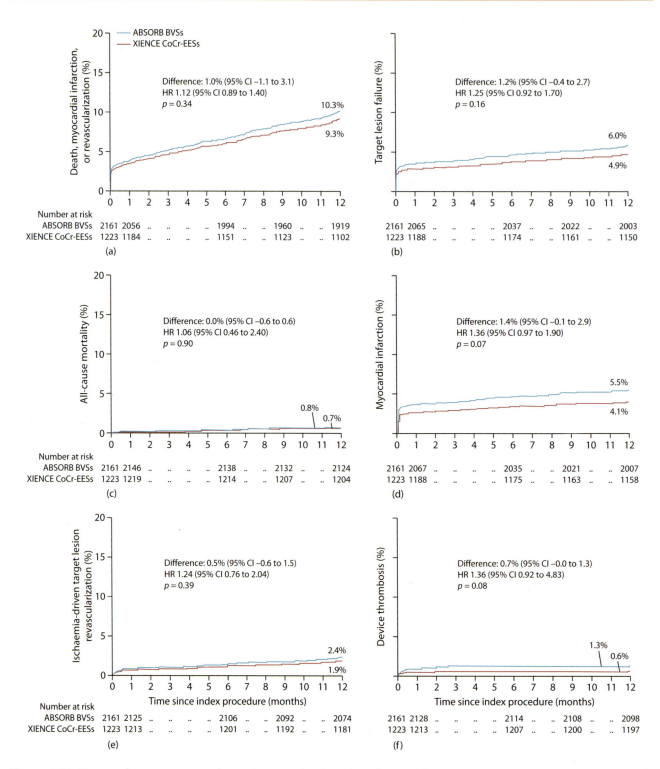

**Figure 6.6.1** Time-to-first event curves for patients randomly assigned to ABSORB BVSs versus XIENCE CoCr-EESs. **(a)** The patient-oriented composite endpoint of death, myocardial infarction, or any revascularization. **(b)** The device-oriented composite endpoint of target lesion failure (cardiac death, target vessel myocardial infarction, or ischemia-driven target lesion revascularization). **(c)** All-cause mortality. **(d)** All myocardial infarction. **(e)** Ischemia-driven target lesion revascularization. **(f)** Device thrombosis (definite or probable). Note that follow-up is censored at the time of first event or at last follow-up or at exactly 12 months (whichever occurred later). BVSs = bioresorbable vascular scaffold; CoCr-EESs = cobalt-chromium everolimus-eluting stent; HR = hazard ratio. (Reprinted from *Lancet*, 387(10025), Stone et al., 1277–1289. Copyright 2016, with permission from Elsevier.)

| % (n/N) | ABSORB BVSs (n = 2164) | XIENCE CoCr-EESs (n = 1225) | 1-year patient-oriented composite endpoint risk ratio (95% CI) | Relative risk (95% CI) | $P_{interaction}$ |
|---|---|---|---|---|---|
| **Age (years)** | | | | | 0.86 |
| <63 (median) | 47.6% (1610/3384) | 11.5% (115/1002) | 10.3% (61/591) | 1.06 (0.79–1.42) | |
| ≥63 (median) | 52.4% (1774/3384) | 12.2% (140/1145) | 11.0% (68/621) | 1.12 (0.86–1.48) | |
| **Sex** | | | | | 0.79 |
| Female | 27.5% (932/3384) | 12.9% (76/589) | 11.0% (37/335) | 1.14 (0.79–1.65) | |
| Male | 72.5% (2452/3384) | 11.5% (179/1558) | 10.5% (92/877) | 1.08 (0.85–1.37) | |
| **Diabetes** | | | | | 0.03 |
| Present | 30.1% (1019/3382) | 13.8% (89/647) | 16.3% (59/363) | 0.84 (0.62–1.13) | |
| Absent | 69.9% (2363/3382) | 11.0% (165/1498) | 8.2% (70/849) | 1.32 (1.01–1.73) | |
| **Previous cardiac intervention** | | | | | 0.76 |
| Yes | 33.7% (1140/3382) | 14.5% (108/746) | 13.6% (52/382) | 1.06 (0.78–1.44) | |
| No | 66.3% (2242/3382) | 10.5% (147/1401) | 9.2% (76/828) | 1.13 (0.87–1.47) | |
| **Presentation** | | | | | 0.36 |
| Acute coronary syndrome | 32.4% (1097/3383) | 10.8% (71/660) | 10.6% (45/423) | 0.97 (0.68–1.38) | |
| Stable coronary artery disease | 67.6% (2286/3383) | 12.6% (184/1486) | 10.6% (84/789) | 1.17 (0.92–1.50) | |
| **Target lesions (n)** | | | | | 0.29 |
| 1 | 94.8% (3207/3383) | 11.9% (242/2032) | 10.4% (120/1152) | 1.13 (0.92–1.39) | |
| ≥2 | 5.2% (176/3383) | 11.3% (13/115) | 15.0% (9/60) | 0.74 (0.33–1.64) | |
| **P2Y12 loading** | | | | | 0.06 |
| Clopidogrel/ticlopidine | 77.0% (2560/3323) | 11.2% (180/1606) | 10.9% (102/939) | 1.01 (0.80–1.27) | |
| Prasugrel/ticagrelor | 23.0% (763/3323) | 14.1% (72/510) | 8.5% (21/246) | 1.64 (1.04–2.61) | |
| **Reference vessel diameter (mm)** | | | | | 0.045 |
| <2.65 (median) | 50.9% (1716/3372) | 13.0% (144/1108) | 14.1% (84/596) | 0.93 (0.73–1.20) | |
| ≥2.65 (median) | 49.1% (1656/3372) | 10.7% (111/1034) | 7.4% (45/611) | 1.40 (1.00–1.95) | |
| **Minimum luminal diameter (mm)** | | | | | 0.67 |
| <0.93 (median) | 51.4% (1734/3372) | 13.9% (152/1095) | 12.9% (81/627) | 1.07 (0.83–1.38) | |
| ≥0.93 (median) | 48.6% (1638/3372) | 9.8% (103/1046) | 8.3% (48/581) | 1.14 (0.82–1.58) | |
| **Lesion length (mm)** | | | | | 0.99 |
| <12.16 (median) | 48.7% (1643/3371) | 11.9% (124/1040) | 10.6% (62/587) | 1.10 (0.82–1.46) | |
| ≥12.16 (median) | 51.3% (1728/3371) | 11.9% (131/1101) | 10.6% (66/620) | 1.11 (0.84–1.46) | |
| **ACC/AHA lesion class** | | | | | 1.00 |
| B2/C | 68.7% (2320/3376) | 13.1% (191/1455) | 11.7% (100/853) | 1.11 (0.88–1.39) | |
| A/B1 | 31.3% (1056/3376) | 9.3% (64/690) | 8.2% (29/355) | 1.08 (0.71–1.65) | |
| **Left anterior descending coronary artery lesion** | | | | | 0.07 |
| Yes | 47.9% (1619/3383) | 10.3% (107/1040) | 11.2% (64/569) | 0.90 (0.67–1.21) | |
| No | 52.1% (1764/3383) | 13.4% (148/1107) | 10.1% (65/643) | 1.30 (0.99–1.72) | |
| **Lesion calcification** | | | | | 0.99 |
| Moderate/severe | 28.0% (943/3369) | 13.6% (82/605) | 12.3% (41/334) | 1.10 (0.78–1.57) | |
| None/mild | 72.0% (2426/3369) | 11.2% (172/1535) | 10.1% (88/873) | 1.09 (0.85–1.39) | |
| **Bifurcation lesion** | | | | | 0.59 |
| Yes | 35.0% (1178/3368) | 13.1% (96/735) | 10.8% (47/437) | 1.18 (0.85–1.64) | |
| No | 65.0% (2190/3368) | 11.2% (158/1406) | 10.5% (81/768) | 1.05 (0.82–1.36) | |

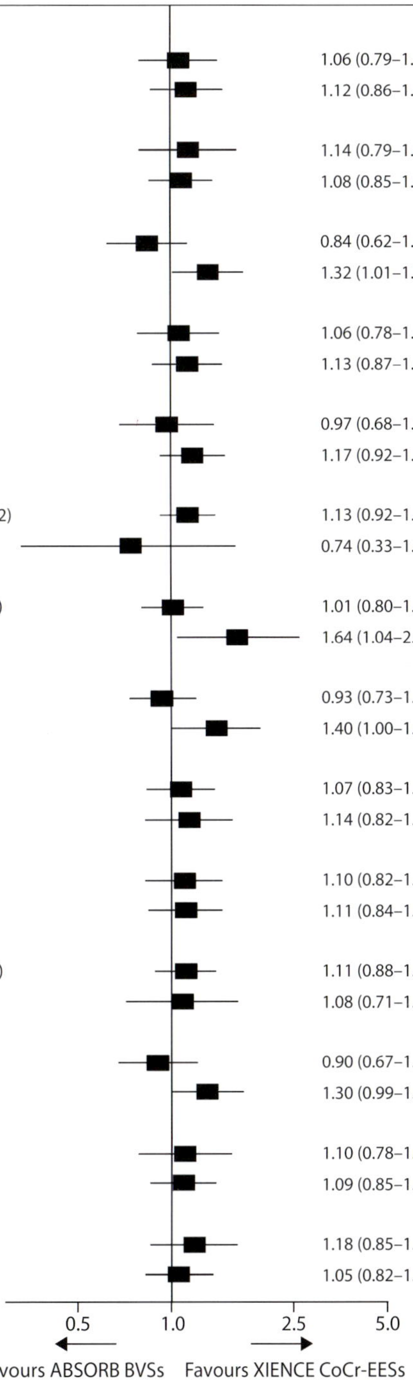

0.5    1.0    2.5    5.0

← Favours ABSORB BVSs    Favours XIENCE CoCr-EESs →

**Figure 6.6.2** Subgroup analyses for the pooled 1-year rates of the patient-oriented composite endpoint of all-cause mortality, all myocardial infarction, or all revascularization in patients randomly assigned to BVSs versus CoCr-EESs. The p value for interaction represents the likelihood of interaction between the variable and the relative treatment effect. ACC = American College of Cardiology; AHA = American Heart Association; BVSs = bioresorbable vascular scaffolds; CoCr-EESs = cobalt-chromium everolimus-eluting stents. (Reprinted from *Lancet*, 387(10025), Stone et al., 1277–1289. Copyright 2016, with permission from Elsevier.)

| | % (n/N) | ABSORB BVSs (n = 2164) | XIENCE CoCr-EESs (n = 1225) | 1-year patient-oriented composite endpoint risk ratio (95% CI) | Relative risk (95% CI) | $p_{interaction}$ |
|---|---|---|---|---|---|---|
| **Age (years)** | | | | | | 0.79 |
| <63 (median) | 47.6% (1610/3384) | 6.3% (63/1002) | 5.1% (30/591) | | 1.16 (0.76–1.78) | |
| ≥63 (median) | 52.4% (1774/3384) | 6.8% (78/1145) | 5.3% (33/621) | | 1.27 (0.86–1.89) | |
| **Sex** | | | | | | 0.79 |
| Female | 27.5% (932/3384) | 7.6% (45/589) | 5.7% (19/335) | | 1.28 (0.76–2.15) | |
| Male | 72.5% (2452/3384) | 6.2% (96/1558) | 5.0% (44/877) | | 1.19 (0.84–1.69) | |
| **Diabetes** | | | | | | 0.13 |
| Present | 30.1% (1019/3382) | 8.2% (53/647) | 8.5% (31/363) | | 0.94 (0.61–1.43) | |
| Absent | 69.9% (2363/3382) | 5.8% (87/1498) | 3.8% (32/849) | | 1.51 (1.01–2.25) | |
| **Previous cardiac intervention** | | | | | | 0.58 |
| Yes | 33.7% (1140/3382) | 8.0% (60/746) | 7.1% (27/382) | | 1.12 (0.73–1.74) | |
| No | 66.3% (2242/3382) | 5.8% (81/1401) | 4.2% (35/828) | | 1.33 (0.90–1.96) | |
| **Presentation** | | | | | | 0.27 |
| Acute coronary syndrome | 32.4% (1097/3383) | 5.5% (36/660) | 5.2% (22/423) | | 0.95 (0.56–1.60) | |
| Stable coronary artery disease | 67.6% (2286/3383) | 7.1% (105/1486) | 5.2% (41/789) | | 1.37 (0.96–1.94) | |
| **Target lesions (n)** | | | | | | 0.84 |
| 1 | 94.8% (3207/3383) | 65% (132/2032) | 5.1% (59/1152) | | 1.24 (0.92–1.67) | |
| ≥2 | 5.2% (176/3383) | 7.8% (9/115) | 6.7% (4/60) | | 1.01 (0.33–3.09) | |
| **P2Y12 loading** | | | | | | 0.26 |
| Clopidogrel/ticlopidine | 77.0% (2560/3323) | 6.4% (102/1606) | 5.3% (50/939) | | 1.15 (0.83–1.60) | |
| Prasugrel/ticagrelor | 23.0% (763/3323) | 7.3% (37/510) | 4.1% (10/246) | | 1.77 (0.90–3.51) | |
| **Reference vessel diameter (mm)** | | | | | | 0.33 |
| <2.65 (median) | 50.9% (1716/3372) | 7.9% (88/1108) | 7.2% (43/596) | | 1.08 (0.76–1.54) | |
| ≥2.65 (median) | 49.1% (1656/3372) | 5.1% (53/1034) | 3.3% (20/611) | | 1.52 (0.91–2.53) | |
| **Minimum luminal diameter (mm)** | | | | | | 0.62 |
| <0.93 (median) | 51.4% (1734/3372) | 7.8% (85/1095) | 6.5% (41/627) | | 1.15 (0.81–1.65) | |
| ≥0.93 (median) | 48.6% (1638/3372) | 5.4% (56/1046) | 3.8% (22/581) | | 1.38 (0.85–2.24) | |
| **Lesion length (mm)** | | | | | | 0.22 |
| <12.16 (median) | 48.7% (1643/3371) | 6.9% (72/1040) | 4.4% (26/587) | | 1.48 (0.96–2.29) | |
| ≥12.16 (median) | 51.3% (1728/3371) | 6.3% (69/1101) | 5.8% (36/620) | | 1.05 (0.71–1.55) | |
| **ACC/AHA lesion class** | | | | | | 0.03 |
| B2/C | 68.7% (2320/3376) | 7.1% (103/1455) | 6.6% (56/853) | | 1.05 (0.77–1.44) | |
| A/B1 | 31.3% (1056/3376) | 5.5% (38/690) | 2.0% (7/355) | | 2.62 (1.18–5.81) | |
| **Left anterior descending coronary artery lesion** | | | | | | 0.07 |
| Yes | 47.9% (1619/3383) | 6.0% (62/1040) | 6.2% (35/569) | | 0.92 (0.62–1.38) | |
| No | 52.1% (1764/3383) | 7.1% (79/1107) | 4.4% (28/643) | | 1.61 (1.06–2.45) | |
| **Lesion calcification** | | | | | | 0.17 |
| Moderate/severe | 28.0% (943/3369) | 7.8% (47/605) | 8.1% (27/334) | | 0.95 (0.61–1.50) | |
| None/mild | 72.0% (2426/3369) | 6.1% (93/1535) | 4.1% (36/873) | | 1.41 (0.97–2.05) | |
| **Bifurcation lesion** | | | | | | 0.93 |
| Yes | 35.0% (1178/3368) | 7.2% (53/735) | 5.7% (25/437) | | 1.21 (0.76–1.92) | |
| No | 65.0% (2190/3368) | 6.3% (88/1406) | 4.9% (38/768) | | 1.22 (0.85–1.77) | |

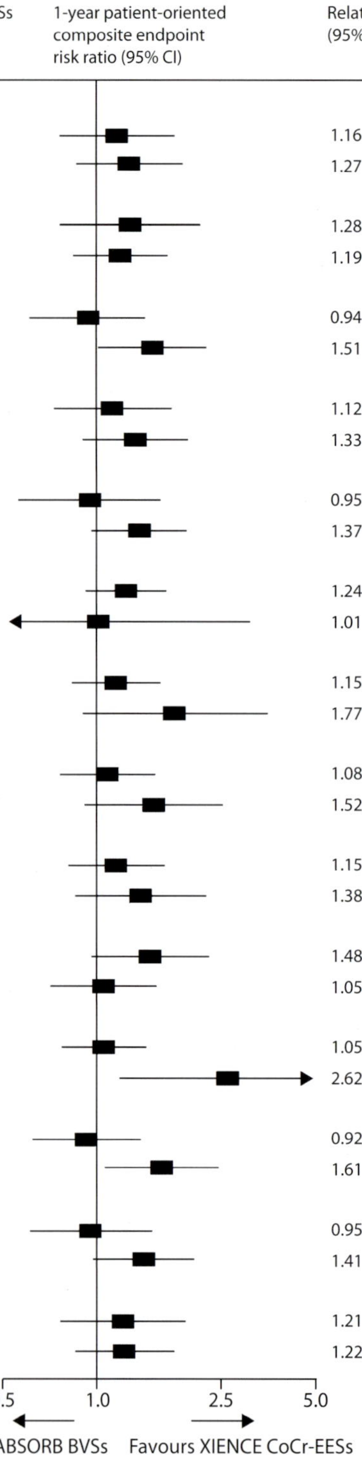

0.5   1.0   2.5   5.0

← Favours ABSORB BVSs    Favours XIENCE CoCr-EESs →

**Figure 6.6.3** Subgroup analyses for the pooled 1-year rates of the device-oriented composite endpoint of target lesion failure (cardiac mortality, target vessel-related myocardial infarction, or ischemia-driven target lesion revascularization) in patients randomly assigned to BVSs versus CoCr-EESs. The p value for interaction represents the likelihood of interaction between the variable and the relative treatment effect. ACC = American College of Cardiology; AHA = American Heart Association; BVSs = bioresorbable vascular scaffolds; CoCr-EESs = cobalt-chromium everolimus-eluting stents. (Reprinted from *Lancet*, 387(10025), Stone et al., 1277–1289. Copyright 2016, with permission from Elsevier.)

implantation, routine high-pressure noncompliant balloon postdilatation to ensure adequate scaffold expansion, and more frequent use of intravascular imaging to optimize lesion coverage and scaffold dimensions) might further reduce thrombosis rates. Nonetheless, neither cardiac nor all-cause mortality were increased with BVSs, and all measures of clinical effectiveness at 1-year were similar with BVSs and CoCr-EESs which is reflective of the similar in-segment luminal dimensions achieved [11]. Combined with the overall similar rates of the patient-oriented composite endpoint and device-oriented composite endpoint, these findings support the safety and effectiveness of BVSs use at 1 year for treatment of patients with stable coronary artery disease and stabilized acute coronary syndromes.

## SCAFFOLD THROMBOSIS

Recently, a systematic review and meta-analysis focusing only on the incidence of scaffold thrombosis in randomized clinical trials and observational studies (59 studies, $n = 16,830$) reported a cumulative rate of acute, subacute, and late definite and probable scaffold thrombosis of 0.4%, 1.1%, and 1.6%, respectively [12]. Of note, in 10 studies ($n = 2331$) with at least 24-months of follow-up, a weighted rate of very late scaffold thrombosis of 1.0% [95% CI 0.6% to 1.5%] was found.

## CONCLUSION

In the present chapter, we overviewed several meta-analyses and one single patient-level meta-analysis. For treatment of simple and moderately complex lesions in patients with stable coronary artery disease and stabilized ACS, the BVSs, compared to the CoCr-EESs, resulted in: (1) similar rates of the patient-oriented and device-oriented composite endpoints, consistent with comparable overall outcomes at 1 year; (2) nonstatistically significant different rates of major safety outcomes, including death, myocardial infarction, and device thrombosis; (3) no significant difference in periprocedural myocardial infarction, but a small increase in target vessel myocardial infarction; (4) comparable measures of efficacy, including ischemia driven-target lesion revascularization, ischemia driven-target vascular revascularization, and all revascularization. The most recent meta-analysis focusing on scaffold thrombosis would remind us of the importance of deep understanding on the mechanisms underlying early, late, and very late scaffold thrombosis. Further investigation with long-term and sequential imaging observation would be warranted.

## REFERENCES

1. Stone GW, Gao R, Kimura T, Kereiakes DJ, Ellis SG, Onuma Y and Cheong WF. 1-year outcomes with the Absorb bioresorbable scaffold in patients with coronary artery disease: A patient-level, pooled meta-analysis. *Lancet (London, England)*. 2016;387:1277–89.

2. Cassese S, Byrne RA, Ndrepepa G, Kufner S, Wiebe J, Repp J, Schunkert H et al. Everolimus-eluting bioresorbable vascular scaffolds versus everolimus-eluting metallic stents: A meta-analysis of randomised controlled trials. *Lancet (London, England)*. 2016;387:537–44.

3. Banach M, Serban MC, Sahebkar A, Garcia-Garcia HM, Mikhailidis DP, Martin SS and Brie D. Comparison of clinical outcomes between bioresorbable vascular stents versus conventional drug-eluting and metallic stents: A systematic review and meta-analysis. *EuroIntervention. Journal of EuroPCR in Collaboration with the Working Group on Interventional Cardiology of the European Society of Cardiology*. 2016;12:e175–89.

4. Bangalore S, Toklu B and Bhatt DL. Outcomes with bioabsorbable vascular scaffolds versus everolimus eluting stents: Insights from randomized trials. *Int J Cardiol*. 2016;212:214–22.

5. Kang SH, Chae IH, Park JJ, Lee HS, Kang DY, Hwang SS, Youn TJ and Kim HS. Stent thrombosis with drug-eluting stents and bioresorbable scaffolds: Evidence from a network meta-analysis of 147 trials. *JACC Cardiovasc Interv*. 2016;9:1203–12.

6. Lipinski MJ, Escarcega RO, Baker NC, Benn HA, Gaglia MA, Jr., Torguson R and Waksman R. Scaffold thrombosis after percutaneous coronary intervention with ABSORB bioresorbable vascular scaffold: A systematic review and meta-analysis. *JACC Cardiovasc Interv*. 2016;9:12–24.

7. Mukete BN, van der Heijden LC, Tandjung K, Baydoun H, Yadav K, Saleh QA, Doggen CJ et al. Safety and efficacy of everolimus-eluting bioresorbable vascular scaffolds versus durable polymer everolimus-eluting metallic stents assessed at 1-year follow-up: A systematic review and meta-analysis of studies. *Int J Cardiol*. 2016;221:1087–1094.

8. Capodanno D. Overlapping meta-analyses of bioresorbable vascular scaffolds versus everolimus-eluting stents: Bringing clarity or confusion? *J Thorac Dis*. 2016;8:1366–1370.

9. Palmerini T, Benedetto U, Biondi-Zoccai G, Della Riva D, Bacchi-Reggiani L, Smits PC, Vlachojannis GJ et al. Long-term safety of drug-eluting and bare-metal stents: Evidence from a comprehensive network meta-analysis. *J Am Coll Cardiol*. 2015;65:2496–507.

10. Moussa ID, Klein LW, Shah B, Mehran R, Mack MJ, Brilakis ES, Reilly JP et al. Consideration of a new definition of clinically relevant myocardial infarction after coronary revascularization: An expert consensus document from the Society for Cardiovascular Angiography and Interventions (SCAI). *J Am Coll Cardiol*. 2013;62:1563–70.

11. Pocock SJ, Lansky AJ, Mehran R, Popma JJ, Fahy MP, Na Y, Dangas G et al. Angiographic surrogate end points in drug-eluting stent trials: A systematic evaluation based on individual patient data from 11 randomized, controlled trials. *J Am Coll Cardiol.* 2008;51:23–32.

12. Collet C, Asano T, Sotomi Y, Cavalcante R, Miyazaki Y, Zeng Y, Tummala K et al. Early, late and very late incidence of bioresorbable scaffold thrombosis: A systematic review and meta-analysis of randomized clinical trials and observational studies. *Minerva Cardioangiol.* 2017;65(1):32–51.

# Summary of investigator-driven registries on ABSORB bioresorbable vascular scaffolds

ANNA FRANZONE, RAFFAELE PICCOLO, AND STEPHAN WINDECKER

## THE ROLE OF INVESTIGATOR-DRIVEN REGISTRIES IN CLINICAL RESEARCH

Once safety and feasibility of coronary devices have been assessed in first-in-man studies, data from postmarket clinical registries play a pivotal role to confirm initial findings, to evaluate their performance in a broader range of patient and lesion subsets, and to obtain information on the long-term performance.

As a general rule, registries aim to evaluate the *effectiveness* of a specific device; that is, how well it performs in a population closely reflecting routine clinical practice. Registries and randomized trials are complementary to build clinical evidence with their own specific advantages and limitations. The efficacy tested in randomized trials determines whether an intervention produces the expected results under ideal circumstances whereas effectiveness measures the degree of beneficial effects in "real-world" clinical settings [1]. The added benefit of registries is the potential to address questions and needs that are unmet by randomized trials, to obtain information in larger cohorts during long-term follow-up and to test device iterations and technical aspects of device implantation [2]. Other potential goals of registries are summarized in Figure 6.7.1. Therefore, investigator-initiated studies (designed and managed typically independent from industry) constitute important sources of data providing guidance in the implementation of novel technology in clinical practice and identifying shortcomings in need of further improvement [3].

### ABSORB bioresorbable vascular scaffold registries

Table 6.7.1 provides an overview of current registries that evaluated the performance of the ABSORB bioresorbable vascular scaffold (BVS) in various clinical settings. All studies employed the second generation scaffold (BVS 1.1) with a modified design providing greater temporary arterial wall support, more consistent drug delivery, and storage at room temperature compared with the previous iteration (BVS 1.0). The following paragraphs provide a detailed description for each study. Currently, clinical results for seven investigator-initiated registries with a total number of 1897 patients are available: three of them completed the planned follow-up (BVS STEMI First, AMC, Polar ACS), whereas interim analyses have been reported in the remaining studies (ASSURE, BVS-EXPAND, GOSTH EU, PRAGUE 19). In most instances, enrollment occurs at multiple sites to ensure wider generalizability. The GOSTH-EU registry is the largest multicenter registry performed to date.

In general, studies included patients and lesions with higher complexity compared with the ABSORB Cohort A [4] and B [5] registries. Despite minor differences in terms of endpoint definitions, outcomes usually focused on device performance (procedural and angiographic success) and adverse events specific for percutaneous coronary intervention (PCI) at a medium follow-up of seven months. Patients with acute coronary syndromes (ACSs) are generously represented owing to the all-comer design of the majority of the studies. Furthermore, BVS STEMI First and Prague 19 included exclusively patients with ST-segment elevation myocardial infarction (STEMI) ($n = 49$ and $n = 40$, respectively). A preliminary analysis of the 6-month outcomes of STEMI patients ($n = 74$) including the ongoing RAI registry is also available.

The considerable number of ongoing or planned registries is summarized in Table 6.7.2.

## INVESTIGATOR-DRIVEN STUDIES

### ASSURE (NCT01583608)

#### STUDY DESIGN AND ENDPOINTS

The ASSURE (ABSORB postmarketing surveillance registry to monitor the everolimus-eluting BVS in patients with coronary artery disease) registry enrolled 183 consecutive

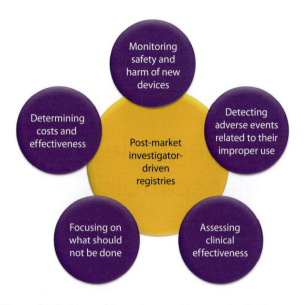

**Figure 6.7.1** Aims of investigator-driven registries in post-market research.

patients aged between 18 and 75 years, with one or more *de novo* coronary lesions at six German centers (from April 2012 to March 2013). The ABSORB BVS was implanted without the mandatory use of intracoronary imaging [6].

Study outcomes were the composite of cardiovascular death, myocardial infarction (MI) and ischema-driven target lesion revascularization (TLR) (MACE), target vessel failure (TVF), target vessel revascularization (TVR) coronary artery bypass grafting (CABG), stroke/TIA, procedural success (achievement of <50% residual stenosis and TIMI flow 3 without the occurrence of MACE during hospital stay), functional outcome (defined as the proportion of patients presenting angina pectoris), and acute gain (assessed with QCA).

## RESULTS

Baseline clinical and angiographic characteristics of included patients are shown in Tables 6.7.3 and 6.7.4. Acute procedural success was recorded for all patients. At 1 year, follow-up was available in 180 patients (98.3%). The overall MACE rate was 5.0%, driven by one death (because of gastrointestinal bleeding), three MI (not related to the target lesion), and five TLR (two involving long lesions and three complex lesions such as vein graft, bifurcation, and proximal lesion). TVR occurred in four patients (2.2%). No patient experienced scaffold thrombosis (ST). Despite a higher lesion complexity compared with ABSORB Cohort A, Cohort B, and ABSORB EXTEND, acute gain (1.54 mm) was somewhat higher in this registry. The mean residual diameter stenosis (16.1%) is comparable with that in patients treated with the metallic XIENCE everolimus-eluting stent in the SPIRIT II trial (13%).

## BVS EXPAND

### STUDY DESIGN AND PRELIMINARY RESULTS

BVS EXPAND is a prospective, single arm, single-center registry (Thoraxcentre, Erasmus MC, Rotterdam, the

Netherlands), including patients with stable coronary artery disease (CAD) and ACS except for STEMI. Enrollment commenced in September 2012 and 5-year follow-up is planned [7].

Patients with bifurcation lesions, high degree of calcification, and long lesions (>32 mm) were also included. Major exclusion criteria were previous CABG or metallic stent in the target vessel, cardiogenic shock, bifurcation lesions requiring kissing balloon postdilatation, allergy, or contraindications to dual antiplatelet therapy (DAPT).

Baseline features of the first 200 included patients with 275 lesions are shown in Tables 6.7.3 and 6.7.4. Procedural success was 98.2% using radial access in 76.6% of patients. At 6-month follow-up, clinical outcomes showed a MACE rate of 3.3%. Rates of cardiac death, MI, and TLR were 1.5%, 1.7%, and 2.2%, respectively. Four patients (2.2%) experienced definite ST.

## GHOST-EU

### STUDY DESIGN AND ENDPOINTS

The GHOST-EU (Gauging coronary Healing with biOresorbable Scaffolding plaTforms in EUrope) registry is currently the largest registry involving 10 European centers with retrospective data collection [8]. The safety and clinical performance of the ABSORB BVS were investigated in a broad patient and lesion population including patients with ACS, moderate and severe chronic kidney failure, poor ventricular function, bifurcation and ostial lesions, in-stent restenosis, chronic total occlusions, and left main disease. The primary endpoint was TLF (device-oriented composite endpoint) defined as the combination of cardiac death, target vessel MI, and clinically driven TLR. Secondary endpoints included each component of TLF, TVF (defined as the composite of cardiac death, target vessel MI, or clinically driven TVR), and ST.

### RESULTS

Between November 2011 and January 2014, 1189 patients were enrolled. According to the protocol, it was possible to implant both a BVS and a metallic drug-eluting stents (DESs) in individual patients and 18.4% of patients received both the ABSORB BVS and metallic stents. Demographic and angiographic characteristics are summarized in Tables 6.7.3 and 6.7.4. Thirty-day and 6-month follow-up were available for 94% and 76% of patients, respectively.

At 6 months, the rates of adverse events were 4.4% for TLF (5.6% among patients also receiving a metallic stent), 1.0% for cardiac death, 2.0% for target vessel MI, 4.0% for TVR, and 2.5% for TLR. Using multivariable analysis, the only independent predictor of TLF was the presence of diabetes mellitus (HR 2.41, 95% CI: 1.28–4.53; $p = 0.006$). The annualized TLF and TVF rates amounted to 10.1% and 11.9%, respectively.

This was the first report showing a considerable rate of ST with the use of the ABSORB BVS: The overall rate of ST was 1.5% at 30 days and 2.1% at 6 months, exceeding the

Table 6.7.1 Overview of ABSORB BVS investigator-initiated registries

| Study name | Population and design | Number of patients (planned) | Primary endpoint | Planned follow-up | Notes | Status |
|---|---|---|---|---|---|---|
| ASSURE | All-comers Multicenter -Germany- | 180 | • Procedural success; acute gain<br>• MACE (cardiac death, MI, TLR); TVF; TVR; CABG; stroke/TIA | 3 years | *De novo* lesions | 1-year outcomes reported [6] |
| BVS EXPAND | Stable angina; ACS Single-center -The Netherlands- | 300 | • Acute clinical device and procedure success<br>• Death, MI, TLR, TVR, ST | 5 years | STEMI not included | 6-month outcomes reported [7] |
| GOSTH-EU | All-comers Multicenter -Germany, Italy, Poland, United Kingdom- | 1189 | • TLF (cardiac death, target vessel-MI, TLR)<br>• Success device (procedural and clinical) | 1 year | | 6-month outcomes reported [8] |
| BVS STEMI FIRST | STEMI Single-center -The Netherlands- | 49 | • Death, MI, TLR, TLF, TVF | 30 days | | Completed [9] |
| Prague 19 | STEMI Multicenter -Czech Republic- | 40 | • Device success<br>• Death, MI, TVR | 3 years | Killip I/II only included | Early procedural results and 6-month clinical outcomes reported [10] |
| AMC | All-comers Single-center -The Netherlands- | 135 | • Angiographic and procedural success<br>• TVF (death, MI, TVR) | 6 months | | Completed [11] |
| POLAR ACS | ACS Multicenter -Poland- | 100 | • Device and procedural success<br>• In-hospital death, MI, TVR, TLR | 1 year | | Completed [12] |

*Abbreviations:* ACS = acute coronary syndromes; CABG = coronary artery bypass grafting; MACE = major adverse cardiac events; MI = myocardial infarction; ST = scaffold thrombosis; STEMI = ST-segment elevation myocardial infarction; TIA = transient ischemic attack; TLF = target lesion failure; TLR = target lesion revascularization; TVR = target vessel revascularization.

rate typically observed with new-generation DES and rather resembling the performance of first generation DES.

The majority of the events (70% of cases) occurred within 30 days of the procedure (most cases resulting in death or MI). Investigators explored the impact of the learning curve on clinical outcomes: patients treated after the first 50 cases were more likely to feature more complex clinical and angiographic presentations (acute coronary syndromes, ostial or thrombotic lesions) and underwent less frequently implantation guided by intravascular imaging. This pattern was, however, associated with a higher number of TLF and ST. These findings prompted a more cautionary attitude calling for meticulous lesion preparation and careful device implantation to obtain optimal angiographic outcomes. Moreover, it has been speculated that the relatively thick strut architecture of the current device and insufficient inhibition of platelet aggregation may have contributed to the predominantly early ST cases.

Table 6.7.2 Ongoing or planned ABSORB BVS investigator-initiated registries

| Study name (ClinicalTrials.gov Identifier) | Patient population | Number of patients (planned) | Primary endpoint | Planned follow-up | Notes |
|---|---|---|---|---|---|
| ASSURE ROT (NCT01915420) | All-comers | 42 | • Cardiac death, MI, TLR | 3 years | One or more complex lesions |
| CTO-ABSORB | CTO | 35 | • Procedural outcomes<br>• ST, death, MI, TLR | 2 years | |
| PABLOS | Bifurcation lesions | 30 | • Procedural and device success | 2 years | |
| IT-DISAPPEARS (NCT02004730) | All-comers | 1000 | • Cardiac death, MI (target vessel), TLR | 5 years | Long (>24 mm) single-vessel or multivessel disease |
| GABI-R (NCT02066623) | All-comers | 5000 | • Death, MI, TVR, stroke | 5 years | |
| REPARA (NCT02256449) | All-comers | 1500 | • Cardiac death, MI, TLR,ST | 1 year | De novo lesions |
| | All-comers | 2000 | • Death, MI, TLR, CABG | 5 years | De novo lesions |
| BVS-RAI (NCT02298413) | All-comers | 2000 | • Procedural success<br>• Cardiac death, TLR, ST | 5 years | |
| ABSORB-ACS (NCT02071342) | ACS | 300 | • Death, MI, TLR, TVR | 2 years | |

Abbreviations: ACS = acute coronary syndromes; CABG = coronary artery bypass grafting; CTO = chronic total occlusion; MI = myocardial infarction; ST = scaffold thrombosis; TLF = target lesion failure; TLR = target lesion revascularization; TVR = target vessel revascularization.

Table 6.7.3 Baseline demographic and clinical characteristics of patients in ABSORB BVS investigator-initiated registries

| | ASSURE (n = 183) | BVS EXPAND (n = 200) | GOSTH-EU (n = 1189) | BVS STEMI FIRST (n = 49) | AMC (n = 135) | POLAR ACS (n = 100) | PRAGUE 19 (n = –41) |
|---|---|---|---|---|---|---|---|
| **Demographics** | | | | | | | |
| Age | 65 ± 9.3 | 60.5 | 62.2 ± 11 | 58.9 ± 10.5 | 59 ± 11 | 63 ± 11 | 58.9 |
| Male | 79.8% | 75% | 79.4% | 77.6% | 73% | 73% | 77.5% |
| Diabetes | 25.7% | 19% | 24.8% | 8.2% | 20% | 27% | 25% |
| Hypertension | 82% | 58% | 73.5% | 38.8% | 50% | 78% | NA |
| Smoke | NA | 57.5% | 29.5% | 69.2% | 29% | 43% | 62.5% |
| Dyslipidemia | 76% | 50.5% | 52.9% | 22.4% | 43% | 71% | NA |
| Prior MI | 27.1% | 17.5% | NA | 2% | 25% | 16% | 2.5% |
| Prior CABG | NA | 0% | 4.6% | 0% | 2% | 8% | 0% |
| Renal disease | NA | 5.5% | 14.9% | 2% | 8% | NA | NA |
| **Clinical Presentation** | | | | | | | |
| Stable angina or silent ischemia | 35.5% | – | 52.6% | – | 47% | – | – |
| Unstable angina | 21.3% | – | 13.2% | – | 10% | 46% | – |
| Non-ST-segment elevation MI | NA | 100% | 18.0% | – | 27% | 38% | – |
| ST-segment elevation MI | – | – | 16.1% | 100% | 13% | 16% | 100% |

Abbreviations: CABG = coronary artery bypass grafting; MI = myocardial infarction; PCI = percutaneous coronary intervention.

Table 6.7.4 Angiographic and procedural characteristics of patients in ABSORB BVS investigator-initiated registries

| | ASSURE (n = 183) | BVS EXPAND (n = 200) | GOSTH-EU (n =1 189) | BVS STEMI FIRST (n = 49) | AMC (n = 135) | POLAR ACS (n = 100) | PRAGUE 19 (n = 41) |
|---|---|---|---|---|---|---|---|
| Target vessel | | | | | | | |
| Left anterior descending | 42.4% | NA | 46.8% | 42.9% | 60% | 46% | 50% |
| Left circumflex | 22.2% | NA | 24.8% | 12.2% | 15% | 20% | 27.5% |
| Right coronary artery | 23.7% | NA | 25.2% | 44.9% | 23% | 26% | 22.5% |
| ACC/AHA lesion class | | NA | | NA | | | NA |
| B1 | 22.2% | | 26.8% | | 16% | 31% | |
| B2 | 43.4% | | 23.6% | | 42% | 38% | |
| C | 21.2% | | 27.6% | | 25% | 20% | |
| Bifurcation | 14.1% | 29.1% | 26.7% | NA | 15% | NA | NA |
| Chronic total occlusion | NA | 12% | 7.8% | NA | 8% | NA | NA |
| Mean reference vessel diameter (mm) | 2.6 ± 0.5 | NA | 3.0 ± 0.5 | NA | NA | 2.8 ± 0.5 | NA |
| Minimum lumen diameter (mm) | 0.9 ± 0.5 | NA | NA | NA | NA | 1.0 ± 0.5 | NA |
| Planned overlap | NA | NA | 32% | NA | 24.5% | NA | NA |

## BVS STEMI FIRST

### STUDY DESIGN AND ENDPOINTS

This investigator initiated, prospective, single arm, single-center study (Thoraxcentre, Erasmus MC, Rotterdam, the Netherlands) was conceived to assess the feasibility and performance of the ABSORB BVS for the treatment of patients presenting with STEMI [9]. Inclusion and exclusion criteria are listed in Table 6.7.5. Study endpoints were based on clinical and angiographic data and acute results evaluated with optical coherence tomography (OCT). The investigators reported various measures of success including device success (the attainment of <30% final diameter stenosis of the segment of the culprit lesion covered by the BVS by visual estimate), procedure success (device success without major periprocedural complications), and clinical success (procedural success without in-hospital MACE). Clinical outcomes were assessed according to the composite endpoint TLF (cardiac death, target-vessel MI, or ischemia-driven TLR), MACE (cardiac death, any reinfarction emergent bypass surgery or clinically driven TLR), and TVF (cardiac death, target-vessel MI, or clinically driven TVR).

### RESULTS

A total of 49 patients with STEMI undergoing BVS implantation were enrolled between November 2012 and April 2013, representing approximately 38% of the total number of eligible patients.

Baseline clinical and angiographic data are reported in Tables 6.7.3, 6.7.4, and 6.7.6. Angiographic analysis revealed post-PCI TIMI-flow grade 3 of 91.7%. OCT findings were comparable with metallic stents showing a rate of malapposed struts of 2.8 ± 3.9%. There were no clinical adverse events related to the treated vessel within the first 30 days after BVS implantation (rate of TLF = 0%). The MACE rate was 2.6% as one patient, after discharge, developed a non-Q-wave MI related to a non-target-vessel lesion and underwent non-target-vessel revascularization.

## Prague 19

### STUDY DESIGN AND ENDPOINTS

Prague 19 is a prospective, multicenter, open-label study with the aim to analyze the performance of BVS implanted during primary PCI and to address the question of which proportion of STEMI patients are eligible for BVS implantation.

Patients are included on the basis of inclusion and exclusion criteria listed in Table 6.7.7. The planned follow-up amounts to 3 years with clinical and CT coronary angiography follow-up after 1 year and invasive coronary angiography with OCT evaluation after 3 years. Preliminary procedural findings and early clinical outcomes have been reported [10].

Study endpoints include device success (defined as the delivery and deployment of BVS at the target lesion with a

Table 6.7.5 BVS STEMI first study: inclusion and exclusion criteria

| Inclusion criteria | Exclusion criteria |
|---|---|
| **Clinical** | |
| • Age >18 years old | • Pregnancy |
| • STEMI, defined as at least 1 mm ST-segment elevation in two or more standard leads or at least 2 mm in two or more contiguous precordial | • Known intolerance to contrast medium |
| | • Uncertain neurological outcome after cardiopulmonary resuscitation |
| • Willing to comply with specified follow-up evaluation and to be contacted by telephone | • Age >75 years |
| | • Participation to another investigational drug or device study before reaching the primary endpoints. |
| **Angiographic** | |
| • Culprit lesions located in vessels within the upper limit of 3.8 mm and the lower limit of 2.0 mm by online quantitative coronary angiography | • Previous percutaneous coronary intervention with the implantation of a metal stent |
| | • Left main (LM) disease |
| | • Previous coronary artery by pass grafting |

*Abbreviation:* STEMI = ST-segment elevation myocardial infarction.

Table 6.7.6 Details of the procedure in primary PCI studies using BVSs

| | BVS STEMI First (n = 49) | PRAGUE 19 (n = 40) |
|---|---|---|
| Mean door to reperfusion (min) | 31.3 ± 19.5 | 29.9 |
| Manual thrombectomy, n (%) | 38 (77.5) | 15 (37.5%) |
| Predilatation, n (%) | 33 (67.3) | 34 (85.0%) |
| Postdilatation, n (%) | 10 (20.4) | 13 (32.5%) |
| Mean scaffolds per-lesion, n | 1.35 ± 0.60 | 1.2 |
| Mean scaffold diameter per-lesion (mm) | 3.2 | 3.3 |
| Mean scaffold length per-lesion (mm) | 26.40 ± 13.86 | 23.2 ± 10.4 |
| TIMI flow pre | | |
| 0 | 50.0% | 55.5% |
| 1 | 15.2% | 5.0% |
| 2 | 21.7% | 27.5% |
| 3 | 13.0% | 12.5% |
| TIMI flow post | | |
| 0 | 0% | 0% |
| 1 | 0% | 2.5% |
| 2 | 8.3% | 2.5% |
| 3 | 91.7% | 95% |

final residual stenosis ≤20% by visual estimate) and a composite clinical endpoint (death, any MI, and TVR).

## RESULTS

From December 2012 to August 2013, 29% of all consecutive STEMI patients (41 of 142 patients) underwent primary PCI with BVS implantation. Baseline and procedural characteristics are described in Tables 6.7.3, 6.7.4, and 6.7.6. The principal reasons to preclude BVS implantation were related to clinical or technical factors: short life expectancy; contraindication for DAPT or indication for oral anticoagulation; vessel diameter outside the recommended 2.3–3.7 mm range; severe calcification and vessel tortuosity.

Device success was 98%, TIMI flow 3 was restored in 95% of patients at the end of the procedure, and acute scaffold recoil was 9.7%. In a subgroup of 21 patients undergoing OCT at the end of the procedure, scaffold strut malapposition and edge dissections were present in 38% of patients but were small and clinically silent. Noteworthy, the RVD measured by QCA was significantly lower than that measured by OCT. Event-free survival was 95% for the BVS, which was comparable to a nonrandomized control group treated with the metallic DES (93%, $p = 0.67$).

Table 6.7.7 Prague 19 study: inclusion and exclusion criteria

| Inclusion criteria | Exclusion criteria |
|---|---|
| **Clinical** | |
| • STEMI <24 h from symptom onset | • Killip III–IV class |
| | • Any other disease with probable prognosis <3 years |
| | • Indication for oral anticoagulation |
| | • Contraindication to prolonged dual antiplatelet therapy |
| **Angiographic** | |
| | • Infarct artery reference diameter <2.3 or >3.7 mm |
| | • Lesion length >24 mm |
| | • Extensive infarct artery calcifications or severe tortuosity |
| | • STEMI caused by in-stent restenosis or stent thrombosis |

*Abbreviation:* STEMI = ST-segment elevation myocardial infarction.

## RAI registry

### STUDY DESIGN AND ENDPOINTS

The RAI ("Registro ABSORB Italiano") registry is an ongoing, multicenter, prospective registry collecting data on patients undergoing unrestricted BVS implantation at several institutions throughout Italy. It is planned to enroll up to 2000 patients and perform 5-year follow-up. Immediate and midterm outcomes of the STEMI cohort have been reported [13]. Patients were eligible for BVS implantation if they had symptom onset <24 hours from hospital admission, suitable anatomy (no tortuosity or severe calcification, reference diameter of infarct artery ≥2.3 mm and ≤3.7 mm), and absence of severe comorbidities. Stent thrombosis at the culprit lesion was an exclusion criterion.

The primary study endpoint was procedural success, defined as <30% final diameter stenosis and TIMI 3 flow without in-hospital major adverse cardiovascular events (MACE: cardiac death, MI, or need for emergent revascularization). The occurrence of cardiac death, MI, TLR, and BVS thrombosis was also assessed at follow-up.

### RESULTS

A total of 1232 STEMI patients underwent primary PCI at the participating centers between December 2012 and February 2014. Among these, 74 (6.0%) underwent primary PCI with implantation of BVS (56 single, 18 at least two overlapping). Procedural success was obtained in 72 (97.3%) cases. Six-month follow-up was available for 68 (91.9%) patients. No cardiac death occurred, while two patients experienced reinfarction (2.7%), three patients (4.1%) underwent TLR. ST was reported in three patients (two receiving single BVS [3.6%] and one overlapping BVS [5.6%], $p = 0.5$).

## AMC

### STUDY DESIGN AND ENDPOINTS

The AMC registry assessed procedural success, acute angiographic results, and 6-month clinical outcomes of the ABSORB BVS 1.1 in a patient population treated at a high-volume tertiary care center (Academic Medical Center, Amsterdam) between August 2012 and August 2013 [12]. Patients with stable CAD or ACS and a wide range of lesion characteristics underwent implantation of the ABSORB BVS 1.1 according to operator's discretion.

Angiographic success (defined as <30% residual stenosis in the target lesion on QCA with TIMI 3 flow in the intended target vessel), and procedural success (defined as angiographic success in the absence of in-hospital TVF) were the major study endpoints. TVF was defined as a composite of all-cause mortality, any MI, and TVR.

### RESULTS

A total of 135 patients with 159 lesions were included in the registry: 39% underwent PCI in the setting of ACS and 13% of patients presented with STEMI. Baseline and angiographic characteristics are depicted in Tables 6.7.3 and 6.7.4. Angiographic and procedural success were 96% and 95%, respectively. Six-month follow-up was available in 97% of the entire cohort and showed a cumulative TVF rate of 8.5%: rates of MI, cardiac death, TLR, and ST were 3.0%, 0.8%, 6.3%, and 3.3%, respectively.

## POLAR-ACS

The POLAR-ACS is a single-arm, prospective, observational study including 100 ACS patients treated with ABSORB BVS 1.1 implantation at 12 centers in Poland between November 2012 and September 2013 [12].

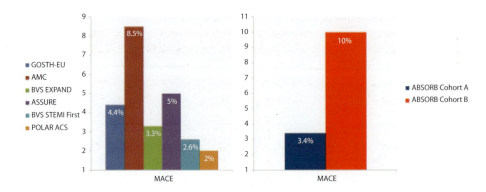

**Figure 6.7.2** Rates of MACE in ABSORB BVS investigator-driven registries and ABSORB Cohort A and Cohort B studies. *30 days outcomes.

The major study endpoint was the 12-month rate of MACE, defined as death, MI, and clinically driven-TLR. Procedural (achievement of final in-scaffold/stent residual stenosis of <50% by QCA with successful delivery and deployment of at least one study scaffold/stent at the intended target lesion and successful withdrawal of the delivery system for all target lesions without the occurrence of MACE during the hospital stay) and device success (successful delivery and deployment of the first study scaffold in the intended target lesion and attainment of final in-scaffold residual stenosis of <50% by QCA) were also assessed.

## RESULTS

Procedural success was achieved in all but one patient and device success in all patients. MACE occurred during the hospital stay in 2% of patients, and there was one case of scaffold thrombosis at 1-year follow-up.

## CONCLUSION

Data from the presented, observational studies demonstrate that the implantation of the ABSORB BVS 1.1 is technically feasible in a wide range of clinical settings and lesions subsets (Figure 6.7.2). They also highlight that meticulous attention to lesion preparation and careful device implantation aiming at an optimal postprocedural outcome are of importance to mitigate the risk of periprocedural complications. These registries provide a valuable basis to compare future device iterations.

## REFERENCES

1. Gartlehner G, Hansen RA, Nissman D, Lohr KN, Carey TS. Criteria for Distinguishing Effectiveness from Efficacy Trials in Systematic Reviews. Rockville, MD: Agency for Healthcare Research and Quality (AHRQ Publication No. 060046). Technical Review 12. 2006.
2. Johnston BC, Vohra S. Investigator-initiated trials are more impartial. *Nature*. 2006;443(7108):144.
3. Tavazzi L. Do we need clinical registries? *Eur Heart J.* 2014;35(1):7–9.
4. Serruys PW, Ormiston JA, Onuma Y, Regar E, Gonzalo N, Garcia-Garcia HM et al. A bioabsorbable everolimus-eluting coronary stent system (ABSORB): 2-year outcomes and results from multiple imaging methods. *Lancet*. 2009;373(9667):897–910.
5. Okamura T, Garg S, Gutierrez-Chico JL, Shin ES, Onuma Y, Garcia-Garcia HM et al. In vivo evaluation of stent strut distribution patterns in the bioabsorbable everolimus-eluting device: An OCT ad hoc analysis of the revision 1.0 and revision 1.1 stent design in the ABSORB clinical trial. *EuroIntervention. Journal of EuroPCR in Collaboration with the Working Group on Interventional Cardiology of the European Society of Cardiology*. 2010;5(8):932–8.
6. Wohrle J, Naber C, Schmitz T, Schwencke C, Frey N, Butter C et al. Beyond the early stages. Insights from the ASSURE registry on bioresorbable vascular scaffolds. *EuroIntervention. Journal of EuroPCR in Collaboration with the Working Group on Interventional Cardiology of the European Society of Cardiology*. 2014.
7. van Geuns RJ. BVS Expand: 6-month results, *euroPCR* 2014.
8. Capodanno D, Gori T, Nef H, Latib A, Mehilli J, Lesiak M et al. Percutaneous coronary intervention with everolimus-eluting bioresorbable vascular scaffolds in routine clinical practice: Early and midterm outcomes from the European multicentre GHOST-EU registry. *EuroIntervention. Journal of EuroPCR in Collaboration with the Working Group on Interventional Cardiology of the European Society of Cardiology*. 2015;10(10):1144–53.
9. Diletti R, Karanasos A, Muramatsu T, Nakatani S, Van Mieghem NM, Onuma Y et al. Everolimus-eluting bioresorbable vascular scaffolds for treatment of patients presenting with ST-segment elevation myocardial infarction: BVS STEMI first study. *Eur Heart J.* 2014;35(12):777–86.

10. Kocka V, Maly M, Tousek P, Budesinsky T, Lisa L, Prodanov P et al. Bioresorbable vascular scaffolds in acute ST-segment elevation myocardial infarction: A prospective multicentre study 'Prague 19'. *Eur Heart J.* 2014;35(12):787–94.

11. Kraak RP, Hassell ME, Grundeken MJ, Koch KT, Henriques JP, Piek JJ et al. Initial experience and clinical evaluation of the Absorb bioresorbable vascular scaffold (BVS) in real-world practice: The AMC Single Centre Real World PCI Registry. *EuroIntervention. Journal of EuroPCR in Collaboration with the Working Group on Interventional Cardiology of the European Society of Cardiology.* 2015;10(10):1160–8.

12. Dudek D, Rzeszutko L, Zasada W, Depukat R, Siudak Z, Ochala A et al. Bioresorbable vascular scaffolds in patients with acute coronary syndromes: The POLAR ACS study. *Pol Arch Med Wewn.* 2014;124(12):669–77.

13. Ielasi A, Cortese B, Varricchio A, Tespili M, Sesana M, Pisano F et al. Immediate and midterm outcomes following primary PCI with bioresorbable vascular scaffold implantation in patients with ST-segment myocardial infarction: Insights from the multicentre 'Registro ABSORB Italiano' (RAI registry). *EuroIntervention. Journal of EuroPCR in Collaboration with the Working Group on Interventional Cardiology of the European Society of Cardiology.* 2014.

# Investigator-driven randomized trials

DANIELE GIACOPPO, ROISIN COLLERAN, AND ADNAN KASTRATI

## OVERVIEW

Over the past decade, newer generation metallic drug-eluting stents using more biocompatible or bioresorbable polymer coatings have been shown to improve vascular healing after coronary stenting. These high-performing devices currently represent the gold standard for the treatment of coronary artery disease across a broad spectrum of clinical and anatomic subsets [1–9]. More recently, drug-eluting bioresorbable scaffolds have attracted substantial interest. Indeed, a drug-eluting bioresorbable scaffold may exhibit several desirable properties, providing not only short-term vessel scaffolding and, through local drug delivery, similar antirestenotic effectiveness to current-generation metallic drug-eluting stents, but also, by fully resorbing, may facilitate enhanced vessel healing, allowing restoration of vasomotion and a potential reduction in the risk of late and very late stent thrombosis [10–13]. Although a number of bioresorbable scaffolds are currently under investigation, to date, only two devices have received CE mark approval [10]. Of these, only the ABSORB bioresorbable scaffold (Abbott Vascular, Abbott Park, IL) has been extensively tested in clinical trials. A number of recent clinical investigations assessing the performance of the ABSORB bioresorbable vascular scaffold in large populations of patients with coronary artery disease have generated enthusiasm for the device as a promising therapeutic alternative to metallic drug-eluting stents (DESs) [14–16].

Evidence recently provided by randomized trials including ABSORB II, ABSORB III, ABSORB Japan, and ABSORB China in support of ABSORB bioresorbable scaffolds is not generalizable to all patient and lesion subsets. Although comprehensive meta-analyses and several reports have confirmed comparable mid- and long-term cardiovascular outcomes between the ABSORB bioresorbable scaffold and the everolimus-eluting metallic stent, they have also highlighted some important limitations related to its use in more complex patients, in addition to revealing a small, but significant increase in scaffold thrombosis compared with new generation metallic DES [17–20]. Furthermore, since clinically relevant benefits of the bioresorbable scaffold will only become apparent in the very long-term, currently available follow-up data from large randomized trials are not sufficient to provide definitive answers at present.

Such unanswered questions, in addition to the several still underexplored patient subgroups (Table 6.8.1), have prompted further trials of the bioresorbable scaffold—mostly investigator-initiated—in specific clinical scenarios of interest. Two such examples are in the treatment of acute coronary syndromes and of intermediate vulnerable plaque. Although a non-randomized, single-arm study previously reported feasibility of bioresorbable scaffold implantation for the treatment of ST-elevation myocardial infarction, inclusion and exclusion criteria were very selective, making it difficult to draw definitive conclusions [21]. In this chapter, available data and first results from both ongoing and completed investigator-initiated randomized clinical trials exploring the bioresorbable scaffold in various clinical and angiographic subsets will be presented and reviewed where results have been reported (Table 6.8.2).

## ACUTE MYOCARDIAL INFARCTION

### ABSORB-STEMI TROFI II

The ABSORB-STEMI TROFI II (Comparison of the ABSORB Everolimus Eluting Bioresorbable Vascular Scaffold System With a Drug-Eluting Metal Stent in Acute ST-Elevation Myocardial Infarction; NCT01986803) trial was a multicenter, single-blind, noninferiority, investigator-initiated randomized clinical trial. A total of 191 patients experiencing ST-elevation myocardial infarction (STEMI) were allocated in a 1:1 ratio to everolimus-eluting bioresorbable scaffold (ABSORB, Abbott Vascular, Abbott Park, IL) or new generation metallic everolimus-eluting stent (XIENCE Expedition, Abbott Vascular, Abbott Park, IL) implantation [22]. The ABSORB-STEMI TROFI II is one of the two investigator-driven randomized clinical trials on the ABSORB bioresorbable scaffold with available primary results. The trial

Table 6.8.1 Underexplored patient and lesion subsets and unanswered questions regarding bioresorbable scaffolds

| Subset of interest | Investigator-driven randomized controlled trial |
|---|---|
| Very long-term effectiveness and safety | The large investigator-initiated AIDA and COMPARE ABSORB trials seek to assess and compare very long-term outcomes of patients assigned to receive the bioresorbable versus the everolimus-eluting metallic stent. |
| ST-elevation myocardial infarction | The ABSORB-STEMI TROFI II and BVS in STEMI trials address the subset of patients with ST-elevation myocardial infarction, whereas the ISAR-ABSORB MI trial includes patients with acute myocardial infarction (with or without ST-elevation). |
| Diabetes mellitus | No randomized clinical trials at the moment are specifically addressing this subset, but particular focus is given to this high-risk condition in the COMPARE ABSORB trial. |
| Vulnerable plaque/optimal medical therapy | The PREVENT and PROSPECT ABSORB trials are specifically addressing treatment of this condition. |
| Myocardial blood flow improvement | The VANISH trial is specifically addressing this issue. |
| Left main coronary artery disease | To date, no randomized data are available pertaining to this lesion subset on account of concerns regarding the systematic feasibility of a bioresorbable scaffold-based strategy in left main coronary artery disease. |
| Bifurcation | To date, no randomized clinical data examining this lesion subset are available on account of concerns regarding the systematic feasibility of a bioresorbable scaffold-based two-stent strategy in "true" bifurcation coronary lesions. |
| Small vessels/distal disease | To date, no randomized clinical data on this lesion subset are available on account of concerns regarding the effectiveness of the bioresorbable scaffold in small vessels due to lower anti-restenotic proprieties and higher strut thickness compared with current-generation drug-eluting stents. |
| High bleeding risk/oral anticoagulation | To date, no randomized clinical data are available on this patient subset as there is no available robust information about bioresorbable scaffold safety and very short dual antiplatelet therapy/triple antithrombotic therapy. |
| Different devices | The EVERBIO II trial compared the bioresorbable scaffold with a platinum-chromium everolimus-eluting stent and a stainless steel biolimus-eluting stent. The ISAR-RESORB trial is comparing the bioresorbable scaffold with a new-generation platinum-chromium everolimus-eluting stent. |
| Coronary artery bypass grafting | The RELEASE-BVS trial is comparing percutaneous coronary intervention using the bioresorbable scaffold with surgical revascularization. |

was sponsored by the European Cardiovascular Research Institute (ECRI), but Abbott Vascular and Terumo Europe were collaborators [22].

Patients presenting within 24 hours of symptom-onset undergoing primary percutaneous coronary intervention (PCI) to a native target vessel with a visual reference vessel diameter of 2.5 mm to 3.8 mm with one or more de novo stenoses were included. Exclusion criteria included cardiogenic shock; unprotected left main coronary artery stenosis; fibrinolyses prior to PCI; distal occlusion of the target vessel; acute myocardial infarction secondary to stent thrombosis; and severely tortuous, angulated, or calcified vessels with suboptimal imaging or excessive risk of complication from placement of an optical frequency domain imaging (OFDI) catheter.

The aim of the trial was to compare the short-term arterial healing response after bioresorbable scaffold and everolimus-eluting metallic stent implantation in coronary artery lesions with relevant thrombotic burden and a large necrotic core. The primary endpoint was the healing score

in 6-month OFDI calculated by assessment of the following four device-related parameters: (1) presence of intraluminal mass (weight of 4 points); (2) presence of both malapposed and uncovered struts (3 points); (3) presence of uncovered struts alone (2 points); and (4) presence of malapposed struts alone (1 point). Stent area and derived measures were based on the abluminal stent contour. This endpoint was considered an acceptable surrogate for device efficacy and safety. Secondary endpoints included: (1) a device-oriented composite endpoint of cardiac death, target vessel myocardial infarction, or clinically driven target lesion revascularization at 1, 6, and 36 months; (2) the assessment of each individual component of the composite endpoint; (3) clinically driven and non-clinically driven target vessel revascularization; (4) stent thrombosis according to Academic Research Consortium (ARC) criteria [23]; and (5) angina status at 6 months according to Canadian Society of Cardiology (CCS) criteria [24]. Device success was defined as postprocedural residual stenosis <30% at the stented site. Procedure success was defined as device success and the

Table 6.8.2 Ongoing and completed investigator-driven randomized clinical trials assessing the effectiveness and safety of the bioresorbable scaffold

| | Comparison | Patients | Clinical presentation | Primary outcomes completion date | Primary endpoint[a] | Registration |
|---|---|---|---|---|---|---|
| ABSORB-STEMI TROFI II | BRS vs. EES | 191 (95 vs. 96) | Acute ST-elevation myocardial infarction | Completed | Healing score at 6 months[a] | NCT01986803 |
| AIDA | BRS vs. EES | 2690 | All-comers | December 2017 | Target vessel failure at 24 months | NCT01858077 |
| BVS in STEMI | BRS vs. EES | 120 | Acute ST-elevation myocardial infarction | August 2016 | Healing index at 12 months[a] | NCT02067091 |
| COMPARE ABSORB | BRS vs. EES | 2100 | All-comers | March 2018 | Target lesion failure • 12 months • 1–5 years • 5 (or 7) years | NCT02486068 |
| EVERBIO II | BRS vs. EES vs. BES | 240 (80 vs. 80 vs. 80) | • Silent ischemia • Stable angina • Non-ST-elevation acute coronary syndrome | Completed | Late lumen loss at 9 months | NCT01711931 |
| ISAR-ABSORB MI | BRS vs. EES | 260 | Acute Myocardial Infarction | Not available | Diameter stenosis at 6–8 months | NCT01942070 |
| ISAR-RESORB | BRS vs. EES | 230 | • Silent ischemia • Stable angina • Non-ST-elevation acute coronary syndrome | December 2016 | Diameter stenosis at 6–8 months | NCT02442016 |
| PREVENT | BRS+OMT vs. OMT | 1600 | Symptomatic or asymptomatic coronary artery disease associated with fractional flow reserve ≥0.80 and IVUS or OCT criteria of significance or plaque instability | January 2019 | At 24 months: • Cardiovascular death • Non-fatal myocardial infarction • Unstable angina leading to rehospitalisation | NCT02316886 |
| PROSPECT ABSORB | BRS+OMT vs. OMT | NR | Non-significant stenosis by angiography and fractional flow reserve/instantaneous wave-free ratio with a plaque burden ≥70% in at least one frame by IVUS | December 2018 | Minimum lumen diameter at 2 years | NCT02171065 |
| RELEASE-BVS | BRS vs. CABG | 140 | Elective patients with symptomatic or asymptomatic three-vessel and/or left main coronary artery disease associated with ischemia at cardiac magnetic resonance imaging | September 2017 | Extent of myocardial ischemia and left ventricular ejection fraction assessed by cardiac magnetic resonance imaging at 12 months | NCT02334826 |
| VANISH | BRS vs. EES | 60 | Elective patients with documented myocardial ischemia and stable coronary artery disease | June 2018 | Myocardial blood flow at 3 years | NCT01876589 |

Abbreviations: BRS = bioresorbable scaffold; CABG = coronary artery bypass grafting; EES = everolimus-eluting stent (metallic); NR = not reported; OCT = optical coherence tomography; OMT = optimal medical therapy.

[a] Assessment by optical coherence tomography (OCT).

absence of postprocedural occurrence of any component of the primary endpoint. Clinical follow-up was scheduled at 1, 6, 12, 24, and 36 months. Angiography and optical frequency domain imaging recordings were analyzed in an independent core laboratory (Cardialysis, Rotterdam, the Netherlands). The primary PCI was performed according to standard practice, although manual thrombectomy was mandatory to reduce thrombotic burden. Although careful lesion predilation is strongly recommended before bioresorbable scaffold implantation, direct stenting was performed in almost 45% of patients assigned to bioresorbable scaffold implantation on account of a heavy thrombotic burden and evident necrotic core with the attendant higher risk of embolism, spasm, and no reflow. Rate of procedural success was numerically lower with the bioresorbable scaffold compared with the metallic stent (95.8% vs. 100%, $p = 0.059$).

Quantitative coronary angiography at 6-month follow-up revealed a mild but significant increase in in-device late lumen loss ($0.17 \pm 0.24$ mm vs. $0.08 \pm 0.28$ mm, $p = 0.024$) and in-device percentage diameter stenosis ($17.3 \pm 7.4\%$ vs. $14.5 \pm 9.3\%$, $p = 0.02$) in the bioresorbable scaffold group compared with the everolimus-eluting metallic stent group, but this difference did not translate into any increase in in-segment binary restenosis, which did not occur at all in this group during the follow-up period (0% vs. 1.1%). The healing score—as assessed by OFDI at 6 months—showed noninferiority ($p < 0.001$) in patients who received the bioresorbable scaffold over those who received the everolimus-eluting metallic stent with a borderline p value for superiority ($p = 0.053$). This result was mainly driven by a higher incidence of covered and malapposed struts ($p = 0.011$) in the everolimus-eluting metallic stent group. Accordingly, incomplete strut apposition volume and incomplete stent apposition area were lower in bioresorbable scaffold patients. The abluminal mean stent areas amounted to 8.73 mm$^2$ and 8.19 mm$^2$ for the bioresorbable scaffold and everolimus-eluting metallic stent, respectively ($p = 0.07$), while the neointimal area was significantly greater in the bioresorbable scaffold compared with the everolimus-eluting metallic stent (1.52 mm$^2$ vs. 1.35 mm$^2$, $p = 0.018$). As a consequence of these counterbalancing effects, the mean luminal area (7.06 mm$^2$ vs. 7.02 mm$^2$, $p = 0.89$), minimum stent area (7.30 mm$^2$ vs. 7.04 mm$^2$, $p = 0.34$), and minimum luminal area (5.40 mm$^2$ vs. 5.53 mm$^2$, $p = 0.65$) were similar between groups.

Although the healing score used has not been robustly validated, the elegant intracoronary imaging evaluation of the ABSORB-STEMI TROFI II trial did not reveal an overall significant difference in performance of the bioresorbable scaffold and everolimus-eluting metallic stent in complex thrombotic lesions in the high-risk clinical subset of patients with STEMI. The ABSORB-STEMI TROFI II is the first trial showing almost complete arterial healing associated with the bioresorbable scaffold in the scenario of the ruptured plaque, which has been shown to be prone to delayed arterial healing. However, the ABSORB-STEMI

TROFI II trial was unpowered for clinical outcomes precluding detection of some important differences between devices. In addition, very late effects of bioresorbable scaffold implantation on complex thrombotic lesions resulting in STEMI remain unknown, although several years after the index procedure the potential advantages of this therapy should be manifest.

## BVS in STEMI

The BVS in STEMI (Performance of Bioresorbable Scaffold in Primary Percutaneous Intervention of ST Elevation Myocardial Infarct; NCT02067091) trial is a multi-center, open-label, randomized clinical trial sponsored by the Haukeland University Hospital. The trial was initiated in August 2014 and is currently ongoing with primary outcome assessment expected in August 2016. In brief, a total of 120 patients with acute STEMI requiring primary PCI will be randomized after thrombus aspiration with restoration of TIMI 2-3 flow to treatment with either the everolimus-eluting bioresorbable scaffold (ABSORB, Abbott Vascular, Abbott Park, IL) or everolimus-eluting metallic stent (XIENCE, Abbott Vascular, Abbott Park, IL). Exclusion criteria include severe impairment of blood flow or persistent occlusion following thrombectomy (TIMI flow 0) or anatomic limitations preventing advancement of the thrombectomy catheter. Angiographic exclusion criteria are heavy calcification, tortuosity, and bifurcation lesion with side branch >2.5 mm. Key clinical exclusion criteria include cardiac arrest or refractory cardiogenic shock; eGFR <45 mL/min; and contraindication to long-term dual antiplatelet therapy.

Clinical follow-up is to be performed at 12 months. Optical coherence tomography (OCT) is performed pre- and poststenting during the index procedure and at 12-months follow-up to evaluate the primary endpoint of Coronary Stent Healing Index. This index includes several parameters, each with its own severity score, as follows: uncovered struts (2% = 1, 5% = 2, 10% = 3, 15% = 4, 20% = 5, 25% = 6, 30% = 7, 35% = 8, 40% = 9); uncovered struts in front of side branch on acquired or persistent malapposed struts (1 point for every 10% increase to 100%); persistent malapposition ($\geq 2$ adjacent struts of at least 1 mm in length = 1; $\geq 2$ mm = 3; $\geq 3$ mm = 3); acquired malapposition ($\geq 2$ adjacent struts of at least 1 mm in length = 2; $\geq 2$ mm = 4; $\geq 3$ mm = 6); neointimal thickness in one frame (>200 UNIT = 1; >300 = 2; >400 = 3) or diameter stenosis (>50% = 4; >75% = 5); cumulative extra-stent lumen increase at cross-sectional analysis ($\geq 0.2$ mm$^2$ = 1; $\geq 0.4$ mm$^2$ = 2; $\geq 0.6$ mm$^2$ = 3; $\geq 0.8$ mm$^2$ = 4; $\geq 1.0$ mm$^2$ = 5; $\geq 1.2$ mm$^2$ = 6). Multislice computed tomography coronary angiography is planned at 12 and 24 months follow-up in a prespecified substudy. The following secondary outcomes will be assessed at 5 years: (1) all-cause death; (2) cardiac death; (3) myocardial infarction; (4) stent thrombosis (ARC criteria) [23]; (5) target lesion revascularization; (6) target vessel revascularization; (7) PCI; (8) coronary artery bypass grafting; (9) nontarget vessel revascularization; (10) CCS angina class [24]; (11) cerebro-vascular events; (12) and readmission for congestive heart failure or arrhythmia.

## ISAR-ABSORB MI

The ISAR-ABSORB MI (Intracoronary Scaffold Assessment a Randomized Evaluation of ABSORB in Myocardial Infarction; NCT01942070) trial is a prospective, multi-center, non-inferiority, randomized clinical trial comparing the performances of the everolimus-eluting bioresorbable scaffold (ABSORB, Abbott Vascular, Abbott Park, IL) and durable polymer metallic everolimus-eluting stent (XIENCE, Abbott Vascular, Abbott Park, IL) in the setting of acute myocardial infarction, both with and without ST-elevation. Patients presenting with a *de novo* coronary artery stenosis located in a native vessel or coronary bypass graft with a reference vessel diameter of ≥2.5 mm and ≤3.9 mm are eligible for inclusion. Key exclusion criteria include culprit lesion located in the left main trunk; or at a bifurcation with a side branch diameter >2.0 mm; in-stent restenosis or severe calcification. Angiographic data are assessed offline by quantitative coronary angiography performed in an independent core laboratory (ISAResearch, Munich, Germany).

The primary endpoint of the ISAR-ABSORB MI is the percentage diameter stenosis of the treated lesion at 6–8 months angiographic follow-up. Secondary endpoints will be assessed at 12 months and include: (1) a device-oriented composite endpoint consisting of cardiac death, target vessel-myocardial infarction, or target lesion revascularization; (2) a patient-oriented composite endpoint consisting of death, any myocardial infarction, or any revascularization; (3) a composite endpoint consisting of death or myocardial infarction; and (4) stent thrombosis.

## ALL-COMERS

### AIDA

The AIDA (Amsterdam Investigator-Initiated ABSORB Strategy All-Comers; NCT01858077) trial is a prospective, single-center, single-blind, all-comers, randomized clinical trial comparing the everolimus-eluting bioresorbable scaffold (ABSORB, Abbott Vascular, Abbott Park, IL) with an everolimus-eluting metallic stent (XIENCE PRIME or XIENCE Xpedition, Abbott Vascular; Abbott Park, IL) in patients requiring PCI for one or more coronary lesions suitable for drug-eluting stent implantation [25]. This investigator-driven clinical trial is currently ongoing and a total of 2690 subjects are planned to be enrolled. The trial is supported by the Academisch Medisch Centrum, Universiteit van Amsterdam, but since trial initiation, a restricted grant by Abbott has been provided. The first patient was enrolled in August 2013 and the estimated date for final data collection for the primary outcome measure is December 2017. To date, approximately 1850 patients have been enrolled but no preliminary results have yet been made available.

Clinical and angiographic eligibility criteria are broadly inclusive. All adult patients capable of providing informed consent are eligible for enrolment, with the following key exclusion criteria: "true" bifurcation lesion requiring *a priori* a double-scaffold/stent strategy; in-stent restenosis; reference vessel diameter <2.5 mm or >4.0 mm; and lesion requiring overlapping scaffolds/stents for a total length of >70 mm or a total number ≥4. Patients are randomized after wiring and predilation of the target lesion. As such, unsuccessful lesion predilation is also an exclusion criterion. All additional lesions, either at index PCI or at subsequent staged procedure, are treated with the same type of device according to previous random assignment. In the AIDA trial, target lesion predilation is performed by conventional angioplasty balloon with a diameter 0.5 mm smaller than that of the assigned study device. Treatment with cutting balloon or rotational atherectomy prior to predilation is allowed at the operators' discretion.

The primary endpoint of the AIDA trial is target vessel failure (TVF), a composite of cardiac death, myocardial infarction not clearly attributable to a nontarget vessel lesion, or target vessel revascularization defined according to Academic Research Consortium (ARC) criteria, at 2 years' follow-up [23]. The Third Universal Myocardial Infarction definitions are used [26]. Secondary endpoints include acute angiographic and clinical outcomes at prespecified follow-up times: (1) device success is defined as successful delivery and deployment of the first study scaffold/stent at the target lesion followed by successful withdrawal of the delivery system with a residual in-scaffold/in-stent residual stenosis <20% by quantitative coronary angiography (QCA) and a TIMI 3 flow grade; (2) procedural success is defined as device success for all the target lesions without the occurrence of cardiac death, target vessel myocardial infarction or repeat target lesion revascularization during the hospital stay. Clinical secondary endpoints include the following: (1) target vessel failure at 2 years; (2) target lesion failure, a composite of cardiac death, myocardial infarction not clearly attributable to a nontarget vessel, or target lesion revascularization; (3) major adverse cardiac events, including all-cause death, any myocardial infarction, or repeat revascularization; (4) death (cardiac, vascular, noncardiovascular); (5) any myocardial infarction; (6) any revascularization, target lesion revascularization, target vessel revascularization, nontarget vessel revascularization; and (7) definite or probable scaffold/stent thrombosis (acute, subacute, and late). Finally, quality of life (EQ-5D) and subjective perception of cardiovascular symptoms (SAQ) at 1 year and 2 years are also being evaluated as secondary endpoints.

Follow-up is obtained by phone at 30 days, 6 months, 1 year, and yearly up to 5 years. The EuroQol (EQ-5D) and Seattle Angina Questionnaire (SAQ) are obtained at baseline, 1 year, and 2 years. Data from the AIDA trial will be analyzed on an intention-to-treat basis. However, an as-treated analysis will also be reported.

## COMPARE ABSORB

The COMPARE ABSORB (ABSORB Bioresorbable Scaffold vs. XIENCE Metallic Stent for Prevention of Restenosis in Patients at High Risk of Restenosis; NCT02486068) is a prospective, multi-center, single-blind, randomized clinical trial comparing the everolimus-eluting bioresorbable scaffold (ABSORB, Abbott Vascular, Abbott Park, IL) with a cobalt-chromium everolimus-eluting stent (XIENCE PRIME, Abbott Vascular, Abbott Park, IL). The trial is investigator-driven and financial support is provided by the European Cardiovascular Research Center. The estimated date for primary outcome measure analysis is March 2018.

In a population of 2100 patients undergoing emergent or elective PCI in 42 sites across Europe, the aim is to investigate the effectiveness and safety of the bioresorbable scaffold as compared with the everolimus-eluting metallic stent at 1-year follow-up and at very long-term follow-up.

Patients aged between 18 and 80 years are deemed eligible when at least one of the following risk factors for restenosis are present: diabetes; multi-vessel disease with more than one de novo target lesion; and/or patients must have at least one complex de novo lesion satisfying one or more of the following criteria: lesion length >28 mm, reference vessel diameter 2.25–2.75 mm ("small vessel"), lesion with pre-existing total occlusion (TIMI-flow grade 0), or bifurcation lesion requiring a single-stent strategy. Randomization sequence is stratified for STEMI and diabetes. Exclusion criteria include the following: left ventricular ejection fraction <30%, renal insufficiency with eGFR <45 mL/min; known comorbidities making it unlikely for patients to complete 5-year follow-up; known nonadherence to dual antiplatelet therapy; patients on oral anticoagulation; cardiogenic shock; reference vessel diameter <2.25 mm and >4.0 mm or >3.5 mm in the setting of STEMI; target lesion located in a graft, ostial left main lesion, bifurcation requiring a two-scaffold/-stent strategy; in-scaffold/stent thrombosis; in-scaffold/stent restenosis; and severe target-vessel tortuosity.

The aim of the trial is to assess noninferiority of the bioresorbable scaffold to the everolimus-eluting stent in terms of the primary endpoint of target lesion failure (TLF) at 1 year, and to assess superiority of the bioresorbable scaffold to the everolimus-eluting stent in terms of target lesion failure at both landmark analysis between 1 and 5 years and at cumulative analysis at 5 years. Secondary endpoints include: (1) individual components of the primary endpoint; (2) all-cause death; (3) target lesion revascularization; (4) definite or probable stent/scaffold thrombosis; (5) angina score; (6) anti-anginal medication use; and (7) chest pain.

Prespecified subgroup analyses include: (1) acute coronary syndrome vs. nonacute coronary syndrome; (2) diabetes; (3) multi-vessel disease vs. single-vessel disease; (4) long lesions (>28 mm); (5) bifurcation lesions; and (6) chronic total occlusion. Planned substudies include: (1) 61 diabetic patients undergoing 5-year angiographic follow-up with intravascular ultrasound (IVUS) imaging; (2) 50 patients undergoing ischemia and vasomotion testing by positron-emission tomography (PET) assessment; (3) angina and cost-effectiveness analyses at 1, 2, and 5 years; (4) a secondary cohort of 300 patients undergoing web-based self-follow-up evaluation ("Smart Follow-Up"). In addition to patients undergoing randomization, the COMPARE ABSORB investigators also plan to enroll a secondary observational cohort of 100 patients with in-stent restenosis.

# BIORESORBABLE SCAFFOLDS VERSUS CURRENT-GENERATION BIODEGRADABLE POLYMER DRUG-ELUTING STENTS

## EVERBIO II

The EVERBIO II (Comparison of Everolimus- and Biolimus-Eluting Stents With Everolimus-Eluting Bioresorbable Vascular Scaffold Stents II; NCT01711931) trial was a prospective, single-center, assessor-blind, randomized clinical trial. Between November 2012 and November 2013, 240 patients aged 18–70 years undergoing elective PCI for symptomatic or silent coronary artery disease were assigned in a 1:1:1 ratio to receive the bioresorbable scaffold (ABSORB, Abbott Vascular, Abbott Park, IL), everolimus-eluting stent (Promus Element, Boston Scientific, Natick, MA), or biolimus-eluting stent (Biomatrix Flex, Biosensors International Ltd., Morges, Switzerland) [27,28]. The EVERBIO II trial is the second investigator-driven randomized clinical trial investigating the ABSORB bioresorbable scaffold with reported primary endpoint data. The EVERBIO II trial was supported by the University of Freiburg. Patients were randomized after successful lesion predilation. Outcome assessors and data analysts were blinded to the intervention; however, patients and operators were not. Although inclusion criteria were extremely broad, exclusion criteria included STEMI in the previous 48 hours; moderate-to-severe kidney failure (creatinine clearance ≤60 mL/min); reference vessel diameter >4.0 mm; and known or presumed hypersensitivity to heparin or antiplatelet therapy.

The primary endpoint was in-device late lumen loss at 9 months as assessed by QCA. Secondary angiographic endpoints at 9-months follow-up included: (1) in-segment late lumen loss; (2) binary restenosis; (3) acute gain; (4) minimum lumen diameter; and (5) percentage diameter stenosis. Secondary clinical endpoints were assessed at 12 months and included: (1) a device-oriented composite endpoint of cardiac death, myocardial infarction, or target lesion revascularization; (2) a patient-oriented composite endpoint of death, myocardial infarction, or any revascularization; and (3) ARC-defined stent thrombosis. Patients were followed every 3 months within the first year postprocedure. Additional follow-up is planned at 2 and 5 years.

Baseline angiographic and procedural characteristics were generally well balanced. However, preprocedural dimensions showed a lower reference vessel diameter in the everolimus-eluting/biolimus-eluting metallic stent group as compared with everolimus-eluting bioresorbable scaffold group (2.39 ± 0.70 mm vs. 2.53 ± 0.84 mm vs. 2.77 ± 0.60 mm). Given that PCI technique was at the discretion of the treating physician, significant differences in technique between the bioresorbable scaffold and metallic stent groups were observed. Specifically, patients assigned to receive the bioresorbable scaffold received direct stenting less frequently (3% vs. 17%, $p < 0.01$), more frequent concomitant implantation of a study stent and a non-study stent for the same lesion (4% vs. 1%, $p = 0.03$), a trend toward longer device implantation (22.8 ± 8.8 mm vs. 20.7 ± 12.1 mm, $p = 0.08$), and greater device size (3.13 ± 0.37 mm vs. 2.99 ± 0.82 mm, $p = 0.03$) as compared with patients allocated to receive the everolimus-/biolimus-eluting metallic stent. Importantly, due to more acute recoil, postprocedural in-stent diameter tended to be lower with the everolimus-eluting bioresorbable scaffold compared with the everolimus-/biolimus-eluting metallic stent (9.5 ± 6.5% vs. 6.6 ± 4.7%, $p < 0.01$).

The primary endpoint of 9-month in-stent late lumen loss was similar across devices with a difference of 0.04 mm between the everolimus-eluting bioresorbable scaffold and the everolimus-eluting metallic stent/biolimus-eluting metallic stent (0.28 ± 0.39 mm vs. 0.25 ± 0.36 mm, respectively; 95% CI −0.06 to 0.13, $p_{superiority} < 0.001$, $p_{noninferiority} = 0.30$). Stratified analysis according to the presence or absence of diabetes mellitus ($p = 0.33$), acute coronary syndrome ($p = 0.28$), and high lesion complexity ($p = 0.94$) did not influence the main conclusions.

The secondary angiographic endpoint of 9-month in-segment late-lumen loss showed a mild but significant increase in the bioresorabable scaffold group compared with the everolimus-eluting metallic stent/biolimus-eluting metallic stent group (0.30 ± 0.44 mm vs. 0.19 ± 0.42 mm, $p = 0.03$). There were no differences in the secondary clinical endpoints of 9-month device-oriented composite of major adverse cardiac events (9% vs. 12%, $p = 0.60$) and patient-oriented composite of major adverse cardiac events (27% vs. 26%, $p = 0.83$). Clinically driven target lesion revascularization was also similar, occurring in 8% of patients receiving bioresorbable scaffold and in 6% of those receiving everolimus-eluting metallic stent/biolimus-eluting metallic stent ($p = 0.54$), as well as clinically driven target vessel revascularization (10% vs. 8%, $p = 0.59$) and nontarget vessel revascularization (12% vs. 11%, $p = 0.83$). There were no target vessel-related myocardial infarctions and overall mortality was 2% with comparable incidence for both devices. Only one case of possible stent thrombosis was observed and this occurred in the bioresorbable scaffold group.

The major finding of the EVERBIO II trial was noninferiority of the everolimus-eluting bioresorbable scaffold to the everolimus-eluting metallic stent and biolimus-eluting metallic stents in terms of the primary angiographic endpoint of in-stent late lumen loss at 9 months. Both scaffold bioabsorption kinetics and animal models suggest that the failure risk of bioresorbable scaffolds would be higher between 6 and 12 months following implantation and that in-stent late lumen loss should peak during this period [28,29]. Finally, clinical outcomes were overall comparable

and no alarming findings were noticed in patients treated with the bioresorbable scaffold.

These results should, however, be interpreted in the context of some important limitations of the EVERBIO II trial. Although a 9-month follow-up is sufficient to detect a potential restenotic propensity of the bioresorbable scaffold, and in-stent late lumen loss is a robust measure of the performance of new coronary stents, angiographic endpoints cannot substitute for clinical endpoints. Moreover, occurrence of the secondary angiographic endpoint of in-segment late lumen loss at 9-months follow-up was significantly higher in patients receiving the bioresorbable scaffold, indicating slightly lower antirestenotic efficacy compared with new-generation metallic drug-eluting stents.

## ISAR-RESORB

The ISAR-RESORB (A Prospective, Randomized Trial of SYNERGY Bioresorbable Polymer Coated Stents Versus ABSORB Bioresorbable Backbone Stents in Patients Undergoing Coronary Stenting; NCT02421016) trial is a prospective, open-label, superiority, randomized clinical trial comparing a thin-strut platinum-chromium bioresorbable abluminal polymer everolimus-eluting stent (SYNERGY, Boston Scientific, Natick, MA) with an everolimus-eluting bioresorbable scaffold in patients undergoing PCI for *de novo* lesions sponsored by the Deutsches Herzzentrum München [30]. The aim of the ISAR-RESORB study is to test the effectiveness and the safety of the ABSORB bioresorbable scaffold against a new-generation high-performance bioresorbable polymer everolimus-eluting metallic stent. Estimated completion date is April 2017.

According to the sample size estimation, 230 patients are required to show superiority in percentage diameter stenosis of the SYNERGY device over the metallic stent. Adult patients with symptoms or evidence of myocardial ischemia in the presence of one or two (in separate vessels) ≥50% *de novo* stenoses located in native coronary vessels are randomized in a 1:1 treatment allocation to either the everolimus-eluting bioresorbable scaffold or the platinum-chromium everolimus-eluting stent. Angiographic inclusion criteria include reference diameter 2.5–3.9 mm, lesion length <28 mm, severe calcification, left main trunk or bypass graft target lesion, ostial lesion, and bifurcation lesion with involvement of a side branch with a diameter ≥2 mm. Key clinical exclusion criteria include cardiogenic shock, STEMI within 48 hours of symptom onset, advanced chronic kidney disease (serum creatinine >2.0 mg/dL or >177 μmol/L within 72 hours before the procedure), and inability to take antiplatelet medications for at least 6 months.

The primary endpoint of the trial is the percentage diameter stenosis assessed by QCA performed in a core laboratory (ISAResearch Center, Munich, Germany) at protocol-mandated 6–8 month angiographic follow-up. Secondary clinical endpoints are assessed at 12 months and include three composite endpoints: (1) cardiac death, target vessel-related myocardial infarction, or target lesion revascularization (device-oriented composite endpoint); (2) all-cause death, any myocardial infarction, or any revascularization (patient-oriented composite endpoint); and (3) cardiovascular death or myocardial infarction. Aside from the latter, the other safety endpoint is ARC-defined definite/probable stent thrombosis [23] at 12 months.

# BIORESORBABLE SCAFFOLDS VERSUS OPTIMAL MEDICAL THERAPY

## PREVENT

The PREVENT (Preventive Implantation of Bioresorbable Vascular Scaffold on Functionally Insignificant Stenosis With Vulnerable Plaque Characteristics; NCT02316886) trial is an open-label, randomized clinical trial testing the prognostic impact and the clinical improvement associated with the everolimus-eluting bioresorbable scaffold (ABSORB, Abbott Vascular, Abbott Park, IL) and optimal medical therapy versus optimal medical therapy alone in patients with functionally nonsignificant coronary stenosis with vulnerable plaque. The study is supported by CardioVascular Research Foundation, Korea. It is planned to enroll a total of 1600 patients, with planned completion in January 2019.

Adult subjects with coronary artery disease—symptomatic or asymptomatic—with at least one coronary artery stenosis associated with a fractional flow reserve (FFR) value >0.80 and possessing at least two of the four following morphological risk factors are considered for inclusion in the trial: minimal luminal area <4 mm² by intravascular ultrasound (IVUS), plaque burden >70% by IVUS, lipid-rich plaque by intracoronary near-infrared spectroscopy (NIRS), thin-cap fibroatheroma by optical coherence tomography (OCT) or virtual histology-intravascular ultrasound (VH-IVUS), respectively, defined as fibrous cap thickness <65 μm plus arc >90° and ≥10% confluent necrotic core protruding >30° into the lumen in three consecutive cross-sectional images. Additional inclusion criteria include reference vessel diameter of 2.75–4.0 mm, and lesion length ≤40 mm. Angiographic exclusion criteria include more than two discrete target vulnerable lesions or two target vulnerable lesions in the same coronary territory, in-stent restenosis lesions, bypass graft lesions, heavily calcified or angulated lesions, and bifurcation lesions requiring a dual-stent technique.

Primary outcome measures at 24 months include cardiovascular death, nonfatal myocardial infarction, and unstable angina requiring unplanned hospitalization. Secondary outcome measures are all-cause death at 24 months, target vessel failure (composite of cardiovascular death, target vessel-related myocardial infarction, or target vessel revascularization) at 24 months, major adverse cardiovascular events (composite of all-cause death, any myocardial infarction, and any repeat revascularization), and the composite of death or myocardial infarction at 1, 6, 12, and 24 months; nonurgent revascularization procedures at 1, 6, 12, and 24 months; CCS anginal class [24] at 1, 6, 12, and 24 months; anti-anginal medication use at 1, 6, 12, and 24 months; and any cerebrovascular event at 1, 6, 12, and 24 months.

## PROSPECT ABSORB

The PROSPECT ABSORB (A Multi-Center Prospective Natural History Study Using Multimodality Imaging in Patients With Acute Coronary Syndromes, Combined With a Randomized, Controlled, Intervention Study) trial is a randomized, open-label, substudy of the PROSPECT II trial, which is an all-comers prospective observational study using multimodality imaging. PROSPECT ABSORB is supported by Uppsala University, but Abbott Vascular, InfraReDx, and The Medicines Company are reported as collaborators. Evaluation of the primary endpoint is planned in December 2018.

The purpose of the PROSPECT ABSORB trial is to examine minimum lumen diameter at 2 years from enrollment in the study. Patients with vulnerable plaques—defined by intravascular ultrasound (IVUS) and near infrared spectroscopy (NIRS) as lesions with a plaque burden ≥70%—are randomly assigned to treatment with either the everolimus-eluting bioresorbable scaffold (ABSORB, Abbott Vascular, Abbott Park, IL) plus optimal medical therapy or optimal medical therapy alone.

Patients must present with de novo lesions with an angiographic diameter <70% and no conventional indication for PCI determined by angiographic qualitative criteria or fractional flow reserve/instantaneous wave-free ratio (FFR/iFR) values. Additional eligibility criteria are a visually estimated reference vessel diameter ≥2.5 mm and ≤4.0 mm and a visually estimated lesion length ≤50 mm, capable of being treated by no more than two overlapping bioresorbable scaffolds. There must be a 10 mm distance between this device and any previously implanted stent/scaffold and this intervening 10 mm segment must not have a plaque burden >50%. Bifurcation lesions are only eligible for inclusion if the side branch is ≤2.5 mm in diameter and has either no lesion requiring treatment or atherosclerotic disease limited to within 5 mm of its origin from the parent vessel, is amenable to balloon angioplasty alone, and if a stent subsequently becomes necessary, only a metallic drug-eluting stent (use of XIENCE, Abbott Vascular, Abbott Park, IL, is strongly recommended) is allowed (using a T-stenting technique). Exclusion criteria are target lesion located in the left main coronary artery or at the ostium of one of the main epicardial vessels (left anterior descending, left circumflex, right coronary artery) or within 10 mm from a lesion previously treated by PCI; severe calcification and/or marked tortuosity; and anatomic conditions which make advancement of the bioresorbable scaffold across the lesion or adequate expansion unlikely.

## BIORESORBABLE SCAFFOLDS VERSUS SURGICAL REVASCULARIZATION

### RELEASE-BVS

The RELEASE-BVS (Revascularization With the Use of Biodegradable Scaffolds Compared to Coronary Artery Bypass Grafting in Patients With Advanced Stable Ischemic Heart Disease; NCT02334826) trial is, to date, the only investigator-driven randomized trial comparing bioresorbable scaffold-based PCI with coronary artery bypass grafting. This open-label, single-center, randomized trial is supported by the Poznan University of Medical Sciences. The expected date for primary outcome assessment is September 2017.

The primary endpoint is the extent of ischemia and left ventricular ejection fraction at 12 months as assessed by cardiovascular magnetic resonance imaging, while the secondary endpoints are patency of coronary arteries and grafts at 12 months as assessed by computed tomography angiography and cumulative incidence of the composite outcome of major adverse cardiac and cerebrovascular events (all-cause death, cardiac death, myocardial infarction, stroke, stent thrombosis, or repeat revascularization) over 5 years.

Adult patients with symptomatic stable angina or silent ischemia due to three-vessel coronary artery disease and/or significant stenosis of the left main coronary artery and documented ischemia evaluated by stress cardiac magnetic resonance are randomized after heart team evaluation to treatment with PCI using bioresorbable scaffolds or coronary artery bypass grafting. Exclusion criteria include prior coronary artery bypass grafting, concomitant valve disease requiring cardiac surgery, acute coronary syndrome within 2 weeks prior to revascularization or stroke/transient ischemic attack within 3 months prior to revascularization, significant stenosis of any vessel (including LM) with a reference diameter >4 mm, left ventricular ejection fraction <35%, estimated glomerular filtration (eGFR) <30 mL/min/1.73 m², contraindication to stress magnetic resonance examination, computed tomography or 12 months dual antiplatelet therapy, chronic oral anticoagulation therapy or bleeding history, life expectancy <12 months, and planned noncardiac surgery within 12 months after randomization.

## MYOCARDIAL BLOOD FLOW IMPROVEMENT

### VANISH

The VANISH (Impact of Vascular Reparative Therapy on Vasomotor Function and Myocardial Perfusion; NCT01876589) trial compares the everolimus-eluting bioresorbable scaffold (ABSORB, Abbott Vascular, Abbott Park, IL) with an everolimus-eluting metallic stent (XIENCE Prime, Abbott Vascular, Abbott Park, IL) in terms of the primary endpoint of improvement in myocardial blood flow 3 years post-device implantation as assessed using positron emission tomography. This is a prospective, single-center, single-blind, randomized trial. The assumption is that patients who receive the bioresorbable scaffold regain vasomotor functions within the stented segment with a resulting long-term beneficial effect on myocardial blood flow. The secondary endpoint is the angiographic assessment of restenosis at 3 years. The VANISH trial is currently ongoing with an expected date for primary outcome evaluation in June 2018. The trial is supported by the VU University Medical Center.

Eligibility criteria for inclusion in the VANISH trial are extremely selective in order to limit conditions which may influence myocardial blood flow assessment. Briefly, a total of 60 patients 18–65 years old with angiographic evidence of a single de novo noncomplex (type A or B1) ≥50% coronary artery stenosis, resulting in TIMI-flow grade ≥2 and myocardial ischemia, assessed by invasive (FFR) or noninvasive means (e.g., exercise ECG, myocardial perfusion imaging, or inducibility of wall motion abnormalities during dobutamine stress) are randomly assigned to receive either an everolimus-eluting bioresorbable scaffold or an everolimus-eluting metallic stent. Coronary lesions meet inclusion criteria if amendable to successful treatment with one of the following BRS device dimensions: length of 18 or 28 mm and diameter of 3.0 or 3.5 mm. Only placement of a single stent is allowed and patients receiving bailout stenting after placement of the study device are excluded. Angiographic exclusion criteria include total occlusion, TIMI-flow grade 0-1, ≥2 lesions, left main coronary artery disease, bifurcation lesions involving a side branch with a diameter >2 mm, and the presence of thrombus. Patients with baseline abnormal echocardiographic findings which could independently influence coronary blood flow, such as wall motion abnormalities, ventricular hypertrophy, and valvular diseases, are excluded. Clinical exclusion criteria include eGFR <30 mL/min, asthma or chronic obstructive pulmonary disease, and heart rhythm other than sinus rhythm.

## REFERENCES

1. Byrne RA, Joner M, Kastrati A. Stent thrombosis and restenosis: What have we learned and where are we going? The Andreas Gruntzig Lecture ESC 2014. *Eur Heart J.* 2015;36:3320–31.
2. Stone GW, Rizvi A, Newman W et al. Everolimus-eluting versus paclitaxel-eluting stents in coronary artery disease. *N Engl J Med.* 2010;362:1663–74.
3. Stefanini GG, Kalesan B, Serruys PW et al. Long-term clinical outcomes of biodegradable polymer biolimus-eluting stents versus durable polymer sirolimus-eluting stents in patients with coronary artery disease (LEADERS): 4 year follow-up of a randomized non-inferiority trial. *Lancet.* 2011;378:1940–8.
4. Maeng M, Tilsted HH, Jensen LO et al. Differential clinical outcomes after 1 year versus 5 years in a randomized comparison of zotarolimus-eluting and

sirolimus-eluting coronary stents (the SORT OUT III study): A multicentre, open-label, randomized superiority trial. *Lancet*. 2014;383:2047–56.

5. Räber L, Magro M, Stefanini GG et al. Very late coronary stent thrombosis of a newer-generation everolimus-eluting stent compared with early-generation drug-eluting stents: A prospective cohort study. *Circulation*. 2012;125:1110–21.

6. Sabate M, Brugaletta S, Cequier A et al. Clinical outcomes in patients with ST-segment elevation myocardial infarction treated with everolimus-eluting stents versus bare-metal stents (EXAMINATION): 5-year results of a randomized trial. *Lancet*. 2016;387:357–66.

7. von Birgelen C, Basalus MW, Tandjung K et al. A randomized controlled trial in second-generation zotarolimus-eluting Resolute stents versus everolimus-eluting XIENCE V stents in real-world patients: The TWENTE trial. *J Am Coll Cardiol*. 2012;59:1350–61.

8. Stefanini GG, Serruys PW, Silber S et al. The impact of patient and lesion complexity on clinical and angiographic outcomes after revascularization with zotarolimus- and everolimus-eluting stents: A substudy of the RESOLUTE All Comers Trial (a randomized comparison of a zotarolimus-eluting stent with an everolimus-eluting stent for percutaneous coronary intervention). *J Am Coll Cardiol*. 2011;57:2221–32.

9. Kaul U, Bangalore S, Seth A et al. Paclitaxel-eluting versus everolimus-eluting coronary stents in diabetes. *N Engl J Med*. 2015;373:1709–19.

10. Iqbal J, Onuma Y, Ormiston J, Abizaid A, Waksman R, Serruys P. Bioresorbable scaffolds: Rationale, current status, challenges, and future. *Eur Heart J*. 2014;35:765–76.

11. Karanasos A, Simsek C, Gnanadesigan M et al. OCT assessment of the long-term vascular healing response 5 years after everolimus-eluting bioresorbable vascular scaffold. *J Am Coll Cardiol*. 2014;64:2343–56.

12. Ormiston JA, Serruys PW, Onuma Y et al. First serial assessment at 6 months and 2 years of the second generation of absorb everolimus-eluting bioresorbable vascular scaffold: A multi-imaging modality study. *Circ Cardiovasc Interv*. 2012;5:620–32.

13. Räber L, Brugaletta S, Yamaji K et al. Very late scaffold thrombosis: Intracoronary imaging and histopathological and spectroscopic findings. *J Am Coll Cardiol*. 2015;66:1901–14.

14. Serruys PW, Chevalier B, Dudek D et al. A bioresorbable everolimus-eluting scaffold versus a metallic everolimus-eluting stent for ischaemic heart disease caused by de-novo native coronary artery lesions (ABSORB II): An interim 1-year analysis of clinical and procedural secondary outcomes from a randomized controlled trial. *Lancet*. 2015;385:43–54.

15. Ellis SG, Kereiakes DJ, Metzger DC et al. Everolimus-eluting bioresorbable scaffolds for coronary artery disease. *N Engl J Med*. 2015;373:1905–15.

16. Kimura T, Kozuma K, Tanabe K et al. A randomized trial evaluating everolimus-eluting Absorb bioresorbable scaffolds vs. everolimus-eluting metallic stents in patients with coronary artery disease: ABSORB Japan. *Eur Heart J*. 2015;36:3332–42.

17. Cassese S, Byrne RA, Ndrepepa G et al. Everolimus-eluting bioresorbable vascular scaffolds versus everolimus-eluting metallic stents: A meta-analysis of randomized controlled trials. *Lancet*. 2016;387:537–44.

18. Brugaletta S, Gori T, Low AF et al. Absorb bioresorbable vascular scaffold versus everolimus-eluting metallic stent in ST-segment elevation myocardial infarction: 1-year results of a propensity score matching comparison: The BVS-EXAMINATION Study (bioresorbable vascular scaffold—A clinical evaluation of everolimus eluting coronary stents in the treatment of patients with ST-segment elevation myocardial infarction). *JACC Cardiovasc Interv*. 2015;8:189–97.

19. Cassese S, Kastrati A. Bioresorbable vascular scaffold technology benefits from healthy skepticism. *J Am Coll Cardiol*. 2016;67:932–5.

20. Puricel S, Cuculi F, Weissner M et al. Bioresorbable coronary scaffold thrombosis: Multicenter comprehensive analysis of clinical presentation, mechanisms, and predictors. *J Am Coll Cardiol*. 2016;67:921–31.

21. Kočka V, Malý M, Toušek P et al. Bioresorbable vascular scaffolds in acute ST-segment elevation myocardial infarction: A prospective multicentre study 'Prague 19'. *Eur Heart J*. 2014;35:787–94.

22. Sabate M, Windecker S, Iniguez A et al. Everolimus-eluting bioresorbable stent vs. durable polymer everolimus-eluting metallic stent in patients with ST-segment elevation myocardial infarction: Results of the randomized ABSORB ST-segment elevation myocardial infarction-TROFI II trial. *Eur Heart J*. 2016;37:229–40.

23. Cutlip DE, Windecker S, Mehran R et al. Clinical end points in coronary stent trials: A case for standardized definitions. *Circulation*. 2007;115:2344–51.

24. Campeau L. Letter: Grading of angina pectoris. *Circulation*. 1976;54:522–3.

25. Woudstra P, Grundeken MJ, Kraak RP et al. Amsterdam Investigator-initiateD Absorb strategy all-comers trial (AIDA trial): A clinical evaluation comparing the efficacy and performance of ABSORB everolimus-eluting bioresorbable vascular scaffold strategy vs. the XIENCE family (XIENCE PRIME or XIENCE Xpedition) everolimus-eluting coronary stent strategy in the treatment of coronary lesions in consecutive all-comers: Rationale and study design. *Am Heart J*. 2014;167:133–40.

26. Thygesen K, Alpert JS, Jaffe AS et al. Third universal definition of myocardial infarction. *Eur Heart J.* 2012;33:2551–67.

27. Arroyo D, Togni M, Puricel S et al. Comparison of everolimus-eluting and biolimus-eluting coronary stents with everolimus-eluting bioresorbable scaffold: Study protocol of the randomized controlled EVERBIO II trial. *Trials.* 2014;15:9.

28. Puricel S, Arroyo D, Corpataux N et al. Comparison of everolimus- and biolimus-eluting coronary stents with everolimus-eluting bioresorbable vascular scaffolds. *J Am Coll Cardiol.* 2015;65:791–801.

29. Otsuka F, Pacheco E, Perkins LE et al. Long-term safety of an everolimus-eluting bioresorbable vascular scaffold and the cobalt-chromium XIENCE V stent in a porcine coronary artery model. *Circ Cardiovasc Interv.* 2014;7:330–42.

30. Meredith IT, Verheye S, Dubois CL et al. Primary endpoint results of the EVOLVE trial: A randomized evaluation of a novel bioabsorbable polymer-coated, everolimus-eluting coronary stent. *J Am Coll Cardiol.* 2012;59:1362–70.

6.9

# The DESolve scaffold

STEFAN VERHEYE, NAGARAJAN RAMESH, LYNN MORRISON, AND SARA TOYLOY

Conceptually, bioresorbable scaffolds (BRSs) were developed as an alternative to metallic stents to provide temporary vascular support, prevent vessel recoil, and avoid late events such as thrombosis, and restenosis. To date, several polymeric and metallic bioresorbable scaffolds have been clinically tested and the initial results with poly-L-lactic-acid (PLLA) scaffolds appear promising [1–5]. Still, the impact of device design, materials, drug, degradation and resorption kinetics on vessel restoration and long-term outcomes remains unclear.

The first absorbable scaffold implanted in humans was the non-drug-eluting Igaki-Tamai PLLA scaffold [4]. The scaffold thickness of 170 μm was greater than the newer generation bioresorbable scaffolds such as ABSORB and DESolve. The late lumen loss (LLL) for the Igaki-Tamai device was >0.90 mm at 6 months in keeping with a non-drug-eluting device. Interestingly, there was a trend toward increase in the in-scaffold area by IVUS between baseline and 6 months. The maintenance of lumen diameter over the 10-year follow-up period supports long-term safety of the polymeric material [6].

The DESolve Novolimus Eluting Bioresorbable Coronary Scaffold System is comprised of a PLLA-based polymer scaffold (150 μm strut thickness) and the drug Novolimus shown in Figure 6.9.1. Novolimus is an active metabolite of rapamycin (sirolimus) which belongs to the family of compounds of macrocyclic lactones with immunosuppressive and antiproliferative properties. The chemical structure of Novolimus is shown in Figure 6.9.2. Novolimus is loaded at approximately 5 μg per mm of scaffold length (85 μg for an 18 mm scaffold) with approximately 80% of the drug being eluted *in vivo* over 4 weeks. The scaffold incorporates two platinum-iridium markers at each end of the scaffold to aid in angiographic assessment of scaffold placement. The DESolve scaffold has several unique differentiating characteristics when compared with other clinically tested bioresorbable devices. These include: (1) its ability to self-correct to the vessel wall in cases of minor malapposition when expanded to the nominal diameter addressing the inherent "sagging" of bioresorbable scaffolds postprocedure

thus maintaining the acute results; (2) short bioresorption time (90% degradation within 6 months, 70% resorption in 1 year and fully bioresorbed within 2 years), addressing potential late or very late events due to the persistent presence of the scaffold; (3) the ability of the scaffold to maintain radial strength and provide vessel support for the critical 3–4 month period of vessel healing despite the shorter polymer degradation time; (4) the ability to expand the scaffold without strut fracture—a 3.0 mm scaffold can be expanded to 4.5 mm. Figures 6.9.3, 6.9.4, and 6.9.5 depict some of these unique characteristics. (Testing on file at Elixir Medical.)

Differing chemical properties of polymers result in differing mechanical capabilities including fracture resistance as compared to metallic stents. The overexpansion (beyond nominal diameter) and through-strut expansion capabilities of the DESolve scaffold were assessed by Ormiston et al. [7] employing independent bench testing methods. The DESolve scaffold was deployed unconstrained in the water bath at 37°C, postdilated with noncompliant (NC) balloons increasingly sized up and inflated to 20 atmospheres of pressure. The results showed that the scaffold did not fracture at diameters up to 5.0 mm. Visible straightening and stretching of the sinusoidal hoops of the scaffold was observed before any fracture thus corroborating the observations from Elixir Medical testing. Similarly, no fractures were observed during through-strut expansion, simulating side branch dilatation, with a 3.0 mm NC balloon at 22 atm. The self-correction characteristic of the DESolve scaffold was also tested by Ormiston et al. [7]. Following deployment of a 3.0 mm diameter DESolve scaffold, recoil of approximately 0.1 mm was seen; however, within 10 to 60 min the scaffold increased in diameter to baseline dimensions. Elixir Medical performed bench testing using OCT imaging at multiple time points with a DESolve scaffold intentionally underdeployed resulting in suboptimal strut apposition as shown in Figure 6.9.3. This model showed that the scaffold self-corrected resulting in full apposition by 30 min. Evidence for self-correction has also been demonstrated *in vivo* with the DESolve scaffold by Wiebe

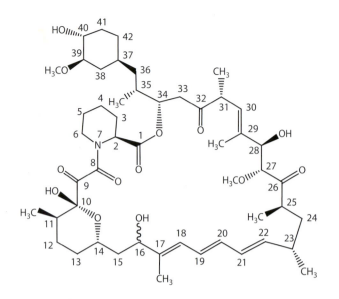

Figure 6.9.1 Chemical structure of novolimus.

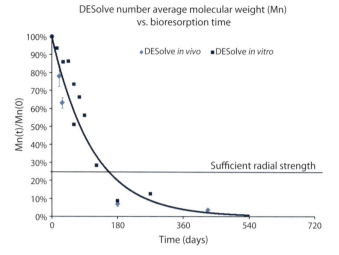

Figure 6.9.4 DESolve bioresorption profile showing *in vitro* and *in vivo* molecular weight measurements by gel permeation chromatography.

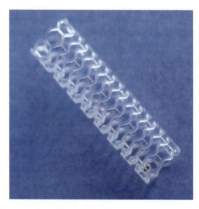

Figure 6.9.2 DESolve® scaffold.

et al. [8] wherein a .5 × 28 mm DESolve was implanted in a mid-circumflex stenosis but which showed some malapposition at baseline. Over a period of 15 minutes, the malapposition was measurably reduced. Thus, the reduced risk of strut fracture and the self-correction characteristic of the DESolve scaffolds affords the interventionalist greater confidence in scaffold expansion and apposition capabilities.

The DESolve scaffold system has been evaluated in two clinical trials. In the first study, a Myolimus (a sirolimus analog) eluting DESolve scaffold was investigated in a multicenter DESolve first-in-man (FIM) trial in which 15 patients with single *de novo* lesions were treated [5]. In the second study, following refinement of the DESolve scaffold which included the use of Novolimus instead of Myolimus along with a broader spectrum of device sizes, was investigated in the DESolve Nx pivotal study.

## DESolve FIM

The DESolve FIM trial was a prospective multicenter study enrolling 16 patients of whom 15 received a study device. The study outline is shown in Figure 6.9.6. The principal safety endpoint was the composite endpoint of major adverse cardiac events (MACE) comprised of: cardiac death, target vessel myocardial infarction (MI), and clinically indicated target lesion revascularization (TLR). The principal imaging endpoint was in-scaffold LLL assessed by quantitative coronary angiography (QCA) at 6 months. Intravascular ultrasound (IVUS) and optical coherence tomography (OCT) imaging was also performed at baseline and 6 months; multi slice computed tomography

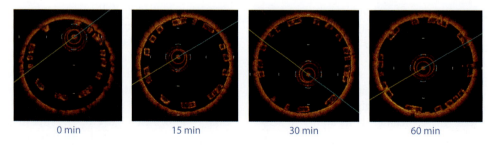

0 min          15 min          30 min          60 min

Figure 6.9.3 Intentionally created suboptimal strut apposition of a DESolve scaffold and progression over time until full self-correction as imaged by OCT.

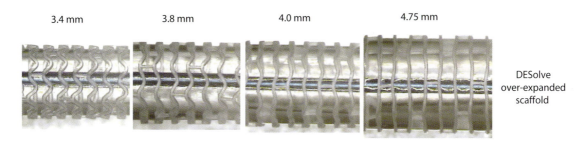

3.4 mm    3.8 mm    4.0 mm    4.75 mm

DESolve over-expanded scaffold

**Figure 6.9.5** Bench testing demonstrating the expansion properties and fracture resistance of the DESolve scaffold.

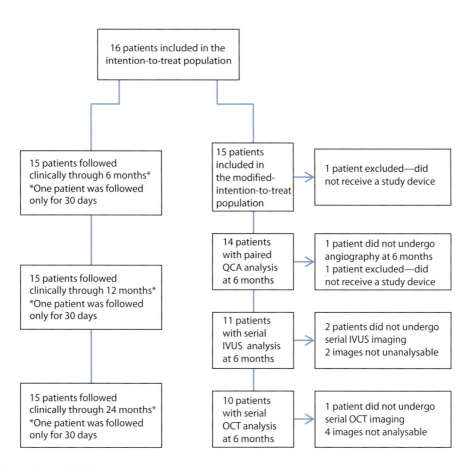

16 patients included in the intention-to-treat population

15 patients followed clinically through 6 months*
*One patient was followed only for 30 days

15 patients included in the modified-intention-to-treat population → 1 patient excluded—did not receive a study device

14 patients with paired QCA analysis at 6 months → 1 patient did not undergo angiography at 6 months
1 patient excluded—did not receive a study device

15 patients followed clinically through 12 months*
*One patient was followed only for 30 days

11 patients with serial IVUS analysis at 6 months → 2 patients did not undergo serial IVUS imaging
2 images not unanalysable

15 patients followed clinically through 24 months*
*One patient was followed only for 30 days

10 patients with serial OCT analysis at 6 months → 1 patient did not undergo serial OCT imaging
4 images not analysable

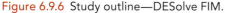

**Figure 6.9.6** Study outline—DESolve FIM.

(MSCT) was performed at 12 months. Eligibility criteria were evidence of myocardial ischemia; a single, *de novo* native coronary artery lesion; reference vessel diameter ≤3.0 mm; lesion length ≤10 mm; and a target lesion percentage diameter stenosis (%DS) <80%. Key exclusion criteria were recent (<3 days) myocardial infarction (MI); left ventricular ejection fraction <30%; left main coronary artery or restenotic lesions; lesions involving a side branch >2 mm; and the presence of thrombus or calcium.

The patient demographics for the DESolve FIM trial are shown in Table 6.9.1. Procedural success was achieved in 15 of 15 patients receiving a scaffold. One acute event was adjudicated by the clinical events committee as a non–Q-wave MI related to a target vessel revascularization (non-target lesion) with no evidence of scaffold thrombosis.

Between 30 days and 6 months, one TLR treated with a drug eluting stent (DES) was reported for a proximal left circumflex stenosis (85.9% diameter stenosis [DS]) located adjacent to the widely patent scaffold (5.9% DS). Between 6 and 12 months, one cardiac death was reported following nontarget vessel coronary artery bypass grafting and aortic valve replacement. There were no cases of scaffold thrombosis (ST) as adjudicated by the clinical events committee through the 12-month time period. Between 12 and 24 months, two TLR procedures were reported for in-scaffold restenosis; there was no ST reported.

Angiographic results at the 6-month time point showed a mean in-scaffold angiographic LLL of 0.19 ± 0.19 mm, a mean in-segment (including the proximal and distal 5 mm segments) LLL of 0.31 ± 0.54 mm and an in-scaffold %DS of

Table 6.9.1 DESolve FIM—Baseline characteristics of the intention-to-treat and modified-intention-to-treat patient population

| Baseline characteristics | Intention to treat population (n = 16) |
|---|---|
| Age (years) | 69.3 (8.4) |
| Gender (% male) | 10 (62.5%) |
| History of smoking | 11 (68.8%) |
| Diabetes Mellitus | 1 (6.3%) |
| Hypertension | 10 (62.5%) |
| Hypercholesterolemia | 11 (68.8%) |
| Family history of CAD | 6 (37.5%) |
| Prior myocardial infarction | 4 (25.0%) |
| Stable angina | 11 (68.8%) |
| Unstable angina | 0 (0.0%) |
| QCA baseline analysis | Modified-intention-to-treat paired (n = 14) |
| Target vessel | |
| Left anterior | 3 (21.4%) |
| Left circumflex | 5 (37.5%) |
| Right coronary artery | 6 (42.9%) |
| AHA/ACC lesion classification | |
| A | 5 (37.5%) |
| B1 | 4 (28.6%) |
| B2 | 5 (37.5%) |
| C | 0 (0.0%) |
| Mean reference vessel diameter (mm) | 2.65 ± 0.32 |
| Minimum lumen diameter (mm) | 0.81 ± 0.29 |
| Diameter stenosis (%) | 69.98 ± 10.49 |
| Lesion length (mm) | 8.95 ± 2.64 |
| Acute gain (mm) | 1.54 ± 0.36 |
| Acute recoil (%) | 6.42 ± 4.63 |

*Note:* Data presented as mean (SD), or N (%).

12.63 ± 11.37% (Table 6.9.2). Serial IVUS demonstrated an average scaffold area increase from 5.35 ± 0.78 mm to 5.61 ± 0.81 mm whereas the lumen area was slightly reduced from 5.35 ± 0.78 mm² to 5.10 ± 0.78 mm² with neither result being significant (Table 6.9.3). The analysis methodology for OCT is shown in Figure 6.9.7. Imaging showed a nonsignificant increase in scaffold area between baseline and follow-up (6.57 ± 0.68 mm² and 6.80 ± 0.85 mm², p = 0.2), similar to the IVUS results. The struts were covered by a thin, uniform layer of neointima in 98.7% of patients (Table 6.9.4; Figure 6.9.8). MSCT imaging at the 12-month time point demonstrated sustained luminal patency with a %DS of 15.9 ± 10% (Table 6.9.5).

## DESolve Nx TRIAL

The DESolve Nx Trial was a prospective, multicenter, nonrandomized study, evaluating the performance, safety, and efficacy of the DESolve scaffold in the treatment of patients with native coronary lesions. The DESolve scaffold evaluated in this study was coated with a matrix of the drug Novolimus and the PLLA-based polymer. In order to accommodate a wide range of expansion diameters, the DESolve scaffold was made available in patterns differentiated by the number of crowns. The DESolve scaffold was available in diameters ranging from 3.0–3.5 mm with lengths of 14 and 18 mm.

The primary (efficacy) endpoint of the trial was in-scaffold LLL, as assessed by QCA at 6 months. Clinical endpoints were assessed at 1 and 6 months and annually to 5 years and included: MACE, target lesion and target vessel failure, and scaffold thrombosis. The same definition of MACE was used in this study as well as the previously mentioned FIM study. Target vessel failure was the composite of cardiac death, myocardial infarction, or clinically indicated target vessel revascularization. Myocardial infarction was defined as new pathologic Q waves in two or more contiguous leads and elevation of two times upper normal limit of CK with elevation of

Table 6.9.2 DESolve FIM—Results of subsegmental quantitative coronary angiographic analysis

| QCA characteristic | In-scaffold | | | In-segment | | |
|---|---|---|---|---|---|---|
| | Postprocedure | 180 days | p-value* | Postprocedure | 180 days | p-value* |
| Mean reference vessel diameter (mm) | 2.84 ± 0.23 | 2.78 ± 0.27 | 0.036 | 2.77 ± 0.25 | 2.71 ± 0.27 | 0.028 |
| Minimum lumen diameter (mm) | 2.60 ± 0.19 | 2.41 ± 0.28 | <0.0001 | 2.35 ± 0.14 | 2.05 ± 0.55 | 0.003 |
| Diameter stenosis (%) | 8.05 ± 7.90 | 12.63 ± 11.37 | 0.049 | 14.64 ± 7.06 | 23.84 ± 22.05 | 0.267 |
| Acute gain (mm) | 1.54 ± 0.36 | | | | | |
| Acute recoil (%) | 6.42 ± 4.63 | | | | | |
| Late lumen loss (mm) | – | 0.19 ± 0.19 | | | 0.31 ± 0.54 | |

*Note:* Data presented as mean (SD) unless stated otherwise.
*Abbreviation:* QCA = qualitative coronary angiography.
*p values are for exploratory information only and between postprocedure and 180-day follow-up.

Table 6.9.3 DESolve FIM—Serial intravascular ultrasound (IVUS) measurement at baseline and 6-months follow-up

| IVUS characteristics | Modified-intention-to-treat paired analysis (n = 11) | | | |
| | Baseline | 180 days | Difference (95% CI) (follow-up—baseline) | p value* |
| --- | --- | --- | --- | --- |
| Mean scaffold area (mm²) | 5.35 ± 0.78 | 5.61 ± 0·81 | 0.26 (−0.06, 0.59) | 0.11 |
| Minimum scaffold area (mm²) | 4.46 ± 0.65 | 4.62 ± 0.75 | 0.16 (−0.34, 0.67) | >0.99 |
| Lumen area (mm²) | 5.34 ± 0.78 | 5.10 ± 0.78 | −0.24 (−0.65, 0.16) | >0.99 |
| Minimum lumen area (mm²) | 4.46 ± 0.65 | 3.92 ± 0.57 | −0.54 (−0.99, −0.08) | 0.23 |
| Plaque area (mm²) | 5.33 ± 2.09 | 5.38 ± 1.97 | 0.05 (−0.53, 0.63) | 0.23 |
| Lumen area stenosis (%) | 16.47 ± 4.56 | 22.46 (10.34) | 5.99 (0.20, 11.7) | 0.23 |
| Neointimal hyperplasia area (mm²) | n/a | 0.4 ± 0.2 | – | – |
| Neointimal obstruction (%) | n/a | 7.18 ± 3.37 | – | – |
| Malapposition | 0 | 0 | – | – |

*Note:* Data are mean (SD) unless stated otherwise.
*p values are for exploratory information only and are between postprocedure and 180-day follow-up.

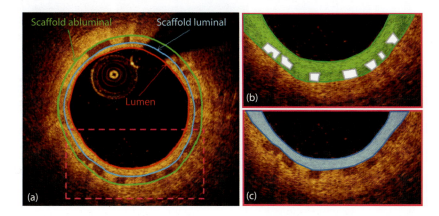

Figure 6.9.7 OCT analysis methodology: **(a)** Demonstrates the lumen and scaffold measurements with the red line depicting the lumen area, the blue line the luminal scaffold border, and the green line the abluminal scaffold border; **(b)** the total neointimal (NI) area including NI in between the struts; and **(c)** the obstructive NI area including the NI on the luminal side of the struts.

Table 6.9.4 DESolve FIM—Serial optical coherence tomography (OCT) measurement at baseline and 6-month follow-up

| OCT characteristics cross-section level | Modified-intention-to-treat paired analysis (n = 10) | | | |
| | Postprocedure | 180 days | Difference (95% CI) (follow-up—baseline) | p value* |
| --- | --- | --- | --- | --- |
| Number of cross-sections analyzed per scaffold | 25.60 ± 2.63 | 23.70 ± 4.99 | −1.90 (−5.03, 1.23) | 0.45 |
| Mean scaffold area, (mm²) | 6.57 ± 0.68 | 6.80 ± 0.85 | 0.23 (−0.16, 0.64) | 0.34 |
| Minimum scaffold area, (mm²) | 5.55 ± 0.56 | 5.45 ± 0.60 | −0.10 (−0.52, 0.32) | 0.76 |
| Mean neointimal area, (mm²) | N/A | 0.71 ± 0.36 | – | – |
| Percent volume obstruction, (%) | N/A | 13.16 ± 5.59 | – | – |
| Frequency of cross-sections with malapposition, (%) | 37/256 (14.45%) | 1/237 (0.04%) | – | 0.01 |
| Mean malapposition area, (mm²) | 0.03 ± 0·04 | 0.0 ± 0.01 | −0.02 (−0.05, 0.001) | 0.02 |
| **Strut-Level** | | | | |
| Total number of struts analyzed (n) | 2984 | 2575 | – | – |
| Number of struts analyzed per scaffold | 298.10 ± 26.93 | 257.50 ± 63.08 | −40.60 (−86.06, 4.86) | 0.11 |
| Number of struts analyzed per cross-section | 11.68 ± 0.80 | 10.79 ± 0 ± 94 | −0.89 (−1.50, 0.27) | 0.02 |
| Frequency of covered struts per scaffold, (%) | N/A | 98.68 (2.44) | – | – |
| Mean neointimal thickness of covered struts, (mm) | N/A | 0.12 ± 0.04 | – | – |
| Frequency of malapposed struts per scaffold, (%) | 2.01 ± 2.75 | 0.04 ± 0.12 | −1.97 (−3.95, 0.004) | 0.02 |

*Note:* Data are mean (SD) unless stated otherwise.
*p values are for exploratory information only and are between postprocedure and 180-day follow-up.

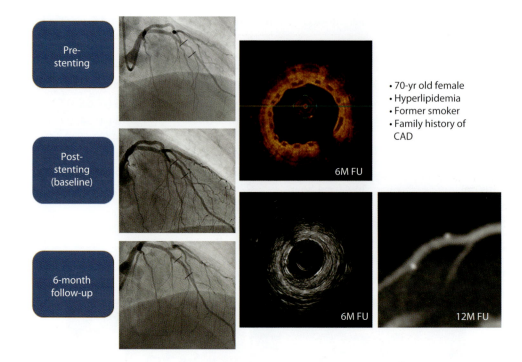

Figure 6.9.8 Case example from the DESolve FIM study. The scaffold implanted in the mid-LAD can be seen on the angiogram (between markers). OCT and IVUS show 6 months outcome. A photograph of the MSCT shows the two markers of the scaffold with a widely patent lumen.

Table 6.9.5 DESolve FIM—Multislice computed tomography (MSCT) analysis at 12-month follow-up

| MSCT in-scaffold analysis | 12 months (n = 12) |
| --- | --- |
| Reference diameter (mm) | 2.9 ± 0.5 |
| Minimal lumen diameter (mm) | 2.4 ± 0.4 |
| Mean diameter stenosis (%) | 15.9 ± 10.0 |
| Lumen area (mm²) | 6.7 ± 2.5 |
| Minimum lumen area (mm²) | 5.1 ± 2.3 |

Note: Data are mean (SD) unless stated otherwise.

CK-MB, or elevation of two times upper normal limit of CK with elevation of CK-MB in the absence of new pathological Q waves. Scaffold thrombosis was to be reported both according to the protocol definition and to the Academic Research Consortium criteria [9]. Device success was defined as successful delivery and deployment of the study device at the target site and attainment of final residual stenosis <50%.

All patients were assigned to angiographic re-evaluation at 6 months; in addition, serial evaluations with IVUS and OCT were performed at postprocedure and 6 months in a subset of approximately 40 patients at select sites. Clinical outcomes up to 24 months are provided along with serial imaging modality analyses. Clinical outcomes were reported by the intention-to-treat (ITT) or the modified-ITT (patients who received the scaffold at the target lesion without major protocol deviations). This was an observational study evaluating the performance, safety, and efficacy of the DESolve scaffold, with the intent to generate hypotheses for future trials. Categorical variables are presented as counts and percentages (%). Overall, continuous variables are presented as mean (standard deviation) and 95% confidence intervals (CI).

A total of 126 patients were enrolled at 13 clinical sites. Figure 6.9.9 outlines the study follow-up. Table 6.9.6 outlines the patient demographics. Overall, the mean age was 62 years, 21% had diabetes, and the majority of patients presented with stable angina. The study device was successfully implanted in 97% of the patients. The cumulative MACE rate at six months was 3.3%, including one cardiac death with probable stent thrombosis occurring in a patient with IVUS-identified proximal undersizing; one target vessel myocardial infarction due to an iatrogenic event, which occurred during the protocol-required IVUS re-evaluation, and two target lesion revascularizations (TLR) (Table 6.9.7); in both cases, the patients had stenoses involving mainly the 5 mm edges outside of the scaffold. Events between 6 and 12 months included: one cardiac death occurring in a patient with multiple co-morbidities and two TLRs involving the scaffold outside edge in one patient, and within the scaffold in the second patient. Between 12 and 24 months, there was one cardiac death in a patient undergoing an urgent procedure for a nontarget vessel intervention; the target lesion was patent and one additional TLR in a patient

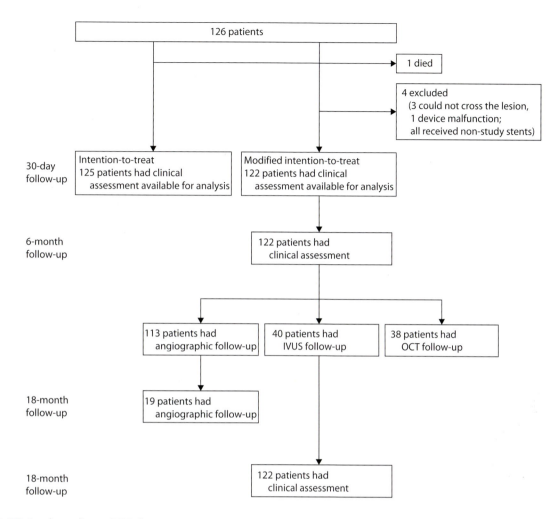

Figure 6.9.9 Study outline—DESolve Nx.

with significant in-scaffold stenosis. Clinical events are summarized in Table 6.9.7.

Serial QCA evaluation postprocedure and at 6-month follow-up are shown in Table 6.9.8. At the end of the procedure acute recoil was observed to be low (6.6%). Overall, 93% of patients complied with angiographic follow-up, and results demonstrated a mean in-scaffold late lumen loss of 0.20 ± 0.32 mm. In-segment binary restenosis was 3.5% with four cases of focal lesions of which three were considered a "geographic miss" wherein the scaffold did not sufficiently cover the original lesion. Also, there was no thrombus or aneurysm formation, nor exaggerated neointimal hyperplasia formation at the outside edges of the scaffold. A subset analysis involving 19 patients treated at a single center demonstrated a minor change of 0.07 mm in LLL from 6 to 18 months (Figure 6.9.10).

Paired analyses for IVUS and OCT were completed in a subset of 40 and 38 patients, respectively (Tables 6.9.9 and 6.9.10). By IVUS, there were three cases of acute incomplete strut apposition; at the 6-month follow-up, two resolved and one persisted. Importantly, there was no evidence of late acquired incomplete strut apposition. Neointimal

hyperplasia was low and by IVUS the neointimal percentage volume obstruction was 5.1%. The OCT imaging at 6-month follow-up showed excellent coverage of the scaffold struts with a frequency of covered struts per patient of 98.8 ± 1.7%; with a mean thickness of tissue covering the struts measuring 100.5 ± 30.6 μm. Similar to the IVUS results, there was no evidence of late-acquired incomplete strut apposition. In this study, the scaffold demonstrated lumen enlargement of approximately 9% by IVUS at 6 months, never before seen with either BRS or DES.

Ongoing/future studies with the DESolve scaffold include a postmarketing clinical follow-up which enrolled 100 patients at multiple sites in Europe using the DESolve 150 μm scaffold, and a 50-patient evaluation of a thinner 120 μm strut DESolve Cx device which is in the imaging follow-up phase. Initial results are very promising.

Both the DESolve FIM and DESolve Nx studies demonstrated the safety and efficacy of the DESolve scaffold which appears to be comparable with the second generation ABSORB PLLA bioresorbable vascular scaffold (BVS 1.1) (Abbott Vascular, Santa Clara, CA). In the studies to date, we found low numbers of events and no safety concerns.

290 The DESolve scaffold

Table 6.9.6 DESolve Nx—Baseline characteristics of the intention-to-treat patient population

| Baseline characteristics | (n = 126) |
|---|---|
| Age (years) | 62 (10) |
| Female gender | 40 (32%) |
| Diabetes mellitus | 27 (21%) |
| Hypertension | 89 (71%) |
| Dyslipidemia | 89 (71%) |
| Smoking (current) | 49 (39%) |
| Family history of coronary artery disease | 45 (36%) |
| Prior myocardial infarction | 56 (44%) |
| Prior percutaneous coronary intervention | 45 (36%) |
| Peripheral vascular disease | 10 (8%) |
| Clinical presentation | |
| – Silent ischemia | 8 (7%) |
| – Stable angina | 95 (75%) |
| – Unstable angina | 16 (13%) |
| – Asymptomatic post-myocardial infarction* | 7 (6%) |
| Target vessel | |
| – Left anterior descending | 48 (38%) |
| – Left circumflex | 39 (31%) |
| – Right coronary artery | 39 (31%) |
| AHA/ACC lesion type A/B1/B2/C | 27 (26%)/41 (40%)/32 (31%)/3 (3%) |
| Lesion length (mm) | 11.23 (3.75) |
| Reference diameter (mm) | 3.00 (0.30) |
| Minimum lumen diameter (mm) | 0.91 (0.38) |
| Diameter stenosis (%) | 70 (12) |

Note: Data are % (number of patients).

Stent thrombosis rates, defined as definite or probable [9], were low with 0% ST in the DESolve FIM [5] and one probable ST (0.8%) in the DESolve Nx study. One patient experienced a non-Q wave periprocedural myocardial infarction in each study by ITT, but there were no spontaneous myocardial infarctions reported, and only one "iatrogenic" event occurring in the DESolve Nx study. Clinical follow-up is ongoing and results continue to demonstrate excellent long-term safety even after the complete resorption of the scaffold at 2 years including no late or very late scaffold thrombosis unlike other BRS. Efficacy was shown as evidenced by the QCA, IVUS, OCT, and MSCT finding in both studies.

Recently published data from the Ghost EU registry suggests that "real-world" use of the ABSORB scaffold resulted in higher rates of definite and probable stent thrombosis (2.1% at 6 months) than previously reported in controlled randomized studies [10]. The latter includes the ABSORB II interim analyses that showed a scaffold thrombosis rate of 1% at 12 months, which is lower than in Ghost EU registry but higher than the metallic control stent arm (0% at 12 months) [11]. The ABSORB Extend study interim analysis also demonstrated a 1.0% thrombosis rate at 12 months [12]. In the DESolve Nx study, there was only one probable scaffold thrombosis (0.8%) through 24 months. The greater fracture resistance and the self-correction ability of the DESolve Scaffold [5] may provide advantages with respect to stent thrombosis but long-term comparative data will be needed to determine any true differences.

Table 6.9.7 DESolve Nx—Cumulative clinical outcomes up to 24 months—Modified-ITT population (n = 122)[a]

| | In-hospital | 30 days | 6 months | 12 months | 24 months |
|---|---|---|---|---|---|
| Major adverse cardiac events[a] | 0% | 0.8% (1) | 3.3% (4) | 5.7% (7) | 7.4% (9) |
| Cardiac death | 0% | 0.8% (1) | 0.8% (1) | 1.6% (2) | 2.5% (3) |
| Non-cardiac death | 0% | 0% | 0% | 0% | 1.6% (2) |
| Myocardial infarction | 0% | 0% | 0.8% (1) | 0.8% (1) | 0.8% (1) |
| Target lesion revascularization[b] | 0% | 0% | 1.6% (2) | 3.3% (4) | 4.1% (5) |
| Target vessel revascularization[b] | 0% | 0% | 1.6% (2) | 3.3% (4) | 4.1% (5) |
| Target lesion failure[c] | 0% | 0.8% (1) | 3.3% (4) | 5.7% (7) | 7.4% (9) |
| Target vessel failure[c] | 0% | 0.8% (1) | 3.3% (4) | 5.7% (7) | 7.4% (9) |
| Stent thrombosis (ARC defined) | 0% | 0.8% (1) | 0.8% (1) | 0.8% (1) | 0.8% (1) |

Note: Data are % (number of patients).
Abbreviations: ARC = Academic Research Consortium; ITT = intention-to-treat.
[a] Excludes 4 patients who received nonstudy stents to treat the target lesion at index procedure.
[b] Clinically indicated revascularization.
[c] Includes clinically indicated revascularization procedure.

Table 6.9.8 QCA results at postprocedure and 6 months

| QCA (paired) | Post-procedure | Post-procedure[b] | 6 months[b] | Difference post-procedure vs. 6 months (95% CI)[b] | p value[b] |
|---|---|---|---|---|---|
| n | 122[a] | 113[b] | 113[b] | – | – |
| In-scaffold reference diameter (mm) | 3.05 (0.25) | 3.05 (0.25) | 2.96 (0.28) | –0.09 (–0.11 to –0.06) | <0.001 |
| In-scaffold minimum lumen diameter (mm) | 2.64 (0.28) | 2.64 (0.28) | 2.44 (0.43) | –0.20 (–0.26 to –0.14) | <0.001 |
| In-scaffold mean diameter (mm) | 2.97 (0.24) | 2.97 (0.23) | 2.84 (0.30) | –0.14 (–0.18 to –0.10) | <0.001 |
| In-scaffold diameter stenosis (%) | 13% (8) | 13% (8) | 18% (13) | 4.37% (2.42 to 6.32) | <0.001 |
| In-scaffold acute gain (mm) | 1.72 (0.43) | 1.72 (0.43) | – | – | – |
| In-scaffold late lumen loss (mm) | – | – | 0.20 (0.32) | – | – |
| In-scaffold binary restenosis (%) | – | – | 3.5% (4/113) | – | – |
| Proximal edge minimum lumen diameter (mm) | 2.90 (0.37) | 2.89 (0.37) | 2.68 (0.42) | –0.21 (–0.26 to –0.16) | <0.001 |
| Proximal edge mean diameter (mm) | 3.08 (0.37) | 3.07 (0.37) | 2.91 (0.39) | –0.16 (–0.20 to –0.12) | <0.001 |
| Proximal edge diameter stenosis (%) | 8% (7) | 8% (8) | 13% (10) | 4.37% (–2.80 to 5.93) | <0.001 |
| Proximal edge late lumen loss (mm) | – | – | 0.21 (0.27) | – | – |
| Distal edge minimum lumen diameter (mm) | 2.72 (0.36) | 2.72 (0.36) | 2.54 (0.37) | –0.17 (–0.22 to –0.13) | <0.001 |
| Distal edge mean diameter (mm) | 2.90 (0.34) | 2.90 (0.34) | 2.76 (0.35) | –0.14 (–0.10 to –0.18) | <0.001 |
| Distal edge diameter stenosis (%) | 8% (7) | 8% (7) | 11% (9) | 2.98% (1.64 to 4.31) | <0.001 |
| Distal edge late lumen loss (mm) | – | – | 0.17 (0.24) | – | – |
| In-segment reference diameter (mm) | 3.04 (0.26) | 3.04 (0.26) | 2.96 (0.27) | –0.08 (–0.11 to –0.06) | <0.001 |
| In-segment minimum lumen diameter (mm) | 2.53 (0.31) | 2.52 (0.31) | 2.31 (0.43) | –0.21 (–0.27 to –0.15) | <0.001 |
| In-segment diameter stenosis (%) | 17% (7) | 17% (7) | 22% (12) | 4.77% (2.97 to 6.57) | <0.001 |
| In-segment acute gain (mm) | 1.61 (0.43) | 1.61 (0.43) | – | – | – |
| In-segment late lumen loss (mm) | – | – | 0.21 (0.31) | – | – |
| In-segment binary restenosis (%) | – | – | 3.5% (4/113) | – | – |

*Note:* Data are mean (SD) or number (%), unless otherwise indicated.

*Abbreviations:* CI = confidence interval; QCA = quantitative coronary angiography.

[a] Modified-ITT population (122/126), excludes 4 patients who received nonstudy stents to treat the target lesion at index procedure.

[b] Subset with paired analysis (n = 113) with serial QCA analysis at postprocedure and 6 months follow-up.

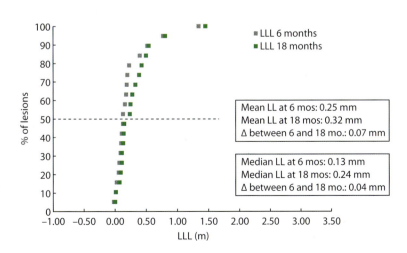

Figure 6.9.10 DESolve Nx—18-months QCA analysis of a single-center patient subset.

Table 6.9.9 DESolve Nx—IVUS results after procedure and at 6 months

| IVUS (paired) | Postprocedure | 6 months | Difference after procedure vs. 6 months (95% CI) | p value |
|---|---|---|---|---|
| n | 40 | 40 | – | – |
| Vessel diameter (mm) | 3.74 (0.64) | 3.67 (0.63) | –0.03 (–0.12 to 0.04) | 0.36 |
| Vessel area (mm²) | 11.21 (3.76) | 10.79 (3.70) | –0.19 (–0.59 to 0.22) | 0.35 |
| Vessel volume (mm³) | 216.28 (67.32) | 234.52 (74.52) | 17.98 (5.83 to 31.13) | 0.005 |
| Lumen diameter (mm) | 2.74 (0.27) | 2.86 (0.31) | 0.12 (0.05 to 0.19) | 0.001 |
| Minimum lumen area (mm²) | 4.84 (1.09) | 4.77 (1.11) | 0.07 (–0.42 to 0.56) | 0.78 |
| Minimum lumen diameter (mm) | 2.08 (0.28) | 2.16 (0.30) | 0.08 (–0.02 to 0.17) | 0.099 |
| Lumen area (mm²) | 5.93 (1.17) | 6.51 (1.43) | 0.58 (0.26 to 0.90) | <0.001 |
| Lumen volume (mm³) | 98.58 (24.97) | 109.99 (33.46) | 11.41 (3.86 to 18.95) | 0.004 |
| Plaque burden (%) | 52% (7) | 52% (7) | 0.00% (–0.02 to 0.01) | 0.68 |
| Plaque area (mm²) | 6.96 (2.56) | 7.25 (2.35) | 0.29 (0.04 to 0.63) | 0.086 |
| Plaque volume (mm³) | 115.21 (49.39) | 124.63 (46.09) | 9.42 (0.41 to 18.44) | 0.04 |
| Scaffold diameter (mm) | 2.75 (0.27) | 2.94 (0.32) | 0.19 (0.12 to 0.27) | <0.001 |
| Scaffold area (mm²) | 5.94 (1.18) | 6.87 (1.55) | 0.93 (0.58 to 1.27) | <0.001 |
| Scaffold volume (mm³) | 98.55 (25.00) | 115.44 (35.16) | 16.89 (9.30 to 24.48) | <0.001 |
| NIH area (mm²) | – | 0.36 (0.34) | – | – |
| NIH volume (mm³) | – | 6.32 (6.60) | – | – |
| NIH volume obstruction (%) | – | 5.13 (4.19) | – | – |

*Note:* Data are mean (SD).
*Abbreviations:* CI = confidence interval; ISA = incomplete stent apposition; IVUS = intravascular ultrasound; NIH = neointimal hyperplasia; OCT = optical coherence tomography.

Table 6.9.10 DESolve Nx—OCT results after procedure and at 6 months

| OCT (paired) | Postprocedure | 6 months | Difference after procedure vs. 6 months (95% CI) | p value |
|---|---|---|---|---|
| n | 38 | 38 | – | – |
| Mean lumen area, mm² | 6.89 ± 1.29 | 5.81 ± 1.18 | –1.07 [–1.34; –0.80] | <0.001 |
| Minimum lumen area, mm² | 5.61 ± 1.10 | 4.20 ± 1.04 | –1.41 [–1.72; –1.11] | <0.001 |
| Mean lumen diameter, mm | 2.93 ± 0.27 | 2.68 ± 0.27 | –0.24 [–0.30; –0.18] | <0.001 |
| Lumen volume, mm³ | 109.59 ± 27.46 | 91.22 ± 24.93 | –18.37 [–22.57; –14.16] | <0.001 |
| Mean scaffold area, mm² | 7.04 ± 1.26 | 8.17 ± 1.34 | 1.13 [0.86; 1.40] | <0.001 |
| Minimum scaffold area, mm² | 5.81 ± 1.09 | 6.31 ± 1.16 | 0.50 [0.20; 0.79] | 0.002 |
| Mean scaffold diameter, mm² | 2.96 ± 0.26 | 3.20 ± 0.26 | 0.24 [0.18; 0.29] | <0.001 |
| Scaffold volume, mm³ | 112.05 ± 27.16 | 128.55 ± 32.33 | 16.50 [11.66; 21.33] | <0.001 |
| NIH area, mm² | – | 0.70 ± 0.26 | – | – |
| NIH volume, mm³ | – | 11.15 ± 5.06 | – | – |
| NIH volume obstruction,% | – | 11.27 ± 4.19 | – | – |
| NIH thickness, μm | – | 100.53 ± 30.58 | – | – |

*Abbreviations:* NIH = neointimal hyperplasia; OCT = optical coherence tomography.

## CONCLUSION

In conclusion, the novel DESolve scaffold demonstrated promising outcomes in the treatment of patients with *de novo* noncomplex coronary lesions, including high device and procedural success, overall low rates of adverse events, and sustained safety up to 24 months in two clinical studies. The DESolve scaffold has demonstrated excellent safety and effectiveness. In addition, the scaffold thrombosis rate was low with no late or very late thrombosis differentiating it from other BRS. Using multi-imaging modality assessment at follow-up, effective scaffolding of the vessel over time, efficacy with respect to the inhibition of neointimal hyperplasia, and a high percentage of strut coverage without signs of local inflammatory reaction or toxicity was detected. These findings warrant further confirmation in larger and broader patient populations.

A criticism of currently available scaffolds is the strut thickness which is close to two times that of the market leading metallic DES (≥150 μm vs. 81 μm). To address this, Elixir has developed and received CE approval for the DESolve Cx scaffold that has a 20% thinner strut (120 μm) scaffold design with the same drug dose, radial strength, and degradation rate as the DESolve Nx (150 μm) design. This reduction in the strut width has the potential to significantly improve scaffold delivery performance as well as reendothelialization following implantation. A registry evaluating the DESolve Cx is in the 6 month follow-up phase and initial clinical and imaging results are very promising. Elixir Medical is developing and testing multiple scaffold designs to address the clinical need currently not satisfied by other bioresorbable scaffolds.

# REFERENCES

1. Haude M, Erbel R, Erne P, Verheye S, Degen H, Bose D, Vermeersch P et al. Safety and performance of the drug-eluting absorbable metal scaffold (DREAMS) in patients with de-novo coronary lesions: 12 month results of the prospective, multicentre, first-in-man BIOSOLVE-I trial. Lancet. 2013; 381:836–844.
2. Ormiston JA, Serruys PW, Regar E, Dudek D, Thuesen L, Webster MW, Onuma Y et al. A bioabsorbable everolimus-eluting coronary stent system for patients with single de-novo coronary artery lesions (ABSORB): A prospective open-label trial. Lancet. 2008; 371:899–907.
3 Serruys PW, Onuma Y, Ormiston JA, de Bruyne B, Regar E, Dudek D, Thuesen L et al. Evaluation of the second generation of a bioresorbable everolimus drug-eluting vascular scaffold for treatment of de novo coronary artery stenosis: Six-month clinical and imaging outcomes. Circulation. 2010; 122:2301–2312.
4. Tamai H, Igaki K, Kyo E, Kosuga K, Kawashima A, Matsui S, Komori H et al. Initial and 6-month results of biodegradable poly-l-lactic acid coronary stents in humans. Circulation. 2000; 102:399–404.
5. Verheye S, Ormiston JA, Stewart J, Webster M, Sanidas E, Costa R, Costa JR Jr et al. A next-generation bioresorbable coronary scaffold system: From bench to first clinical evaluation: 6- and 12-month clinical and multimodality imaging results. JACC Cardiovasc Interv. 2014; 7:89–99.
6. Nishio S, Kosuga K, Igaki K, Okada M, Kyo E, Tsuji T, Takeuchi E et al. Longterm (10 Years) clinical outcomes of first-in-human biodegradable poly-L-lactic acid coronary stents: Igaki-Tamai stents. Circulation. 2012; 125:2343–2353.
7. Ormiston JA, Webber B, Ubod B, Darremont O and Webster MWI. An independent branch comparison of two bioresorbable drug-eluting coronary scaffolds (Absorb and DESolve) with a durable metallic drug-eluting stent (ML8/Xpedition). EuroIntervention. 2015 May; 11(1):60–7.
8. Wiebe J, Bauer T, Dorr O, Mollmann H, Hamm CW and Nef HM. Implantation of Novolimus-eluting bioresorbable scaffold with a strut thickness of 100 μm showing evidence of self-correction. EuroIntervention. 2015 Jun; 11(2):204.
9. Cutlip DE, Windecker S, Mehran R, Boam A, Cohen DJ, van Es GA, Steg PG et al. Clinical end points in coronary stent trials: A case for standardized definitions. Circulation. 2007; 115:2344–51.
10. Capodanno D, Gori T, Nef H, Latib A, Mehilli J, Lesiak M, Caramanno G et al. Percutaneous coronary intervention with everolimus-eluting bioresorbable vascular scaffolds in routine clinical practice: Early and midterm outcomes from the European multicentre GHOST-EU registry. EuroIntervention. 2015 Feb; 10(10):1144–53.
11. Serruys PW. ABSORB II: What has the randomized trial taught us beyond the registries? TCT. 2014.
12. Abizaid A, Costa Jr JR, Bartorelli AL, Whitbourn R, Jan van Geuns R, Chevalier B, Patel T et al. The ABSORB EXTEND study: Preliminary report of the twelve-month clinical outcomes in the first 512 patients enrolled. EuroIntervention. 2015 Apr; 10(12):1396–401.

# Results of clinical trials with BIOTRONIK magnesium scaffolds

MICHAEL HAUDE, DANIEL LOOTZ, RAIMUND ERBEL, JACQUES KOOLEN, AND RON WAKSMAN

## INTRODUCTION

The innovation of the bioresorbable scaffold for intracoronary implantation in patients with coronary artery disease attempts to overcome the limitations of conventional permanent stents. As with stents designed to keep treated vessel segments patent, absorbable vascular scaffolds are implanted in a similar way and for similar indications, but unlike stents, scaffolds degrade over time and allow the vessel to resume its natural physiological state including vasomotion and remodeling without the permanent presence of foreign materials, exposing the artery wall to long-term inflammatory and mechanical stress [1–3]. There are several putative clinical advantages of such novel absorbable scaffolds over permanent stents: less frequent late and very late stent thrombosis and the associated requirement of prolonged dual antiplatelet therapy, uncaging of the target vessel segment allowing the vessel to reshape to its original configuration, elimination of chronic vessel wall inflammation and its consequences, improved ability for non-invasive vessel lumen imaging by computed tomography or magnetic resonance imaging, and easier facilitation of percutaneous or surgical reinterventions because of the absence of foreign material in the target vessel [1,2,4].

A magnesium-based scaffold (BIOTRONIK, Bülach, Switzerland) has been designed and incrementally improved over three product innovation steps [5,6]. In a Chapter 3.3, the rationale for selecting magnesium as the most suitable material for an absorbable metal scaffold was described.

The first-generation absorbable metal scaffold (AMS) was clinically investigated beginning in December 2003 for vascular interventions below the knee [7] and from July 2004 on for coronary interventions [8]. The first-generation drug-eluting absorbable metal scaffold (DREAMS, also subsequently called DREAMS-1G) offered incremental

improvements including paclitaxel drug elution; it was first evaluated in human coronary arteries starting in August 2010 [4]. The second-generation drug-eluting absorbable metal scaffold (DREAMS-2G, commercially available as Magmaris) offers sirolimus elution and has been evaluated since October 2013 [9]. The goal of this chapter is to summarize the main design features and clinical trial results for the AMS, DREAMS-1G, and DREAMS-2G absorbable magnesium scaffolds.

## AMS, THE FIRST-GENERATION MAGNESIUM SCAFFOLD

The first-generation magnesium scaffold (**A**bsorbable **M**etal **S**caffold or AMS, BIOTRONIK, Bülach, Switzerland) is a tubular, laser-cut, balloon-expandable, non-drug-eluting scaffold made of WE43 alloy (93% magnesium and 7% rare earth elements) [6,8]. The scaffold was premounted on a low-compliance balloon catheter. The AMS scaffold was available for the studies in lengths of 10 and 15 mm and with diameters of 3.0 and 3.5 mm. As illustrated in Figure 6.10.1, AMS struts have a rectangular cross-sectional profile (80 × 165 μm). The mechanical characteristics of the AMS are similar to those of permanent stainless-steel stents, including sufficient collapse pressure (0.8 bar), low elastic recoil (<8%), and a minimal amount of foreshortening after inflation (<5%) [1,8].

## PROGRESS-AMS: The first-in-man trial of an absorbable coronary metal scaffold

The Clinical Performance and Angiographic Results of Coronary Stenting with Absorbable Metal Stents (PROGRESS-AMS) study, a multicenter prospective single-arm study, evaluated the safety and feasibility of the use of

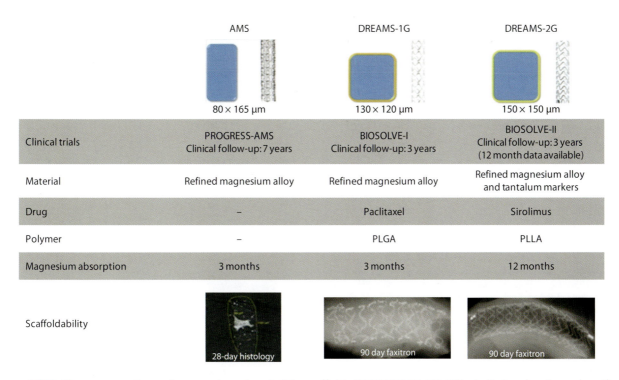

**Figure 6.10.1** Three generations of magnesium absorbable scaffolds (BIOTRONIK AG, Bülach, Switzerland) are described. Schematic cross-sectional profile of struts appears in blue; the polymer coating is depicted as a thin yellow layer around the strut. Note that histology findings at 28 days after AMS implantation in a porcine coronary model show the appearance of struts under the light microscope (unstained ground sections, archive data). Faxitron images illustrate the fracture rate of implanted scaffolds DREAMS-1G and DREAMS-2G at 28 days in a porcine model. AMS = absorbable metal stent (product name); DREAMS = drug-eluting absorbable metal scaffold (product name); PLGA = poly(lactitde-*co*-glycolide) acid; PLLA = poly-L-lactic acid.

AMS in human coronary arteries [8]. The primary endpoint was major adverse cardiac events (MACE) after four months, defined as a composite endpoint of cardiac death, Q-wave myocardial infarction, or clinically driven target lesion revascularization (TLR). Clinically driven TLR was defined as a repeated percutaneous intervention of the target lesion or bypass surgery involving the target lesion, necessitated by an in-lesion diameter stenosis of 50–70% combined with angina symptoms or a positive functional test or by stenosis ≥70%, irrespective of symptoms and ischemia status.

Secondary endpoints of the study included MACE after 6 and 12 months; TLR after 4, 6, and 12 months; procedural and device success; evidence of scaffold degradation; and the in-scaffold and in-segment LLL, percentage diameter stenosis, and binary restenosis at 4 months [8,10].

As reported by Erbel et al. [8], 63 patients received a total of 71 AMS scaffolds. Patients were eligible for inclusion in the study if they had a single, discrete, *de novo* lesion in a coronary artery with a reference vessel diameter between 3.0 and 3.5 mm, lesion length ≤13 mm, and stenosis diameter 50–99%. Patients were excluded if they had extensive calcification, intraluminal thrombus, bifurcation lesions, ostial lesions, or a left-ventricular ejection fraction (LVEF) <30% [8]. A summary of selected baseline patient characteristics appears in Table 6.10.1.

AMS scaffolds were implanted after mandatory predilatation. Two radiopaque markers at the balloon ends were used for precise positioning of the radiolucent AMS. Post-dilatation was optional and carried out in 67% of patients at the operator's discretion. Procedural and device success was 100%, defined as residual target segment stenosis of <50% without in-hospital MACE after any percutaneous method (procedural success) or after AMS deployment (device success, acute). Diameter stenosis was reduced from 61.5% to 12.6% after scaffold implantation, with an acute lumen gain of 1.41 mm [8].

The clinically driven TLR rate after 4 months was 23.8%. No myocardial infarction, scaffold thrombosis, or death occurred during follow-up. Thus, the MACE rate after 4 months was also 23.8% [8].

At 4 months, the in-scaffold LLL was 1.08 ± 0.49 mm, with a net lumen gain of 0.33 ± 0.60 mm.

Contributing factors to restenosis were identified on serial intravascular ultrasonography (IVUS) as a combination of neointimal growth and the decrease of external elastic membrane volume, resulting from the inability of the degrading AMS to counteract constrictive vessel remodeling. There was no substantial change in the original plaque [8]. At 4 months, only small remnants of the original struts embedded into the intima were visible by IVUS [8].

Overall, the PROGRESS-AMS trial showed that absorbable magnesium scaffolds can achieve an immediate angiographic result similar to that obtained with other metal stents in atherosclerotic coronary arteries and that the

Table 6.10.1 Baseline characteristics of patients enrolled in trials of absorbable magnesium scaffolds

| | PROGRESS-AMS n = 63 (%) | BIOSOLVE-I n = 46 (%) | BIOSOLVE-II n = 123 (%) |
|---|---|---|---|
| Scaffold used in study | AMS | DREAMS-1G | DREAMS-2G |
| Age (years) | 61.3 ± 9.5 | 65.3 ± 9.7 | 65.2 ± 10.3 |
| Men | 44 (69.8) | 34 (73.9) | 78 (63) |
| History of myocardial infarction | 26 (41.3) | 15 (32.6) | 29 (24) |
| Previous PCI | 15 (23.8) | 27 (58.7) | 44 (36) |
| Previous CABG | 3 (4.8) | Not reported | 8 (7) |
| Hyperlipidaemia | 39 (61.2) | 41 (89.1) | 74 (60) |
| Hypertension | 41 (65.1) | 40 (87.0) | 101 (82) |
| Smoking | 30 (47.6) | 17 (37.0) | 67 (54) |
| Diabetes | 11 (17.4) | 7 (15.2) | 36 (29) |
| Stable angina | 52 (82.6) | 43 (93.5) | 88 (72) |
| Unstable angina | 6 (9.5) | 2 (4.3) | 17 (14) |
| Target coronary artery | Of 63 lesions | Of 47 lesions | Of 123 lesions |
| Left anterior descending | 22 (34.9) | 16 (34.0) | 47 (38) |
| Left circumflex artery | 18 (28.6) | 16 (34.0) | 29 (24) |
| Right coronary artery | 23 (36.5) | 15 (32.0) | 45 (37) |
| **ACC/AHA Lesion Classification** | | | |
| Type A | 31 (49.2) | 12 (25.5) | 1 (<1) |
| Type B1 | 27 (42.8) | 31 (66.0) | 68 (56) |
| Type B2 | 5 (7.9) | 4 (8.5) | 51 (42) |
| Moderate to severe calcification | 8 (12.7) | 7 (14.9) | 13 (11) |

Note: Data are presented mean ± standard deviation (SD) or n (%).

Abbreviations: ACC/AHA = American College of Cardiology/American Heart Association's system for lesion morphology classification; AMS = absorbable metal stent; CABG = coronary artery bypass graft surgery; DREAMS = Drug-Eluting Absorbable Metal Scaffold study; PCI = percutaneous coronary intervention.

scaffold safely degrades after 4 months [8]. The absence of documented embolization of scaffold material during the short absorption period of 4 months indirectly confirmed that the degradation of the alloy occurs within the vessel wall after rapid re-endothelialization and strut coverage, rather than in the vessel lumen. Compared to permanent bare metal stents, the overall incidence of TLR was quite high, [11], indicating the need for slower scaffold degradation and additional antiproliferative drug elution [1,5,8].

## Angiographic and IVUS follow-up to 28 months

To further evaluate the natural history of vascular response to AMS, Waksman et al. [12] conducted a substudy (n = 9) of patients who had no clinical events and no revascularization through 28 months of follow-up; this population had serial IVUS data postprocedure, at 4 months and late data (at 12 to 28 months). In these patients, paired IVUS analysis demonstrated complete scaffold degradation at 4 months and results were shown to be durable, without any early or late adverse events.

While there was no evidence of recoil or neointimal proliferation after 4 months in these patients, neointimal regression and lumen diameter were observed to increase during long-term follow-up. Overall, from 4 months to late follow-up, a reduction of neointima (by 3.6 ± 5.2 mm³) and of LLL (from median 0.62 to 0.40 mm) were observed, along with an increase of scaffold cross-sectional area (by 0.5 ± 1.0 mm²) and of in-scaffold minimal lumen diameter (from median 1.87 to 2.17 mm) [12]. The long-term IVUS evaluation depicted in Figure 6.10.2 illustrates the disappearances of the scaffold struts and the preservation of the vessel wall.

## AMS vasomotion testing

In a study from the United Kingdom, Ghimire et al. compared the endothelium-independent coronary smooth muscle vasomotor function in patients with no angiographic restenosis at 4 months after AMS implantation (AMS patients, n = 5) to those with no angiographic restenosis at over 1 year following permanent metal stent (PMS) implantation (PMS patients, n = 10) [14]. Vessel diameters were measured by quantitative coronary angiography at 0.2 mm longitudinal intervals in the scaffolded or stented segment and at 1 cm proximal to the reference segment, both before and after the intracoronary administration of 2 mg of isosorbide dinitrate (a vasodilator). Vasodilation after isosorbide dinitrate administration was then quantified by calculating the percentage of change in the mean cross-sectional area of the vessel. The scaffolded segments

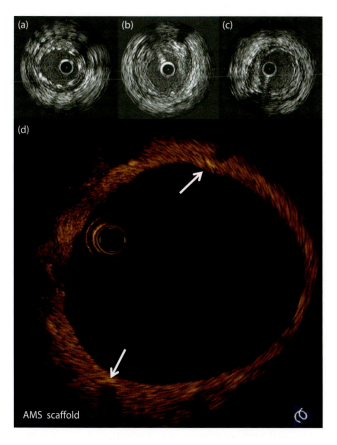

Figure 6.10.2 IVUS follow-up immediately after (a), at 4 months (b), and at 16 months (c) after AMS implantation from the PROGRESS-AMS substudy [12]. In a different patient OCT at 15 months following AMS implantation (d) shows strut remnants. ([a,b,c] From Waksman R et al. *JACC Cardiovasc Interv.* 2009;2(4):312–20; [d] Barlis P et al. *Eur Heart J.* 2007;28(19):2319.)

showed vasodilatation in the AMS group (mean dilation +6.8% vs. −1.3%, *p* = 0.003) while the stented segments remained unchanged. The reference segments showed vasodilatation in all patients (mean dilation +13.3% vs. +17.2% for the AMS and PMS groups, respectively, *p* = 0.39) [14].

## DREAMS-1G, THE FIRST DRUG-ELUTING MAGNESIUM SCAFFOLD

To reduce the coronary revascularization rate associated with AMS, DREAMS-1G (**Dr**ug-**e**luting **a**bsorbable **m**etal **s**caffold, first generation) was made of a refined, more slowly degrading magnesium alloy (BIOTRONIK, Bülach, Switzerland) and had a six-crown, three-link design with higher collapse pressure (1.5 bar for DREAMS-1G vs. 0.8 bar for AMS) [6,15]. Strut thickness was reduced by 27%, from 165 μm in AMS to 120 μm in DREAMS-1G.

The DREAMS-1G scaffold is coated with a 1 μm bioresorbable polylactic-*co*-glycolic acid (PLGA) polymer matrix coating. The PLGA coating is loaded with 0.07 μg/

mm² of paclitaxel, one of the most-studied antiproliferative drugs in coronary angioplasty [3,4,6,15,16]. The scaffold was designed to provide controlled paclitaxel release during the first 3 months with subsequent absorption of the PLGA [4,6,15]. For the clinical study it was available in 16 mm length with diameters of 3.25 and 3.5 mm premounted on a semicompliant rapid-exchange balloon catheter [5]. This device was tested in the first-in-man BIOSOLVE-I trial.

## BIOSOLVE-I: The first-in-man clinical trial of DREAMS-1G

This multicenter, prospective, single-arm **BIO**TRONIK **S**afety and Clinical Performance **of** the First Drug-Eluting Generation Absorbable Metal Stent in Patients with *de novo* **L**esions in Nati**ve** Coronary Arteries (BIOSOLVE-I) study attempted to assess the safety and performance of the DREAMS-1G scaffold [4]. In this trial, the first 22 patients had a planned invasive follow-up at 6 months, the remaining 24 patients at 12 months. The primary endpoint of the study was target lesion failure (TLF) after 6 months (Cohort 1) and 12 months (Cohort 2), where TLF was a composite of cardiac death, TV-MI, or clinically driven TLR, as defined in the literature [17,18]. Secondary endpoints included TLF after 1, 24, and 36 months, scaffold thrombosis, procedural and device success, in-scaffold and in-segment LLL, percentage diameter restenosis, and binary restenosis at 6 and 12 months [17]. Device success was defined as successful scaffold delivery and deployment followed by appropriate removal of the delivery system. Procedural success was defined as device success plus residual target lesion stenosis of less than 50% without in-hospital MACE [4].

As reported by Haude and colleagues [4], the study enrolled 46 patients with 47 lesions treated. Patients were eligible for inclusion if they presented with stable or unstable angina or documented silent ischemia and had a maximum of two single *de novo* lesions in two separate coronary arteries with a reference vessel diameter between 3.0 mm and 3.5 mm, lesion length ≤12 mm, and a diameter stenosis of 50–99%. Patients were excluded if they had severe calcification, thrombus in the target vessel, bifurcation lesions, ostial lesions, previous bypass surgery supplying the perfusion bed distal to the target lesion, LVEF <30%, and several other conditions [4]. As shown in Table 6.10.1, the BIOSOLVE-I patients had a markedly higher rate of prior percutaneous coronary intervention (PCI), hyperlipidemia, hypertension, and Type B1 lesions compared to the patients in the PROGRESS-AMS study.

Target lesions were scaffolded (DREAMS-1G scaffolds with 16 mm length and 3.25 or 3.5 mm diameter) after mandatory predilatation. The premounted, radiolucent scaffold was centered between two radiopaque markers of the balloon catheter to ease fluoroscopic visualization and positioning. Postdilatation was performed in the event of incomplete scaffold expansion or residual stenosis at the operator's discretion. Device and procedural success rates were 100%, as in the PROGRESS-AMS study. Post-implantation, in-scaffold diameter stenosis and lumen gain were 6.8% and 1.35 mm, respectively. The acute recoil was $9.2 \pm 7.2\%$. All patients were recommended dual antiplatelet therapy for at least 12 months. Three patients were lost to follow-up between 6 and 12 months due to consent withdrawal ($n = 2$) and non-cardiac death ($n = 1$) [4].

Of the 46 patients in the study, 2 had TLF at 6 months and 1 additional patient had TLF at 12 months (4.3% and 6.8%, respectively), with no reported cardiac deaths or definite or probable scaffold thrombosis [4]. The two TLF after 6 months were clinically driven TLR, which were then treated with drug-eluting stents. The third case of TLF was a perioperative TV-MI at 12 months follow-up due to a target vessel, but not target lesion, PCI.

There was a significant improvement in efficacy between the AMS device and the DREAMS-1G. Indeed, the ci-TLR of the AMS was reported to be 23.8% at 4 months follow-up, whereas the ci-TLR of DREAMS-1G was only 4.3% at 6 months (see Table 6.10.2). Three-year data was available for 44 patients and found no further TLF and stated the 3-year rate as 6.6% [18].

The mean in-scaffold LLL was $0.65 \pm 0.50$ mm at 6 months and $0.52 \pm 0.39$ mm at 12 months. This difference was not statistically significant, nor was the difference between 6-month and 12-month in-scaffold diameter stenosis ($25.01 \pm 21.07\%$ vs. $20.92 \pm 16.70\%$, respectively). There was no significant difference between the minimum lumen diameters at 6 and 12 months (1.95 ±

0.59 mm vs. $2.06 \pm 0.47$ mm, respectively). The minimum in-segment lumen diameter was $2.34 \pm 0.40$ mm (2.22–2.46) after the procedure, $1.84 \pm 0.52$ mm (1.66–2.01) at 6 months and $1.96 \pm 0.43$ mm (1.81–2.11) at 12 months ($p < 0.0001$ for after procedure vs. 6 months, $p = 0.0001$ for after procedure vs. 12 months and $p = 0.2682$ for 6 vs. 12 months).

No significant difference appeared for the minimum lumen diameter, which was $1.95 \pm 0.59$ mm at 6 months and $2.06 \pm 0.47$ mm at 12 months ($p = 0.37$). IVUS data at both 6 and 12 months were available for 21 patients, which showed a reduction in the cross-sectional area of scaffolding ($7.29 \pm 1.39$ mm$^2$ after procedure vs. $6.49 \pm 2.11$ mm$^2$ at 6 months and $6.40 \pm 2.04$ mm$^2$ at 12 months) along with an increase in in-scaffold neointimal hyperplasia (0 immediately after procedure vs. $0.30 \pm 0.41$ mm at 6 months vs. $0.40 \pm 0.32$ mm at 12 months), with the net effect that the mean lumen area reduced at both 6 and 12 months versus the immediate postprocedural value ($7.31 \pm 1.42$ mm$^2$ after the procedure vs. $6.19 \pm 1.93$ mm$^2$ at 6 months and $6.02 \pm 1.94$ mm$^2$ at 12 months). This reduction was significant when compared to the after-procedure value ($p = 0.002$ for postprocedure vs. 6 months and $p = 0.0008$ for postprocedure vs. 12 months) but there was no statistically significant difference between the values for 6 vs. 12 months ($p = 0.42$). Of the original patient population, seven patients underwent additional angiography at $28 \pm 4$ months, at which time it was determined that in-scaffold LLL had improved from the 12-month value of $0.51 \pm 0.56$ mm (median 0.28 mm) to $0.32 \pm 0.32$ mm (median 0.20 mm) [18].

Table 6.10.2 Summary of clinical, angiographic, and procedural trial results for the three generations of magnesium absorbable scaffolds (AMS in PROGRESS AMS, DREAMS-1G in BIOSOLVE-I, and DREAMS-2G in BIOSOLVE-II)

| | PROGRESS-AMS Reported at 4-month follow-up (N = 63) | BIOSOLVE-I Reported at 6-month follow-up (N = 46) | BIOSOLVE-II Reported at 6-month follow-up (N = 123) |
|---|---|---|---|
| Cardiac death (%) | 0.0 | 0.0 | 0.8 |
| Target vessel MI (%) | 0.0 | 0.0 | 0.8 |
| Clinically driven target lesion revascularization (%) | 23.8 | 4.3 | 1.7 |
| TLF (%) | N/A | 4.3 | 3.3 |
| MACE (%) | 23.8 | N/A | N/A |
| Definite scaffold thrombosis (%) | 0.0 | 0.0 | 0.0 |
| Probable/possible scaffold thrombosis (%) | N/A | 0.0 | 0.0 |
| Minimal lumen diameter (mean ± STD, in mm) | 1.38 ± 0.51 | 1.95 ± 0.59 | 2.00 ± 0.44 |
| In-segment LLL (mean ± STD, in mm) | 0.83 ± 0.51 | 0.52 ± 0.48 | 0.27 ± 0.37 |
| In-scaffold LLL (mean ± STD, in mm) | 1.08 ± 0.49 | 0.65 ± 0.50 | 0.44 ± 0.36 |
| In-segment binary restenosis (%) | 47.5 | 19.4 | 5 |
| In-scaffold binary restenosis (%) | 47.5 | 16.7 | 5 |
| Procedural success (%) | 100 | 100 | 99 |
| Device success (%) | 100 | 100 | 93 |

Source: Haude M, Erbel R, Erne P, Verheye S, Degen H, Bose D et al. Lancet. 2013;381(9869):836–44. Erbel R, Di Mario C, Bartunek J, Bonnier J, de Bruyne B, Eberli FR et al. Lancet. 2007;369(9576):1869–75. Haude M, Ince H, Abizaid A, Toelg R, Lemos PA, von Birgelen C et al. Lancet. 2015.

Abbreviations: LLL = late lumen loss; MACE = major adverse cardiac events; TLF = target lesion failure.

The mean cross-sectional LLL of 1.30 mm² at 12 months was driven by the combination of neointimal proliferation (relative contribution 31%) and compression of the scaffold by an increasing extra-scaffold plaque area (69%). Since the vessel area did not change significantly over time, chronic recoil and negative remodeling were not important contributors to the decrease in in-scaffold area [4]. Table 6.10.2 summarizes the studies' results.

Overall, the BIOSOLVE-I trial demonstrated that the DREAMS-1G scaffold was associated with target lesion failure rates (safety performance) similar to that of contemporary permanent drug-eluting stents or absorbable everolimus-eluting scaffolds. Indeed, at 3 years, no cardiac deaths or scaffold thrombosis has been reported [18].

On the other hand, the DREAMS-1G did not offer excellent LLL results compared to other drug-eluting stents or scaffolds. This led to a redesign of DREAMS-1G for the next-generation scaffold, DREAMS-2G.

## DREAMS-1G: Intracoronary imaging

Haude et al. [4] proved that with the virtual histology IVUS technology magnesium backscatters as dense calcium. The 6-month virtual histology IVUS analysis for DREAMS-1G, similar to the bare AMS version, showed a significant 39.5% decrease in dense calcium area of the misclassified struts ($p = 0.0015$), which then remained stable between 6 and 12 months. This decrease was interpreted by Haude et al. as a signal of the progressive bioresorption of the magnesium component of DREAMS-1G.

Seven patients underwent serial optical coherence tomography (OCT) postprocedure at 6 and 12 months ($n = 5791$ assessable struts). The rate of apposed struts was 95.9% postprocedure, 97.2% at 6 months, and 99.8% at 12 months, when only 0.1% of struts exhibited persistent incomplete apposition and 0.1% late acquired incomplete apposition [4]. The high rates of strut apposition at all time-points demonstrate the good conformability of the DREAMS-1G scaffold.

As reported by Waksman and colleagues [19], the BIOSOLVE-I substudy included patients who at 6 and 12 months underwent serial invasive imaging, such as quantitative coronary angiography for detailed vessel geometry evaluation, IVUS for echogenicity evaluation, OCT for analysis of the degradation process and corresponding vessel dimensions, or vasomotion testing. Parameters of vessel geometry were assessed as curvature and angulation of the in-scaffold segment. Curvature was defined as the infinitesimal rate of change in the tangent vector at each point of a center-line as configured by a software application capable of automatically detecting lumen contours. A perfect circle was fitted through the centerline of the vessel and the curvature was calculated as 1/radius of the circle. Angulation was defined as the angle that the tip of an intracoronary guidewire would need to reach the distal part of a coronary bend. The cardiac-contraction-induced cyclic changes in vessel curvature and angulation were estimated as absolute differences between the curvatures/angles at the end of both diastole and systole [19].

Both curvature and angulation were significantly increased by the degradation process. The greatest increase was observed in the period from postimplantation to 6 months. The median curvature changed from 0.41 cm⁻¹ (preimplantation) to 0.31 cm⁻¹ (postimplantation, $p < 0.0001$ vs. preimplantation value) and to 0.45 cm⁻¹ (at 6 months, $p < 0.0001$ vs. postimplantation value) and to 0.41 cm⁻¹ (at 12 months, $p = 0.56$ vs. 6 months). The median angulation changed from 40.2° (preimplantation) to 22.4° (postimplantation, $p < 0.0001$ vs. preimplantation) and 33.4° (6 months, $p < 0.0001$ vs. postimplantation) to 43.4° (12 months, $p = 0.60$ at 6 months). The systolic-diastolic changes of the curvature and angulation restored gradually, starting from 0.13 cm⁻¹ to 0.08 cm⁻¹ to 0.11 cm⁻¹ and from 7.6° to 4.5° to 6.4° for preimplantation, postimplantation, and 12 months, respectively [19].

Echogenicity data were used to quantify the changes in strut structure as the decrease in intensity of the ultrasound signal. The mean percentage of hyperechogenic tissue between the lumen and media contour within the scaffolded segment decreased continuously over time, most pronouncedly between postimplantation (22.1 ± 7.0%) and 6 months (15.8 ± 3.7%) ($p < 0.001$) and to a lesser degree until 12 months (12.9 ± 3.3%) and 18 months (11.6 ± 4.3%) [19].

Struts still discernible on OCT at 6 and 12 months showed full neointimal coverage and a stable mean scaffold area between 6 and 12 months. The mean neointimal areas (1.55 ± 0.51 mm² vs. 1.58 ± 0.34 mm², $p = 0.79$) remained unchanged from 6 to 12 months.

## DREAMS-1G: Vasomotion testing

At 6 months, vasoconstriction after administration of acetylcholine (reduction in mean lumen diameter −10.0% ± 20.3%, $p = 0.0008$) followed by vasodilatation after intracoronary nitroglycerin administration (increase in mean lumen diameter, +8.7 ± 10.1%, $p < 0.0001$) of the scaffolded segment demonstrated the uncaging aspect of DREAMS-1G absorption. There were no notable changes at 12 months. Figure 6.10.3 shows similar vasoreactivity in the scaffolded, proximal, and distal segments at 6 months.

## DREAMS-2G: THE SECOND-GENERATION DRUG-ELUTING MAGNESIUM SCAFFOLD

The DREAMS-2G (**Dr**ug-**E**luting **M**etal **S**caffold, **2**nd **G**eneration) is a sirolimus-eluting scaffold made of the same refined magnesium alloy as the DREAMS-1G scaffold. In addition to the magnesium properties, DREAMS-2G offers a six-crown, two-link design, a slightly larger strut cross-sectional profile (see Figure 6.10.1) with a strut thickness of 150 µm to prolong scaffolding time [6]. Radiopaque tantalum markers have been added at both scaffold ends

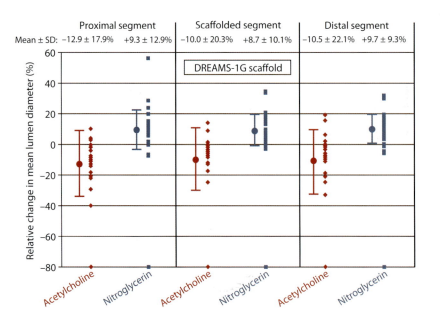

**Figure 6.10.3** Vasomotion test results at 6 months after implantation of DREAMS-1G in the BIOSOLVE-I study. Percentage changes in the mean lumen diameter are presented after acethylcholine and nitroglycerin administration to the target coronary artery. The distance of proximal and distal segments from the scaffolded segment was 5 mm. (Adapted from Waksman R, Prati F, Bruining N, Haude M, Bose D, Kitabata H et al. *Circ Cardiovasc Interv.* 2013;6(6):644–53, with permission.)

to permit more precise implantation and postdilatation visibility. The scaffold is coated with a 7-µm thick absorbable PLLA polymer loaded with 1.4 µg/mm² sirolimus, an agent considered to have a more potent antiproliferative effect than paclitaxel [6]. The dose density and release rate of sirolimus and the biodegradable polymer coating (BIOlute®, BIOTRONIK AG, Bülach, Switzerland) are identical to those used in the drug-eluting stent Orsiro® (BIOTRONIK AG, Bülach, Switzerland), which has recently been reported as having excellent clinical performance [20]. The rapid-exchange delivery system used for DREAMS-2G is based on the same platform used for the Orsiro stent. DREAMS-2G scaffolds, for the clinical study, were available in lengths of 20 and 25 mm and in diameters of 2.5, 3.0, and 3.5 mm and tested in the first-in-man BIOSOLVE-II trial.

## BIOSOLVE-II: The first-in-man clinical trial of DREAMS-2G

The BIOSOLVE-II clinical study is a prospective, multicenter, non-randomized, first-in-man trial that enrolled 123 patients with *de novo* lesions (*n* = 123 target lesions). Patients were included if they had stable or unstable angina or documented silent ischemia, and a maximum of two *de novo* lesions in two separate coronary arteries with a reference vessel diameter in the range of 2.2 to 3.7 mm [21]. Patients were followed at 1, 6, 12, 24, and 36 months post-implantation with mandatory angiographic imaging at 6 months. The

primary endpoint was angiographic in-segment LLL at 6 months. Patient characteristics at baseline are presented in Table 6.10.1. While patients in the PROGRESS-AMS, BIOSOLVE-I, and BIOSOLVE-II studies were similar in many ways, patients in BIOSOLVE-II had more Type B2 lesions (42%) than patients in other studies, PROGRESS-AMS, or BIOSOLVE-I (8% and 9%, respectively). While BIOSOLVE-II could include patients with two *de novo* lesions, all patients (*n* = 123) had one lesion each (*n* = 123 lesions). The DREAMS-2G device could not be implanted in two patients (2/123) because of insufficient predilatation. The rates of procedural and device success were 99% and 93%, respectively.

At 6 months, the mean in-segment LLL was 0.27 ± 0.37 mm [21]. Paired data from 6- and 12-month observations found in-segment LLL was 0.20 ± 0.21 mm (95% confidence interval [CI], 0.13–0.26) at 6 months and 0.25 ± 0.22 mm (95% CI, 0.29–0.45) at 12 months [22].

At 6 months, the in-scaffold LLL was reported as 0.44 ± 0.36 mm [21]. Paired data at 6 and 12 months found the in-scaffold LLL was 0.37 ± 0.25 mm (95% CI, 0.29–0.45) and 0.39 ± 0.27 mm (95% CI, 0.31–0.48), *p* = 0.446 [22]. For the overall study population and in patients without target lesion revascularization, the in-segment and in-scaffold LLL values were 0.27 ± 0.37 mm and 0.44 ± 0.36 mm, respectively, at 6 months. At 12 months, these values were 0.21 ± 0.28 mm and 0.37 ± 0.28 mm, respectively [22]. Figure 6.10.4 compares the in-segment LLL in PROGRESS-AMS, BIOSOLVE-I, and BIOSOLVE-II.

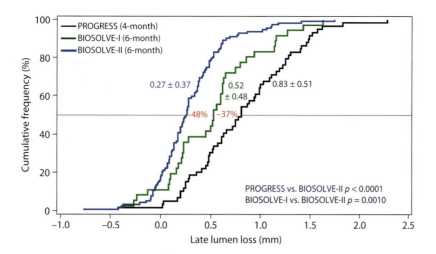

**Figure 6.10.4** Cumulative frequency distributions of the in-segment LLL for AMS after 4 months (PROGRESS-AMS study), DREAMS-1G after 6 months (BIOSOLVE-I study), and DREAMS-2G after 6 months (BIOSOLVE-II study). Mean and standard deviation values are indicated. The mean value for DREAMS-1G was 37% lower than that for AMS. Similarly, the mean value for DREAMS-2G was 48% lower than that of DREAMS-1G.

DREAMS-2G reduced the in-segment LLL by 48% compared to the DREAMS-1G.

Target lesion failure occurred in 3.3% of patients ($n = 4$) [21] at 6 months; no target lesion failure occurred after the 6-month period [22]. Within the first 6 months, one patient died of cancer and one died of unknown causes, whose death was classified as a cardiac death. One patient experienced a periprocedural myocardial infarction, and two had clinically driven TLR procedures within the first 6 months. No definite or probable scaffold thrombosis was observed in any patient at 6 and 12 months [21,22].

## DREAMS-2G: Intracoronary imaging

After the procedure, in IVUS the mean scaffold area was $6.24 \pm 1.15$ mm² and decreased to $6.21 \pm 1.22$ mm² at 6 months (not significant). The minimum scaffold area was $5.41 \pm 1.16$ mm² after the procedure and decreased significantly to $4.62 \pm 0.99$ mm² at 6 months ($p < 0.0001$). At 6 months, the neointimal hyperplasia area was $0.08 \pm 0.09$ mm² and no intraluminal mass could be detected on optical coherence tomography with excellent scaffold strut apposition immediately after implantation and during the absorption process [21]. Figure 6.10.5 illustrates the variation of lumen, scaffold, vessel, and plaque area after implantation of DREAMS-2G in the 11 subjects who underwent serial IVUS analysis at baseline, 6, and 12 months.

Figure 6.10.6 shows the variation of fibrous tissue, fibrous fatty tissue, necrotic core tissue, and calcium after implantation of DREAMS-2G in the 11 subjects who underwent serial IVUS analysis. Interestingly, the magnesium signal is backscattered at the same frequency of the calcium signal and appears white as well. As documented for all magnesium scaffold generations, the reduction of calcium in

virtual histology is considered in this case as a surrogate parameter for the scaffold degradation.

## DREAMS-2G: Vasomotion testing

Vasomotion testing was performed at 6 months in a subset of patients ($n = 25$) and documented a mean lumen diameter of $2.60 \pm 0.29$ mm in the treated segment, which acetylcholine decreased to $2.49 \pm 0.3$ mm ($-0.10$ mm difference, $p = 0.014$) and nitroglycerine dilated to $2.66 \pm 0.33$ mm (difference compared to the postacetylcholine value is 0.17 mm, $p < 0.001$). A change in mean lumen diameter of 3.0% or greater at the scaffold site occurred with vasodilation or vasoconstriction (using acetylcholine or nitroglycerin, respectively) in 80% of the patients tested (20/24) showing the uncaging of the scaffolded vessel segment already at the 6-month time point. Similar results were documented also at 12 months.

## CONCLUSION

The AMS, DREAMS-1G, and DREAMS-2G represent an iterative progression of absorbable metal scaffolds, with each successive generation implementing changes to improve device performance, efficacy, and safety. Results from the BIOSOLVE-II study demonstrate contemporary LLL at 6 and 12 months, favorable clinical outcome data with respect to low target lesion failures and ischemia-driven TLR rates and no definite or probable scaffold thrombosis up to the thus far reported follow-up period of 12 months. In June 2016, the DREAMS-2G obtained its CE mark for market release to the European Union as the first bioresorbable drug-eluting metal scaffold and the third drug-eluting scaffold device (including the two prior PLLA-based ABSORB BVS and DeSolve scaffolds).

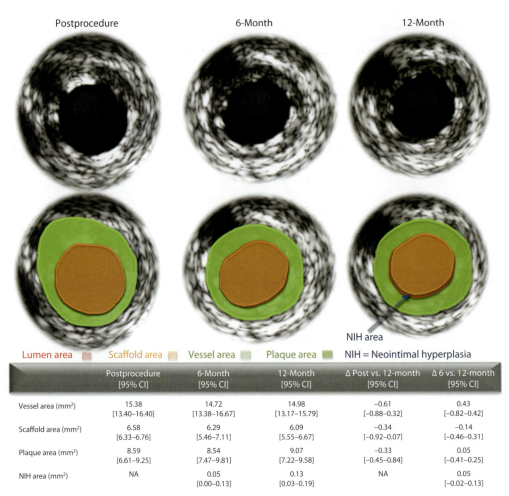

Lumen area ▮   Scaffold area ▮   Vessel area ▮   Plaque area ▮   NIH = Neointimal hyperplasia

|  | Postprocedure [95% CI] | 6-Month [95% CI] | 12-Month [95% CI] | Δ Post vs. 12-month [95% CI] | Δ 6 vs. 12-month [95% CI] |
|---|---|---|---|---|---|
| Vessel area (mm²) | 15.38 [13.40–16.40] | 14.72 [13.38–16.67] | 14.98 [13.17–15.79] | −0.61 [−0.88–0.32] | 0.43 [−0.82–0.42] |
| Scaffold area (mm²) | 6.58 [6.33–6.76] | 6.29 [5.46–7.11] | 6.09 [5.55–6.67] | −0.34 [−0.92–0.07] | −0.14 [−0.46–0.31] |
| Plaque area (mm²) | 8.59 [6.61–9.25] | 8.54 [7.47–9.81] | 9.07 [7.22–9.58] | −0.33 [−0.45–0.84] | 0.05 [−0.41–0.25] |
| NIH area (mm²) | NA | 0.05 [0.00–0.13] | 0.13 [0.03–0.19] | NA | 0.05 [−0.02–0.13] |

Data presented as median [Interquartile range: Q1, Q3], there was no significant difference in outcomes between 6 and 12-months

**Figure 6.10.5** Serial IVUS analysis in 11 subjects at baseline, 6, and 12 months follow-up after implantation of DREAMS-2G.

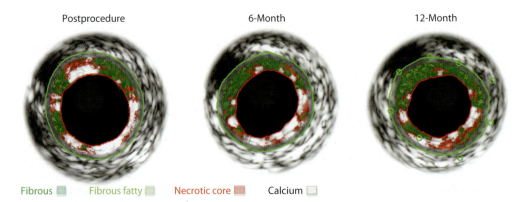

Fibrous ▮   Fibrous fatty ▮   Necrotic core ▮   Calcium ▯

|  | Postprocedure | 6-Month | 12-Month | Δ Post vs. 12-month (p value) | Δ 6 vs. 12-month (p value) |
|---|---|---|---|---|---|
| Fibrous (%) | 31.29 | 46.52 | 43.68 | 12.39 (<0.001) | −2.84 (0.24) |
| Fibrous fatty (%) | 4.57 | 10.27 | 6.77 | 2.2 (0.22) | 5.7 (0.004) |
| Necrotic core (%) | 29.27 | 25.96 | 28.64 | −0.63 (0.76) | 2.68 (0.20) |
| Calcium (%) | 34.88 | 17.25 | 20.91 | −13.97 (<0.001) | 3.66 (0.12) |

**Figure 6.10.6** Serial IVUS virtual histology analysis in 11 subjects at baseline, 6, and 12 months after DREAMS-2G implantation. IVUS virtual histology analysis is based on raw data from Figure 6.10.5.

## ACKNOWLEDGMENTS

The author would like to acknowledge Jo Ann LeQuang and Ludovica Visciola for their assistance in manuscript preparation and review.

## REFERENCES

1. Onuma Y, Serruys PW. Bioresorbable scaffold: The advent of a new era in percutaneous coronary and peripheral revascularization? *Circulation.* 2011;123(7):779–97.
2. Serruys PW, Garcia-Garcia HM, Onuma Y. From metallic cages to transient bioresorbable scaffolds: Change in paradigm of coronary revascularization in the upcoming decade? *Eur Heart J.* 2012;33(1):16–25b.
3. Daemen J, Serruys PW. Drug-eluting stent update 2007: Part I. A survey of current and future generation drug-eluting stents: Meaningful advances or more of the same? *Circulation.* 2007;116(3):316–28.
4. Haude M, Erbel R, Erne P, Verheye S, Degen H, Bose D et al. Safety and performance of the drug-eluting absorbable metal scaffold (DREAMS) in patients with de-novo coronary lesions: 12 month results of the prospective, multicentre, first-in-man BIOSOLVE-I trial. *Lancet.* 2013;381(9869):836–44.
5. Waksman R. Current state of the absorbable metallic (magnesium) stent. *EuroIntervention. Journal of EuroPCR in Collaboration with the Working Group on Interventional Cardiology of the European Society of Cardiology.* 2009;5 Suppl F:F94–7.
6. Campos CM, Muramatsu T, Iqbal J, Zhang YJ, Onuma Y, Garcia-Garcia HM et al. Bioresorbable drug-eluting magnesium-alloy scaffold for treatment of coronary artery disease. *Int J Mol Sci.* 2013;14(12):24492–500.
7. Bosiers M, Deloose K, Verbist J, Peeters P. First clinical application of absorbable metal stents in the treatment of critical limb ischemia: 12-month results. *Vasc Dis Manag.* 2005;2(4):86–91.
8. Erbel R, Di Mario C, Bartunek J, Bonnier J, de Bruyne B, Eberli FR et al. Temporary scaffolding of coronary arteries with bioabsorbable magnesium stents: A prospective, non-randomised multicentre trial. *Lancet.* 2007;369(9576):1869–75.
9. Haude M, Ince H, Abizaid A, Toelg R, Lemos PA, von Birgelen C et al. Safety and performance of the second-generation drug-eluting absorbable metal scaffold in patients with de-novo coronary artery lesions (BIOSOLVE-II): 6 month results of a prospective, multicentre, non-randomised, first-in-man trial. *Lancet.* 2016;387:31–9.
10. Heublein B, Rohde R, Kaese V, Niemeyer M, Hartung W, Haverich A. Biocorrosion of magnesium alloys: A new principle in cardiovascular implant technology? *Heart (British Cardiac Society).* 2003;89(6):651–6.
11. Morice M, Serruys P, Sousa J, Fajadet J, Ban Hayashi E, Perin M et al. A randomized comparison of a sirolimus-eluting stent with a standard stent for coronary revascularization. *New Engl J Med.* 2002;346(1773–1780).
12. Waksman R, Erbel R, Di Mario C, Bartunek J, de Bruyne B, Eberli FR et al. Early- and long-term intravascular ultrasound and angiographic findings after bioabsorbable magnesium stent implantation in human coronary arteries. *JACC Cardiovasc Interv.* 2009;2(4):312–20.
13. Barlis P, Tanigawa J, Di Mario C. Coronary bioabsorbable magnesium stent: 15-month intravascular ultrasound and optical coherence tomography findings. *Eur Heart J.* 2007;28(19):2319.
14. Ghimire G, Spiro J, Kharbanda R, Roughton M, Barlis P, Mason M et al. Initial evidence for the return of coronary vasoreactivity following the absorption of bioabsorbable magnesium alloy coronary stents. *EuroIntervention. Journal of EuroPCR in Collaboration with the Working Group on Interventional Cardiology of the European Society of Cardiology.* 2009;4(4):481–4.
15. Wittchow E, Adden N, Riedmuller J, Savard C, Waksman R, Braune M. Bioresorbable drug-eluting magnesium-alloy scaffold: Design and feasibility in a porcine coronary model. *EuroIntervention. Journal of EuroPCR in Collaboration with the Working Group on Interventional Cardiology of the European Society of Cardiology.* 2013;8(12):1441–50.
16. Grube E, Silber S, Hauptmann KE, Mueller R, Buellesfeld L, Gerckens U et al. TAXUS I: Six- and twelve-month results from a randomized, double-blind trial on a slow-release paclitaxel-eluting stent for de novo coronary lesions. *Circulation.* 2003;107(1):38–42.
17. Cutlip DE, Windecker S, Mehran R, Boam A, Cohen DJ, van Es GA et al. Clinical end points in coronary stent trials: A case for standardized definitions. *Circulation.* 2007;115(17):2344–51.
18. Haude M, Erbel R, Erne P, Verheye S, Degen H, Vermeersch P et al. Safety and performance of the DRug-Eluting Absorbable Metal Scaffold (DREAMS) in patients with de novo coronary lesions: 3-year results of the prospective, multicentre, first-in-man BIOSOLVE-I trial. *EuroIntervention. Journal of EuroPCR in Collaboration with the Working Group on Interventional Cardiology of the European Society of Cardiology.* 2016;12(2):e160–e6.

19. Waksman R, Prati F, Bruining N, Haude M, Bose D, Kitabata H et al. Serial observation of drug-eluting absorbable metal scaffold: Multi-imaging modality assessment. *Circ Cardiovasc Interv.* 2013;6(6):644–53.

20. Windecker S, Haude M, Neumann FJ, Stangl K, Witzenbichler B, Slagboom T et al. Comparison of a novel biodegradable polymer sirolimus-eluting stent with a durable polymer everolimus-eluting stent: Results of the randomized BIOFLOW-II trial. *Circ Cardiovasc Interv.* 2015;8(2):e001441.

21. Haude M, Ince H, Abizaid A, Toelg R, Lemos PA, von Birgelen C et al. Safety and performance of the second-generation drug-eluting absorbable metal scaffold in patients with de-novo coronary artery lesions (BIOSOLVE-II): 6 month results of a prospective, multicentre, non-randomised, first-in-man trial. *Lancet.* 2016;387(10013):31–9.

22. Haude M, Ince H, Abizaid A, Toelg R, Lemos P, Von Birgelen C et al. Sustained safety and performance of the second-generation drug-eluting absorbable metal scaffold (DREAMS 2G) in patients with de novo coronary lesions: 12 month clinical results and angiographic findings of the BIOSOLVE-II first-in-man trial. *Eur Heart J* 2016, in press.

# The REVA Medical Program: From *ReZolve*® to *Fantom*®

ALEXANDRE ABIZAID AND J. RIBAMAR COSTA JR.

## REVA'S SCAFFOLDS MAIN FEATURES

REVA Medical, Inc. (San Diego, CA) took a unique approach to fully integrate both a novel design and material in developing a sirolimus-eluting bioresorbable coronary scaffold.

A major drawback of contemporary polymers is that they lack intrinsic radiopacity. REVA, in collaboration with Drs. Kohn and Bolikal at Rutgers University in New Jersey, developed a proprietary inherently radiopaque polymer comprised of tyrosine analogs and other natural metabolites. Additionally, iodine is incorporated into the polymer backbone, which allows the device to be visualized using conventional angiography. Iodine atoms are covalently bound directly to the backbone of the desaminotyrosine (DAT) component and, due to their greater mass, scatter x-rays and impart radiopacity [1,3].

REVA's polymer was engineered to have a degradation profile that supports the vessel during the initial healing and remodeling process prior to significant degradation of the scaffold. This polymer is used both for the structure of the scaffold and for the drug delivery coating.

The REVA Scaffolds "family" includes two expansion designs, the *Slide & Lock* design as found in the *ReZolve*® scaffold series and the *Deformable* design used in the *Fantom*® scaffold series (Figures 6.11.1 and 6.11.2).

Unlike traditional deformable metal stent designs, the *Slide & Lock* design deploys by sliding open and locking into place [4,5]. This novel scaffold design eliminates the need to significantly deform the device during deployment, making it ideally suited for use with polymers, which are inherently not as amenable to deformation as metals. The *Slide & Lock ReZolve* design has a series of 15 individual components that are assembled into a single scaffold. These components are made up of two primary elements, which include 12 U-shaped 120 μ struts and three sinusoidal backbone components that are approximately 230 μ in thickness (Figure 6.11.3). As the U-shape component passes through the backbone element, it transitions through a series of mechanical locks until the final desired diameter is achieved.

In addition to the *Slide & Lock* design, REVA scaffold is also available in a *Traditional, Deformable Design*. The Deformable design expands in a similar manner to traditional metal drug-eluting stents and other bioresorbable scaffolds with a clinically significant expansion range of more than 1 mm from the nominal size. The *Deformable Fantom* platform is a single element device that contains a uniform thickness of approximately 125 μ across the full length of the scaffold. While the *ReZolve* scaffold is 6Fr guiding-catheter compatible, the *Fantom* scaffold is compatible with a 5Fr guiding-catheter, with an overall nominal profile of 1.27 mm. Figure 6.11.4 is a comparison of the *Fantom* scaffold profile to the commercially available ABSORB scaffold (Abbott Vascular, Santa Clara, CA) (Test performed by REVA Medical. Data on company files.).

Besides the complete scaffold visibility (Figure 6.11.5), both REVA designs allow for standard handling and use techniques. Neither device requires any special storage requirements such as refrigeration, and both devices are delivered and implanted using the exact techniques that are employed in traditional metal drug-eluting stents. Once the scaffold is delivered to the target lesion, both designs can be fully expanded to the intended clinical diameter in a single continuous inflation. There is no need to pause at designated pressures when expanding either REVA BRS design.

The *ReZolve* and *Fantom* are both sirolimus-eluting scaffolds. In each case, the device is coated with a combination of the base polymer mixed with sirolimus. The nominal dose on a 3.0 × 18 mm device is 115 μg of sirolimus. Greater

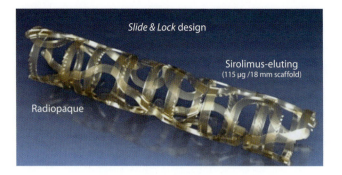

**Figure 6.11.1** *ReZolve* scaffold design: This system has a unique slide and lock design aimed to increase radial force preventing acute "recoil."

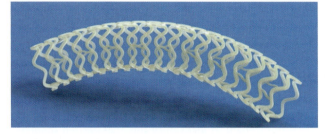

**Figure 6.11.2** Novel *Fantom* scaffold.

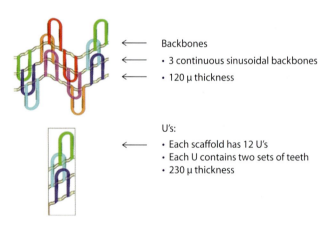

**Figure 6.11.3** Schematic representation of the main components of the *ReZolve* scaffold.

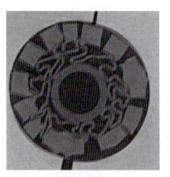
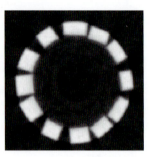

PLLA scaffold
1.4 mm (.55")

Fantom
<1.27 mm (.50")

**Figure 6.11.4** Comparison of the "crimped" profile between the commercially available ABSORB scaffold and the novel *Fantom* scaffold: a reduction in strut-thickness of only 25–30 μm achieves >10% decrease in profile.

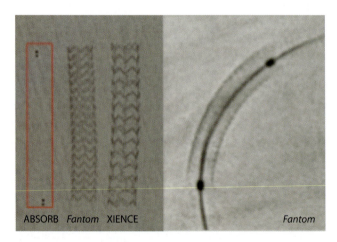

**Figure 6.11.5** Scaffold X-ray visibility comparison: As noticed, the *Fantom* scaffold had a radiopacity profile comparable to metallic platforms, which might facilitate the identification of its boundaries preventing "geographical miss" and edge dissections during scaffold deployment and postdilatation.

than 80% of the total sirolimus load is eluted within the first 90 days.

REVA has designed both scaffolds to maintain full mechanical functionality through the critical vessel-healing period. After the artery has healed, the scaffold will gradually degrade and the treated vessel is expected to return to a natural state of normal vasomotion. As the scaffold degrades and is resorbed, there will be a seamless integration of arterial tissue into the space previously occupied by the scaffold. The mechanism for degradation of their scaffolds is primarily hydrolysis. The structure of the polymer consists of a diester of iodinated desaminotyrosine along with common non-radiopaque biodegradable components. On absorption of water, the diester hydrolyzes to form two molecules of the iodinated desaminotyrosine along with other resorbable natural products. On absorption of the iodinated desaminotyrosine into the blood, it is eliminated rapidly through the kidneys. The iodine component of the polymer remains bound to the desaminotyrosine molecule so it is not free and is excreted from the body through the normal degradation process. In addition, the amount of iodine bound in the desaminotyrosine molecule is less than 1% of the amount contained in a single milliliter of contrast solution. Figure 6.11.6 represents a typical *in vitro* degradation profile for the REVA scaffolds.

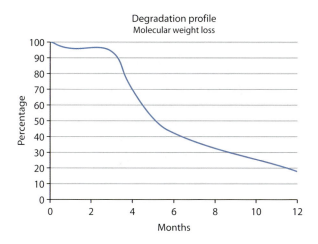

Degradation profile
Molecular weight loss

**Figure 6.11.6** REVA scaffolds degradation profile: Both systems are engineered to maintain at least 75% of their initial mechanical strength to support the vessel through the most critical healing and remodeling phase (up to 4 months). After this initial period, the lost of molecular weight speeds up considerably, with the full resorption process completed up to 24 months.

## CLINICAL EXPERIENCE WITH *ReZolve* AND *ReZolve2* SCAFFOLDS

### *ReZolve* scaffold and phase I of the RESTORE clinical trial

The RESTORE clinical trial (pilot study of the **Re**Zolve **S**irolimus-Elu**t**ing Bi**ore**sorbable coronary scaffold) is a prospective, multi-center study evaluating the safety and performance of the *ReZolve* scaffold. The *ReZolve* scaffold system has a 7 French profile (Fr). The balloon catheter for delivery had a retractable-sheathed system, which was implemented to enhance retention and delivery.

In the first phase of RESTORE there were 26 patients enrolled in the RESTORE I study; of these, 22 patients were successfully treated with a *ReZolve* scaffold. Implants were performed in Brazil, Germany, Poland, and Austria. All patients in this ongoing trial have completed a 1-year angiographic follow-up and will be followed for 5 years. The primary study endpoints are freedom from ischemic-driven target lesion revascularization at 6 months and quantitative measurements at 12 months (QCA: quantitative coronary angiography/IVUS: intravascular ultrasound).

Technical success, defined as delivery and deployment of the device, was achieved in 85% of the cases. Four patients were not implanted due to the relatively high system profile (7 Fr), which caused some difficulty when traversing moderately tortuous anatomy. When the device was deployed, acute procedural success (residual stenosis <20%) was obtained in 100% of the cases. Clinical procedural success, defined as acute procedure success without the occurrence of major adverse cardiac events (MACE) through 1 month, was also 100%.

At 12 months, one patient declined invasive follow-up and there were four study-related TLRs and one death, in a patient who had successfully completed the 6-month follow-up (no angiographic restenosis) with a negative stress test within 1 month of the fatal event. The late lumen loss at 12 months for nonretreated patients ($n = 14$) was 0.29 ± 0.33 mm with a percentage of in-scaffold stenosis of 20.2 ± 15.4%. The interim results of this trial were presented in the Transcatheter Therapeutics (TCT) Meeting, San Francisco, CA, in 2013.

In the first phase of the RESTORE trial there was a successful demonstration of *ReZolve* platform as the acute recoil had a low average of 3.8%. Additionally, the device had several ease-of-use features (e.g., radiopacity, single-step inflation, no special storage considerations, and relevant clinical sizing.) The deliverability was marked as a specific feature for improvement. The findings from this first phase of the RESTORE clinical trial were rapidly incorporated into *ReZolve2* program.

### *ReZolve2* scaffold and the RESTORE clinical trial

The RESTORE clinical trial was amended for a phase II pilot study of the *ReZolve2* scaffold. The primary differences between the *ReZolve* Scaffold and the *ReZolve2* scaffold were a reduction in profile from a 7Fr-compatible device to a 6 Fr-compatible device, elimination of the retractable sheath, and a minor revision to the polymer formulation.

After completion of the initial pilot enrollment, the clinical program for the *ReZolve2 scaffold* was once again expanded into RESTORE II trial, a prospective, multicenter study evaluating the safety and performance of the *ReZolve2* scaffold.

Patients were enrolled at 23 clinical sites across Brazil, Australia, New Zealand, Poland, Slovenia, and Germany. The *ReZolve2* scaffold had a marked improvement in the acute performance, achieving a technical success rate of 96% for device delivery and deployment (107 patients successfully treated with the study device out of 112 enrolled in the study). This outcome is equivalent to that which has been reported for the current commercially available ABSORB™ Bioresorbable Vascular Scaffold by Abbott Vascular [6].

All patients have completed 6-month clinical follow-up and greater than 90% have completed their 12-month visit. Patients with the *ReZolve2* scaffold will be followed for 5 years. The primary study endpoints for the *ReZolve2* analyses are freedom from ischemic-driven target lesion revascularization at 6 months and quantitative QCA/IVUS measurements at a later date.

MACE was obtained in all cases. The final safety and efficacy results through 12 months as well as core lab data (QCA, IVUS, OCT) are currently in the analysis phase and will be presented in the near future. Figure 6.11.7 depicts a case from our experience at Dante Pazzanese.

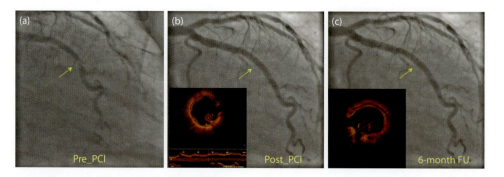

**Figure 6.11.7** Example of a patient treated with the *ReZolve2* scaffold at Dante Pazzanese: Panel **(a)** shows the presence of a severe de novo stenosis in the circumflex artery. Panel **(b)** shows the result immediately after the implant of the scaffold. At the left bottom of the picture there is an OCT image showing the slide and lock mechanism of the *ReZolve* device with its unique "semi-colon" appearance. Panel **(c)** shows the 6-month angiographic result. Note the excellent angiographic and OCT appearance of the device, with minimum, homogenous NIH tissue formation (small picture at the left bottom of the panel).

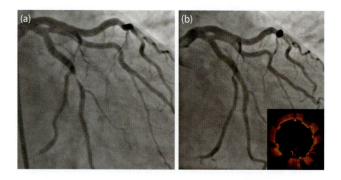

**Figure 6.11.8** Example of a patient treated with the *Fantom* scaffold at Dante Pazzanese: Panel **(a)** shows the presence of a severe de novo stenosis in the OM branch of the circumflex artery. Panel **(b)** shows the result immediately after the implant of the scaffold. At the right bottom of the picture, there is an OCT image showing the low profile of the scaffold struts which, contrary to the usual PLLA devices, does not have the shape of a box.

## *Fantom* clinical program

In parallel to the *ReZolve* clinical program, REVA has initiated a human clinical trial with the *Fantom Sirolimus-Eluting Bioresorbable Scaffold*. The initial implants have demonstrated that the *Fantom* deformable design performed as intended with all of the ease-of-use features currently found in metal drug-eluting stents, such as nonspecial handling or storage, continuous inflation to intended diameter at implant, and complete visibility under standard x-ray imaging. The *Fantom* clinical program is intended to enroll up to 125 patients in centers in Europe and Brazil. The primary endpoint is the QCA assessment of in-scaffold late loss at 6 months. Furthermore, patients will be clinically followed for 5 years. Figure 6.11.8 shows an example of patients treated with the *Fantom* device in our center.

## REFERENCES

1. Shymko MJ. Reactions to iodinated contrast. *Radiol Technol.* 2001;72:381–2.
2. Christiansen C, Pichler WJ, Skotland T. Delayed allergy-like reactions to X-ray contrast media: Mechanistic considerations. *Eur Radiol.* 2000;10:1965–75.
3. Hash RB. Intravascular radiographic contrast media: Issues for family physicians. *J Am Board Fam Pract.* 1999;12:32–42.
4. Zeltinger J, Schmid E, Brandom D, Bolikal D, Pesnell A, Kohn J. Advances in the development of coronary stents. *Society for Biomaterials, Biomaterials Forum.* 2004;26:8,9,24.
5. Kohn J, Zeltinger J. Resorbable, drug-eluting stents: A new frontier in the treatment of coronary artery disease. *Expert Rev Med Devices.* 2005;2:667–71.
6. Serruys PW, Chevalier B, Dudek D, Cequier A, Carrié D, Iniguez A, Dominici M et al. A bioresorbable everolimus-eluting scaffold versus a metallic everolimus-eluting stent for ischaemic heart disease caused by de-novo native coronary artery lesions (ABSORB II): An interim 1-year analysis of clinical and procedural secondary outcomes from a randomised controlled trial. *Lancet.* 2015 Jan 3;385(9962):43–54.

# 6.12

# The Amaranth bioresorbable vascular scaffold technology

ALAIDE CHIEFFO, JUAN F. GRANADA, AND ANTONIO COLOMBO

## TECHNOLOGY BACKGROUND

One of the major challenges in the BRS field has been the development of scaffolds displaying optimal mechanical strength and resistance to the compressive load imposed by the vessel components following acute deployment in challenging anatomical conditions (i.e., calcification). In the first generation BRS, polymer orientation and crystallinity determine the mechanical strength of the scaffold. In turn, the polymer's ability to orient and gain crystallinity depends on its molecular weight and the tube manufacturing process. These first generation BRS technologies utilize lower molecular weight polymers, which can be readily oriented resulting in a substantial increase of their crystallinity. Highly crystalline polymer structures, however, significantly limit the scaffold's resistance to fracture especially under high stress conditions (i.e., overexpansion). Then, despite the fact current generation BRS have achieved biomechanical performances equivalent to metallic stents, BRS are still limited by their capacity to overexpand beyond predetermined limits and to resist vascular recoil under extreme conditions [1–5]. The Amaranth polymer technology improves on the biomechanical properties of the current generation BRS, which rely on polymer orientation and crystallinity, due to the intrinsic material properties uniquely associated with ultra-high molecular weight polymer and the proprietary manufacturing methodology. *Ex vivo* studies have shown that this type of noncrystalline polymer dramatically improves overexpansion capabilities and resistance to fracture under static and dynamic loading conditions compared to other BRS [6].

## TECHNOLOGY DESCRIPTION

The Amaranth's BRS (Amaranth Medical Inc., Mountain View, CA) is a novel Sirolimus-eluting, fully bioresorbable coronary scaffold. The technology comprises a PLLA scaffold

and a Sirolimus drug coating matrix that is mounted on a dedicated balloon-catheter delivery system. Two generations of scaffolds have been developed to date displaying different strut thicknesses: FORTITUDE® (~150 microns, first generation scaffold) and APTITUDE™ (~120 microns, current generation technology). Both devices display a zig-zag helical design (Figure 6.12.1). In their expanded state, both scaffolds cover less than 25% of the total vessel surface area. The core technology involves a proprietary process of high molecular weight polymer synthesis and processing technology designed to achieve a balance between strength, flexibility, and high resistance to fracture. Tube manufacturing is achieved by a proprietary multilayer deposition process, enabling significant dimensional accuracy and stability.

The biomechanical properties of the polymer, from PLLA tubing fabrication to final sterile device, are fully preserved throughout the entire manufacturing cycle, with negligible reduction of molecular weight and no alteration of thermal properties. Both FORTITUDE and APTITUDE scaffolds are inherently isotropic with a highly balanced response to application of an external load, virtually eliminating strut distortions associated with crimping and expansion of scaffolds. This minimizes stress concentrations and susceptibility to fractures. It also provides for a symmetrical scaffold structure during expansion and implantation, which results in significant flexibility and conformability to the arterial wall.

## BIOMECHANICAL PROPERTIES

### Radial strength

Radial strength is essential for the acute performance of BRS and to achieve optimal clinical outcomes. The Amaranth's scaffold is designed to have a circumferential radial force equivalent to metallic stents in a wide variety

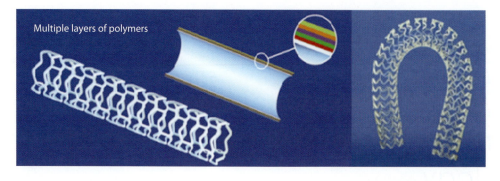

**Figure 6.12.1** Amaranth BRS displaying a zigzag helical design, cut from a multilayer PLLA tube.

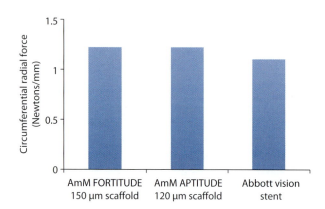

**Figure 6.12.2** Amaranth's FORTITUDE (150 μm) and APTITUDE (120 μm) scaffold normalized radial strength is, at minimum, equivalent to conventional metallic stents. The circumferential radial force (Newton) is divided by the scaffold or stent length (mm) to give the normalized radial strength.

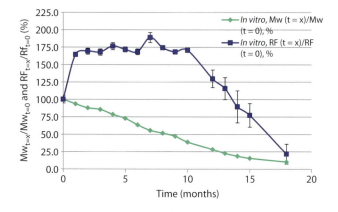

**Figure 6.12.3** *In vitro* scaffold radial force and polymer molecular weight change over time for the Amaranth scaffold.

of scaffold wall thicknesses (Figure 6.12.2). For the 150 μm and 120 μm wall thickness, the normalized radial strength (circumferential force divided by scaffold length) is, at minimum, equivalent to conventional metallic stents. The high radial strength of the Amaranth scaffold is maintained for an extended period of time (up to 10 months following implantation), fully supporting the treated vessel during the healing period, and then gradually ceasing to provide luminal support when it is no longer needed. This strength is maintained during the early phases of the degradation process and gradually decreases as the polymer is predictably reabsorbed (Figure 6.12.3).

## Fracture resistance and ductility

The scaffold is cut from a specially manufactured PLLA tube. Unlike other PLLA-based scaffolds, the specialized tube-manufacturing processes used to make the Amaranth's scaffolds result in optimized properties of the PLLA material. PLLA used to manufacture first generation scaffolds elongates to ~5%, whereas the Amaranth proprietary PLLA can elongate to 45–50% (at minimum), before breaking. The unique

tube manufacturing methods, in tandem with the scaffold design, provide the Amaranth scaffold with intrinsic strength while maintaining ductility. The Amaranth scaffold can be overexpanded beyond its normal operating diameters without fracturing, yet still maintain superior radial strength and minimum recoil across a variety of diameters (Figure 6.12.4). These favorable biomechanical characteristics are especially important in the situation in which polymer expansion is needed such as side branch dilatation following scaffold implantation. As seen in Figure 6.12.5, the Amaranth scaffolds can withstand overexpansion between, or within, rings, which allows for easier side branch access and postdilatation.

## Scaffold surface area

In order to maximize radial force, many BRS are required to increase the scaffold surface area (footprint) to make up for their inherent limited material strength. The inherent strength of the Amaranth's scaffolds results in radial forces that are equivalent to metallic stents; however, material thickness and overall surface area are less compared to other BRS (Figure 6.12.6). Then, the percentage surface area exposed to the vessel wall is considerably less than that of other BRS.

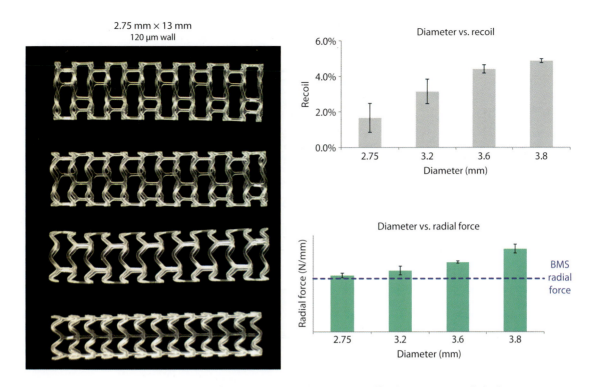

2.75 mm × 13 mm
120 µm wall

Figure 6.12.4 Fracture resistance (toughness) for the 2.75 mm diameter scaffold at 120 µm wall thickness.

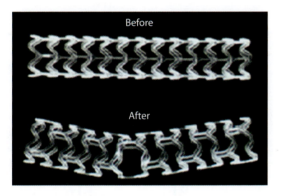

Figure 6.12.5 Amaranth 120-micron scaffold overexpanded between rings and within a ring allowing side branch access.

## EXPERIMENTAL VALIDATION STUDIES

The safety and performance of the Amaranth's Sirolimus-eluting bioresorbable coronary scaffold and delivery system has been tested through extensive preclinical studies. A series of *in vivo* animal studies have been performed using the porcine model to characterize the biocompatibility, pharmacokinetics, and healing response of all Amaranth BRS systems. In addition, multimodality imaging and histology have been performed in order to evaluate the healing response and resorption pattern of all drug eluting Amaranth scaffolds. In total, 16 studies, involving 148 animals implanted with 300 Amaranth scaffolds and 144 control devices (either bare metal stents or Abbott BVS) have been performed to date. A description of the typical

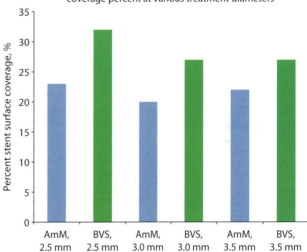

Figure 6.12.6 Comparative scaffold surface coverage data of the Amaranth BRS versus the BVS (Abbott Vascular) scaffold. The Amaranth's BRS has 28% less scaffold surface coverage area at 2.5 mm vessel treatment diameter, 26% less at 3.0 mm, and 19% less at 3.5 mm. Analysis was based on light microscopy (40×) and includes strut width and number of rings. The Amaranth BRS data was compared to previously published data of the Absorb BVS.

healing response up to 6 months of 120-micron BRS is presented in Figure 6.12.7. As shown in the figure, the lumen and device areas remained stable over time proving the biomechanical stability of the scaffold even at advanced stages of polymer degradation. Also, the low inflammatory scores

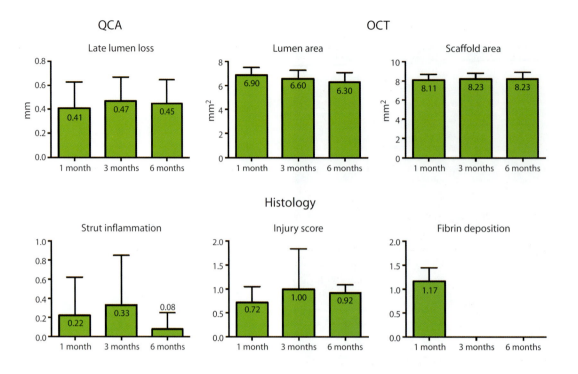

**Figure 6.12.7** Healing response of the APTITUDE scaffold (120-micron) evaluated by angiography, OCT, and histology up to 6 months.

shown over time is a reflection of the high vascular compatibility displayed by the polymer at different degradation phases.

## Vascular healing data

Evaluation of vascular healing was conducted by implanting scaffolds delivering no drug (bare scaffold), nominal dose (1×), and twice the dose (2×), both in the acute and chronic setting postimplantation. Studies were performed in the nondiseased porcine coronary artery model. Scaffold safety has been evaluated through the characterization of thrombosis and neointimal formation. Longitudinal imaging and histology have been used to assess *in vivo* thrombogenicity, inflammation, and strut healing characteristics. Long-term biocompatibility studies showed that the Amaranth's polymer elicited comparable levels of inflammation and neointimal formation compared to bare metal stent controls in the absence of antiproliferative drugs. In the evaluation of the scaffold at no dose, nominal dose (1×), and 2× the dose, strut-associated inflammation was minimal as observed at 28, 90, and 180 days post-implant. Strut coverage and endothelialization was complete (100%) in all BRS devices at 28 days. A mature neointima was seen at 90 days and small amounts of fibrin deposits were still present up to 180 days. There were no observations of leukocyte margination, hemorrhage, occlusion, thrombosis, or aneurysmal formation. With the absence of the drug (bare scaffold), neointimal formation was characterized as a thick, mature layer by 28 days with no uncovered struts or thrombosis. Representative

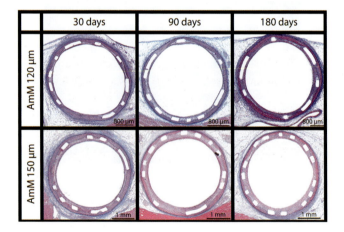

**Figure 6.12.8** Representative histological thumbnails of the FORTITUDE (150 μm) and APTITUDE (120 μm) scaffolds up to 180 days.

histological pictures of the healing response up to 6-months with the nominal dose are presented in Figure 6.12.8.

## *In vivo* imaging analysis

Angiographic and OCT images for vessels treated at nominal doses showed patent lumens and no evidence of restenosis for all scaffolds at 28, 90, and 180 days follow-up. There were no observed intraluminal filling defects, negative distal flow characteristics, malapposition, or side branch occlusions with the implant. Average in-scaffold late lumen loss (ISLL) indicated that the Amaranth scaffold performed as intended compared to control and with no reported complications during the survival periods. Neointimal thickness (NIT) and lumen areas as observed via OCT assessments were favorable in that the NIT was consistent over time with no abrupt changes. The percentage area stenosis (% AS) remained low over time as well.

## Pharmacokinetic studies

The active pharmaceutical ingredient chosen for the AmM bioresorbable coronary scaffold is the antiproliferative drug Sirolimus (rapamycin). *In vivo* porcine studies of the pharmacokinetic characterization for the AmM bioresorbable drug-eluting coronary scaffold consisted of local, regional, and systemic assessments. Characterization of local effects evaluated drug content from excised vessels up to 90 days. Drug remaining in tissue from the implant site (including proximal and distal region of stented segment) was determined. The study showed that approximately 75% of the drug was released by 28 days, and about 90% of the drug was released by 90 days.

Regional effects were characterized by drug concentrations in various organs following the implantation of two overlapping Amaranth scaffolds (2× dose). Tissue samples were collected from the myocardium, liver, lung, kidney, and spleen at 28, 90, and 180 days postimplant. For all time points, Sirolimus levels in these tissues were well below the limit of quantification. Systemic assessment of drug released by the implanted AmM scaffold at nominal dose was evaluated with the collection of whole blood collected for the first 24 hours of implant through 7 days postimplant. Sirolimus concentrations in blood were quantifiable for up

to 3 days postimplant with peak drug concentrations measured at 0.5–1 hour postimplant. The average peak blood concentration was approximately 3 ng/mL, which was well below the peak blood levels of >200 ng/mL found to be safe and well tolerated in humans following a single intravenous dose administration [7]. Sirolimus blood concentrations declined quickly, and were not measurable at 7 days postimplant. Average terminal half-life is estimated to be 39 hours.

## CLINICAL DATA

Several clinical studies have been completed to evaluate the safety and efficacy of the Amaranth fully bioresorbable scaffolds in patients undergoing elective percutaneous coronary intervention in single *de novo*, native coronary lesions. Patients were enrolled if clinical and angiographic criteria were met and written informed consent was provided. The study protocols were approved by the local ethics committees. The primary endpoint was the freedom from target vessel failure, which was defined as no occurrence of cardiac death, target vessel myocardial infarction, or ischemia driven target vessel revascularization at 6–9 months. Clinical device success was defined as the successful deployment of the scaffold at the intended location with a postimplantation diameter stenosis of <50%. Clinical procedure success was defined as device success without the occurrence of major adverse clinical events related to ischemia up to 7 days after the index procedure and allowed the use of an adjunctive device. All patients underwent elective percutaneous coronary intervention with mandatory predilatation of the target lesion. Table 6.12.1 provides an overview of these studies.

Table 6.12.1 Summary of clinical studies using the FORTITUDE (150 μm) and APTITUDE (120 μm) scaffolds to date including study design and clinical end points

| Study | MEND | MEND II and RENASCENT | RENASCENT II |
|---|---|---|---|
| Study device | FORTITUDE Bare Scaffold (non drug-eluting) 150–200 μm PLLA bioresorbable scaffold mounted on a RX delivery balloon catheter | FORTITUDE Sirolimus-eluting 150 μm PLLA bioresorbable scaffold mounted on a RX delivery balloon catheter | APTITUDE Sirolimus-eluting 120 μm PLLA bioresorbable scaffold mounted on a RX delivery balloon catheter |
| Study design | Prospective, nonrandomized, first-in-man study | Prospective, nonrandomized, multicenter, noninferiority study | Prospective, nonrandomized, multicenter, noninferiority study |
| Primary safety endpoint | Freedom from target vessel failure (TVF) at 6 months | Freedom from target vessel failure (TVF) at 9 months | Freedom from target vessel failure (TVF) at 9 months |
| Primary performance endpoint | Device success Procedure success | In-scaffold late lumen loss (LLL) by QCA at 9 months | In-scaffold late lumen loss (LLL) by QCA at 9 months |
| Secondary endpoints | – | Device success Procedure success Vessel patency at 2 years | Device success Procedure success Vessel patency at 2 years |
| Clinical follow-up | 30, 180, 270 days, and 1, 2 years | 30 days, 270 days, and 2 years | 30 days, 270 days, and 2 years |
| Non-office follow-up | 3, 4, and 5 years | 180 days; 3, 4, and 5 years | 3, 4, and 5 years |

Table 6.12.2 Safety endpoints for all clinical studies of Amaranth's BRS

| Clinical outcome % (n) | MEND (150–200 μm, Bare) (n = 13) | | MEND II + RENASCENT (150 μm, Sirolimus) (n = 49) | RENASCENT II (120 μm, Sirolimus) (n = 20) |
|---|---|---|---|---|
| | 1 year | 2 years | 9 months | 30 days |
| Target vessel failure | 7.7% (1) | 7.7% (1) | 6.1% (3) | 0% (0) |
| – Cardiac death | 0% (0) | 0% (0) | 0% (0) | 0% (0) |
| – Target vessel MI | 0% (0) | 0% (0) | 4.1% (2) | 0% (0) |
| – Ischemia driven TVR/TLR | 7.7% (1) | 7.7% (1) | 2.0% (1) | 0% (0) |
| Scaffold thrombosis | 0% (0) | 0% (0) | 0% (0) | 0% (0) |

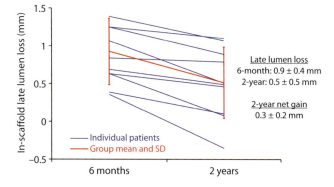

Late lumen loss
6-month: 0.9 ± 0.4 mm
2-year: 0.5 ± 0.5 mm

2-year net gain
0.3 ± 0.2 mm

Figure 6.12.9 Angiographic late loss analysis at 2 years in the MEND-I trial including the FORTITUDE (Bare) Amaranth's BRS.

The MEND study was performed to assess the biomechanical features and polymer biocompatibility of the FORTITUDE BRS (150 μm) in the absence of antiproliferative drugs in 13 patients. All patients have been followed up to 2 years with angiography and OCT. At this time point, only one restenosis has been reported and angiographic lumen gain has been observed in 10 patients (average of 54% of late gain). QCA images for three patients were not analyzable. Table 6.12.2 shows that freedom from target vessel failure was 92.3% at 2 years. IVUS and QCA analyses at 6 months were performed at an independent core laboratory. The angiographic follow-up at 6 months revealed an in-scaffold late loss of 0.92 mm ± 0.44 mm (mean ± standard deviation for 13 subjects), which was comparable to that seen with non-drug-eluting bare metal stents [8]. The analysis of IVUS imaging revealed successful scaffold deployment with no dissections. Two-year follow-up QCA data for the 10 subjects with analyzable angiographic imaging demonstrated late lumen gain in all patients, averaging 0.3 ± 0.2 mm compared to 6 months (Figure 6.12.9).

Two separate trials with virtually identical protocols evaluated the safety and efficacy of the 150 μm Sirolimus-eluting version of the FORTITUDE scaffold, and are combined for the purposes of this report. The MEND II (enrolling subjects in Colombia, South America) and the RENASCENT (enrolling subjects in Italy) studies evaluated a total of 63 patients who underwent elective PCI and met the same clinical and angiographic criteria defined for the MEND study. High rates of clinical device and procedural success were achieved based on improved deliverability and visibility compared to currently available BRS (see Table 6.12.3). Freedom from target vessel failure was 93.9% at 9 months for the first 49 patients analyzed. This included two periprocedural myocardial infarctions in patients with elevated cardiac enzymes postprocedure following the successful treatment of dissections with a DES, and one ischemia driven target lesion revascularization at 9 months in a patient with a scaffold that had been

Table 6.12.3 Efficacy endpoints for all clinical studies of Amaranth's BRS

| Effectiveness endpoints | MEND (150–200 μm, Bare) (n = 13) | MEND II + RENASCENT (150 μm, Sirolimus) (n = 63) | RENASCENT II (120 μm, Sirolimus) (n = 22) |
|---|---|---|---|
| Clinical device success<br>Defined as successful delivery and deployment of the AmM scaffold at the intended target lesion with final residual stenosis of <50% of the target lesion by QCA after the index procedure. | 84.6% (11/13) | 98.4% (62/63) | 100% (22/22) |
| Clinical procedure success<br>Defined as clinical device success with any adjunctive device without the occurrence of major adverse clinical events related to ischemia up to day of discharge. | 92.3% (12/13) | 98.4% (62/63) | 100% (22/22) |

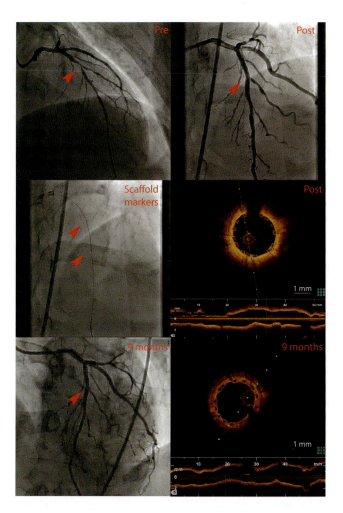

**Figure 6.12.10** Angiography and OCT imaging pre- and postimplantation and at 9 months follow-up in the MEND II Study (150 μm Sirolimus-Eluting FORTITUDE Scaffold).

greatly overexpanded at implantation. Nine-month clinical and imaging follow-up is still ongoing for the remaining patients, and will be completed at the end of June 2016. A representative sample of the angiographic and OCT imaging of a patient pre- and post-treatment and at the 9-month follow-up is shown in Figure 6.12.10. Efficacy will be assessed through the measure of in-scaffold late lumen loss at 9 months. Safety (incidence of target vessel failure) will be monitored throughout the study.

The RENASCENT II study is currently evaluating the safety and efficacy of the 120 μm sirolimus-eluting APTITUDE scaffold in clinical sites in Colombia and Italy, and enrollment is expected to be completed by the end of May 2016. Safety and efficacy of the device for the initially analyzed subjects returning for follow-up visits are included in Tables 6.12.2 and 6.12.3.

In summary, the early clinical experience with the Amaranth BRS demonstrated that the polymer is highly biocompatible and it is safe and effective in improving coronary luminal diameter in patients undergoing elective percutaneous coronary intervention. The ongoing studies of the sirolimus eluting Amaranth BRS will determine the long-term safety and efficacy of the technology in a more complex anatomical setting.

## REFERENCES

1. Ormiston JA, De Vroey F, Serruys PW, Webster MWI. Bioresorbable polymeric vascular scaffolds: A cautionary tale. *Circ Cardiovasc Interv.* 2011;4:535–538.
2. Stankovic G, Darremont O, Ferenc M, Hildick-Smith D, Louvard Y, Albiero R, Pan M et al. Percutaneous coronary intervention for bifurcation lesions: 2008 consensus document from the fourth meeting of the European Bifurcation Club. *EuroIntervention.* 2009;5:39–49.
3. Foin N, Mari JM, Davies JE, Di Mario C, Girard M. Imaging of coronary artery plaques using contrast-enhanced optical coherence tomography. *Eur Heart J Cardiovasc Imaging.* 2013;14:85.
4. Rzeszutko L, Depukat R, Dudek D. Biodegradable vascular scaffold ABSORB BVS™ – Scientific evidence and methods of implantation. *Postepy Kardiol Interwencyjnej (Advances in Interventional Cardiology).* 2013;9:22–30.
5. Džavík V, Colombo A. The absorb bioresorbable vascular scaffold in coronary bifurcations: Insights from bench testing. *JACC Cardiovasc Interv.* 2014;7:81–88.
6. Granada JF. Amaranth: Differentiating features and clinical update. Oral presentation. *Transcatheter Cardiovascular Therapeutics.* 2015.
7. CYPHER Sirolimus-eluting Stent PMA #P020026 presentation by Dennis Donohoe, MD, slide #9; http://www.fda.gov/ohrms/dockets/ac/02/slides/3905s1-01-sponsor.pdf.
8. Mauri L, Orav EJ, Kuntz RE. 2005 Late loss in lumen diameter and binary restenosis for drug-eluting stent comparison. *Circulation.* 111:3435–3442.

# The Mirage microfiber sirolimus eluting coronary scaffold

TEGUH SANTOSO, LIEW HOUNG BANG, RICARDO COSTA, DANIEL CHAMIÉ,
SOLOMON SU, ALEXANDER ABIZAID, YOSHINOBU ONUMA, AND PATRICK W.J.C. SERRUYS

## INTRODUCTION

Bioresorbable scaffolds (BRSs) may potentially overcome the many pitfalls related to drug eluting stents (DESs). Following CE mark approval, the rapid adoption of this novel treatment has led to its use in all comers with complex lesion morphology even without randomized comparison with the DESs. The only published randomized clinical study thus far is the ABSORB II. However, the current generation (ABBOTT Bioresorbable Vascular Scaffold, BVSs™) still has a lot of limitations. The Mirage Microfiber Sirolimus Eluting Coronary Scaffold (MMSES™, Manli Cardiology™) is designed to address the concerns of BVSs, such as improved vessel wall conformability, reduced strut protrusion into lumen, fracture resistance allowing rapid deployment until rated burst pressure, excellent deliverability, faster degradation time, ability to store at ambient room temperature <25°C, and no restriction on size availability. In contrast to the BVSs, the MMSES struts are round and thinner with less protrusion into the lumen. This streamlined geometry results in lesser activation of coagulation cascade and better promotion of endothelialization. This feature is interesting, especially in view of recent reports of somewhat higher BVSs thrombosis as compared to DESs.

The primary objective of this study was to evaluate the safety and effectiveness of the MMSES compared to the BVSs in the treatment of stenotic target lesions located in native coronary arteries, ranging from ≥2.27 mm to ≤4.0 mm in diameter. The secondary objectives of this study were to establish the long-term safety, effectiveness, and performance of the MMSES , assessed at multiple time points through assessment of clinical and/or angiographic, OCT, and IVUS data.

## METHODS

### Study design and population

We undertook a prospective, single blinded, randomized clinical investigation in two centers that enrolled 60 cases from Jakarta and Kota Kinabalu. Patients with coronary artery disease undergoing scaffold implantation who fulfill the eligibility criteria were randomly allocated in a 1:1 ratio to treatment with a MMSES and BVSs. A *run-in* cohort of five patients receiving the MMSES was conducted prior to start of trial randomization to allow investigators to learn the implant characteristics of the investigational device. These five patients were included in the randomized trial analysis but still were followed clinically and angiographically/OCT at the time points indicated further below. The primary endpoint of the MMSES Feasibility Clinical Investigation was the in-scaffold late lumen loss as assessed by QCA in subjects undergoing angiographic follow-up at 12 months postprocedure.

Eligibility criteria included the following: The subject was 18 years of age or older and was an acceptable candidate for PTCA, stenting, and emergent CABG. If the subject was female, she was either not of childbearing potential or had a negative pregnancy test done within 7 days prior to the index procedure and effective contraception had been used during participation in the clinical investigation. The subject or the subject's legal representative had provided written informed consent. Overlapping was allowed with a maximum of two scaffolds per lesion. Patients had up to two *de novo* lesions in a native coronary artery, located in different vessel segments only. Target lesion was less than 24 mm length. The target vessel reference diameter was

≥2.27 mm and ≤4.0 mm by visual estimate or online QCA. Target lesion was in a major artery or branch with a visually estimated stenosis of more than 50% and less than 100% with a TIMI flow of 1 or more. If two treatable lesions met the inclusion criteria, they were in separate major epicardial vessels (LAD with septal and diagonal branches, LCX with obtuse marginal and/or ramus intermedius branches, and RCA and any of its branches). Percutaneous interventions for lesions in a nontarget vessel were done ≥30 days prior to or 6 months after the index procedure.

Exclusion criteria included: (1) Known hypersensitivity or contraindication to aspirin, heparin, bivalirudin, ticlopidine and clopidogrel, poly (L-lactide), poly (DL-lactide), sirolimus, everolimus or sensitivity to contrast media which could not be adequately premedicated, (2) any contraindications as mentioned in the BVSs instructions for use, (3) in-stent restenosis, (4) lesion(s) located in the left main vessel, (5) lesion(s) involving a bifurcation with side branch vessel ≥2 mm in diameter and/or ostial lesion >40% stenoses by visual estimation or side branch requiring predilatation, (6) the patient was experiencing clinical symptoms consistent with an acute myocardial infarction (AMI), (7) concurrent medical condition with a life expectancy of less than 18 months, (8) currently participating in an investigational drug or another device study, (9) left ventricular ejection fraction (LVEF) <30%, (10) elective surgery was planned within the first 6 months after the procedure that required discontinuing either aspirin or clopidogrel, (11) renal insufficiency (e.g., serum creatinine level of more than 2.5 mg/dL, or patient on dialysis), (12) total occlusion (TIMI flow 0), prior to wire passing, (13) target lesions contained a visible thrombus, (14) another clinically significant lesion was located in the same epicardial vessel (including side branch) as the target lesion(s), (15) subject had received brachytherapy in any epicardial vessel (including side branches), moderate to severe calcifications, and tortuosity of target vessel.

The clinical endpoints were assessed at 30 days, 3, 6, 12 months, and 2, 3, 4, and 5 years. Angiographic, intravascular ultrasound (IVUS), and optical coherence tomographic endpoints were assessed at pre- and postscaffold implantation and at 6 and 12 months. The pilot cases only underwent angiographic and OCT investigations. All study patients underwent angiographic and OCT investigations, but IVUS was done in 15 randomized patients of each group. All major adverse events were adjudicated by an independent clinical event committee and a data safety monitoring board monitored patient safety. All angiographic, IVUS, and OCT data were analyzed by an independent core laboratory (Brazil).

## Study device

The MMSES is a coil-like structure with three longitudinal supporting monofilaments. It is made of mechanically strengthened polylactide (PLA) monofilament. The high mechanical strength of PLA monofilament results in the high radial strength of MMSES. Circular monofilaments in diameter of 125 and 150 μm are used for building

scaffolds with diameter less or equal to 3.0 mm and greater or equal to 3.5 mm, respectively. Circular geometry of PLA monofilament is also well preserved in MMSES. MMSES has a circular strut that is believed to accelerate the re-endothelialization process and minimize the risk for scaffold thrombosis [1]. PLA monofilament technology offers great flexibility in manufacturing bioresorbable scaffolds. MMSES was made into various sizes that were virtually the same as those in DESs. In this study, MMSES were used for lesions with reference diameters from 2.27 to 4.0 mm and length ≤48 mm. Scaffolds of 10 sizes, i.e., 2.5 × 18, 2.5 × 28, 2.75 × 18, 2.75 × 28, 3.0 × 18, 3.0 × 28, 3.5 × 18, 3.5 × 28, 4.0 × 18, and 4.0 × 28 mm, were supplied for this trial.

## Definitions

The primary endpoint of the trial was the in-scaffold late lumen loss as assessed by QCA at 12 months' postprocedure. The secondary endpoints were: (1) **Clinical:** Myocardial infarction (MI) (q-wave and non-q-wave), clinically driven target vessel revascularization (TVR), and cardiac death (major adverse cardiac event [MACE #1] or all death [MACE#2]), definite stent thrombosis according to the Academic Research Consortium (ARC) definitions, ischemia driven MACE, target vessel failure, ischemia driven target lesion and target vessel revascularization, and acute success (clinical device and clinical procedural success), (2) **Angiographic/OCT/IVUS endpoint**s: angiographic in-segment late loss, proximal late loss (proximal defined as within 5 mm of tissue proximal to scaffold placement), distal late loss (distal defined as within 5 mm of tissue distal to scaffold placement), in-scaffold and in-segment angiographic binary restenosis rate, in-scaffold percentage volume obstruction, acute and persisting incomplete apposition, late incomplete apposition, aneurysm, thrombus, and persisting dissection, all at index procedure and at 6 and 12 months, OCT strut coverage, OCT lumen symmetry, in-segment/proximal/distal late loss, in-scaffold and in-segment angiographic binary restenosis, in-scaffold percentage volume obstruction, incomplete apposition, aneurysm, thrombus, persisting dissection, all at 6 and 12 months, acute and late recoil postprocedure at 1, 3, 6, 12 months on angiography, postprocedure side branch patency on angiography, percentage scaffold obstruction on IVUS at 6 months, and scaffold strut apposition on IVUS.

## Study procedure, analysis and reporting

After signing informed consent, subjects were randomized in a blinded fashion in a 1:1 ratio of MMSES to BVSs. Randomized subjects who were not treated with the assigned study scaffold were followed for safety purposes through the 12 months' primary endpoint period and were included in the intent-to-treat analysis and underwent the same follow-up assessments. For all subjects, a baseline electrocardiogram, white blood cell count, and platelet count were obtained within 7 days of the procedure. A creatine kinase (CK) and creatine kinase myocardial-band (CK-MB) isoenzyme test were obtained within 72 hours of the procedure. The antiplatelet regimen for this study required that all patients were already on daily aspirin therapy at the time of recruitment or were given at least 300 mg of aspirin 6 hours before the procedure. Furthermore, the patients were pretreated with a 600 mg loading dose of clopidogrel, at least within 2 hours postprocedure.

After introducer sheath and catheter introduction, heparin or bivalirudin with or without a glycoprotein IIb/IIIa (GPIIb/IIIa) receptor blocker were administered and supplemented as needed to maintain anticoagulation throughout the procedure. Following intracoronary injection of nitroglycerin (institution standard dose), baseline angiography of the vessel was performed in at least two near-orthogonal views that showed the target lesion free of foreshortening or vessel overlap, using a 6 French or larger guiding catheter. The target lesion was always pretreated with standard percutaneous transluminal balloon angioplasty. In general, a predilatation ratio of 1:1 between the balloon and the reference vessel with a balloon shorter than the MMSES or BVSs was required. Pretreatment therapies other than PTCA (such as excimer laser, rotational atherectomy, etc.) were not permitted in this trial. Patients having additional vessels with lesions were treated by another DESs preferably a sirolimus eluting DESs or with a bare metal stent at the discretion of the operator. The scaffolding procedure was performed according to the Instructions for Use. Postdilation was performed in all cases. Overlapping was allowed with a maximum of two scaffolds to treat the lesion. However, in the case of a bailout procedure or geographical miss, additional study scaffolds of the same type as first implanted may be used. Bailout procedures, which required additional scaffold of the same type or DESs, were performed if a study subject experienced a major dissection or an occlusive complication manifested as decreased target vessel flow, chest pain, or ischemic ECG changes that did not respond to repeat balloon inflations, intracoronary vasodilators (nitroglycerin, verapamil, diltiazem, nitroprusside), or fibrinolytic agents. If more than one scaffold was required to avoid the potential for gap restenosis, the scaffolds were adequately overlapped (e.g., overlap by 1 to 3 mm). Serial coronary angiography, OCT, and IVUS obtained at baseline, final, and follow-up were obtained after intracoronary nitrate administration. All patients received dual antiplatelet therapy for a minimum of 6 months. Thereafter, aspirin was continued indefinitely at a dose of 81 mg per day.

Analysis was independently performed "off-line" at the core laboratory of the Cardiovascular Research Institute in São Paulo, Brazil. It consisted of: (1) qualitative analysis including lesion location, vessel morphology, lesion characteristics, blood flow, and angiographic complications; and (2) quantitative analysis including standard measures for analysis of drug eluting stents—QCA analysis was performed at: (a) "in-stent," within the stented segment; (b) "in-segment," spanning the stented segment plus the 5-mm proximal and distal peristent areas; and (c) individually in the 5-mm proximal and distal peristent areas. Angiographic analysis was performed with the latest version of a validated software: QAngio XA™ system version 7.3 from Medis, Leiden, the Netherlands.

Adverse events were reported according to the ISO 14155:2011 Clinical Investigation of Medical Devices For Human Subjects–Good Clinical Practice Guidelines, while recognizing and following other specific laws, regulations, directives, standards, and/or guidelines as appropriate and as required by the countries in which the study was conducted.

## Statistical analysis

Within an equivalence hypothesis framework, statistical calculations were done with a 5% two-tailed alpha and 80% power. This allowed the trial to demonstrate, with a 5% risk of type I error and 20% risk of type II error, that the difference between BVSs and MMSES was not greater than the chosen equivalence margin. Statistical computation indicated that enrollment of 60 patients (30 patients in each group with an allocation ratio of 1:1) would enable hypothesis testing for equivalence, assuming similar point estimate and SD in the two groups, with a ±0.17 mm equivalence margin for late lumen loss at QCA and a ±8.1 mm$^2$ late lumen loss at OCT after 6 months, and, respectively, ±0.17 mm and ±11.0 mm$^2$ at 12 months. The equivalence margin was comparable with the standard deviation reported in the reference trials.

## REFERENCE

1. Otsuka, F. et al. The importance of the endothelium in atherothrombosis and coronary stenting. *Nat. Rev. Cardiol.* 2012; doi:10.1038/nrcardio.2012.64.

# The Igaki–Tamai stent: The legacy of the work of Hideo Tamai

SOJI NISHIO, KUNIHIKO KOSUGA, EISHO KYO, TAKAFUMI TSUJI, MASAHARU OKADA, SHINSAKU TAKEDA, YASUTAKA INUZUKA, TATSUHIKO HATA, YUZO TAKEUCHI, JUNYA SEKI, AND SHIGERU IKEGUCHI

## THE IGAKI–TAMAI STENT

The objective for developing bioresorbable scaffolds (BRSs) devices has been to overcome the limitations of permanent metallic stents [1]. Metallic stents are effective for preventing acute occlusion and late restenosis following angioplasty. As these adverse events commonly occur within 1 year, the clinical need for scaffolding is reduced after this time. Considering the need for temporary scaffolding for atherosclerotic lesions, scaffolds made of a bioresorbable material have the potential to be preferable alternatives. The essential requirements for an ideal BRSs include those having sufficient radial force with minimum radial recoil, an appropriate bioresorption period for temporary scaffolding, antithrombogenic properties, and biocompatibility, which will collectively provide both short-term and long-term safety.

In the 1990s, the biocompatibility of polymers for BRSs, including poly-l-lactic acid (PLLA), was controversial. Zidar et al. [2] reported minimal inflammatory reaction and minimal neointimal hyperplasia with the use of PLLA stents in canine femoral arteries. On the other hand, Van der Giessen et al. [3] observed a marked inflammatory response after implantation of each of five different bioresorbable polymer stents (polyglycolic acid [PGA]/polylactic acid, polycaprolactone, polyhydroxybutyrate valerate, polyorthoester, and polyethyleneoxide/polybutylene terephthalate), in a porcine coronary artery model. Finally, in 1999, the issue of the biocompatibility of polymers was resolved by the development of the Igaki–Tamai stent (Kyoto Medical Planning Co, Ltd, Kyoto, Japan) (Figure 6.14.1) [4]. This was the first-in-human fully BRSs constructed of PLLA. Its development was the successful outcome of a continuous process of trial and error.

The history of the Igaki–Tamai stent goes back to 1990, when Dr. Keiji Igaki, an engineer, and Dr. Hideo Tamai [5], an interventional cardiologist who died on February 10, 2009, started to develop this technology. Initially, there were two major problems to overcome: the scaffold material and the design. At that time, the candidates for the scaffold material were PGA and PLLA, which were already being used clinically in orthopedics. PGA usually degrades in 6–12 months in human coronary arteries, whereas PLLA takes 24–36 months for bioresorption [6]. Considering that the requirement of temporary scaffolding for atheromatous lesions is no more than 1 year, PGA was initially regarded as the ideal material from the perspective of its bioresorption period. Although these bioresorption periods were not accurately known at the outset, Dr. Igaki and Dr. Tamai recognized that PGA degraded faster than PLLA. However, our preliminary unpublished data showed that severe inflammation occurred in porcine coronary arteries after implantation of the PGA stent. In general, a higher bioresorption (degradation) speed evokes a more severe inflammatory reaction [7]. Therefore, as PGA provokes greater inflammation than PLLA, we concluded that the latter was preferable for a BRSs, in spite of its longer bioresorption period.

The second problem was that of stent design. At first, it was thought that a PLLA scaffold was unlikely to produce a sufficient radial force with minimum radial recoil when deployed in atheromatous lesions. The initial design of the Igaki–Tamai stent was the knitted type (Figure 6.14.2), and a marked inflammatory response with neointimal hyperplasia was observed after its implantation in porcine coronary arteries. Additionally, this stent design could not exert a sufficiently high radial force. In order to acquire sufficient force, a high molecular weight PLLA (183 kDa) was adopted. Furthermore, the PLLA was stretched into a monofilament,

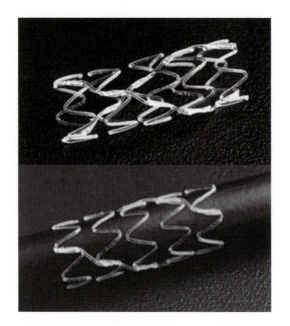

Figure 6.14.1 The Igaki–Tamai stent.

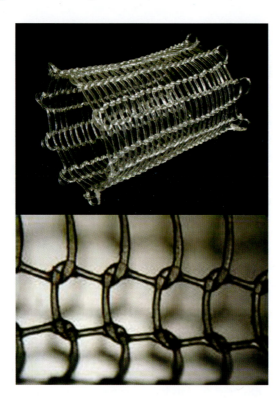

Figure 6.14.2 The initial design of the Igaki–Tamai stent (knitted type). A marked inflammatory response with neointimal hyperplasia was observed after implantation in porcine coronary arteries. This design could not achieve a sufficiently high radial force, and it had no self-expanding property.

which enabled it to have highly orientated reinforced properties. As oversizing the stent also achieved a greater radial force, the Igaki–Tamai stent was made by looping a PLLA monofilament around a tube of greater diameter. This stent also had self-expanding capability, which could minimize

the radial recoil of the scaffold. During the PLLA monofilament-making process, the monofilament acquired a temperature-dependent shape-memory property, such that a zigzag PLLA monofilament recovered its original linear shape when exposed to the glass-transition temperature. Our preliminary study showed that the PLLA stent expanded to its original size in 0.2 seconds when heated to 70°C, in 13 seconds at 50°C, and in 20 minutes at 37°C [4]. By means of this novel technology, the Igaki–Tamai stent produced a high radial force with minimal radial recoil. The radial force of the stent was 11.9%/0.006MPa, which was comparable with that of 15.4%/0.006MPa with a Radius stent (Boston Scientific, Natick, MA).

Finally, the Igaki–Tamai stent came to its fruition. Its properties have been described elsewhere [1,4,8,9]. Briefly, the stent was composed of a non–drug-eluting, high-molecular-weight PLLA monofilament (183 kDa) with a zigzag helical coil design (Figure 6.14.1). The stent strut thickness was 0.17 mm (0.007 inch); its diameter was 3.0, 3.5, and 4.0 mm; and its length was 12 mm. As the stent structure was not radiopaque, gold markers were implanted at each end. The stent was deployed with a balloon-expandable 5F covered sheath system through an 8F guiding catheter. The balloon inflation was performed using contrast medium heated to 80°C for 30 seconds inflation at 6–14 atm (the latest Igaki–Tamai stents can be implanted with normal contrast media through a 6F guiding catheter without a covered sheath system). The stent had a self-expanding property, and dilatation continued until equilibrium was attained between the circumferential elastic resistance of the artery wall and the dilating force of the PLLA stent.

## ANIMAL STUDY

Before performing clinical trials in humans, the safety and efficacy of the Igaki–Tamai stents were studied in porcine coronary arteries [8]. Fourteen PLLA stents were implanted in six normocholesterolaemic pigs, and nine Palmaz-Schatz half stents in nine normocholesterolaemic pigs. There were no significant differences between the groups in minimal lumen diameter (MLD) at 2 and 6 weeks. Histological analyses at 2, 6, and 16 weeks revealed no inflammation and minimal neointimal coverage on the PLLA stent struts. These results suggested that the biocompatibility, safety, and efficacy of the Igaki–Tamai stent were comparable to those of the bare metal stent (BMS) in porcine coronary arteries.

## INITIAL CLINICAL RESULTS WITH THE IGAKI–TAMAI STENT

Based on the animal study, the safety, feasibility, and efficacy of this stent in humans were evaluated in 15 patients, in whom 19 lesions were treated with 25 Igaki–Tamai stents [4]. In this first-in-human study, all stents were successfully implanted. The clinical results were encouraging with a target lesion revascularization (TLR) rate of 6.7% at 6 months.

Intravascular ultrasound (IVUS) revealed no significant stent recoil at one day, and continued stent expansion at follow-up, suggesting there is no reason for concern regarding significant scaffold collapse after PLLA scaffold implantation. Furthermore, no major adverse cardiac event (MACE), apart from one repeat angioplasty, was recorded within 6 months.

In a larger cohort of 50 patients, 63 lesions were treated electively with 84 Igaki–Tamai stents [9]. The average lesion length was 13.5 ± 5.7 mm, and the reference diameter was 2.95 ± 0.46 mm. Multiple stenting was performed in 18 lesions (29%), of which 25% were AHA/ACC classification type B1, 57% were type B2, and 18% were type C. As the lesions were relatively complicated (75% being type B2 or C), debulking before stenting was performed in 25% of the lesions (rotablator 3%, directional coronary atherectomy 22%). All stents were successfully implanted with good angiographic results. At one year, the TLR rate in this cohort was 16%, and the MACE free rate was 84.2%, results comparable with those obtained with conventional BMS. One case, subacute scaffold thrombosis was observed at day five, which resulted in Q-wave myocardial infarction (MI). This was probably due to discontinuation of antiplatelet therapy secondary to an acute hemorrhagic gastric ulcer. This was the first reported case of polymer scaffold thrombosis in humans, indicating that antiplatelet therapy is essential, as it also is with metallic stents.

## LONG-TERM OUTCOME OF THE IGAKI–TAMAI STENT

We have also reported long-term (>10 years) clinical outcomes with this BRSs [9]. During the total clinical follow-up period (121 ± 17 months), there were 1 cardiac death (sudden death at 57 months), 6 noncardiac deaths, and 4 MIs. Survival rates free from cardiac death, all cause death, and MACEs at 10 years were 98%, 87%, and 50%, respectively (Figure 6.14.3). The high survival rate free from cardiac death confirmed the long-term safety of this BRSs. Two definite scaffold thromboses were recorded: one subacute and one very late. The former was probably due to discontinuation of antiplatelet therapy, as previously mentioned. The latter was related to a sirolimus-eluting stent, which was implanted for a lesion proximal to an Igaki–Tamai stent. Therefore, this case of very late scaffold thrombosis was not related directly to the Igaki–Tamai stent. The cumulative rates of TLR (target vascular revascularization; TVR) were 16% (16%) at one year, 18% (22%) at five years, and 28% (38%) at 10 years. During the process of bioresorption (1 to 3 years), TLR and TVR almost reached plateaus, suggesting that the process of PLLA bioresorption did not correlate with an increased risk of clinical events. In serial quantitative analyses of 18 lesions without TLRs (Figure 6.14.4), the late loss was 0.69 ± 0.48 mm at 6 months, with improvement at 3 years (0.51 ± 0.33 mm). Quantitative IVUS analysis also showed that minimal lumen area (MLA) had a minimum value of 4.23 ± 1.82 mm² at 6 months, after which MLA improvement was observed (4.57 ± 1.70 mm² at 1 year,

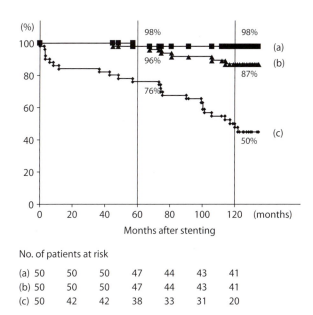

**Figure 6.14.3** Kaplan–Meier curves showing survival rates free from **(a)** cardiac death, **(b)** all cause death, and **(c)** major adverse cardiac events.

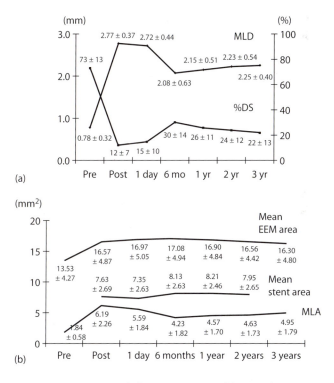

**Figure 6.14.4 (a)** Serial changes in minimal lumen diameter (MLD) and percentage diameter stenosis (%DS) of 18 lesions without target lesion revascularization (TLR). **(b)** Changes in cross-sectional areas of 18 lesions without TLR. EEM = external elastic membrane; MLA = minimal lumen area.

and 4.95 ± 1.79 mm² at 3 years). These angiographic and IVUS results could be explained by the phenomenon of late lumen enlargement, which was not seen in any vessel with metal stent implantation. The stent area and external elastic membrane area did not change over time, suggesting that stent recoil and vessel remodeling did not occur during bioresorption.

IVUS-derived quantitative echogenicity has been shown to be valuable for monitoring the degradation and bioresorption processes of PLLA scaffolds [10]. Serial IVUS echogenicity analyses in 13 lesions showed that a significant increase in hyperechogenicity of the scaffolded segment occurred after stent implantation, followed by a significant reduction beginning at 12 months, such that the value at 36 months was comparable to that recorded before stent implantation. This IVUS echogenicity analysis suggested that the Igaki–Tamai stent required 3 years for complete resorption. This finding suggests a different bioresorption period between the Igaki–Tamai stent and the ABSORB BVSs (Abbott Vascular, Santa Clara, CA). In the ABSORB trial, the expected period by IVUS echogenicity analysis was 2 years [11]. This difference can be explained by the differences in the manufacturing process of the PLLA. Of note, whereas the Igaki–Tamai stent consists of PLLA (183 KDa), the BVSs consists of PLLA (molecular weight is confidential) for the backbone and a copolymer of D- and L-lactic acid (PDLLA) for the coating, which includes an antiproliferative drug. PDLLA degrades faster than PLLA, as it has lower crystallinity.

Although IVUS is useful for acquiring such information, other procedures such as optical coherence tomography (OCT) may provide greater detail. Onuma and colleagues reported serial angiographic and OCT images of the Igaki–Tamai stent throughout 10 years of follow-up in one anecdotal case [12]. In this patient, coronary angiography revealed no restenosis, and there was complete resorption of the PLLA struts in OCT images. The endoluminal lining of the vessel was circular and smooth.

## HISTOLOGICAL ANALYSIS

Histological analysis of the PLLA scaffold struts in the long-term period is of great interest, and we had the opportunity to do this in two cases. In the first case, directional atherectomy was performed to excise a lesion that had been scaffolded 42 months previously (Figure 6.14.5) [9]. The specimen demonstrated intimal thickening composed of completed fibrosis with scant fibroblasts and few inflammatory cells. The remnants of polymeric struts were also identified. Around the remnants, there was almost no inflammatory cell infiltration or foreign body reaction, suggesting that PLLA is biocompatible with human coronary arteries. The space previously occupied by PLLA was stained by Alcian blue, suggesting it had been replaced by proteoglycan.

The second was an autopsy case, analyzed 12 years after the implantation of the Igaki–Tamai stent [13]. The histology showed that the spaces previously occupied by PLLA struts had disappeared, suggesting complete bioresorption of the PLLA (Figure 6.14.6g, j, and m). This was the first human histology case to show complete bioresorption of

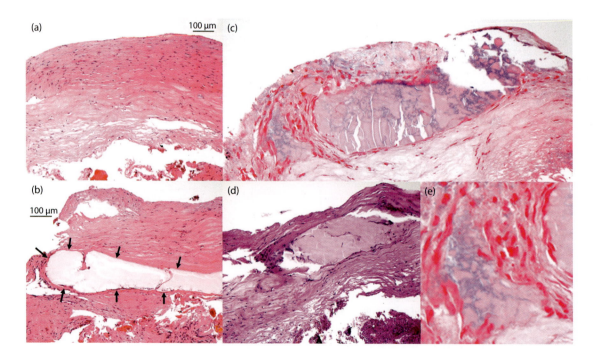

Figure 6.14.5 Histological features of specimens excised by directional atherectomy 42 months after implantation of an Igaki–Tamai stent. **(a)** Resected intima with fibrous thickening without inflammatory cell infiltration. The upper side is the luminal surface (hematoxylin and eosin stain). **(b)** Remnants of polymeric struts are observed in a deeper layer of thickened intima (arrows). Note the minimal inflammation around the remnants (hematoxylin and eosin stain). The space previously occupied by poly-*l*-lactic acid was stained by Alcian blue **(c)**, but not by periodic acid–Schiff **(d)**. **(e)** Magnified area of Alcian blue staining.

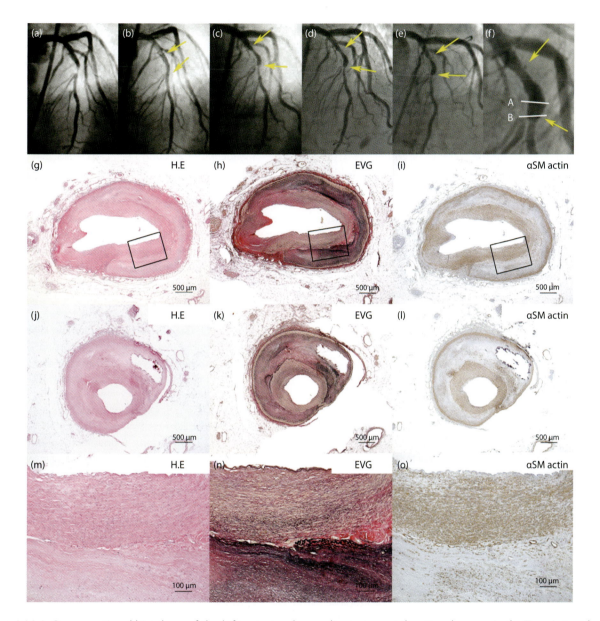

Figure 6.14.6 Cross-sectional histology of the left anterior descending artery at the site where an Igaki–Tamai stent had been implanted. The index lesion (a). One 4 ×12 mm Igaki–Tamai stent had been implanted (b). Follow-up angiography 6 months (c), 2 years (d), and 6 years (e) after implantation of the stent. Although restenosis was observed at the distal edge of the stent (c), late lumen enlargement was observed after 2 and 6 years of follow-up (d and e). The yellow arrows indicate the radiopaque gold markers at the edges of the stent. Panel g corresponds to the white line A in Panel f, and Panel j corresponds to the white line B in Panel f. The spaces previously occupied by PLLA had completely disappeared (g, j). Inflammatory cell infiltration, foreign body reaction, and thrombus were not observed. The stable neointimal layer sealed off old pre-existing atherosclerotic plaques. The phenomenon of so-called "neoatherosclerosis" was not observed. Magnified histology of the neointima (m, n, o). In the neointima, proliferation of connective tissue and smooth muscle cells are shown using Elastiva van Gieson (EVG) staining (h, k, n) and α-smooth muscle actin staining (i, l, o), respectively.

PLLA. Inflammatory cell infiltration, foreign body reaction, and thrombus formation were not observed. The neointima consisted of connective tissue (Figure 6.14.6h, k, and n) and smooth muscle cells (Figure 6.14.6i, l, and o). This stable neointimal layer sealed off old pre-existing atherosclerotic plaques. The phenomenon of so-called neoatherosclerosis [14] (i.e., neointimal atherosclerotic change after metallic stent implantation, which usually occurs beyond 5 years with BMS) was not observed. Although these histological descriptions were only anecdotal case reports, they provide encouragement that PLLA may have good biocompatibility over the long term in human coronary arteries.

## CONCLUSION

The pioneering Igaki–Tamai stent technology marks a milestone in the history of interventional cardiology. It has shown for the first time that polymers can be applied to coronary stents, whose safety, feasibility, and effectiveness have been demonstrated in both the short term and long term (>10 years).

Despite controversy and debate on the biocompatibility of PLLA in the 1990s, this technology has raised hope that polymers, especially PLLA, are safe and can be used as the material of BRSs. However, the biocompatibility of a polymer depends on its molecular weight, manufacturing process, scaffold design, and the presence or absence of drugs. Therefore, it is necessary for each new polymer scaffolding device to undergo evaluation for biocompatibility.

The thrombogenicity of polymers remains to be resolved. In this study [9], scaffold thrombosis occurred in two cases, and notably only one case was associated with the Igaki–Tamai stent. However, it is too soon to draw any conclusions regarding the thrombogenicity of PLLA without results from a larger cohort.

The Igaki–Tamai stent is the prototype of PLLA stents. With this non- drug-eluting stent, the MACE rate was comparable to conventional BMS. Currently, an Igaki–Tamai stent for peripheral artery diseases, sold under the trade name REMEDY™, is clinically available [15]. The possibility of scaffold polymers being used as vehicles for drug delivery in the coronary artery has also been discussed [16]. By polymerizing with another polymer, adding antiproliferative drugs, or making PLLA struts thinner with novel technologies, improved or modified PLLA scaffolds should soon be available as the main workhorse for the treatment of coronary artery disease.

# REFERENCES

1. Tamai H. Igaki-Tamai Stent. In: Serruys PW, MJB Kutryk, Eds. *Handbook of Coronary Stents*. 3rd ed. Martin Dunitz, London; 2000:297–303.

2. Zidar J, Lincoff A, Stack R. Biodegradable stents. In: Topol EJ, Ed. *Textbook of Interventional Cardiology*. 2nd ed. Philadelphia, PA: Saunders; 1994:787–802.

3. Van der Giessen WJ, Lincoff AM, Schwartz RS, van Beusekom HM, Serruys PW, Holmes DR Jr, Ellis SG et al. Marked inflammatory sequelae to implantation of biodegradable and nonbiodegradable polymers in porcine coronary arteries. *Circulation*. 1996; 94:1690–1697.

4. Tamai H, Igaki K, Kyo E, Kosuga K, Kawashima A, Matsui S, Komori H et al. Initial and 6-month results of biodegradable poly-*l*-lactic acid coronary stents in humans. *Circulation*. 2000; 102:399–404.

5. Katoh O, Suzuki T, Reifart N, Margolis J. Hideo Tamai memorial. *EuroIntervention*. 2009; 5:15–17.

6. Onuma Y, Serruys PW. Bioresorbable scaffold: The advent of a new era in percutaneous coronary and peripheral revascularization? *Circulation*. 2011; 123:779–797.

7. Jiang WW, Su SH, Eberhart RC, Tang L. Phagocyte responses to degradable polymers. *J Biomed Mater Res A*. 2007; 82:492–497.

8. Tamai H, Igaki K, Tsuji T, Kyo E, Kosuga K, Kawashima A, Matsui S et al. A biodegradable poly-*l*-lactic acid coronary stent in the porcine coronary artery. *J Interv Cardiol*. 1999; 12:443–450.

9. Nishio S, Kosuga K, Igaki K, Okada M, Kyo E, Tsuji T, Takeuchi E et al. Long-term (>10 years) clinical outcomes of first-in-human biodegradable poly-*l*-lactic acid coronary stents: Igaki-Tamai stents. *Circulation*. 2012; 125:2343–2353.

10. Bruining N, de Winter S, Roelandt JR, Regar E, Heller I, van Domburg RT, Hamers R et al. Monitoring in vivo absorption of a drug-eluting bioabsorbable stent with intravascular ultrasound-derived parameters: A feasibility study. *JACC Cardiovasc Interv*. 2010; 3:449–456.

11. Serruys PW, Ormiston JA, Onuma Y, Regar E, Gonzalo N, Garcia-Garcia HM, Nieman K et al. A bioabsorbable everolimus-eluting coronary stent system (ABSORB): 2-year outcomes and results from multiple imaging methods. *Lancet*. 2009; 373:897–910.

12. Onuma Y, Garg S, Okamura T, Ligthart J, van Geuns R, de Feyter, Serruys PW et al. Ten-year follow-up of the IGAKI-TAMAI stent: A posthumous tribute to the scientific work of Dr. Hideo Tamai. *EuroIntervention. Suppl* 2009; 5:F109–111.

13. Nishio S, Takeda S, Kosuga K, Okada M, Kyo E, Tsuji T, Takeuchi E et al. Decade of histological follow-up for a fully biodegradable poly-*l*-lactic acid coronary stent (Igaki-Tamai stent) in humans: Are bioresorbable scaffolds the answer? *Circulation*. 2014; 129:534–535.

14. Nakazawa G, Otsuka F, Nakano M, Vorpahl M, Yazdani SK, Ladich E, Kolodgie FD et al. The pathology of neoatherosclerosis in human coronary implants: Bare metal and drug-eluting stents. *J Am Coll Cardiol*. 2011; 57:1314–1322.

15. Werner M, Micari A, Cioppa A, Vadalà G, Schmidt A, Sievert H, Rubino P et al. Evaluation of the biodegradable peripheral Igaki-Tamai stent in the treatment of de novo lesions in the superficial femoral artery: The GAIA study. *JACC Cardiovasc Interv*. 2014; 7:305–312.

16. Tsuji T, Tamai H, Igaki K, Kyo E, Kosuga K, Hata T, Nakamura T et al. Biodegradable stents as a platform to drug loading. *Int J Cardiovasc Intervent*. 2003; 5:13–16.

# PART 7

# Clinical evidence in specific patient subsets: Personal perspective

# Left main interventions with BRSs

BERT EVERAERT, PIERA CAPRANZANO, CORRADO TAMBURINO, ASHOK SETH, AND ROBERT-JAN M. VAN GEUNS

## INTRODUCTION

Percutaneous coronary intervention (PCI) has become a reliable revascularization option to treat advanced coronary artery disease (CAD) [1]. Several recent trials suggest that PCI with metallic drug-eluting stents (DESs) is feasible and safe and has equivalent long-term outcomes compared to coronary artery bypass grafting (CABG) for the treatment of lesser complex LM stenosis [2,3].

However, these permanent implants continue to remain as a foreign body even after vascular healing following the PCI and this leads to rates of target vessel failure of more than 2% per year [4,5]. To eliminate this and other potential limitations of a permanent metallic implant, bioresorbable coronary stents or "scaffolds" (BRSs) have been developed.

Currently, the use of BRSs for the treatment of left main (LM) coronary artery stenosis is not properly studied and is therefore considered investigational. However, limited evidence from case reports supports the feasibility of BRS implantation in these patients and shows good angiographical and clinical results in the short term. In this chapter we will mainly review the indication and technical considerations of BRS implantation in LM disease and focus on scaffolding strategies for the LM bifurcation.

## INDICATIONS FOR LM REVASCULARIZATION

CABG is still considered the "gold standard" treatment for most patients with LM disease. However, several studies have indicated equally good clinical outcomes while comparing CABG to PCI in selected patient populations [3,5]. Therefore, the 2014 ESC/EACTS Guidelines on myocardial revascularization have upgraded the indication for PCI for LM revascularization in patients with stable CAD to a class I indication in patients with a low SYNTAX score (<22),
a class IIa indication for an intermediate SYNTAX score (23–32), and a class III indication for a high SYNTAX score (>32) [2].

When considering PCI for the treatment of LM CAD, besides the SYNTAX score, other lesion characteristics are predictive of a favorable clinical outcome, such as lesion location (ostial or shaft), isolated LM disease, LM in combination with single vessel disease, plaque distribution pattern favoring a single stent cross-over technique, and limited calcium burden [6]. Importantly, PCI with DES has to be selected as the revascularization strategy only in patients able to comply with dual antiplatelet therapy (DAPT) for several months.

## TECHNICAL CONSIDERATIONS FOR BRS IMPLANTATION IN LM DISEASE

Several technical considerations, pertaining to the current generation of BRS, preclude its broad use in LM PCI (Table 7.1.1).

First and most important is the limited overexpansion capability of the current generation of BRS, impairing adequate stent apposition. As with other stent platforms [7], BRS malapposition and/or incomplete lesion coverage could increase the risk of acute and chronic scaffold thrombosis and in-scaffold restenosis. The largest commercially available ABSORB™ BVS (Abbott Vascular, Santa Clara, CA) is 3.5 mm, which should not be expanded to beyond 4.0 mm as it risks device disruption; hence, vessels with a diameter greater than 4.0 mm (quantitatively measured by IVUS or OCT, and 3.8 mm for QCA) should not be treated because of the high risk of malapposition. The newer, but less extensively tested DESolve Scaffold System (Elixir, Sunnyvale, CA) has a larger expansion capability, up to 5.0 mm with some self-correction after initial acute recoil [8]. The first magnesium alloy based BRS (DREAMS 2G, Biotronik AG, Bulach, Switzerland)

Table 7.1.1 Current limitations of BRS in the setting of LM disease

| Limitations of using BRS in LM disease |
| --- |
| Restricted BRS expansion limit: ≤4.0 mm with BVS (≤4.1 with DREAMS and ≤5.0 mm with DESolve) |
| Lower radial strength off PLLA scaffolds compared to metallic stent platforms |
| Limited side-branch fenestrations capabilities |
| Optimal lesion preparation with extensive balloon dilatation required |

Source: Adapted from EuroIntervention 2015;11: Supplement V, Everaert B, Capranzano P, Tamburino C, Seth A, van Geuns R-J Bioresorbable vascular scaffolds in left main coronary artery disease, V135–V138, Copyright 2015, with permission from Europa Digital & Publishing.

has similar expansion capabilities as most metallic DES and has been tested up to 5.3 mm [9]. As LM diameters are often considerably larger than 4.0 mm, only a small proportion of patients qualify for BRS implantation. In a study using IVUS, Shand et al. [10] showed a mean maximal LM diameter of 5.7 mm (range 4.0–7.4 mm), indicating the requirement for postdilation beyond nominal diameter with current generation permanent BMSs and DESs. The DESolve and DREAMS 2G BRSs have been tested in noncomplex lesions showing results similar to the ABSORB BRS [11,12]. The DREAMS 2G scaffold has been recently commercialized as Magmaris™ in diameters from 2.5 to 3.5 mm and lengths of 14, 18, and 28 mm. Since its introduction some small series of complex patients have been reported but none are published yet. The DREAMS 2G scaffold received CE mark in June and is now tested in a small series of more real-world lesions (BIOSOLVE-III study) with either the 3.0 or 3.5 mm device and a maximum allowed expansion diameter of 3.8 mm. However, the left main coronary artery disease is still an exclusion criteria.

Second, to minimize the risk of BRS malapposition in the LM, correct scaffold sizing based on a reliable assessment of LM dimensions should always include invasive imaging modalities such as IVUS or OCT. These techniques have been proven to be superior to angiography in providing accurate estimation of LM diameter, lesion length, and the involvement of the LM bifurcation and its distal side branches. OCT is particularly suited to visualize BRS struts and their interaction with the vessel wall and can greatly optimize BRS implantation [13]. Before implantation, OCT is indicated to predetermine lesion characteristics, such as lesion length and the amount of calcification, to estimate the optimal scaffold size and length, and to identify the optimal proximal and distal landing zones. OCT after scaffold implantation can be invaluable to guide postdilatation of the scaffold with properly sized noncompliant balloons to optimize strut apposition, taking into account the expansion limits.

Third, the radial strength of all PLLA based scaffold designs is outperformed by cobalt-chromium or especially platinum-chromium stent platforms. LM PCI for ostial disease frequently suffers from acute stent recoil due to the fibroelastic properties of the aortic wall and the increased presence of calcium. The current designs of both ABSORB and DESolve have lower radial strength compared to the XIENCE Xpedition Cobalt chromium stent. DESolve has a little higher radial strength compared to ASBSORB but still less compared to current DES [8]. To attain sufficient radial strength, the strut thickness of the BRS has to be larger which affects the scaffold's crossing profile. However, with adequate predilatation and lesion preparation, this generally does not compromise scaffold deliverability, particularly in LM disease. While there is a concern that aggressive balloon dilatations within a highly calcified LM could potentially result in LM dissection with serious consequences, it must be stated that calcified lesions at non-LM sites have been regularly treated successfully with BRS after adequate lesion preparation by high pressure noncompliant balloon dilatation, cutting balloon dilatation or rotational atherectomy.

Fourth, PLLA-based scaffolds have to be expanded gradually by increasing the inflation pressure by 2 atmospheres (atm) every 5 seconds, and terminating by a long inflation of approximately 30 seconds. Thus, for a 3.5 mm BVS to be expanded to its expansion limit of 4.0 mm at 16 atm, in total approximately 65 s of occlusion of LM is needed. In the setting of LV dysfunction and/or if the right coronary artery is diseased, these prolonged inflation times could result in ischemic complications, severe hypotension, or life-threatening arrhythmias.

Another technical concern, although minor, may be the challenging ostial positioning with these non-radiopaque scaffolds. Like for all stents protrusion of struts into the aorta is necessary to cover the full ostium of the coronary artery with an increased risk of scaffold deformation due to guide catheter manipulation. As most scaffolds are hardly visual on fluoroscopy, this deformation might be more difficult to recognize compared to metallic DES. Also, the final behavior of the protruding struts during the resorption process is unknown and embolization of small particles not omitted.

## LM bifurcation lesions

Bifurcation lesions in appropriately selected patients are potentially good candidates for BRS treatment. However, as most of LM lesions involve the LM bifurcation (40–96% in different series) and 70–80% of LM disease patients present with multivessel disease [14], although theoretically sound, the LM bifurcation is less attractive for BRS treatment. Unprotected distal LM bifurcation PCI is always a challenging procedure and has worse long-term clinical outcome than the more favorable results obtained with ostial- or shaft-LM lesions, especially when a 2-stent approach is used [15]. In the SYNTAX study 63% of LM lesions involved the left main bifurcation and required treatment. Of these,

>90% had plaque extension into the left anterior descending (LAD) coronary artery and about three-fourths into the circumflex (LCx) territory.

At this moment, the data on BRS bifurcation techniques is still limited compared to metallic DES bifurcation techniques, although even for metal DES there is no good systematic data supporting one bifurcation technique over another for LM bifurcation stenting [16]. For use of a BRS in a coronary bifurcation, the European Bifurcation Club (EBC) proposed the strategy of provisional side branch cross-over scaffolding with a proximal optimization technique (POT) for proper apposition, side branch dilatation in case of TIMI flow <2 or symptoms of angina at low pressures (maximum 8 atm), and a second stent (DES or scaffold) as bailout with final POT (Table 7.1.2) [17]. Bench testing using bifurcation phantoms has been performed to assess the safety and efficacy of side branch dilatation through the BRS and main branch postdilatation techniques. Strut fractures were not observed at low inflation pressures, but high inflation pressures or larger side branch balloons frequently caused scaffold fractures and/or lumen compromise using the ABSORB BVS [18]. The DESolve scaffold has a higher safety threshold for side branch dilatation, comparable to that of the XIENCE Xpedition, and was tested up to 22 atm using a 3.0 mm NC balloon without observing evidence of scaffold fractures [8]. When a 2-scaffold strategy has to be used, a provisional T-stenting or TAP technique is recommended in the majority of cases. However, at least in a bifurcation phantom model, also other contemporary bifurcation techniques, such as the culotte, double-crush, or mini-crush performed well using the ABSORB BVS [19]. These techniques are generally not advocated for use with BRS in small vessel bifurcations, as these would result in two or more layers of scaffold struts resulting in a serious luminal reduction and a high chance of delayed vessel healing. However, in particular in the setting of an LM bifurcation with a main branch lumen of >3.5–4.0 mm, such a luminal reduction over a short coronary segment may well be tolerated (Figure 7.1.1). V-stenting may be carried out for LM bifurcation lesions of Medina 0,1,1 type without much deformation to the scaffolds (Figure 7.1.2). Importantly, at least in non-LM bifurcations, treating bifurcation lesions

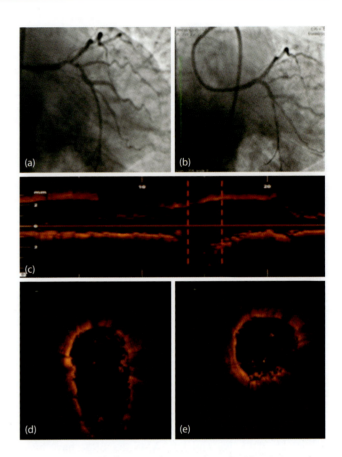

**Figure 7.1.1** LM bifucation lesion treated with mini-crush technique and final kissing balloon postdilatation. Distal LM lesion before **(a)** and after treatment with 2 BRS (LCx and LM-LAD), mini-crush and final kissing balloon postdilatation **(b)**. OCT of LM-LAD showing good stent apposition **(c)**. Red dotted lines: OCT images of LM bifurcation **(d)** and LM carina **(e)**. Three layers of BRS struts are visible at the carina. (Reprinted from *EuroIntervention* 2015;11:Supplement V, Everaert B, Capranzano P, Tamburino C, Seth A, van Geuns R-J Bioresorbable vascular scaffolds in left main coronary artery disease, V135–V138, Copyright 2015, with permission from Europa Digital & Publishing.)

**Table 7.1.2** Current EBC recommendations for BRS use in bifurcations

| Recommendations for using BRS in bifurcation lesions |
| --- |
| Use provisional approach with side branch (SB) crossover scaffolding |
| Proximal optimization technique (POT) with noncompliant (NC) balloon (maximum 0.5 mm above nominal scaffold diameter) is recommended |
| Side branch dilatation only when compromised |
| Second stent (DES or scaffold) in SB only for bailout |
| Final POT after SB dilatation/scaffolding |

with a double-scaffolding strategy tended to result in higher target lesion revascularization rates compared to single scaffolding of the MB and the use of DES for the SB [20]. Whether this also applies to LM bifurcation lesions is uncertain.

As the expansion capabilities of the ABSORB BVS are limited, simultaneous kissing balloon postdilatation is usually not recommended. A strategy of sequential POT, side branch postdilatation and final re-POT was proposed at the last EBC meeting and at least in bench testing this strategy proved to reduce the chance of scaffold strut fracture [21]. However, if a simultaneous kissing balloon dilatation would be performed, with the ABSORB BVS only low inflation pressures (safety threshold of 5 atm) are advised and preferably with the side-branch balloon protruding just outside the side branch, "snuggling" against the main branch balloon [22]. For POT, noncompliant

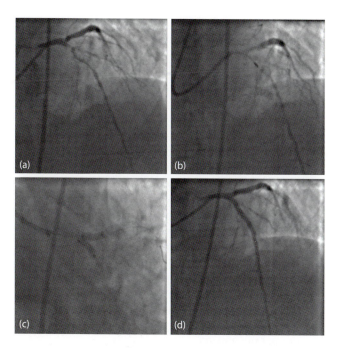

**Figure 7.1.2** LM bifurcation stenosis treated with V-stenting. LM bifurcation stenosis (Medina 0,1,1) and diffuse calcification of the proximal and mid LAD **(a)**. Rotational atherectomy of LAD **(b)**. V-stenting with a 3.5 × 18 mm BVS in both LAD and LCx **(c)**. Final result after implantation of 4 BRS (3 in the LAD, 1 in the LCx) **(d)**. (Reprinted from *EuroIntervention* 2015;11:Supplement V, Everaert B, Capranzano P, Tamburino C, Seth A, van Geuns R-J Bioresorbable vascular scaffolds in left main coronary artery disease, V135–V138, Copyright 2015, with permission from Europa Digital & Publishing.)

balloons with a diameter no greater than 0.5 mm above nominal scaffold diameter should be used.

Also, intracoronary imaging with IVUS or OCT should always be considered to determine optimal stent size and landing zones and is highly recommended to ensure adequate stent expansion and apposition in all LM bifurcation segments after the procedure.

## PATIENT CONSIDERATIONS IN LM DISEASE

Patients presenting with LM disease tend to be older than the average PCI patient population [2], leading to a higher bleeding risk and less preference for long-term DAPT. However, as a shorter DAPT duration for second generation DES was recently shown to be safe [23], DAPT for at least 12 months is still advocated for BRS because of the strut thickness and concerns about stent thrombosis [24], making this technology less appropriate for patients with an increased risk for bleeding complications.

### Case reports on BRS use in LM disease

Several authors have already reported on the successful use of ABSORB BVS in LM disease. However, most of these

cases are only a report of the initial treatment success and information on the long-term follow-up is generally lacking. Fernandez et al. described the case of a 56-year-old male patient with a history of CABG, who presented with an NSTEMI due to a severe lesion in the distal LM. The LAD was protected by a LIMA graft and was ostially occluded. The circumflex territory, however, was not protected. After predilatation, a 3.5 × 18 mm BVS was expanded to 3.94 mm at 14 atm with good final angiographic result and no events at 30-day follow-up [25]. A similar case was reported by Gargiulo et al.; however, this patient developed BVS failure at 13 months due to in-scaffold neoatherosclerosis [26]. Concerning the LM bifurcation, two successful PCI cases, using a bifurcation cross-over technique with stenting from LM toward the LAD and subsequent fenestration of the scaffold struts toward the circumflex artery, were published [27,28]. Additionally, Cortese et al. described nine patients with unprotected LM disease involving the bifurcation and a low SYNTAX score. A single-scaffold strategy was performed in all patients. Invasive imaging with IVUS showed four cases of scaffold underexpansion and one case of acute recoil. One patient developed recurrent angina 12 months after the index-PCI due to late scaffold recoil and underwent CABG [29]. Furthermore, V-stenting with two ABSORB BVS scaffolds for an LM bifurcation lesion was also described [30], but after 5 months the patient presented with in-scaffold restenosis treated by PCI, as reported by Miyazaki et al. [31]. Finally, in the GHOST-EU trial, 17 of the 1189 ABSORB BVS-treated patients (1.2%) received a scaffold for LM disease. One of these patients presented with a scaffold thrombosis at day 84. Unfortunately, no further description of the implantation technique or of the individual patient outcomes was reported for the remaining 16 patients [24].

## CONCLUSIONS

To summarize, currently the use of BRSs for the treatment of LM disease is generally not recommended and considered to be investigational with the present BRS platforms. However, in highly selected cases, the current BRS devices could still be applied with favorable results especially in young patients with noncalcific LM lesions of ≤4.0 mm diameter with ostial or shaft disease or distal LM disease involving the LAD alone where a single crossover scaffold strategy can be applied. More data on long-term safety and efficacy with newer scaffold designs in larger sizes to overcome the above limitations and concerns would be needed before BRS can be recommended for regular treatment of LM disease.

## REFERENCES

1. Deb S, Wijeysundera HC, Ko DT, Tsubota H, Hill S, Fremes SE. Coronary artery bypass graft surgery vs percutaneous interventions in coronary revascularization: A systematic review. *JAMA.* 2013;310(19):2086–95.

2. Authors/Task Force members, Windecker S, Kolh P, Alfonso F, Collet JP, Cremer J et al. 2014 ESC/EACTS Guidelines on myocardial revascularization: The Task Force on Myocardial Revascularization of the European Society of Cardiology (ESC) and the European Association for Cardio-Thoracic Surgery (EACTS) Developed with the special contribution of the European Association of Percutaneous Cardiovascular Interventions (EAPCI). *Eur Heart J*. 2014;35(37):2541–619.

3. Morice MC, Serruys PW, Kappetein AP, Feldman TE, Stahle E, Colombo A et al. Five-year outcomes in patients with left main disease treated with either percutaneous coronary intervention or coronary artery bypass grafting in the synergy between percutaneous coronary intervention with taxus and cardiac surgery trial. *Circulation*. 2014;129(23):2388–94.

4. Simsek C, Magro M, Boersma E, Onuma Y, Nauta ST, Gaspersz MP et al. The unrestricted use of sirolimus- and paclitaxel-eluting stents results in better clinical outcomes during 6-year follow-up than bare-metal stents: An analysis of the RESEARCH (Rapamycin-Eluting Stent Evaluated At Rotterdam Cardiology Hospital) and T-SEARCH (Taxus-Stent Evaluated At Rotterdam Cardiology Hospital) registries. *JACC Cardiovasc Interv*. 2010;3(10):1051–8.

5. Park SJ, Kim YH, Park DW, Yun SC, Ahn JM, Song HG et al. Randomized trial of stents versus bypass surgery for left main coronary artery disease. *N Engl J Med*. 2011;364(18):1718–27.

6. Park SJ, Park DW. Left main stenting: Is it a different animal? *EuroIntervention*. 2010;6 Suppl J:J112–7.

7. Roy P, Waksman R. Intravascular ultrasound guidance in drug-eluting stent deployment. *Minerva Cardioangiol*. 2008;56(1):67–77.

8. Ormiston JA, Webber B, Ubod B, Darremont O, Webster MW. An independent bench comparison of two bioresorbable drug-eluting coronary scaffolds (Absorb and DESolve) with a durable metallic drug-eluting stent (ML8/Xpedition). *EuroIntervention*. 2015;11(1):60–7.

9. Kitabata H, Waksman R, Warnack B. Bioresorbable metal scaffold for cardiovascular application: Current knowledge and future perspectives. *Cardiovasc Revasc Med*. 2014;15(2):109–16.

10. Shand JA, Sharma D, Hanratty C, McClelland A, Menown IB, Spence MS et al. A prospective intravascular ultrasound investigation of the necessity for and efficacy of postdilation beyond nominal diameter of 3 current generation DES platforms for the percutaneous treatment of the left main coronary artery. *Catheter Cardiovasc Interv*. 2014;84(3):351–8.

11. Abizaid A, Costa RA, Schofer J, Ormiston J, Maeng M, Witzenbichler B, Botelho RV et al. Serial multimodality imaging and 2-year clinical outcomes of the novel DESolve novolimus-eluting bioresorbable coronary scaffold system for the treatment of single de novo coronary lesions. *JACC Cardiovasc Interv*. 2016;9:565–74.

12. Haude M, Ince H, Abizaid A, Toelg R, Lemos PA, von Birgelen C et al. Safety and performance of the second-generation drug-eluting absorbable metal scaffold in patients with de-novo coronary artery lesions (BIOSOLVE-II): 6 month results of a prospective, multicentre, non-randomised, first-in-man trial. *Lancet*. 2016;387(10013):31–9.

13. Allahwala UK, Cockburn JA, Shaw E, Figtree GA, Hansen PS, Bhindi R. Clinical utility of optical coherence tomography (OCT) in the optimisation of Absorb bioresorbable vascular scaffold deployment during percutaneous coronary intervention. *EuroIntervention*. 2015;10(10):1154–9.

14. Taggart DP, Kaul S, Boden WE, Ferguson TB, Jr., Guyton RA, Mack MJ et al. Revascularization for unprotected left main stem coronary artery stenosis stenting or surgery. *J Am Coll Cardiol*. 2008;51(9):885–92.

15. Teirstein PS, Price MJ. Left main percutaneous coronary intervention. *J Am Coll Cardiol*. 2012;60(17):1605–13.

16. Chen SL, Zhang Y, Xu B, Ye F, Zhang J, Tian N et al. Five-year clinical follow-up of unprotected left main bifurcation lesion stenting: One-stent versus two-stent techniques versus double-kissing crush technique. *EuroIntervention*. 2012;8(7):803–14.

17. Lassen JF, Holm NR, Stankovic G, Lefevre T, Chieffo A, Hildick-Smith D et al. Percutaneous coronary intervention for coronary bifurcation disease: Consensus from the first 10 years of the European Bifurcation Club meetings. *EuroIntervention*. 2014;10(5):545–60.

18. Ormiston JA, Webber B, Ubod B, Webster MW, White J. Absorb everolimus-eluting bioresorbable scaffolds in coronary bifurcations: A bench study of deployment, side branch dilatation and post-dilatation strategies. *EuroIntervention*. 2015;10(10):1169–77.

19. Dzavik V, Colombo A. The absorb bioresorbable vascular scaffold in coronary bifurcations: Insights from bench testing. *JACC Cardiovasc Interv*. 2014;7(1):81–8.

20. Tanaka A, Latib A, Kawamoto H, Jabbour RJ, Mangieri A, Pagnesi M et al. Clinical outcomes following bifurcation double-stenting with bioresorbable scaffolds. *Catheter Cardiovasc Interv*. 2016 May 17. doi: 10.1002/ccd.26579. [Epub ahead of print]

21. Derimay F, Souteyrand G, Motreff P, Guerin P, Pilet P, Ohayon J et al. Sequential Proximal Optimizing Technique in Provisional Bifurcation Stenting With Everolimus-Eluting Bioresorbable Vascular Scaffold: Fractal Coronary Bifurcation Bench for Comparative Test Between Absorb and XIENCE Xpedition. *JACC Cardiovasc Interv*. 2016;9:1397–406.

22. Seth A, Sengottuvelu G, Ravisekar V. Salvage of side branch by provisional "TAP technique" using Absorb bioresorbable vascular scaffolds for bifurcation lesions: First case reports with technical considerations. *Catheter Cardiovasc Interv.* 2014;84(1):55–61.

23. Colombo A, Chieffo A, Frasheri A, Garbo R, Masotti-Centol M, Salvatella N et al. Second-generation drug-eluting stent implantation followed by 6- versus 12-month dual antiplatelet therapy: The SECURITY randomized clinical trial. *J Am Coll Cardiol.* 2014;64(20):2086–97.

24. Capodanno D, Gori T, Nef H, Latib A, Mehilli J, Lesiak M et al. Percutaneous coronary intervention with everolimus-eluting bioresorbable vascular scaffolds in routine clinical practice: Early and midterm outcomes from the European multicentre GHOST-EU registry. *EuroIntervention.* 2015;10(10):1144–53.

25. Fernandez D, Brugaletta S, Martin-Yuste V, Regueiro A, de Mingo A, Santos A et al. First experience of a bioresorbable vascular scaffold implantation in left main stenosis. *Int J Cardiol.* 2013;168(2):1566–8.

26. Gargiulo G, Longo G, Capodanno D, Francaviglia B, Capranzano P, Tamburino C. Cyphering the mechanism of late failure of bioresorbable vascular scaffolds in percutaneous coronary intervention of the left main coronary artery. *JACC Cardiovasc Interv.* 2015;8:e95–7.

27. Grundeken MJ, Kraak RP, de Bruin DM, Wykrzykowska JJ. Three-dimensional optical coherence tomography evaluation of a left main bifurcation lesion treated with ABSORB(R) bioresorbable vascular scaffold including fenestration and dilatation of the side branch. *Int J Cardiol.* 2013;168(3):e107–8.

28. Miyazaki T, Panoulas VF, Sato K, Naganuma T, Latib A, Colombo A. Bioresorbable vascular scaffolds for left main lesions; a novel strategy to overcome limitations. *Int J Cardiol.* 2014;175(1):e11–3.

29. Cortese B, Orrego PS, Sebik R, Sesana M, Pisano F, Zavalloni D et al. Biovascular scaffolding of distal left main trunk: Experience and follow up from the multicenter prospective RAI registry (Registro Italiano Absorb). *Int J Cardiol.* 2014;177(2):497–9.

30. Sato K, Latib A, Panoulas VF, Naganuma T, Miyazaki T, Colombo A. A case of true left main bifurcation treated with bioresorbable everolimus-eluting stent v-stenting. *JACC Cardiovasc Interv.* 2014;7(8):e103–4.

31. Miyazaki T, Panoulas VF, Sato K, Kawamoto H, Naganuma T, Latib A et al. In-scaffold restenosis in a previous left main bifurcation lesion treated with bioresorbable scaffold v-stenting. *JACC Cardiovasc Interv.* 2015;8(1 Pt A):e7–e10.

# Bioresorbable scaffolds in bifurcations

FILIPPO FIGINI, HIROYOSHI KAWAMOTO, AND AZEEM LATIB

## BACKGROUND

Bioresorbable scaffolds (BRSs) represent one of the most promising innovations in the field of coronary intervention in recent memory. In the first trials investigating their use, only simple lesions were included, and the presence of side branches (SB) ≥2 mm were an exclusion criterion [1–3]; therefore, at present BRS implantation in bifurcations is regarded as an off-label practice. On the other hand, the idea of avoiding a permanent metallic cage seems particularly attractive in the case of a bifurcation lesion [4], because:

- Bifurcations represent a risk factor for stent thrombosis (ST) [5]: A BRS, by "leaving nothing behind," might eliminate the risk of very late ST once the resorption process is completed.
- Normal bifurcation anatomy is expected to be restored, with normalization of shear stress.
- SB jailing could spontaneously resolve once the scaffold is degraded.
- The issue of multiple layers of struts associated with complex stenting techniques (e.g., crush or culotte) would be temporary.

Of note, the advantages would only become apparent after the process of resorption has been completed, which may take several years with current BRS. During the initial phase after the procedure, the increased strut thickness (currently around 150 μm)—approximately twice that of newer generation metallic drug eluting stents (DESs)—may indeed expose the patient to a higher risk of scaffold thrombosis.

Another important issue is that BRS have a larger crossing profile (around 1.4 mm) and reduced deliverability compared to DES, which may hinder their use in complex anatomical settings. Furthermore, BRS struts may be disrupted if exposed to mechanical stress, which often happens if they are dilated beyond their recommended expansion limits.

Currently, postdilatation of the ABSORB BRS (Abbott Vascular, Santa Clara, CA) is only allowed up to 0.5 mm beyond the nominal scaffold size [6]. In bifurcations, overdilatation of stent struts is often required, and considering the discrepancy in diameter between the proximal main branch (MB) and the daughter vessels, particularly during kissing balloon inflation (KBI), the proximal MB struts are exposed to overexpansion, which may result in disruption of the scaffold.

Besides their increased thickness, BRS struts are also wider than metallic DES (190 μm wide struts for 2.5 and 3.0 mm ABSORB, and 216 μm for the 3.5 mm ABSORB). This results in a higher coverage of the vessel wall [7], which may be unfavorable for small SBs. Small-size SB occlusion was indeed more frequent with ABSORB BRS in the ABSORB Extend Study compared to everolimus-eluting metallic stents in the SPIRIT trials (ABSORB BRS 6.0% vs. XIENCE DES 4.1%, $p = 0.09$); on the other hand, in the randomized ABSORB trials no significant difference in the rate of periprocedural myocardial infarction was observed between BRSs and DESs [8]. Several patterns of SB ostium compartmentalization by overhanging struts have been described [9]. Although this pattern is random, the larger the SB ostium, the greater the number of strut segments across it, with increasingly complex patterns, which in turn could have an impact on SB rewiring or induced flow disturbances.

Some reports have questioned the hypothesis that SB jailing may resolve totally after scaffold resorption. Indeed, tissue bridges or membranes grow over the jailing struts, thereby creating a "neo-plastic carina," which has been postulated to be derived from the complex interactions between the BRS struts, the vessel wall, and shear stress [9]. The structure persists as signal-rich structures after polymer resorption as viewed by OCT. Although the neo-carina and neo-intimal bridges are presumably better than a permanent metallic cage, they may have a negative impact on flow patterns at the bifurcation level [10].

Most of the currently available evidence, both from bench testing and clinical trials, is derived from the ABSORB

BRS platform. Presently, another BRS has CE mark approval, the DESolve (Elixir Medical Corp., Sunnyvale, CA) [11], and many new platforms are under development [12]. It must be mentioned that the individual properties of each device may have important advantages or drawbacks over its utilization in bifurcations, and therefore evidence obtained with one platform may not be applicable to the others.

## EVIDENCE FROM BENCH TESTING

According to data provided from the manufacturer, the cell perimeter of ABSORB BRS varies with scaffold size: The theoretical maximum diameter is 3 mm for a 3.0 mm scaffold and 3.6 mm for a 3.5 mm BRS. In an experimental bench model of bifurcation treatment with ABSORB BRS, SB dilatation with a 2.5 or 3.0 mm balloon did not cause any fractures up to a dilatation pressure of 10 atm [13]. Beyond this pressure (up to 14–16 atm), the risk of disruption of hoops or connectors increased, particularly when a 3.0 mm balloon was used. As with DES, SB dilatation effectively displaces struts away from the ostium and results in distortion of the MB stent. This distortion may be corrected by scaffold postdilatation or by kissing balloon inflation (KBI), especially with minimal overlap of the balloons ("mini-KBI") (Figure 7.2.1). Mini-KB I with two 3.0 mm balloons in a 3.0 mm BRS caused no damage of the scaffold up to an inflation pressure of 5 atm, while hoop fractures occurred with higher pressures. No fractures occurred when the main branch (MB) was postdilated after SB dilatation, or after proximal optimization technique (POT) with a 3.5 mm noncompliant balloon inflated to 14 atm in a 3.0 mm scaffold. Importantly, SB ostium size was maintained after MB postdilatation and mini-KBI.

In another bench model, the DESolve device could be dilated toward the SB with a 3.0 mm noncompliant balloon up to 22 atm with no fractures of the scaffold [7]. Moreover, no ruptures occurred when a 3.0 mm DESolve platform was exposed to mini-KBI with two 3.0 mm balloons inflated to 20 atm, and the proximal part of the main branch scaffold could be overexpanded up to 5 mm at 20 atm without damage. In the same study, while the recoil after 1 minute was similar both for ABSORB and DESolve BRS, the latter tended to resume its original diameter after 1 hour. Whether

this "self-correction" phenomenon will translate into an *in vivo* clinical benefit remains to be determined.

Although most bifurcations can be treated with a single stent on the MB, in many cases the SB needs to be stented also either as intention-to-treat or as a bailout after provisional stenting. Data from bench testing showed that T-stenting, crush and culotte techniques are feasible also with BRS [14]. A potential limitation of this approach is represented again by the thick struts of the currently available devices: in the case of the crush technique, the triple plastic layers will approach a thickness of 0.5 mm. It is currently not known how such struts will resorb or how the underlying vessel will heal: Complex stenting therefore appears technically feasible, but must be carefully evaluated. An important insight from bench testing is that BRS fractures are a real concern when treating bifurcations: this phenomenon is not apparent at angiography; intracoronary imaging modalities are therefore strongly recommended in this situation. In particular, optical coherence tomography (OCT) may be preferred over intravascular ultrasound (IVUS) because of higher resolution and the ability to identify struts more precisely.

## EVIDENCE FROM CLINICAL TRIALS

OCT follow-up of ABSORB Cohort A [15] demonstrated that the most proximal struts over the SB ostium were incorporated into the vessel wall, while the most distal were covered by the formation of tissue bridges (Figure 7.2.2). However, as mentioned before, lesions with significant SB (>2 mm) were specifically excluded, similarly to the ABSORB Cohort B, ABSORB II, and ABSORB EXTEND trials.

Despite the lack of data from pivotal trials, experienced operators have started to use BRS in more complex lesions including bifurcations. Capranzano et al. analyzed 46 coronary artery bifurcations treated with the ABSORB BRS in a single center; roughly half of the lesions were true bifurcations. A provisional approach was adopted in 78% of cases, while in 22% a complex, double BRS strategy was performed (mainly with a mini-crush technique). At 6-months follow up, no adverse events occurred, apart from one case of target lesion revascularization [11]. Another study reported clinical outcomes at 1 year following BRS implantation in bifurcation

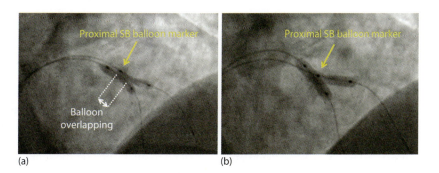

**Figure 7.2.1** T-KBI. **(a)** Coventional kissing balloon. **(b)** T-kissing balloon.

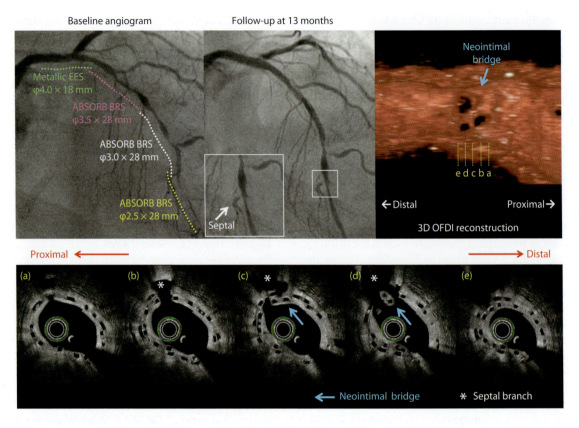

**Figure 7.2.2** Neointimal bridge. Baseline angiogram (top left panel) and follow-up at 13 months (top mid) of a diffusely diseased LAD treated with multiple BRSs. LAD-septal branch bifurcation is magnified in the white square: top right panel shows 3D optical frequency domain imaging (OFDI) reconstruction of the same segment, with Y-shaped neointimal bridge on the origin of the septal branch. Lower panels show cross-sectional OFDI images corresponding to letters **a–e** in the 3D reconstruction; note neointimal bridge in **(c)** and **(d)**.

lesions [16], 99 were treated with a provisional approach and 23 with a planned double stenting strategy. The rate of target lesion revascularization (TLR) was numerically higher in the complex technique group (11.2% vs. 5.5%, $p = 0.49$); however, the limited number of lesions treated with double stenting (and the multiple techniques used in this arm) limit interpretation of the data. In the GHOST-EU multicenter registry, which included 1731 ABSORB BRS implantations in 1189 patients [17], 27% of lesions were bifurcations; almost half of these were true bifurcations.

Left anterior descending artery bifurcations were the most commonly treated lesion. In over 80% of cases, a provisional approach was attempted, with crossover to stenting of the SB in approximately 5% of cases. Final KBI was performed in 18% and sequential SB-MB dilatation in 5%. The incidence of target lesion failure (TLF) in the overall cohort at 6-months follow-up was 4.4%. Univariate analysis demonstrated that bifurcation treatment was not associated with a significant increase in the risk of TLF (HR 1.37; 95% CI: 0.82–2.31, $p = 0.23$). On the other hand, it should be noted that some registries [17–19] and meta-analyses [20,21] have reported a higher risk of device thrombosis with BRS when compared to current generation DES. Future studies are required to further analyze whether this phenomenon is influenced by implantation technique.

## TECHNICAL TIPS AND TRICKS IN BIFURCATIONS STENTING WITH BRS

### Provisional stenting

As reported in the GHOST-EU registry, the provisional approach remains the default strategy for treating bifurcations and can be performed as previously described for metallic stents [22]. With DES, there is no significant concern about postdilatation with a balloon bigger than the nominal size of the stent; therefore, stent size is always based on the distal reference vessel diameter, and the proximal part of the stent is then optimized with adequate postdilatation (proximal optimization technique, POT). Because of the limited postdilatation capability of BRS, it is suggested by some that the scaffold should be selected according to proximal reference vessel diameter. On the other hand, there are other considerations as well:

- The proximal MB diameter is usually within 0.5 mm of the distal MB, thus allowing the performance of a POT without the risk of overdilatation and disruption.
- The scaffold is mounted on compliant balloons which tend to dilate more at the shoulders: there is therefore a concern about the risk of distal edge dissections when the sizing is based on the proximal MB.

- If the scaffold diameter is selected according to the proximal reference vessel diameter, the footprint at the distal MB and SB would be larger.

Therefore, we prefer to select the BRS size based on the distal MB unless there is significant tapering of the vessel and the difference between the proximal and distal MB is >0.5 mm. Moreover, as reported above, bench test data show that the DESolve platform can be safely overdilated well beyond the 0.5 mm limit, making this device an attractive option when there is a significant mismatch between the proximal and distal MB diameter [15]. However, it must be recognized that any data derived from bench tests should be validated *in vivo* before being applied in clinical practice.

SB wires can be jailed as normal and removed without difficulty. Similar to metallic stents, the MB BRS should be recrossed at the most distal part of bifurcation to ensure optimal scaffolding at the SB ostium [14]. Residual SB stenosis after MB stenting can be treated with SB balloon dilatation, followed by MB postdilatation or low-pressure KBI to correct for MB scaffold distortion. As discussed above, limited data are available regarding the necessity of SB dilatation, considering the eventual resorption of jailing struts on one hand and the formation of a neo-carina on the other. Some groups suggest that theoretically dilatation of large SBs can be performed routinely in order to prevent the future formation of neo-intimal bridges.

## Kissing balloon inflation

The majority of bifurcations in the GHOST-EU registry were treated with a simple strategy of MB stenting without any treatment of the SB. However, in selected cases of a suboptimal result at the SB due to plaque or carina shift, KBI was performed. Significant overlapping of the kissing balloons in the MB scaffold should be avoided as it can result in scaffold disruption: therefore, we recommend minimizing the protrusion of the SB balloon into the MB, so that the two balloons should snuggle against each other (called "T-KBI," "mini-KBI," or snuggling/hugging balloons). Ormiston et al. have shown that, when performing T-KBI, 5 atm is a safe threshold for two 3.0 mm noncompliant balloons in a 3.0 mm ABSORB BRS [13].

While KBI inflation is considered mandatory in double stenting with DES, in patients of the GHOST-EU registry treated with complex techniques it was performed in only half of the cases. Some operators, in order to avoid scaffold disruption and excessive elliptical expansion, perform sequential SB and MB dilatation instead of KBI.

## Crossover from provisional to double stenting

The "T and small protrusion" (TAP) technique is the simplest and most predictable way to cross over from single to double stenting [23,24], and has become our default strategy

in bifurcation stenting with a BRS when the result on the SB after dilatation or KBI is not satisfactory (Figure 7.2.3). The TAP technique is easy to perform and results in complete coverage of the ostium without excessive overlapping struts. We have successfully performed TAP stenting with another BRS in some cases with large SBs and favorable anatomy. However, due to the large profile and strut thickness of currently available scaffolds, it is not uncommon to fail to deliver it across the MB BRS struts. Furthermore, the protrusion of thick struts into the MB might result in aggressive neointimal hyperplasia in the MB [10]: therefore, we have performed the TAP technique more commonly with a conventional metallic DES in the SB.

## Elective double stenting techniques

T-stenting techniques are the first choice for planned double stenting with two BRS if possible, while the culotte and crush approaches should be avoided to prevent excessive overlapping of the thick struts and structural deformation of the scaffold [14]. However, T-stenting requires precise SB scaffold placement and a favorable bifurcation angle, close to 90°. In shallow bifurcations, protrusion of the BRS into the MB at the carina level is unavoidable and can result in an inadvertent crushing of the SB scaffold and major scaffold fractures (Figure 7.2.4) [25]. In these cases, an elective TAP can be performed but we prefer to avoid elective double BRS stenting. We use a "hybrid" approach with a DES on the SB and a BRS on the MB [26]. A hybrid mini-crush technique is particularly useful when the bifurcation angle is narrow: a DES is placed at the SB ostium and then crushed. KBI can then be performed and after the MB BRS is implanted, a further second KBI is optional (Figure 7.2.5).

## Scaffold optimization and antithrombotic therapy

The increased strut thickness of BRS carries a concern for a higher risk of thrombosis; therefore, obtaining optimal expansion and apposition is even more important than with metallic DES, particularly in the setting of bifurcations. Optimal lesion preparation, stepwise inflation, and routine high-pressure postdilatation with a noncompliant balloon are mandatory. We also strongly recommend that intravascular imaging be utilized to guide BRS optimization, evaluate malapposition and underexpansion, and identify any protruding ruptured struts.

New adenosine diphosphate P2Y12 receptor antagonists, such as prasugrel and ticagrelor, were only given to a limited number of patients in the GHOST-EU population (26.2%) and the bifurcation subgroup (19%). Although prasugrel and ticagrelor are currently approved for use in patients with acute coronary syndromes, it has become our routine practice to recommend these more potent P2Y12 receptor antagonists in patients with stable coronary artery disease undergoing PCI with BRS of bifurcation lesions,

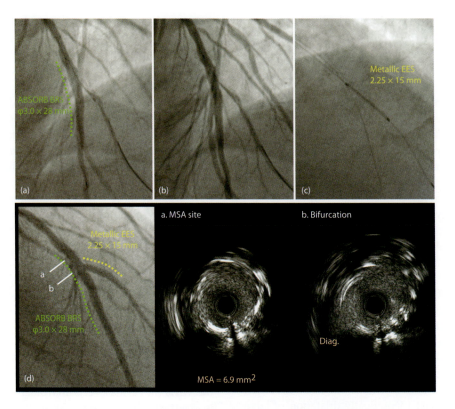

**Figure 7.2.3** Hybrid TAP. **(a)** After MB stenting. **(b)** After SB ballooning. **(c)** SB stenting. **(d)** Final (after final KBI).

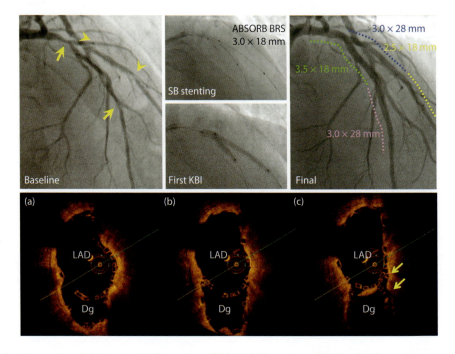

**Figure 7.2.4** Elective T-stenting. **(a)** Proximal bifurcation. **(b)** Mid-bifurcation. **(c)** Distal bifurcation.

particularly if they have undergone complex procedures and are not at high risk of bleeding. Usually, after a course of 1–3 months of prasugrel or ticagrelor treatment, the patient can be switched on clopidogrel ("de-escalation strategy"). However, no data are currently available to support this approach.

## BRSs IN LEFT MAIN LESIONS

Currently available BRSs have a maximum diameter of 3.5 mm and (at least in the case of the ABSORB BRS) can be dilated only up to 4 mm. This feature is a limitation in the treatment of the left main (LM) coronary artery, as LM

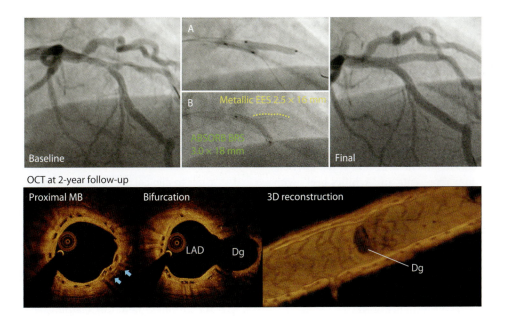

**Figure 7.2.5** Hybrid mini-crush.

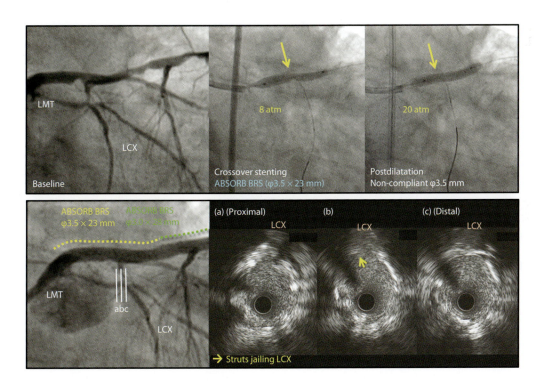

**Figure 7.2.6** LMT single crossover.

diameter often exceeds 4 mm. As a consequence, limited data are available regarding use of BRSs in LM disease. However, we do not consider this a contraindication to BRS use, provided careful baseline assessment by intravascular imaging is performed. As discussed above, other platforms may be postdilated more liberally on bench testing compared to ABSORB BRS [7], but clinical data are lacking.

When considering BRSs in LM, for scaffold sizing we suggest using the maximal lumen diameter at the proximal landing instead of the "media-to-media" measure: this enables adequate scaffold apposition [27]. Regarding the technical aspects of distal LM bifurcation treatment, the same considerations reported above hold true in this situation, with a provisional strategy preferred over complex techniques.

LM bifurcation lesions best suited for BRS implantation include isolated ostial left anterior descending artery lesions (Medina 0,1,0) or lesions not involving the left circumflex (LCx) ostium (Medina 1,0,0 or 1,1,0): all of these situations can be approached with a single stent from distal LM to LAD (Figure 7.2.6). In contrast, we actively discourage single stent crossover from LM to LCx, due to an unfavorable branch angulation and hinge motion, which may result in increased risk of restenosis [28]. When the LCx has a large diameter and requires treatment, treatment with BRS is not advised. Indeed, the LCx ostium represents an "Achilles heel" with conventional DES. In our limited experience, BRS do not show any advantage when compared to conventional DES. The high mechanical stress in this position during the cardiac cycle may instead lead to fracture of the BRS struts. Another technical aspect to be taken into account is the requirement for a long inflation time, which may not be tolerated in unprotected LM: in this case, an alternative is to perform sequential short inflations at progressively higher pressures.

## CONCLUSIONS

BRSs are increasingly being utilized in bifurcation lesions in real-world practice. Specific approaches and modified techniques should be considered taking into account the physical properties of current BRSs. The provisional approach remains the default strategy. However, when a 2-scaffold strategy is necessary, upfront T-stenting or TAP can be performed. The current BRSs are structurally different compared to conventional metallic DESs and thus careful attention should be paid when performing SB dilatation and KBI in order not to damage their structural integrity, which could increase the risk of events such as restenosis and thrombosis. Scaffold optimization with intravascular imaging and appropriate antithrombotic therapy might reduce the risk of early scaffold thrombosis, and therefore is almost mandatory. However, larger studies with longer follow-up are needed for BRS to be routinely recommended in the treatment of bifurcation lesions.

## REFERENCES

1. Abizaid A, Costa JR, Jr., Bartorelli AL, Whitbourn R, van Geuns RJ, Chevalier B et al. The ABSORB EXTEND study: Preliminary report of the twelve-month clinical outcomes in the first 512 patients enrolled. *EuroIntervention. Journal of EuroPCR in Collaboration with the Working Group on Interventional Cardiology of the European Society of Cardiology.* 2014.
2. Ormiston JA, Serruys PW, Regar E, Dudek D, Thuesen L, Webster MW et al. A bioabsorbable everolimus-eluting coronary stent system for patients with single de-novo coronary artery lesions (ABSORB): A prospective open-label trial. *Lancet.* 2008;371(9616):899–907.
3. Serruys PW, Onuma Y, Ormiston JA, de Bruyne B, Regar E, Dudek D et al. Evaluation of the second generation of a bioresorbable everolimus drug-eluting vascular scaffold for treatment of de novo coronary artery stenosis: Six-month clinical and imaging outcomes. *Circulation.* 2010;122(22):2301–12.
4. Latib A, Costopoulos C, Naganuma T, Colombo A. Which patients could benefit the most from bioresorbable vascular scaffold implant: From clinical trials to clinical practice. *Minerva Cardioangiol.* 2013;61(3):255–62.
5. Iakovou I, Schmidt T, Bonizzoni E, Ge L, Sangiorgi GM, Stankovic G et al. Incidence, predictors, and outcome of thrombosis after successful implantation of drug-eluting stents. *JAMA.* 2005;293(17):2126–30.
6. Ormiston JA, De Vroey F, Serruys PW, Webster MW. Bioresorbable polymeric vascular scaffolds: A cautionary tale. *Circ Cardiovasc Interv.* 2011;4(5):535–8.
7. Ormiston JA, Webber B, Ubod B, Darremont O, Webster MW. An independent bench comparison of two bioresorbable drug-eluting coronary scaffolds (Absorb and DESolve) with a durable metallic drug-eluting stent (ML8/Xpedition). *EuroIntervention. Journal of EuroPCR in Collaboration with the Working Group on Interventional Cardiology of the European Society of Cardiology.* 2015.
8. Muramatsu T, Onuma Y, Garcia-Garcia HM, Farooq V, Bourantas CV, Morel MA et al. Incidence and short-term clinical outcomes of small side branch occlusion after implantation of an everolimus-eluting bioresorbable vascular scaffold: An interim report of 435 patients in the ABSORB-EXTEND single-arm trial in comparison with an everolimus-eluting metallic stent in the SPIRIT first and II trials. *JACC Cardiovasc Interv.* 2013;6(3):247–57.
9. Okamura T, Onuma Y, Garcia-Garcia HM, Regar E, Wykrzykowska JJ, Koolen J et al. 3-Dimensional optical coherence tomography assessment of jailed side branches by bioresorbable vascular scaffolds: A proposal for classification. *JACC Cardiovasc Interv.* 2010;3(8):836–44.
10. Karanasos A, Li Y, Tu S, Wentzel JJ, Reiber JH, van Geuns RJ et al. Is it safe to implant bioresorbable scaffolds in ostial side-branch lesions? Impact of 'neo-carina' formation on main-branch flow pattern. Longitudinal clinical observations. *Atherosclerosis.* 2015;238(1):22–5.
11. Capranzano P, Gargiulo G, Capodanno D, Longo G, Tamburino C, Ohno Y et al. Treatment of coronary bifurcation lesions with bioresorbable vascular scaffolds. *Minerva Cardioangiol.* 2014;62(3):229–34.

12. Giacchi G, Ortega-Paz L, Brugaletta S, Ishida K, Sabate M. Bioresorbable vascular scaffolds technology: Current use and future developments. *Med Devices.* 2016;9:185–98.

13. Ormiston JA, Webber B, Ubod B, Webster MW, White J. Absorb everolimus-eluting bioresorbable scaffolds in coronary bifurcations: A bench study of deployment, side branch dilatation and post-dilatation strategies. *EuroIntervention. Journal of EuroPCR in Collaboration with the Working Group on Interventional Cardiology of the European Society of Cardiology.* 2015;10(11):1169–77.

14. Dzavik V, Colombo A. The absorb bioresorbable vascular scaffold in coronary bifurcations: Insights from bench testing. *JACC Cardiovasc Interv.* 2014;7(1):81–8.

15. Lefevre T, Darremont O, Albiero R. Provisional side branch stenting for the treatment of bifurcation lesions. *EuroIntervention. Journal of EuroPCR in Collaboration with the Working Group on Interventional Cardiology of the European Society of Cardiology.* 2010;6 Suppl J:J65–71.

16. Kawamoto H, Latib A, Ruparelia N, Miyazaki T, Sticchi A, Naganuma T et al. Clinical outcomes following bioresorbable scaffold implantation for bifurcation lesions: Overall outcomes and comparison between provisional and planned double stenting strategy. *Cathet Cardiovasc Interv. Official Journal of the Society for Cardiac Angiography & Interventions.* 2015;86(4):644–52.

17. Capodanno D, Gori T, Nef H, Latib A, Mehilli J, Lesiak M et al. Percutaneous coronary intervention with everolimus-eluting bioresorbable vascular scaffolds in routine clinical practice: Early and midterm outcomes from the European multicentre GHOST-EU registry. *EuroIntervention. Journal of EuroPCR in Collaboration with the Working Group on Interventional Cardiology of the European Society of Cardiology.* 2015;10(11):1144–53.

18. Jaguszewski M, Ghadri JR, Zipponi M, Bataiosu DR, Diekmann J, Geyer V et al. Feasibility of second-generation bioresorbable vascular scaffold implantation in complex anatomical and clinical scenarios. *Clin Res Cardiol. Official Journal of the German Cardiac Society.* 2015;104(2):124–35.

19. Kraak RP, Hassell ME, Grundeken MJ, Koch KT, Henriques JP, Piek JJ et al. Initial experience and clinical evaluation of the Absorb bioresorbable vascular scaffold (BVS) in real-world practice: The AMC Single Centre Real World PCI Registry. *EuroIntervention. Journal of EuroPCR in Collaboration with the Working Group on Interventional Cardiology of the European Society of Cardiology.* 2015;10(10):1160–8.

20. Cassese S, Byrne RA, Ndrepepa G, Kufner S, Wiebe J, Repp J et al. Everolimus-eluting bioresorbable vascular scaffolds versus everolimus-eluting metallic stents: A meta-analysis of randomised controlled trials. *Lancet.* 2016;387(10018):537–44.

21. Mukete BN, van der Heijden LC, Tandjung K, Baydoun H, Yadav K, Saleh QA et al. Safety and efficacy of everolimus-eluting bioresorbable vascular scaffolds versus durable polymer everolimus-eluting metallic stents assessed at 1-year follow-up: A systematic review and meta-analysis of studies. *Int J Cardiol.* 2016;221:1087–94.

22. Latib A, Colombo A. Bifurcation disease: What do we know, what should we do? *JACC Cardiovasc Interv.* 2008;1(3):218–26.

23. Burzotta F, Gwon HC, Hahn JY, Romagnoli E, Choi JH, Trani C et al. Modified T-stenting with intentional protrusion of the side-branch stent within the main vessel stent to ensure ostial coverage and facilitate final kissing balloon: The T-stenting and small protrusion technique (TAP-stenting). Report of bench testing and first clinical Italian-Korean two-centre experience. *Cathet Cardiovasc Interv. Official Journal of the Society for Cardiac Angiography & Interventions.* 2007;70(1):75–82.

24. Latib A, Moussa I, Sheiban I, Colombo A. When are two stents needed? Which technique is the best? How to perform? *EuroIntervention. Journal of EuroPCR in Collaboration with the Working Group on Interventional Cardiology of the European Society of Cardiology.* 2010;6 Suppl J:J81–7.

25. Costopoulos C, Naganuma T, Latib A, Colombo A. Optical coherence tomography of a bifurcation lesion treated with bioresorbable vascular scaffolds with the "mini-crush" technique. *JACC Cardiovasc Interv.* 2013;6(12):1326–7.

26. Wiebe J, Hamm C, Nef H. A true bifurcational stenosis treated with a bioresorbable vascular scaffold and a drug-eluting metallic stent: Degradable meets durable. *Cathet Cardiovasc Interv. Official Journal of the Society for Cardiac Angiography & Interventions.* 2015.

27. Miyazaki T, Panoulas VF, Sato K, Naganuma T, Latib A, Colombo A. Bioresorbable vascular scaffolds for left main lesions; a novel strategy to overcome limitations. *Int J Cardiol.* 2014;175(1):e11–3.

28. Naganuma T, Chieffo A, Basavarajaiah S, Takagi K, Costopoulos C, Latib A et al. Single-stent crossover technique from distal unprotected left main coronary artery to the left circumflex artery. *Cathet Cardiovasc Interv: Official Journal of the Society for Cardiac Angiography & Interventions.* 2013;82(5):757–64.

# BVSs in chronic total occlusions: Clinical evidence, tips, and tricks

ANTONIO SERRA

## INTRODUCTION

Coronary chronic total occlusions (CTOs) still remain one of the most challenging scenarios for percutaneous coronary intervention. Cumulative experience over years, development of new treatment strategies, and refinement of specific devices has led to an increasing complexity of CTO lesions treated by PCI. Although success rate has considerably increased, it continues to be low compared to non-CTO PCI lesions [1,2]. At present, successful recanalization of unselected and complex CTO lesions is around 80% in high-volume centers [2]. CTO lesions usually involve long fibrocalcific plaques often treated with a continuous long-segment stenting (>50 mm). Although drug-eluting stents (DESs) have significantly reduced major acute coronary events and second revascularizations, "full metal jacket" stenting of CTOs has major drawbacks. Permanent metallic contact with the arterial wall may cause vascular inflammation, restenosis, thrombosis, and neoatherosclerosis in the late or very late period. Besides, permanent metallic caging of the vessel indefinitely impairs the physiological vasomotor function of the vessel and precludes potential bypass grafting of the stented segment.

The everolimus-eluting bioarsorbable vascular scaffold (BVS) may be an attractive technology in such kind of lesions. The reabsortion of the device on 3+ years may provide theoretical advantages at long-term follow-up when compared with DESs. Liberating the vessel from its cage and restoring pulsatility, cyclic strain, physiological shear stress, and mechanotransduction permits vascular remodeling and late lumen enlargement and future surgical revascularization if needed [3].

## CLINICAL EVIDENCE

Currently there are few isolated case reports in the literature and 5 registries evaluating the safety and feasibility of the BVS in CTO lesions (Table 7.3.1).

All registries included true CTO lesions, defined as a complete obstruction of the vessel with thrombolisis in myocardial infarction (TIMI) flow grade 0 through the affected segment of ≥3 months estimated duration [1]. BVS implant was uniformly done following the recommendations of the manufacturer: accurate selection of scaffold diameter, slow progressive increase of dilatation pressure, overlapping by only 1–2 mm, and postdilatation with a shorter NC balloon at nominal pressure with a maximal increase of the balloon above scaffold size of 0.5 mm. Postdilatation was systematically performed in all patients in 4 registries [4–7], but guided by postimplantation OCT analysis in another one [8]. Procedural success was homogeneously defined as achievement of final in-scaffold residual stenosis of <30% with TIMI 3 grade flow, without in-hospital major clinical complications.

Patients demographic and clinical characteristics are shown in Table 7.3.1. Treated patients in those registries were relatively young, with a mean age around 60 years, and a majority of males. Clinical characteristics revealed a more comorbid population in the registry of La Manna et al. [6] with a higher proportion of diabetic patients, prior myocardial infarction (MI) and prior interventional procedures, although left ventricular ejection fraction was similar in all registries (Table 7.3.1). The most commonly treated vessel was right coronary artery in 3 registries and left anterior descending artery in the remaining two. Reference vessel diameter

Table 7.3.1 Patient demographic and clinical characteristics

| Series | Vaquerizo | Ojeda | Wiebe | La Manna | Goktekin |
|---|---|---|---|---|---|
| Patients/lesions | 33/35 | 42/46 | 23 | 32 | 70/76 |
| Age (years) | 60.7 ± 9.7 | 58 ± 9 | 60.4 ± 9.0 | 62.6 ± 8.1 | 56.9 ± 9.4 |
| Male (%) | 80 | 98 | 83 | 85 | 90 |
| Diabetes (%) | 20 | 33 | 35 | 44 | 21 |
| Hypertension (%) | 60 | 57 | 91 | 84 | 78 |
| Dyslipidemia (%) | 74 | 64 | 65 | 68 | 53 |
| Current smoker | 20 | 19 | NA | 25 | 17 |
| Prior MI (%) | 29 | 28 | NA | 44 | 17 |
| Prior PCI (%) | 37 | 36 | NA | 81 | NA |
| Multivessel disease | 55 | 67 | 82 | 50 | 68 |
| LVEF | <50%; 23% | 54 ± 8% | 54 ± 15% | 52 ± 9% | 52 ± 7% |

*Abbreviations:* LVEF = left ventricular ejection fraction; MI = myocardial infarction; PCI = percutaneous coronary intervention.

Table 7.3.2 Angiographic lesion characteristics

| Series | Vaquerizo | Ojeda | Wiebe | La Manna | Goktekin |
|---|---|---|---|---|---|
| Target vessel | | | | | |
| LAD (%) | 41 | 48 | 43 | 34 | 56 |
| LCx (%) | 11 | 24 | 9 | 28 | 24 |
| RCA (%) | 48 | 28 | 48 | 38 | 33 |
| J-CTO ≥ 2 (%) | 26 | 46 | Mean 1.7 ± 9.0 | 47 | NA |
| RVD (mm) | 2.99 ± 0.34 | 3.03 ± 0.4 | NA | 2.92 ± 0.34 | NA |
| Occlusion length (mm) | 19 ± 12 | NA | NA | 20 ± 13 | NA |
| Lesion length (mm) | 36 ± 16 | 35 ± 19 | NA | NA | NA |

*Abbreviations:* LAD = left anterior descending artery; LCx = left circumflex artery; RCA = right coronary artery; RVD = reference vessel diameter.

was around 3.0 mm in all. According to the Japanese-CTO score complexity, less than 50% of CTO lesions were classified as difficult or very difficult (J-CTO score ≥ 3), reflecting a certain degree of lesion selection (Table 7.3.2). In fact, selection of favorable anatomies for BVS after wire crossing was performed in 4 registries [4,5,7,8], mainly excluding severely calcified lesions and tortuous anatomies.

Antegrade strategy was the predominant route to open the chronically occluded vessel (74–85%). Use of intravascular ultrasound to guide intervention was heterogeneous among registries (Table 7.3.3). A systematic approach was only used in the registry by Vaquerizo, Serra et al. [8],

Table 7.3.3 Procedural characteristics

| Series | Vaquerizo | Ojeda | Wiebe | La Manna | Goktekin |
|---|---|---|---|---|---|
| Bilateral injection | 63 | 56 | 100 | 87 | 53 |
| Antegrade access | 86 | 74 | 96 | 94 | 100 |
| Retrograde | 14 | 26 | 4 | 6 | 5 |
| IVUS Pre-BVS (%) | 100 | 100 | 35 | 66 | NA |
| Predilatation (%) | 100 | 100 | 100 | 100 | 100 |
| Scoring/cutting balloons (%) | 71.4 | NA | NA | 25 | NA |
| Rotablation (%) | 8.6 | 0 | NA | 0 | NA |
| BVS/CTO (n) | 2.2 ± 0.9 | 2.6 ± 1.9 | 2.8 ± 1.0 | 2.8 ± 1.3 | 2.0 ± 1.0 |
| Stent length (mm) | 52.5 ± 22.9 | 43 ± 21 | 64.8 ± 24.2 | 54.9 ± 28.4 | 36.5 ± 19.5 |
| Postdilatation (%) | 63 (OCT guided) | 70 | 100 | >90 | 100 |
| OCT post-BVS (%) | 100 | 30 | 26 | 81 | NA |
| Procedural success (%) | 100 | 95.2 | 100 | 78.1 | 98.7 |

*Abbreviations:* BVS = bioresorbable vascular scaffold; IVUS = intravascular ultrasound; OCT = optical coherence tomography.

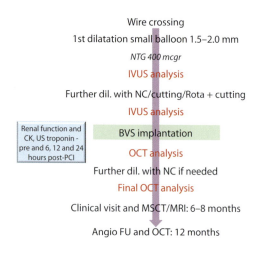

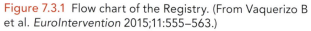

Wire crossing

1st dilatation small balloon 1.5–2.0 mm

*NTG 400 mcgr*

IVUS analysis

Further dil. with NC/cutting/Rota + cutting

IVUS analysis

Renal function and CK, US troponin - pre and 6, 12 and 24 hours post-PCI

BVS implantation

OCT analysis

Further dil. with NC if needed

Final OCT analysis

Clinical visit and MSCT/MRI: 6–8 months

Angio FU and OCT: 12 months

**Figure 7.3.1** Flow chart of the Registry. (From Vaquerizo B et al. *EuroIntervention* 2015;11:555–563.)

following a strict protocol (Figure 7.3.1). In this series, IVUS interrogation was performed after balloon dilatation and before scaffold implantation to analyze vessel size, morphological and anatomical characteristics of the lesion (fibrocalcific or calcified plaque not apparent angiographically, and areas of inadequate expansion). Predilatation was then optimized by either cutting balloon or NC balloons to minimize the risk of underexpansion of the scaffold in any area of the entire plaque. If the predilatation was optimal, BVS was selected according to QCA and IVUS measurements.

IVUS interrogation was also systematically done pre-BVS implant to analyze vessel size in the registry of Ojeda et al. [7], and in a nonpredefined strategy in a variable proportion of patients in the remaining 3 registries [5–7]. Accordingly, predilatation strategy was different among series. Rotablator was used in 8.6% of lesions and scoring/cutting ballons in 71% in the series of Vaquerizo et al. [8], and in 25% in the registry of La Manna et al. [6]. No information about tools for predilation, other than balloons, was reported in the remaining registries.

Total BVS length per lesion was above 50 mm in 3 registries [5,6,8], with a maximum length of 64.8 ± 24.2 mm in the series of Wiebe et al. [5], reflecting a frequent "full plastic jacket" of overlapped scaffolds in these kinds of lesions.

Postdilatation was guided by (OCT) per-protocol in the series of Vaquerizo et al. [8]. The entire treated segment was analyzed, and residual stenosis of more than 30% were postdilated with a shorter NC balloon at nominal pressure in 63% of the lesions. After postdilatation, no areas of underexpansion, malapposition, or stent fracture were found (Figure 7.3.2). Systematic postdilation was the rule in the rest of the registries [5–7].

Procedural success was very high, ranging from 95 to 100% in registries with selected lesions [7–10]. However, in the La Manna et al. [6] series, with a less restrictive lesion selection, BVS implantation was associated with a lower procedural success (78.1%) compared to the other registries. These results were mainly driven by suboptimal scaffold expansion (6 patients; 18.7%) and delivery failure of the

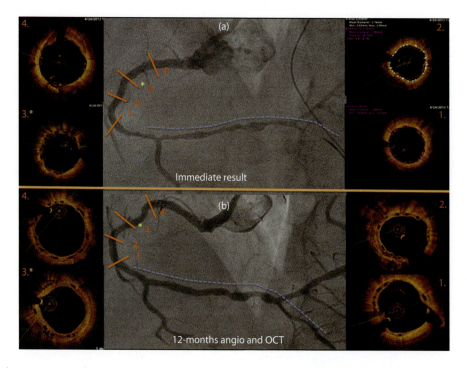

**Figure 7.3.2** Serial assessment of BVS by OCT. Coronary angiography and OCT (1 to 4) immediate postprocedure BVS implantation at the mid-right coronary artery. "*," Indicates position of the radiopaque markers at the level of the overlap. No incomplete apposed struts were detected. **(a)** Coronary angiography 12 months after BVS implantation; 1 to 4 OCT assessment 12 months after BVS implantation. All the struts were covered by neointima **(b)**.

BVS at target site (1 patient). Postprocedural QCA revealed a maximum residual stenosis > 30% within the treated segment in those 6 patients (vs. 3.7% in a historical DES control group), consistent with the quantitative OCT analysis, which revealed a similar incidence of BVS underexpansion (22%). Scaffold underexpansion was mainly related to the presence of heavily calcified plaque. Importantly, these outcomes were achieved despite systematic postdilatation (>90%).

Clinical events during hospitalization and MACE at follow-up are summarized in Table 7.3.4. The in-hospital course was uneventful in all series except in the registry of Ojeda et al. [4], where one non-Q MI occurred (2.3%).

Follow-up was heterogeneous among the registries. Vaquerizo et al. [8,9] performed a systematic clinical and MSCT follow-up at 6 months and clinical and angiographic follow-up with OCT examination at one year [9]. At complete 6-month follow-up, no major adverse events were observed. MSCT identified two cases of asymptomatic scaffold reocclusion that were left untreated. At 1 year, angiography confirmed the previous 2 silent scaffold occlusions detected by MSCT at 6 months. Notably, 1-year in-scaffold late loss was 0.28 ± 0.31 mm and in-stent restenosis was observed in 6%, similar to the ABSORB cohort B trial that reported a 1-year in-scaffold late loss of 0.27 ± 0.32 and binary restenosis of 5.6% [11]. No scaffold thrombosis or other major adverse cardiac events were reported beyond 6 months (MACE 0%). One-year OCT follow-up showed that 94% of struts were well apposed and covered (5% of uncovered struts and 1% of nonapposed struts), and only 0.6% of struts were nonapposed and uncovered (Figure 7.3.2). In the series of Ojeda et al. [4], follow-up by MSCT was obtained at 6 ± 1 month in all patients. One patient with asymptomatic scaffold reocclusion was detected. Coronary angiography was only performed in the presence of clinical recurrence. After 13 ± 5 months of follow-up, 2 reocclusions and a focal restenosis were identified, leading to 2 repeat revascularizations. Neither death nor MI at follow-up was documented (MACE 7.1%). In the series of Wiebe [5], angiographic follow-up was not regularly obtained. During a clinical follow-up of 108 (79.5–214.5) days one in-scaffold thrombosis was noted 4 days after the CTO procedure probably due to a lack of dual antiplatelet therapy. No further major adverse cardiac events occurred (MACE 4.3%). La Manna [6] did not report any follow-up result beyond hospitalization. In the series of Goktekin [7], systematic angiographic follow-up was not performed. Median clinical follow-up was 11 months. Two patients suffered from ischemia-driven TLR because of restenosis within the previously treated segment (MACE 4.3%).

## DISCUSSION, TIPS, AND TRICKS

Although registries on CTO-PCI with BVS involve a small number of patients, they show that bioresorbable scaffolds can be safely and effectively used in such challenging lesions in selected patients. Observed MACE rates are below 10% at 1 year follow-up and are comparable to results observed in the treatment of CTO with second generation metallic DES [12–14].

However, compared to metallic DES, BVS have some limitations. First, stent diameters are not available in all sizes, and restricted to 2.5, 3.0, and 3.5 mm. A technical limitation is the overexpansion capability of the ABSORB, restricted to 0.5 mm. Thus, a vessel with a diameter above 4.0 mm, not uncommon in CTOs of the RCA and proximal LAD, should not be targeted because of the greater risk of extensive malapposition [15].

Second, the crossing profile of BVS is 1.4 mm, 36% greater than the crossing profile of a second generation metallic DES like the XIENCE Prime (1.04 mm). In noncomplex lesions, as those treated in large randomized BVS trials, this compromise in trackability and steerability is not so important, but it becomes of outmost importance when treating CTO lesions where long and fibrocalcific or calcified plaques combined with some degree of tortuosity are not uncommon.

Severely calcified lesions and/or excessive tortuosity either proximal to or at the target lesion represents the worse scenario to ensure a secure delivery and adequate expansion of the scaffold. Patients included in CTO registries were highly selected in the majority of them. In the series of Vaquerizo et al. [8], 22% of eligible patients were rejected for treatment with BVS due to anatomical

Table 7.3.4 Clinical events and MACE

| Series | Vaquerizo, Serra | Ojeda | Wiebe | La Manna | Goktekin |
|---|---|---|---|---|---|
| In-hospital | | | | | |
| MACE | 0 | 1 non-Q MI | 0 | 0 | 0 |
| Follow-up | 1 year | 1 year | 108 days | NA | 11 months |
| Death | 0 | 0 | 0 | NA | 0 |
| MI | 0 | 0 | 0 | NA | 0 |
| TLR | 0 | 2 | 1 | NA | 2 |
| Total MACE (%) | 0 | 4.8 | 4.3 | NA | 4.2 |
| BVS thrombosis | 0 | 0 | 1 | 0 | 0 |

*Abbreviations:* MACE = major adverse coronary events; MI = myocardial infarction; TLR = target lesion revascularization.

considerations and technical success was achieved in 100%. However, in the registry of La Manna et al. [6], involving an all-comer population less restrictive to anatomic characteristics, technical success was lower (78.1%), mainly driven by suboptimal scaffold expansion and delivery failure of the BVS at target site. Scaffold underexpansion was related to the presence of heavily calcified plaque, despite systematic postdilatation.

To overcome difficulties in steerability or trackability of BVS, adequate size and shape of the guiding catheter should be selected for a maximum back-up support. 7Fr is the minimum size recommended for the treatment of CTO with BVS. Amplatz left (AL) 0.75 or AL1 for right coronary artery, Extrabackup (EBU) 3.5/4.0 for the left anterior descending and Amplatz left 2.0 or EBU 4.0 for the left circumflex artery is recommended for adequate back-up support. If other techniques are needed to deliver the scaffold, some advices should be taken into account. With anchoring technique, advancing a BVS into a 7Fr guiding catheter is not feasible due to its crossing profile. An alternative is to retrieve the anchoring balloon temporarily and advance it again, once after BVS is positioned distal to the anchor vessel. However, if an anchoring technique is planned, an 8Fr guiding catheter should be selected from the beginning. A guiding catheter extension (Guideliner, Vascular Solutions) could also be used to increase back-up support. A 6Fr Guideliner (7 Fr guiding catheter) is sufficient for 2.5 or 3.0 mm scaffolds, whereas a 7Fr Guideliner (8 Fr guiding catheter) is required for 3.5 mm scaffolds.

Given the anatomopathology of true CTO lesions, adequate plaque preparation before BVS expansion is of capital importance to ensure proper delivery and expansion of the scaffold. In the series of Vaquerizo et al. [8] IVUS examination was used in all patients to size the vessel and to analyze vessel size, and morphological and anatomical characteristics of the lesion. Predilatation was then more aggressively optimized by cutting the balloon in 71% of cases due to calcified lesions. As a result, scaffolds could be effectively delivered and deployed at the target site in all patients. OCT examination was systematically performed after BVS implantation. Postdilatation with NC balloons 0.5 mm larger than the BVS diameter was done in 63% of cases to correct areas of underexpansion or malapposition. This fact highlights the importance of performing postdilatation in all CTO cases regardless of the lesion anatomy and stent size to minimize underexpansion and malapposition when OCT is not systematically done after BVS implantation. More selective use of intracoronary imaging techniques was done in the other registries, with acceptable results. Systematic use of intracoronary imaging, both IVUS and OCT, translates into optimal immediate and mid-term results CTO-PCIs with BVS, and ideally, may represent the standard of care in such complex lesions. However, due to economical reasons in an era of budget restrictions and the results observed in the registries, selective use of intracoronary imaging seems a reasonable policy. Use of IVUS to

guide BVS implantation should be recommended in difficult or very difficult CTO cases (J-CTO ≥3) or the combination of long (>20 mm) and calcified lesions (moderately to severe calcification). The probability of delivery failure of the scaffold at the target site and, specially, scaffold underexpansion is much higher in these kinds of lesions. On the other hand, the use of OCT may be restricted to the following cases: suspected underexpansion or malapposition of the scaffold, suspected complication (proximal or distal dissection, thrombosis) or when the scaffold has been manipulated (dilatation of the struts in bifurcated lesions, overexpansion > 0.5 mm the size of the scaffold, postdilatation at very high pressures to treat underexpansion), to rule out stent fracture.

Percutaneous treatment of CTOs frequently ends up with a long stented segment (52.5 ± 22.9 mm in the registry of Vaquerizo et al. [8] and 64.8 ± 24.2 mm in the registry of Wiebe et al. [5]). The risks inherent to "full-metal jackets," including late restenosis and thrombosis, turn the concept of a "full plastic jacket" that will subsequently disappear into a very attractive alternative. A BVS-CTO strategy appears even more appealing in young patients, since reabsorption of scaffolds will likely reduce risks for late events and allow future surgical revascularization if needed. Due to the limitation in length of the BVS (maximum 28 mm), overlapping is needed in the vast majority of cases. In an experimental model, overlapping BVSs resulted in delayed strut coverage and higher neo-intimal hyperplasia, which can potentially lead to important clinical consequences [16]. According to this, the technique of BVS implantation should not focus only on proper scaffold expansion and apposition, but also on reducing scaffold overlap area. Enough time and attention should be allocated to overlap BVS scaffolds following the marker-to-marker technique [17] to minimize the number of stacked struts as much as possible. Enhanced stent visualization techniques (Stent Boost) may help to improve BVS edge marker identification, to increase the liability of the overlapping technique [18] (Figure 7.3.3).

Early studies reported a definite thrombosis rate of 0% in ABSORB cohort B [19]. The incidence of scaffold thrombosis in CTO registries are extremely low (only 1 acute scaffold thrombosis, following cessation of dual antiplatelet therapy), and notable in view of the higher rates of scaffold thrombosis (2.1% to 3.0%) reported in nonselected real-world lesions treated with BVSs [20,21], attributed in part to greater strut thickness and lesion/case complexity. Although these results may be purely fortuitous, they are, at least in part, explained by lesion preparation and BVS implantation technique.

Patient and anatomic CTO lesion selection, careful strategy preparation of the CTO case, adequate plaque preparation guided with imaging in most complex cases, correct sizing of the scaffold, exquisite overlapping technique, and systematic postdilatation with NC balloons are the key elements to anticipate good results of the percutaneous treatment of CTO lesions with BVSs at mid-term.

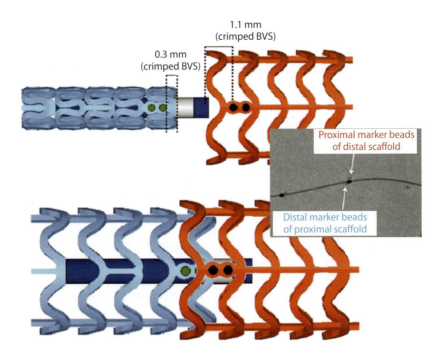

0.3 mm
(crimped BVS)

1.1 mm
(crimped BVS)

Proximal marker beads
of distal scaffold

Distal marker beads
of proximal scaffold

**Figure 7.3.3** Consideration for overlapped ABSORB implantation. To avoid a gap between scaffolds or too much overlap, the following strategy is suggested: (1) Advance the second scaffold system until the distal balloon marker lines up with the proximal marker beads of the implanted scaffold; (2) the markers of the second scaffold will be adjacent to the markers of the deployed scaffold (scaffold marker to scaffold marker); (3) the result will be about 1 mm of BVS overlap.

# REFERENCES

1. Di Mario C, Werner G, Sianos G, Galassi A, Büttner J, Dudek D, Chevalier B et al. European perspective in the recanalisation of chronic total occlusions (CTO): Consensus document from the EuroCTO Club. *EuroIntervention*. 2007;3:30–43.

2. Sianos G, Werner G, Galassi A, Papafaklis M, Escaned J, Hildick-Smith D, Christiansen E et al. Recanalisation of chronic total coronary occlusions: 2012 consensus document from the EuroCTO club. *EuroIntervention*. 2012;8:139–145.

3. Latib A, Costopoulos C, Naganuma T, Colombo A. Which patients could benefit the most from bioresorbable vascular scaffold implant: From clinical trials to clinical practice. *Minerva Cardioangiol*. 2013;61:255–262.

4. Ojeda S, Pan M, Romero M, Suarez de Lezo J, Mazuelos F, Segura J, Espejo S et al. Outcomes and computed tomography scan follow-up of bioresorbable vascular scaffold for the percutaneous treatment of chronic total coronary artery occlusion. *Am J Cardiol*. 2015;115:1487–1493.

5. Wiebe J, Liebetrau C, Dörr O, Most A, Weipert K, Rixe J, Bauer T et al. Feasibility of everolimus-eluting bioresorbable vascular scaffolds in patients with chronic total occlusion. *Int J Cardiol*. 2015;179:90–94.

6. La Manna A, Chisari A, Giacchi G, Capodanno D, Longo G, Di Silvestro M, Capranzano P et al. Everolimus-eluting bioresorbable vascular scaffolds versus second generation drug-eluting stents for percutaneous treatment of chronic total coronary occlusions: Technical and procedural outcomes from the GHOST-CTO registry. *Catheter Cardiovasc Interv*. 2016 Jan 12. doi: 10.1002/ccd.26397. [Epub ahead of print]

7. Goktekin O, Yamac AH, Latib A, Tastan A, Panoulas VF, Sato K, Erdogan E et al. Evaluation of the safety of everolimus-eluting bioresorbable vascular scaffold (BVS) implantation in patients with chronic total coronary occlusions: Acute procedural and short-term clinical results. *J Invasive Cardiol*. 2015;27:461–466.

8. Vaquerizo B, Barros A, Pujadas S, Bajo E, Estrada D, Miranda-Guardiola F, Rigla J et al. Bioresorbable everolimus-eluting vascular scaffold for the treatment of chronic total occlusions: CTO-ABSORB pilot study. *EuroIntervention*. 2015;11:555–563.

9. Vaquerizo B, Barros A, Pujadas S, Bajo E, Jimenez M, Gómez-Lara J, Jacobi F et al. One-year results bioresorbable vascular scaffolds for coronary chronic total occlusions. *Am J Cardiol*. 2016;117:906–917.

10. Morino Y, Abe M, Morimoto T, Kimura T, Hayashi Y, Muramatsu T, Ochiai M et al. Predicting successful guidewire crossing through chronic total occlusion of native coronary lesions within 30 minutes. The

j-CTO (Multicenter CTO registry in Japan) score as a difficulty grading and time assessment tool. *JACC Cardiovasc Interv.* 2011;4:213–221.

11. Diletti R, Farooq V, Girasis C, Bourantas C, Onuma Y, Heo JH, Gogas BD et al. Clinical and intravascular imaging outcomes at 1 and 2 years after implantation of absorb everolimus eluting bioresorbable vascular scaffolds in small vessels. Late lumen enlargement: Does bioresorption matter with small vessel size? Insight from the ABSORB cohort B trial. *Heart.* 2013; 99:98–105.

12. Park HJ, Kim HY, Lee JM, Choi YS, Park CS, Kim DB, Her SH et al. Randomized comparison of the efficacy and safety of zotarolimus-eluting stents vs. sirolimus-eluting stents for percutaneous coronary intervention in chronic total occlusion-CAtholic Total Occlusion Study (CATOS) trial. *Circ J.* 2012;76:868–875.

13. Teeuwen K, Van den Branden BJ, Koolen JJ, van der Schaaf RJ, Henriques JP, Tijssen JG, Kelder JC et al. Three-year clinical outcome in the Primary Stenting of Totally Occluded Native Coronary Arteries III (PRISON III) trial: A randomised comparison between sirolimus-eluting stent implantation and zotarolimus-eluting stent implantation for the treatment of total coronary occlusions. *EuroIntervention.* 2015;10:1272–75.

14. Markovic S, Lützner M, Rottbauer W, Wöhrle J. Zotarolimus compared with everolimus eluting stents-angiographic and clinical results after recanalization of true coronary chronic total occlusions. *Catheter Cardiovasc Interv.* 2016 Mar 4. doi: 10.1002 /ccd.26482. [Epub ahead of print]

15. Everaert B, Felix C, Koolen J, den Heijer P, Henriques J, Wykrzykowska JJ, van der Schaaf R et al. Appropriate use of bioresorbable vascular scaffolds in percutaneous coronary interventions: A recommendation from experienced users: A position statement on the use of bioresorbable vascular scaffolds in the Netherlands. *Neth Heart.* 2015;23:161–65.

16. Farooq V, Serruys PW, Heo JH, Gogas BD, Onuma Y, Perkins LE, Diletti R et al. Intracoronary optical coherence tomography and histology of overlapping everolimus-eluting bioresorbable vascular scaffolds in a porcine coronary artery model: The potential implications for clinical practice. *JACC Cardiovasc Interv.* 2013;6:523–32.

17. Ielasi A, Tespili M. Current status and future perspectives on drug-eluting bioresorbable coronary scaffolds: Will the paradigm of PCI shift? *EMJ Int Cardiol.* 2014;1:81–90.

18. Biscaglia S, Secco GC, Tumscitz C, Di Mario C, Campo G. Optical coherence tomography evaluation of overlapping everolimus-eluting vascular scaffold implantation guided by enhanced stent visualization system. *Inter J Cardiol.* 2015;182:1–3.

19. Zhang YJ, Iqbal J, Nakatani S, Bourantas CV, Campos CM, Ishibashi Y, Cho YK et al. Scaffold and edge vascular response following implantation of everolimus-eluting bioresorbable vascular scaffold: A 3-year serial optical coherence tomography study. *JACC Cardiovasc Interv.* 2014;7:1361–1369.

20. Capodanno D, Gori T, Nef H, Latib A, Mehilli J, Lesiak M, Caramanno G et al. Percutaneous coronary intervention with everolimus-eluting bioresorbable vascular scaffolds in routine clinical practice: Early and midterm outcomes from the European multicentre GHOST-EU registry. *EuroIntervention.* 2015;10:1144–1153.

21. Kraak RP, Hassell ME, Grundeken MJ, Koch KT, Henriques JP, Piek JJ, Baan J Jr et al. Initial experience and clinical evaluation of the Absorb bioresorbable vascular scaffold (BVS) in real-world practice: The AMC Single Centre Real World PCI Registry. *EuroIntervention.* 2015;10:1160–1168.

# Bioresorbable scaffolds in diffuse disease

NEIL RUPARELIA, HIROYOSHI KAWAMOTO, AND ANTONIO COLOMBO

## INTRODUCTION

Patients presenting with diffuse coronary artery disease pose a difficult treatment challenge and a number of different revascularization strategies have been employed with variable success [1–5]. Currently, widely accepted options include coronary artery bypass grafting (CABG), percutaneous coronary intervention (PCI), and medical therapy; however, each of these has limitations.

In up to 25% of patients presenting with diffuse coronary disease, CABG cannot be performed without significant risk to the patient [6] or due to likely suboptimal results due to poor distal anastomosis sites. Furthermore, small disease distal vessels have been shown to be inversely proportional to perioperative mortality [7] and the long-term rate of graft occlusion [8].

PCI for diffuse coronary artery disease is also not without risk. Treatment with bare metal stents (BMS) is associated with high rates of restenosis [9,10]. While outcomes have improved with the use of drug eluting stents (DESs) [11,12], the risk of restenosis [13] and late stent thrombosis [14] still exists, and increases further with longer stent lengths which are commonly required when treating long segments of diffuse disease [15,16]. Placement of a very long permanent foreign body will interfere with vasomotion, preclude the benefits of positive remodeling, and possibly promote neoatherosclerosis. Furthermore, the implantation of a "full metal jacket" also rules out future CABG with the loss of any potential distal grafting location.

The development of bioresorbable scaffolds (BRSs) provides the clinician with an additional management option and has already been demonstrated to be both viable and feasible in this clinical setting [17]. During the course of this chapter, we shall discuss the advantages and disadvantages associated with treating diffuse disease with BRSs and practical aspects that should be considered when deciding on this treatment option.

## ADVANTAGES OF BIORESORBABLE SCAFFOLDS

There are a number of potential advantages of utilizing BRS in the treatment of diffuse coronary artery disease. Their complete reabsorption within 2–3 years of implantation means that it is therefore possible to treat the entire vessel without leaving residual disease while still permitting the potential for future CABG if required as demonstrated in Figure 7.4.1. This approach may also therefore reduce the risk of subsequent restenosis [18]; however, this risk is not completely eliminated (Figure 7.4.2).

BRSs are also associated with favorable effects with regard to the long-term positive remodeling of the target vessel [19], improved vasomotion and endothelialization [20,21], therefore resulting in minimal changes to vessel geometry and local hemodynamics [22]. These advantages may be particularly pronounced when treating long segments of disease when compared to treatment with metallic stents.

One issue that needs early clarification is the duration of dual antiplatelet therapy. The need for mandatory dual antiplatelet therapy is dependent on complete endothelialization which is unlikely to occur faster than new generation metallic DES. Due to the process of scaffold resorption, it may become advantageous in these patients to extend dual antiplatelet therapy beyond 6–12 months [23].

Finally, BRSs may facilitate patient follow-up, many of whom who will present with multivessel coronary disease, enabling the use of noninvasive functional or morphological assessment of the artery (e.g., with multislice computed tomography possibly) which in contrast to metallic stents do not produce artefacts [24,25]. Advantages of BVS in comparison to BMS and DES are summarized in Table 7.4.1.

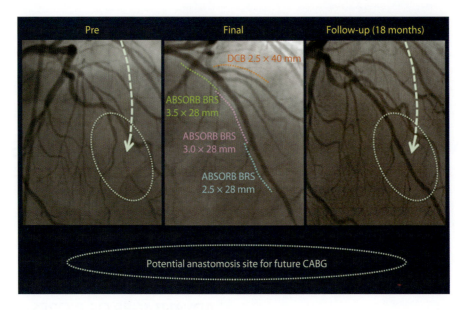

**Figure 7.4.1** Demonstration of treatment of diffuse disease with bioresorbable scaffold that may allow for future surgical grafting. Angiography demonstrated severe diffuse disease in the left anterior descending (LAD) artery and diagonal branch (left panel). The diagonal branch was treated with a drug-coated balloon (DCB). The LAD was treated with three overlapping bioresorbable scaffolds (BRSs) with an excellent final result (middle panel) that was confirmed at 18-month follow-up (right panel). The outlined area (white dotted line) demonstrates a future potential surgical graft anastomosis site at the distal LAD. BRS = bioresorbable scaffold; DCB = drug-coated balloon; CABG = coronary artery bypass grafting.

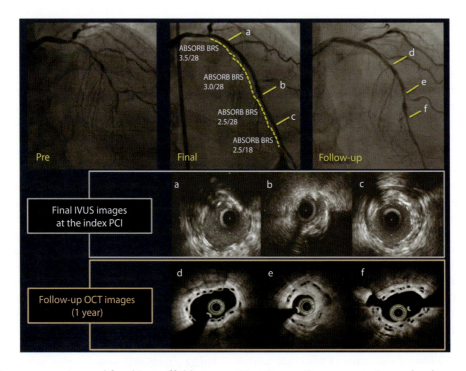

**Figure 7.4.2** LAD reconstruction and focal in-scaffold restenosis at 1 year. Coronary angiography demonstrated a long segment of severe diffuse disease in the left anterior descending artery (LAD) (top left panel). Due to poor distal targets, the patient was turned down for coronary artery bypass grafting. Four ABSORB BRS were implanted with a good final angiographic result (middle top panel). IVUS demonstrated diffuse disease including calcium **(b)** with good scaffold apposition following implantation **(a–c)**. At 1-year follow-up, angiography revealed appearance of focal in-scaffold restenosis (top right panel). OCT demonstrated severe in-scaffold restenosis **(e)** that required further coronary intervention with a drug-coated balloon. LAD = left anterior descending; BRS = bioresorbable scaffold; IVUS = intravascular ultrasound; PCI = percutaneous coronary intervention; OCT = optical coherence tomography.

Table 7.4.1 Potential advantages of bioresorbable scaffolds (BRSs) in comparison to bare metal stents (BMSs) and drug-eluting stents (DESs)

| | BRS | DES | BMS |
|---|---|---|---|
| Positive vessel wall remodeling | Yes | No | No |
| Potential for future CABG of treated segment | Yes | No | No |
| Noninvasive imaging follow-up | Yes | No | No |
| Radial support | Short-term | Long-term | Long-term |
| Late and very late stent thrombosis | No | Yes | Yes |
| Potential recovery of endothelial function | Yes | No | No |

*Abbreviations:* BMS = bare metal stent; BRS = bioresorbable scaffold; CABG = coronary artery bypass grafting; DES = drug-eluting stent.

## LIMITATIONS OF BIORESORBABLE SCAFFOLDS

There are some limitations of current BRS devices that require consideration. Current devices are bulky with thick struts in comparison to current generation DES. Thus, while they may be more flexible than DES, they have a worse crossing profile and are more difficult to deliver. This is particularly true when tackling long segments of disease that are often complicated by tortuosity and calcification. Meticulous attention should therefore be paid to aggressive vessel predilatation, use of the appropriate guiding catheter, and wire selection to facilitate delivery.

The presence of thicker struts is also an important consideration when treating long segments of disease due to the risk of side branch occlusion and iatrogenic plaque rupture with resultant periprocedural myocardial infarction [26].

Due to the limited extensibility and radial strength of BRS, careful attention should be paid to correct vessel sizing and preparation. In contrast to DES that can be overexpanded if they are smaller than the reference vessel diameter, BRS only have limited distensibility due to the risk of scaffold fracture which is particularly relevant to the ABSORB BRS (Abbott Vascular, Santa Rosa, CA) although different designs, for example, the DESolve scaffold (Elixir Medical Corporation, Sunnyvale, CA) may allow for more expansion [27].

Finally, current BRS technology is expensive with the additional requirement of adjunctive tools (e.g., more balloons and intravascular imaging) resulting in increased procedural costs, longer procedure times, and higher radiation and contrast doses administered to the patient.

## CURRENT EVIDENCE OF BRS IN DIFFUSE DISEASE

There are limited data with regard to the use of BRSs in diffuse disease. Initial trials excluded patients with complex coronary lesions [28]; however, with increasing operator experience and follow-up from initial studies, BRSs have been used for a number of different indications [29–31].

In the Gauging coronary Healing with biOresorbable Scaffolding plaTforms in EUrope (GHOST-EU) registry [32], which was the first "real-life" registry of patients treated with BRS during routine clinical evidence, 11.9% (121) of all lesions (1017) were >34 mm in length. While a specific subset analysis of patients with diffuse coronary artery disease was not conducted, the total number of BRS used or total BRS length were not found to be predictors of target lesion failure at 6 months follow-up, supporting the feasibility of this treatment approach. This approach is further supported by a second "all-comer" registry where 67% (106 patients) of all patients enrolled had lesions >20 mm, again no subset analysis was carried out but outcomes with regard to major adverse cardiovascular events were acceptable at a median of 198 days [33]. This has been further supported by a single-center study that demonstrated acceptable short-term outcomes [17], when BRS were used for the treatment of long segments (>60 mm) of diffuse coronary disease and were found to be noninferior when compared to patients treated with DES [34].

Thus, the use of BRSs in complex lesions and specifically in diffuse lesions is feasible. However, specific evidence supporting this approach is currently lacking. More data are required to investigate outcomes with this treatment strategy in comparison to more conventional approaches (e.g., treatment with DES) before it can be recommended as part of routine clinical management.

## PRACTICAL CONSIDERATIONS

Due to current device design and the specific challenges of treating diffuse disease, a number of practical considerations should be taken into account when opting to treat diffuse coronary artery disease with BRS.

As previously mentioned, the use of intravascular imaging (e.g., intravascular ultrasound or optical coherence tomography) is invaluable in treating long segments of disease. Due to current device design, appreciation of plaque composition (e.g., the presence of calcium) and measurement of the reference vessel diameter is essential prior to BRS implantation (Figure 7.4.3). This enables appropriate vessel preparation and BRS sizing considering the limited potential of upsizing following implantation due to the risk

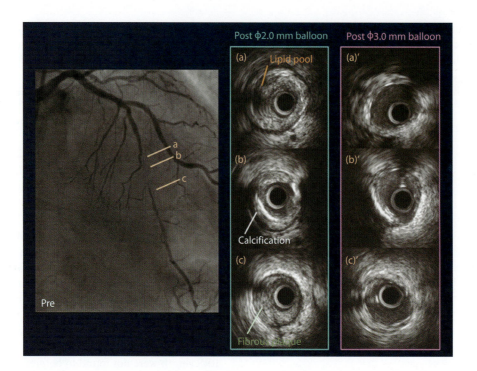

**Figure 7.4.3** Importance of intravascular imaging in treating diffuse disease with bioresorbable scaffold. Intravascular imaging (IVUS) of a long severe diffusely disease segment of a left anterior descending (LAD) artery. IVUS prior to bioresorbable scaffold (BRS) implantation enabled accurate reference vessel sizing and identification of a lipid pool **(a)**, calcification **(b)**, and fibrous plaque **(c)** to facilitate optimal lesion preparation. Following BRS implantation, IVUS confirmed optimal BRS apposition following postdilatation **(a',b',c')**. BRS = bioresorbable scaffold; dist = distal; prox = proximal.

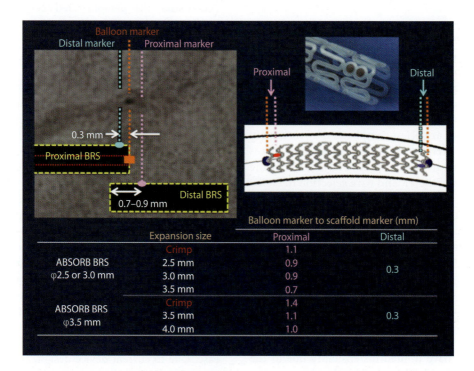

**Figure 7.4.4** Relationship of balloon markers, scaffold markers to the proximal and distal edge of the scaffold. Fluoroscopic image (top left panel) demonstrating the relationship of the distal platinum scaffold marker, the balloon marker, and the scaffold. It can be seen (top right panel) that the BRS edge is at the center of the balloon marker, which is 0.3 mm distal to the distal scaffold platinum marker and between 0.7 and 1.4 mm proximal to the proximal scaffold platinum marker (depending on scaffold and expansion size). BRS = bioresorbable scaffold.

of strut fracture. Finally, to allow adequate expansion and stent apposition, postimplantation intravascular imaging is mandatory to ensure optimal results and the best clinical outcomes. Appropriate postdilatation will facilitate embedment of the struts into the vessel wall partially counteracting the impact of greater strut thickness.

Long segments of disease will inevitably demand multiple BRS that will require overlapping. Based on bench work and on data from animal models, it appears that when two BRS overlap, there is reduced endothelialization of the stacked struts. While the clinical significance of this is unclear currently, extensive overlapping is therefore not recommended [35]. As with all overlapping scaffolds, it is important that the overlap site does not occur at the site of a side branch to minimize the risk of occlusion. The Abbott ABSORB stent (Abbott Vascular, Santa Clara, CA) has two fluoroscopically visible markers: the distal platinum marker is 0.3 mm proximal to the distal end of the BRS and the proximal marker is at least 0.7 mm distal to the proximal end of the BRS. The balloon markers are located at the ends of the BRS as opposed to DES where the stent ends are located within the balloon markers (Figure 7.4.4). To avoid a potential gap between BRS, an overlap of 1 mm ("marker to marker") has been suggested with a maximum of a 4 mm overlap (Figure 7.4.5). More recently we have adopted the technique of BRS abutting rather than overlapping. We

achieve this goal by placing the balloon marker of the more proximal scaffold being deployed proximal to the scaffold marker of the deployed distal scaffold.

When implanting multiple BRS in the same vessel, it is also important to implant distally to proximal due to the risk of not being able to pass a second BRS through the more proximal scaffold, due to the bulky nature of the device. If resistance is felt, when trying to advance a BRS it is important not to push due to the risk of dislodgement from the balloon—there should be a low threshold to taking another device in such instances when there is concern about scaffold distortion.

## CONCLUSION

The treatment of patients presenting with diffuse coronary artery presents a significant challenge. Current options include CABG, which is limited by the risk of incomplete revascularization and poor outcomes; and PCI (with DES), which is limited by the risks of permanent long foreign bodies in the vessel. Treatment of these patients with BRS may overcome many of these limitations. The current experience in this patient group suggests that this approach is feasible; however, larger studies with longer follow-up are required for BRS to be recommended for the routine treatment of diffuse coronary artery disease.

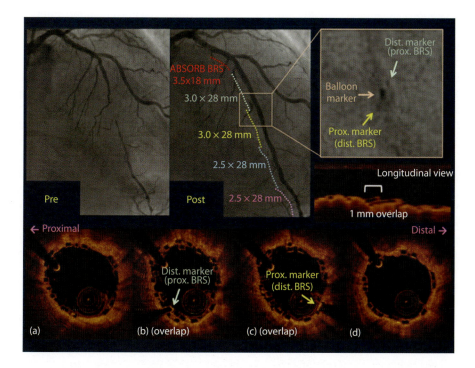

Figure 7.4.5 Overlapping bioresorbable scaffolds. The same patient as demonstrated in Figure 7.4.2. The patient required treatment with multiple overlapping bioresorbable scaffolds (BRSs). The distal marker of ABSORB BRS is 0.3 mm proximal to the distal edge, and the proximal marker is at least 0.7 mm distal to the proximal edge. Lining up the markers on fluoroscopy results in a 1 mm BRS overlap (top right panel). This is demonstrated on optical coherence tomography (OCT) both longitudinally (middle right panel) and also in cross-sectional views with the distal marker of the proximal BRS (b), the proximal marker of the distal BRS (c) visible. OCT shows concentric expansion and well-apposed BRS struts at the proximal (a) and distal (d) part to the overlapping site. BRS = bioresorbable scaffold, dist = distal; prox = proximal.

# REFERENCES

1. Basavarajaiah S, Latib A, Shannon J, Naganuma T, Sticchi A, Bertoldi L, Costopoulos C et al. Drug-eluting balloon in the treatment of in-stent restenosis and diffuse coronary artery disease: Real-world experience from our registry. *J Interv Cardiol.* 2014;**27**(4):348–55.

2. Rosengart TK, Bishawi MM, Halbreiner MS, Fakhoury M, Finnin E, Hollmann C, Shroyer AL et al. Long-term follow-up assessment of a phase 1 trial of angiogenic gene therapy using direct intramyocardial administration of an adenoviral vector expressing the VEGF121 cDNA for the treatment of diffuse coronary artery disease. *Hum Gene Ther.* 2013;**24**(2):203–8.

3. Prieto AR, Przybysz A, Fischell TA. Long balloon angioplasty with focal stenting for the treatment of diffuse coronary artery disease. *Catheter Cardiovasc Interv.* 2002;**57**(4):437–43.

4. Alamanni F, Parolari A, Agrifoglio M, Valerio N, Zanobini M, Repossini A, Arena V et al. Myocardial revascularization procedures on multisegment diseased left anterior descending artery: Endarterectomy or multiple sequential anastomoses (jumping)? *Minerva Cardioangiol.* 1996;**44**(10):471–7.

5. Costopoulos C, Latib A, Naganuma T, Sticchi A, Figini F, Basavarajaiah S, Carlino M et al. The role of drug-eluting balloons alone or in combination with drug-eluting stents in the treatment of de novo diffuse coronary disease. *JACC Cardiovasc Interv.* 2013;**6**(11):1153–9.

6. Sundt TM, 3rd, Camillo CJ, Mendeloff EN, Barner HB, Gay WA, Jr. Reappraisal of coronary endarterectomy for the treatment of diffuse coronary artery disease. *Ann Thorac Surg.* 1999;**68**(4):1272–7.

7. O'Connor NJ, Morton JR, Birkmeyer JD, Olmstead EM, O'Connor GT. Effect of coronary artery diameter in patients undergoing coronary bypass surgery. Northern New England Cardiovascular Disease Study Group. *Circulation.* 1996;**93**(4):652–5.

8. Shah PJ, Gordon I, Fuller J, Seevanayagam S, Rosalion A, Tatoulis J, Raman JS et al. Factors affecting saphenous vein graft patency: Clinical and angiographic study in 1402 symptomatic patients operated on between 1977 and 1999. *J Thorac Cardiovasc Surg.* 2003;**126**(6):1972–7.

9. Oemrawsingh PV, Mintz GS, Schalij MJ, Zwinderman AH, Jukema JW, van der Wall EE. Evaluation TSTa, effects of ultrasound guidance in long intracoronary stent P. Intravascular ultrasound guidance improves angiographic and clinical outcome of stent implantation for long coronary artery stenoses: Final results of a randomized comparison with angiographic guidance (TULIP Study). *Circulation.* 2003;**107**(1):62–7.

10. Kobayashi Y, De Gregorio J, Kobayashi N, Akiyama T, Reimers B, Finci L, Di Mario C et al. Stented segment length as an independent predictor of restenosis. *J Am Coll Cardiol.* 1999;**34**(3):651–9.

11. Tsagalou E, Chieffo A, Iakovou I, Ge L, Sangiorgi GM, Corvaja N, Airoldi F et al. Multiple overlapping drug-eluting stents to treat diffuse disease of the left anterior descending coronary artery. *J Am Coll Cardiol.* 2005;**45**(10):1570–3.

12. Lee CW, Park KH, Kim YH, Hong MK, Kim JJ, Park SW, Park SJ. Clinical and angiographic outcomes after placement of multiple overlapping drug-eluting stents in diffuse coronary lesions. *Am J Cardiol.* 2006;**98**(7):918–22.

13. Sharp AS, Latib A, Ielasi A, Larosa C, Godino C, Saolini M, Magni V et al. Long-term follow-up on a large cohort of "full-metal jacket" percutaneous coronary intervention procedures. *Circ Cardiovasc Interv.* 2009;**2**(5):416–22.

14. Karanasos A, Ligthart JM, Regar E. In-stent neoatherosclerosis: A cause of late stent thrombosis in a patient with "full metal jacket" 15 years after implantation: Insights from optical coherence tomography. *JACC Cardiovasc Interv.* 2012;**5**(7):799–800.

15. Claessen BE, Smits PC, Kereiakes DJ, Parise H, Fahy M, Kedhi E, Serruys PW et al. Impact of lesion length and vessel size on clinical outcomes after percutaneous coronary intervention with everolimus-versus paclitaxel-eluting stents pooled analysis from the SPIRIT (Clinical Evaluation of the XIENCE V Everolimus Eluting Coronary Stent System) and COMPARE (Second-generation everolimus-eluting and paclitaxel-eluting stents in real-life practice) Randomized Trials. *JACC Cardiovasc Interv.* 2011;**4**(11):1209–15.

16. Lee CW, Ahn JM, Lee JY, Kim WJ, Park DW, Kang SJ, Lee SW et al. Long-term (8 year) outcomes and predictors of major adverse cardiac events after full metal jacket drug-eluting stent implantation. *Catheter Cardiovasc Interv.* 2014;**84**(3):361–5.

17. Kawamoto H, Panoulas VF, Sato K, Miyazaki T, Naganuma T, Sticchi A, Latib A et al. Short-term outcomes following "full-plastic jacket" everolimus-eluting bioresorbable scaffold implantation. *Int J Cardiol.* 2014;**177**(2):607–9.

18. Sakurai R, Ako J, Morino Y, Sonoda S, Kaneda H, Terashima M, Hassan AH et al. Predictors of edge stenosis following sirolimus-eluting stent deployment (a quantitative intravascular ultrasound analysis from the SIRIUS trial). *Am J Cardiol.* 2005;**96**(9):1251–3.

19. Karanasos A, Simsek C, Gnanadesigan M, van Ditzhuijzen NS, Freire R, Dijkstra J, Tu S et al. OCT assessment of the long-term vascular healing response 5 years after everolimus-eluting bioresorbable vascular scaffold. *J Am Coll Cardiol.* 2014;**64**(22):2343–56.

20. Barlis P, Regar E, Serruys PW, Dimopoulos K, van der Giessen WJ, van Geuns RJ et al. An optical coherence tomography study of a biodegradable vs. durable polymer-coated limus-eluting stent: A LEADERS trial sub-study. *Eur Heart J.* 2010;**31**(2):165–76.

21. Hamilos MI, Ostojic M, Beleslin B, Sagic D, Mangovski L, Stojkovic S, Nedeljkovic M et al. Differential effects of drug-eluting stents on local endothelium-dependent coronary vasomotion. *J Am Coll Cardiol.* 2008;**51**(22):2123–9.

22. Gomez-Lara J, Garcia-Garcia HM, Onuma Y, Garg S, Regar E, De Bruyne B, Windecker S et al. A comparison of the conformability of everolimus-eluting bioresorbable vascular scaffolds to metal platform coronary stents. *JACC Cardiovasc Interv.* 2010;**3**(11):1190–8.

23. Mauri L, Kereiakes DJ, Yeh RW, Driscoll-Shempp P, Cutlip DE, Steg PG, Normand SL et al. Twelve or 30 months of dual antiplatelet therapy after drug-eluting stents. *N Engl J Med.* 2014.

24. Bourantas CV, Onuma Y, Farooq V, Zhang Y, Garcia-Garcia HM, Serruys PW. Bioresorbable scaffolds: Current knowledge, potentialities and limitations experienced during their first clinical applications. *Int J Cardiol.* 2013;**167**(1):11–21.

25. Onuma Y, Dudek D, Thuesen L, Webster M, Nieman K, Garcia-Garcia HM, Ormiston JA et al. Five-year clinical and functional multislice computed tomography angiographic results after coronary implantation of the fully resorbable polymeric everolimus-eluting scaffold in patients with de novo coronary artery disease: The ABSORB cohort A trial. *JACC Cardiovasc Interv.* 2013;**6**(10):999–1009.

26. Muramatsu T, Onuma Y, Garcia-Garcia HM, Farooq V, Bourantas CV, Morel MA, Li X et al. Incidence and short-term clinical outcomes of small side branch occlusion after implantation of an everolimus-eluting bioresorbable vascular scaffold: An interim report of 435 patients in the ABSORB-EXTEND single-arm trial in comparison with an everolimus-eluting metallic stent in the SPIRIT first and II trials. *JACC Cardiovasc Interv.* 2013;**6**(3):247–57.

27. Verheye S, Ormiston JA, Stewart J, Webster M, Sanidas E, Costa R, Costa JR, Jr. et al. A next-generation bioresorbable coronary scaffold system: From bench to first clinical evaluation: 6- and 12-month clinical and multimodality imaging results. *JACC Cardiovasc Interv.* 2014;**7**(1):89–99.

28. Serruys PW, Ormiston JA, Onuma Y, Regar E, Gonzalo N, Garcia-Garcia HM, Nieman K et al. A bioabsorbable everolimus-eluting coronary stent system (ABSORB): 2-year outcomes and results from multiple imaging methods. *Lancet.* 2009;**373**(9667):897–910.

29. Gori T, Schulz E, Hink U, Wenzel P, Post F, Jabs A, Munzel T. Early outcome after implantation of Absorb bioresorbable drug-eluting scaffolds in patients with acute coronary syndromes. *EuroIntervention.* 2014;**9**(9):1036–41.

30. Grundeken MJ, Kraak RP, de Bruin DM, Wykrzykowska JJ. Three-dimensional optical coherence tomography evaluation of a left main bifurcation lesion treated with ABSORB(R) bioresorbable vascular scaffold including fenestration and dilatation of the side branch. *Int J Cardiol.* 2013;**168**(3):e107–8.

31. Gori T, Guagliumi G, Munzel T. Absorb bioresorbable scaffold implantation for the treatment of an ostial chronic total occlusion. *Int J Cardiol.* 2014;**172**(2):e377–8.

32. Capodanno D, Gori T, Nef H, Latib A, Mehilli J, Lesiak M, Caramanno G et al. Percutaneous coronary intervention with everolimus-eluting bioresorbable vascular scaffolds in routine clinical practice: Early and midterm outcomes from the European multicentre GHOST-EU registry. *EuroIntervention.* 2014.

33. Kraak RP, Hassell ME, Grundeken MJ, Koch KT, Henriques JP, Piek JJ, Baan J, Jr. et al. Initial experience and clinical evaluation of the Absorb bioresorbable vascular scaffold (BVS) in real-world practice: The AMC Single Centre Real World PCI Registry. *EuroIntervention.* 2014.

34. Basavarajaiah S, Naganuma T, Latib A, Hasegawa T, Sharp A, Rezq A, Sticchi A et al. Extended follow-up following "full-metal jacket" percutaneous coronary interventions with drug-eluting stents. *Cath Cardiovasc Interv.* 2014;**84**(7):1042–50.

35. Farooq V, Onuma Y, Radu M, Okamura T, Gomez-Lara J, Brugaletta S, Gogas BD et al. Optical coherence tomography (OCT) of overlapping bioresorbable scaffolds: From benchwork to clinical application. *EuroIntervention.* 2011;**7**(3):386–99.

# Bioresorbable scaffolds in multivessel coronary disease

R.P. KRAAK, MAIK J. GRUNDEKEN, AND JOANNA J. WYKRZYKOWSKA

## INTRODUCTION

Bioresorbable technology has the potential to change the way interventional cardiology is being practiced in the coming years.

Compared with previously used bare metal stents and first generation drug-eluting metallic stents [1,2], second- and third-generation drug-eluting stents (DESs) have shown very low rates of major adverse cardiac events (MACEs) in the treatment of complex patient populations and various coronary artery lesion complexities [3–6]. However, these devices have not resolved all the weaknesses of metallic stents [7–9]. Bioresorbable technology has the potential to overcome these remaining limitations in the treatment of coronary artery lesions with the intuitively attractive advantage of freeing the coronary artery from foreign material after complete resorption of the implanted scaffold. Complete resorption, between 1 to 4 years depending on the bioresorbable scaffold (BRS) device, provides the possibility of implanting a coronary artery bypass graft on previously scaffolded segments in patients suffering from multivessel disease (MVD). Furthermore, restoration of vasomotion of the treated segment after resorption of the implanted scaffold can play an important role in the potential reduction of angina complaints. A reduction of angina complaints has been described after BVS implantation in a post-hoc analysis of the ABSORB II trial. However, no reduction of angina complaints was found in the ABSORB III trial [10,11]. Therefore, the results of the ABSORB IV trial are highly awaited as the primary endpoint of this trial is angina complaints. The above-mentioned potential benefits can lead to a change of treatment strategies, especially in young patients, in whom coronary artery bypass grafting (CABG) can be deferred by an initial strategy of percutaneous coronary intervention (PCI) with a BRS, keeping the opportunity to place bypass grafts on previously treated segments. Moreover, complete resorption of implanted BRS devices can decrease the risk of very late in-stent restenosis and therefore can diminish the risk of long-term repeat revascularizations.

Patients with more complex coronary artery lesions and more extensive coronary artery disease can therefore benefit the most from the potential advantages of BRSs. These patients still have, when treated with second- or third-generation DESs, a higher MACE rate compared with patients with less complex coronary artery lesions [12]. Furthermore, PCI with first- and second-generation DES has not been proven to be superior or equal to CABG in multiple randomized trials, such as the SYNTAX, FREEDOM, and the recent BEST trial in patients with extensive multivessel disease [13–15]. Therefore, the current guidelines of the European Society of Cardiology (ESC) recommend performing CABG in patients with multivessel disease and an intermediate or high SYNTAX score [16].

This chapter will discuss data on BRSs use in patients with MVD and will provide tips and tricks on how to use BRSs in these patients. Not only the implantation technique of BRS differs somewhat from metallic stents, but this technology could also lead to an adjustment in treatment strategies in patients. Finally, implantation techniques may also differ between the various available polylactide based and absorbable metallic-based BRS devices [17].

## CLINICAL EVIDENCE

Data on BRS use in extensively diseased coronary arteries are sparse, as patients suffering from MVD were excluded from most of the previous (randomized) trials. The first-in-human studies, on different polylactic acid and metallic bioresorbable scaffolds, mainly included patients with non-complex *de-novo* single vessel lesions and at maximum two lesions in two different coronary arteries. Table 7.5.1 demonstrates the major inclusion and exclusion criteria of the published ABSORB trials [22,23]. The trials on the ABSORB BVS have shown safety and efficacy in a highly selected patient population, with comparable clinical outcomes at 2-year follow-up between ABSORB BVS and the XIENCE DES (Abbott Vascular, Santa Clara, CA), as shown in the ABSORB II, III, ABSORB Japan, and ABSORB China

randomized controlled trial [10,11,24–26]. However, there seems to be a trend toward a higher ST rate with BVS at 2-year follow-up. These findings need to be further investigated in future trials.

Most data on BRS use in MVD and more complex lesions has been derived from "real-world" clinical registries on the ABSORB BVS which were conducted after the commercial release of the ABSORB BVS, in 2010. In these registries, the use of the ABSORB BVS was evaluated in the setting of daily clinical practice and thus also

**Table 7.5.1** Overview of inclusion and exclusion criteria of the ABSORB randomized controlled trials

| Study | N | Main inclusion criteria | Main exclusion criteria | Primary endpoint |
|---|---|---|---|---|
| ABSORB II [10] | 501 | Age ≥18 and ≤85 years; evidence of myocardial ischemia; ≤2 *de novo* coronary lesions | Acute MI; recent MI without normalized cardiac markers; LVEF ≤30% | 3-year mean lumen diameter change before and after nitrate administration |
| ABSORB Japan [18] | 400 | Age ≥20 years; evidence of myocardial ischemia; ≤2 *de novo* coronary lesions; reference vessel diameter ≥2.5 and ≤3.75 mm; lesion length ≤24 mm | Recent MI; LVEF ≤30%; estimated glomerular filtration rate mL/min/1.73m²; high bleeding risk; restenotic lesion left main stenosis; excessive vessel tortuosity bifurcation lesion with a side branch diameter >2.0 mm; ostial lesion; moderate/heavy calcified lesion; thrombotic lesion | 1 year TLF |
| EVERBIO [19] | 158 | Age ≥18 years; stable or unstable ischemic heart disease | Reference vessel diameter ≥4.0 mm; known or presumed hypersensitivity to heparin, antiplatelet drugs, or contrast dye not controllable with standard premedication | 9-months in-stent LLL |
| ABSORB III [11] | 2008 | Age ≥18 years; evidence of myocardial ischemia; ≤2 *de novo* coronary lesions; reference vessel diameter ≥2.5 and ≤3.75 mm; lesion length ≤24 mm | Acute MI; recent MI without normalized cardiac markers; LVEF ≤30%; previous PCI in the target vessel ≤1 year; left main stenosis; thrombotic lesion; bifurcation lesion with a side branch diameter >2.0 mm; ostial lesion; moderate/heavy calcified lesion | 1 year TLF |
| ABSORB China [20] | 480 | Age ≥18 years; evidence of myocardial ischemia; ≤2 *de novo* coronary lesions; reference vessel diameter ≥2.5 and ≤3.75 mm; lesion length ≤24 mm | Acute MI; recent MI without normalized cardiac markers; LVEF ≤30%; previous PCI in the target vessel ≤1 year; left main stenosis; bifurcation lesion with a side branch diameter >2.0 mm; ostial lesion; moderate/heavy calcified lesion; thrombotic lesion | 1 year in-stent LLL |
| TROFI II [21] | 191 | Age ≥18 years; STEMI ≤24h after the symptoms onset requiring emergent PCI; reference vessel diameter ≥2.25 and ≤3.8 mm | Cardiogenic shock; severe tortuosity or calcification; inadequate vessel size | 6 months healing score on OCT |

*Abbreviations:* LLL = late lumen loss; LVEF = left ventricular ejection fraction; MI = myocardial infarction; OCT = optical coherence tomography; PCI = percutaneous coronary intervention; STEMI = ST-segment elevation myocardial infarction; TLF = target lesion failure.

included patients with MVD. Almost half of the included patient population (47%) of the AMC registry had MVD, while the GHOST-EU registry included 40.9% patients with MVD and the RAI registry included MVD patients in the BVS group in 40.5% of the cases. The ASSURE registry on the other hand only included 13.1% patients with MVD [27–30]. These registries have shown acceptable clinical outcomes at a follow-up of 2 years, although they also raise concerns about a non-negligible increase in scaffold thrombosis (ST) rate (2.1% in GHOST-EU and 3.0% in AMC registry). Regarding the use of BRS in MVD, the GHOST-EU registry investigators demonstrated that there was no difference in clinical event rates at 1-year follow-up if BRS are used in long lesions in an overlapping fashion [31].

In the coming years large all-comer randomized trials, such as the AIDA (NCT01858077), COMPARE-ABSORB (NCT02486068), and SUGAR-EVE (NCT02632292)trials, comparing BRS with second-generation DES in more complex lesions and more complex patient populations, will provide important data on the use of BRS in multivessel disease. The AIDA and COMPARE-ABSORB trials have a prespecified SYNTAX score analysis, which will shed more light on the use of BRSs in MVD and potentially could lead to different SYNTAX score cut off values for BRS usage [32]. Furthermore, the large IT-DISAPPEARS registry [33] and the Korean randomized controlled trial focused on long lesions (NCT02796157) will specifically focus on the procedural and clinical performance of the ABSORB BVS in patients with long (>24 mm) single-vessel coronary artery disease or with MVD and could provide important information on the use of BRSs in patients with high risk diffuse coronary artery disease (Table 7.5.2).

## PRACTICAL TIPS AND TRICKS FOR MULTIVESSEL TREATMENT WITH BRS

When using BRSs in the treatment of coronary artery lesions, especially in patients with diffusely diseased coronary arteries and MVD, there are several considerations the treating physician might have to bear in mind. However, since the data on BRS use in MVD is sparse and randomized data in this specific subgroup is lacking, we do acknowledge that these considerations are not "evidence-based" yet, but rather based on the clinical experience we have with BRS use in our center. The first consideration you might face is whether to use a BRS only strategy, treating all lesions with BRS or use a hybrid approach combining BRSs with metallic permanent stents [34]. Another consideration before starting the procedure is whether to treat the patient in one procedure or whether complete revascularization should be achieved in multiple staged procedures.

The currently available scaffolds are considered to be bulky and have limited expansion limits. So, if a BRS only strategy is planned, the physician should make sure that all lesions and vessels are suitable for BRS implantation. If there is any expectation of a delivery problem, you might want to revise the treatment strategy, renounce the use of BRS, or use a hybrid approach.

When using a BRS only strategy you might consider implanting the most distal scaffold first. The rationale behind this is that implantation of a BRS through a previously implanted BRS located more proximally may lead to delivery problems of the distally placed BRS, while it may damage the previously placed BRS.

Furthermore, the currently available ABSORB BVS have a strut thickness of around 150 μm; therefore, theoretically these devices might be prone to in-scaffold restenosis if they are being used, especially if scaffold overlap is needed,

**Table 7.5.2** Ongoing trials on multivessel disease and complex patients treated with ABSORB BVS

| Study | Patients | N | Comparator | Primary endpoint | Hypothesis | Status | Reveal |
|---|---|---|---|---|---|---|---|
| AIDA | All-comers | 1848 | XIENCE DES | 2 year TVF | Noninferiority | Completed | ~2017 |
| ABSORB COMPARE | More-comers | 2100 | XIENCE DES | 1 year TLF | Noninferiority | Enrolling | ~2018 |
| | | | | 5 year TLF | Superiority | | |
| SUGAR-EVE | Diabetes | 224 | Promus DES | 8–10 months in-stent LLL | Noninferiority | Enrolling | ~2017 |
| Yonsei University | Non-ASC patients Lesion length >28 mm | 950 | XIENCE DES | 1 year MACE | Noninferiority | Enrolling | ~2018 |
| IT-DISAPPEARS | MVD Lesion length >24 mm | 1000 | None | 1–5 years TVF | – | Enrolling | ~2018 |

*Abbreviations:* LLL = late lumen loss; MACE = major adverse cardiac event (composite of cardiac death, non-fatal myocardial infarction, stent thrombosis, and target lesion revascularization) MVD = multivessel disease; TLF = target lesion failure; TVF = target vessel failure.

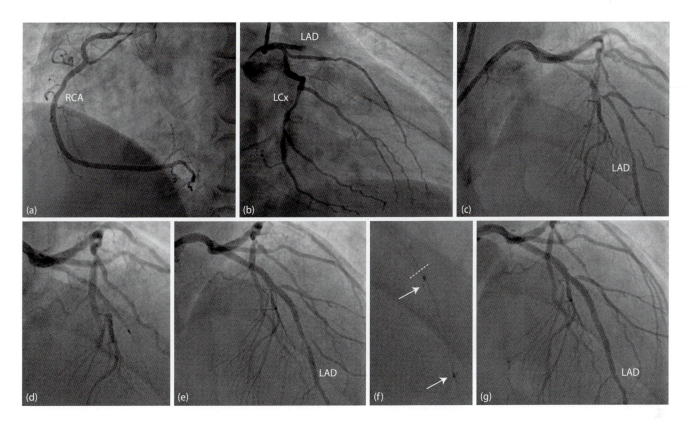

**Figure 7.5.1** Hybrid treatment strategy. Metallic DES in combination with ABSORB BVS. A 51-year-old male was referred to our hospital with ST-segment elevation in the precordial leads. Emergency angiography showed no significant stenosis in the right coronary artery **(a)**, an intermediate stenosis in the mid left circumflex, and a totally occluded left anterior descending artery (LAD) **(b)**. After thrombus aspiration two significant stenosis were observed in the LAD, one proximal and one distal of the second diagonal branch **(c)**. The LAD was wired with a balance middle weight guidewire and a 3.0 × 38 mm XIENCE drug-eluting stent was implanted at 15 atm in the proximal LAD **(d)**. After stenting the first lesion, with a good results **(e)** a 3.0 × 23 mm everolimus-eluting ABSORB bioresorbable vascular scaffold (BVS) was positioned **(f)** distal from the previously placed metallic stent (marked with the dashed line) and inflated at 16 atm. The procedure was finalized with postdilation with a 3.0 × 18 mm noncompliant balloon at 20 atm in both the XIENCE and the ABSORB BVS. Final angiogram showed a good result of both devices in the LAD **(g)**. This hybrid approach was opted for the relative young age of the patient and the potential benefit to keep the possibility of future implantation of a coronary artery bypass graft on the distal LAD after the scaffold has been completely resorbed.

in small (i.e., <2.5 mm) vessels. On the other hand, it has been demonstrated by Diletti et al. [35] that implantation in these small vessels appears to be safe, with similar clinical outcomes compared with those of larger vessels [32]. Therefore, we believe that the use of scaffolds in smaller distal vessels could be attractive in a hybrid approach, for example, a DES is implanted in a large (4.0 mm) proximal left anterior descending (LAD) artery and an ABSORB BVS more distal in the LAD (Figure 7.5.1). Despite the use of DES, this approach could allow a young patient to benefit in the future from biodegradable technology, as a bypass graft could be implanted at the distal LAD after resorption of the BRS. It is important to realize that other potential benefits, such as restoration of vasomotion or the use of noninvasive imaging techniques could be reduced using a hybrid approach.

Once the treatment strategy is chosen, we would recommend starting with the most difficult lesion. This allows a revision of the strategy in the event, for whatever reason, implantation of a BRS turns out to be impossible. Before implanting the scaffold, be sure that optimal pretreatment of the lesion is obtained with the use of predilatation balloons (1:1 predilatation), cutting/scoring balloons, or rotational atherectomy. In diffusely diseased coronary arteries, for example, calcified arteries, it is sometimes also necessary to perform pretreatment of the proximal trajectory or the use of a mother-child catheter technique is needed to allow delivery of the scaffold to the distally located lesions. The use of a mother-child catheter technique is feasible with the ABSORB BVS. However, it is important to know that only the 2.5 mm and the 3.0 mm scaffold are able to be advanced through a 6 French guideliner.

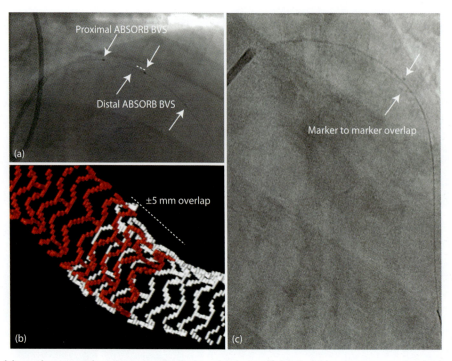

**Figure 7.5.2** Scaffold overlap considerations. Implanting multiple scaffolds in long coronary artery lesions could lead to overlapping scaffolds. The radio-opaque markers, both on the scaffold as on the delivery balloon, could be used in guidance to minimize scaffold overlap. Long overlap, as demonstrated in **(a)** and **(b)**, could lead to more flow disturbance and alterations in shear stress. Therefore, we advise to use the so called "marker to marker" method. This will lead to approximately 1 mm of scaffold overlap **(c)**.

Thereafter, we would recommend first implanting the most distal scaffold in the first target vessel and if needed implant adjacent scaffolds from distal to proximal. Implanting the scaffold from distal to proximal could reduce the risk of delivery problems. On the other hand, implanting the scaffolds from proximal to distal makes minimal overlap between scaffolds easier to accomplish and ensures that the proximal scaffold does not protrude in the left main. If overlap is needed, try using the so-called "marker to marker" overlap (Figure 7.5.2); this will lead to an overlap of approximately 1 mm. Finally, postdilatation of the scaffolded segment with the use of noncompliant (NC) balloons is, according to our experience, highly recommended. The use of NC balloons, when using the ABSORB BVS, could allow postdilatation at relative high pressure (14–18 atm or even higher) without the risk of overexpansion of the scaffold. However, the effect of postdilatation, and the balloon diameters and postdilatation pressures used, could be different in other polylactic acid and metallic scaffolds [17]. In the treatment of multivessel coronary artery disease all procedural steps, including pretreatment, scaffold delivery, and postdilatation, should be repeated in the all subsequent lesions to ensure optimal results. Multiple staged procedures may therefore be needed to achieve complete revascularization, as more excessive predilatation and vessel preparation could lead to more contrast usage, prolonged procedures, and prolonged radiation load for the patient. The use of intravascular imaging, especially optical coherence tomography (OCT) is highly recommended at the early stage of your BRS experience. The use of intravascular imaging may extend the procedure time even further, highlighting the importance of a careful planning of the treatment of MVD with BVS.

Total revascularization versus culprit only in the setting of primary PCI to treat patients presenting with ST-segment elevation myocardial infarction (STEMI) is still a topic of ongoing debate [36,37]. However, when MVD is observed during the emergency angiography including a lesion more distal than the culprit lesion, one might consider, if using BRS, treating not only the culprit lesion but also the lesion more distal in the culprit vessel and to treat this lesion prior to the culprit lesion. As discussed above, this will prevent the second BRS not passing the previously implanted scaffold and damages to the proximal BRS. Other diseased nonculprit vessels could be treated, if needed, during a staged procedure (Figure 7.5.3), in a similar fashion as when DES is used, according to contemporary guidelines [16]. Treatment of bifurcation lesions, often present in multivessel disease patient with ABSORB will be discussed in Chapter 7.2.

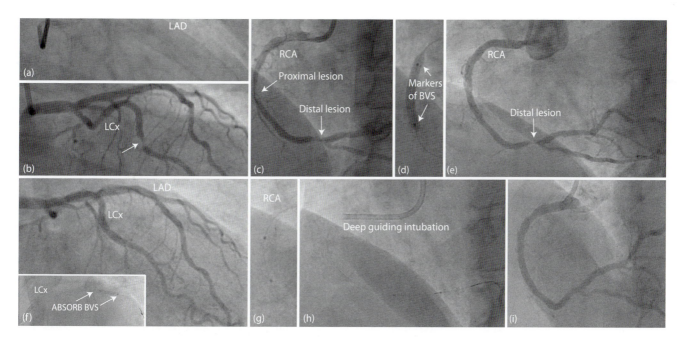

**Figure 7.5.3** Staged procedure in STEMI patient with BRS-only strategy. A 72-year-old female, with a history of diabetes mellitus, hypertension, hypercholesterolemia, and prior PCI in 2004 of the proximal LAD, was presented at our hospital with ST-segment elevation in the inferior leads. Emergency angiography of the left coronary artery showed a patent stent and no significant stenosis in the left anterior descending artery (LAD) **(a)** and a significant stenosis in the mid left circum-flexus (LCx) **(b)**. The right coronary artery (RCA) showed two lesions, one in the mid segment and one more distal **(c)**. After thrombus aspiration and predilatation with a 2.5 × 20 mm semicompliant balloon at 14 atm, a 3.0 × 23 mm ABSORB BVS was implanted at 12 atm in the mid RCA **(d)**. The procedure was finalized postdilatation with a 3.0 × 15 mm semicompliant balloon at 20 atm, because a noncompliant balloon could not be advanced through the implanted scaffold. Final angiography showed a good result of the treated lesion **(e)**. Two weeks later, patient underwent a repeat staged PCI of both the RCA as the LCx. The LCx was treated first and after predilatation a 2.5 × 12 mm ABSORB BVS was implanted at 18 atm with a good angiographic result **(f)**. During this procedure it was difficult to advance a 2.0 × 20 mm and 2.0 × 15 mm semi-compliant balloon through the ABSORB BVS; therefore, no scaffold was implanted in the distal lesion **(g)**. Deep guiding intubation was eventually needed to cross the scaffold, and a 3.0 × 15 mm Paclitaxel-eluting balloon was positioned and inflated at 7 atm **(h)**. Final angiography showed a good result of both treated lesion in the RCA **(i)**. This case demonstrates the potential difficulties accessing a second lesion, located more distally, through a proximal implanted scaffold and the need for careful planning of treatment strategy during the initial procedure.

## CONCLUSION

Despite the current technical limitations of BRSs, implantation in relative simple coronary artery lesions has been proven to be feasible and safe and to have comparable clinical results at 2-year follow-up with DESs. The potential theoretical advantages, after complete resorption of the BRS in MVD, reducing the risk of very-late scaffold thrombosis (after its complete absorption), reduction of anginal complaints, and the potential to perform coronary artery bypass grafting on previously percutaneously treated segments needs to be further investigated in future observational and randomized trials. Before using BRSs in MVD patients, an appropriate treatment strategy should be planned; this could either be a complete BRS strategy or a hybrid approach combining BRSs with (drug-eluting) metallic stents. Finally, we would recommend to first gain experience in its use in more simple lesions before encountering more complex lesions in the setting of MVD.

## REFERENCES

1. Moses JW, Leon MB, Popma JJ, Fitzgerald PJ, Holmes DR, O'Shaughnessy C, Caputo RP et al. Sirolimus-eluting stents versus standard stents in patients with stenosis in a native coronary artery. *New Engl J Med.* 2003;349:1315–23.
2. Grube E, Silber S, Hauptmann KE, Mueller R, Buellesfeld L, Gerckens U, Russell ME. TAXUS I: Six-and twelve-month results from a randomized, double-blind trial on a slow-release paclitaxel-eluting stent for de novo coronary lesions. *Circulation.* 2003;107:38–42.
3. Windecker S, Serruys PW, Wandel S, Buszman P, Trznadel S, Linke A, Lenk K et al. Biolimus-eluting stent with biodegradable polymer versus sirolimus-eluting stent with durable polymer for coronary revascularisation (LEADERS): A randomised non-inferiority trial. *Lancet.* 2008;372:1163–73.

4. Jensen LO, Thayssen P, Hansen HS, Christiansen EH, Tilsted HH, Krusell LR, Villadsen AB et al. Randomized comparison of everolimus-eluting and sirolimus-eluting stents in patients treated with percutaneous coronary intervention: The Scandinavian Organization for Randomized Trials with Clinical Outcome IV (SORT OUT IV). *Circulation.* 2012;125:1246–55.

5. Smits PC, Hofma S, Togni M, Vazquez N, Valdes M, Voudris V, Slagboom T et al. Abluminal biodegradable polymer biolimus-eluting stent versus durable polymer everolimus-eluting stent (COMPARE II): A randomised, controlled, non-inferiority trial. *Lancet.* 2013;381:651–60.

6. Navarese EP, Kowalewski M, Kandzari D, Lansky A, Gorny B, Koltowski L, Waksman R et al. First-generation versus second-generation drug-eluting stents in current clinical practice: Updated evidence from a comprehensive meta-analysis of randomised clinical trials comprising 31 379 patients. *Open Heart.* 2014;1:e000064.

7. Nakazawa G, Otsuka F, Nakano M, Vorpahl M, Yazdani SK, Ladich E, Kolodgie FD et al. The pathology of neoatherosclerosis in human coronary implants bare-metal and drug-eluting stents. *J Am Coll Cardiol.* 2011;57:1314–22.

8. Maier W, Windecker S, Kung A, Lutolf R, Eberli FR, Meier B, Hess OM. Exercise-induced coronary artery vasodilation is not impaired by stent placement. *Circulation.* 2002;105:2373–7.

9. Joner M, Finn AV, Farb A, Mont EK, Kolodgie FD, Ladich E, Kutys R et al. Pathology of drug-eluting stents in humans: Delayed healing and late thrombotic risk. *J Am Coll Cardiol.* 2006;48:193–202.

10. Serruys PW, Chevalier B, Dudek D, Cequier A, Carrie D, Iniguez A, Dominici M et al. A bioresorbable everolimus-eluting scaffold versus a metallic everolimus-eluting stent for ischaemic heart disease caused by de-novo native coronary artery lesions (ABSORB II): An interim 1-year analysis of clinical and procedural secondary outcomes from a randomised controlled trial. *Lancet.* 2015;385:43–54.

11. Ellis SG, Kereiakes DJ, Metzger DC, Caputo RP, Rizik DG, Teirstein PS, Litt MR et al. Everolimus-eluting bioresorbable scaffolds for coronary artery disease. *New Engl J Med.* 2015.

12. Wykrzykowska JJ, Garg S, Girasis C, de Vries T, Morel MA, van Es GA, Buszman P et al. Value of the SYNTAX score for risk assessment in the all-comers population of the randomized multicenter LEADERS (Limus Eluted from A Durable versus ERodable Stent coating) trial. *J Am Coll Cardiol.* 2010;56:272–7.

13. Mohr FW, Morice MC, Kappetein AP, Feldman TE, Stahle E, Colombo A, Mack MJ et al. Coronary artery bypass graft surgery versus percutaneous coronary intervention in patients with three-vessel disease and left main coronary disease: 5-year follow-up of the randomised, clinical SYNTAX trial. *Lancet.* 2013;381:629–38.

14. Farkouh ME, Domanski M, Sleeper LA, Siami FS, Dangas G, Mack M, Yang M et al. Strategies for multivessel revascularization in patients with diabetes. *New Engl J Med.* 2012;367:2375–84.

15. Park SJ Ahn JM, Kim YH, Park DW, Yun SC, Lee JY, Kang SJ et al. Trial of everolimus-eluting stents or bypass surgery for coronary disease. *New Engl J Med.* 2015;372:1204–12.

16. Authors/Task Force m, Windecker S, Kolh P, Alfonso F, Collet JP, Cremer J, Falk V et al. 2014 ESC/EACTS Guidelines on myocardial revascularization: The Task Force on Myocardial Revascularization of the European Society of Cardiology (ESC) and the European Association for Cardio-Thoracic Surgery (EACTS) Developed with the special contribution of the European Association of Percutaneous Cardiovascular Interventions (EAPCI). *Eur Heart J.* 2014;35:2541–619.

17. Ormiston JA, Webber B, Ubod B, Darremont O, Webster MW. An independent bench comparison of two bioresorbable drug-eluting coronary scaffolds (Absorb and DESolve) with a durable metallic drug-eluting stent (ML8/Xpedition). *EuroIntervention. Journal of EuroPCR in Collaboration with the Working Group on Interventional Cardiology of the European Society of Cardiology.* 2015;11:60–7.

18. Stone GW, Gao R, Kimura T, Kereiakes DJ, Ellis SG, Onuma Y, Cheong WF et al. 1-year outcomes with the Absorb bioresorbable scaffold in patients with coronary artery disease: A patient-level, pooled meta-analysis. *Lancet.* 2016;387:1277–89.

19. Puricel S, Arroyo D, Corpataux N, Baeriswyl G, Lehmann S, Kallinikou Z, Muller O et al. Comparison of everolimus- and biolimus-eluting coronary stents with everolimus-eluting bioresorbable vascular scaffolds. *J Am Coll Cardiol.* 2015;65:791–801.

20. Gao R, Yang Y, Han Y, Huo Y, Chen J, Yu B, Su X et al. Bioresorbable vascular scaffolds versus metallic stents in patients with coronary artery disease: ABSORB China Trial. *J Am Coll Cardiol.* 2015;66:2298–309.

21. Sabate M, Windecker S, Iniguez A, Okkels-Jensen L, Cequier A, Brugaletta S, Hofma SH et al. Everolimus-eluting bioresorbable stent vs. durable polymer everolimus-eluting metallic stent in patients with ST-segment elevation myocardial infarction: Results of the randomized ABSORB ST-segment elevation myocardial infarction-TROFI II trial. *Eur Heart J.* 2016;37:229–40.

22. Verheye S, Ormiston JA, Stewart J, Webster M, Sanidas E, Costa R, Costa JR, Jr. et al. A next-generation bioresorbable coronary scaffold system: From bench to first clinical evaluation: 6- and 12-month clinical and multimodality imaging results. *JACC Cardiovasc Interv.* 2014;7:89–99.

23. Haude M, Erbel R, Erne P, Verheye S, Degen H, Bose D, Vermeersch P et al. Safety and performance of the drug-eluting absorbable metal scaffold (DREAMS) in patients with de-novo coronary lesions: 12 month results of the prospective, multicentre, first-in-man BIOSOLVE-I trial. *Lancet.* 2013;381:836–44.

24. Ormiston JA, Serruys PW, Regar E, Dudek D, Thuesen L, Webster MW, Onuma Y et al. A bioabsorbable everolimus-eluting coronary stent system for patients with single de-novo coronary artery lesions (ABSORB): A prospective open-label trial. *Lancet.* 2008;371:899–907.

25. Serruys PW, Onuma Y, Ormiston JA, de Bruyne B, Regar E, Dudek D, Thuesen L et al. Evaluation of the second generation of a bioresorbable everolimus drug-eluting vascular scaffold for treatment of de novo coronary artery stenosis: Six-month clinical and imaging outcomes. *Circulation.* 2010;122:2301–12.

26. Onuma Y, Sotomi Y, Shiomi H, Ozaki Y, Namiki A, Yasuda S, Ueno T et al. Two-year clinical, angiographic, and serial optical coherence tomographic follow-up after implantation of an everolimus-eluting bioresorbable scaffold and an everolimus-eluting metallic stent: Insights from the randomised ABSORB Japan trial. *EuroIntervention. Journal of EuroPCR in Collaboration with the Working Group on Interventional Cardiology of the European Society of Cardiology.* 2016;12.

27. Capodanno D, Gori T, Nef H, Latib A, Mehilli J, Lesiak M, Caramanno G et al. Percutaneous coronary intervention with everolimus-eluting bioresorbable vascular scaffolds in routine clinical practice: Early and midterm outcomes from the European multicentre GHOST-EU registry. *EuroIntervention. Journal of EuroPCR in Collaboration with the Working Group on Interventional Cardiology of the European Society of Cardiology.* 2015;10:1144–53.

28. Kraak RP, Hassell ME, Grundeken MJ, Koch KT, Henriques JP, Piek JJ, Baan J, Jr. et al. Initial experience and clinical evaluation of the Absorb bioresorbable vascular scaffold (BVS) in real-world practice: The AMC Single Centre Real World PCI Registry. *EuroIntervention. Journal of EuroPCR in Collaboration with the Working Group on Interventional Cardiology of the European Society of Cardiology.* 2015;10:1160–8.

29. Wohrle J, Naber C, Schmitz T, Schwencke C, Frey N, Butter C, Brachmann J et al. Beyond the early stages: Insights from the ASSURE registry on bioresorbable vascular scaffolds. *EuroIntervention. Journal of EuroPCR in Collaboration with the Working Group on Interventional Cardiology of the European Society of Cardiology.* 2015;11:149–56.

30. Ielasi A, Cortese B, Varricchio A, Tespili M, Sesana M, Pisano F, Loi B et al. Immediate and midterm outcomes following primary PCI with bioresorbable vascular scaffold implantation in patients with ST-segment myocardial infarction: Insights from the multicentre "Registro ABSORB Italiano" (RAI registry). *EuroIntervention. Journal of EuroPCR in Collaboration with the Working Group on Interventional Cardiology of the European Society of Cardiology.* 2015;11:157–62.

31. Ortega-Paz L, Capodanno D, Giacchi G, Gori T, Nef H, Latib A, Caramanno G et al. Impact of overlapping on 1-year clinical outcomes in patients undergoing everolimus-eluting bioresorbable scaffolds implantation in routine clinical practice: Insights from the European multicenter GHOST-EU registry. *Cath Cardiovasc Interv.* 2016.

32. Woudstra P, Grundeken MJ, Kraak RP, Hassell ME, Arkenbout EK, Baan J, Jr., Vis MM et al. Amsterdam Investigator-initiateD Absorb strategy all-comers trial (AIDA trial): A clinical evaluation comparing the efficacy and performance of ABSORB everolimus-eluting bioresorbable vascular scaffold strategy vs the XIENCE family (XIENCE PRIME or XIENCE Xpedition) everolimus-eluting coronary stent strategy in the treatment of coronary lesions in consecutive all-comers: Rationale and study design. *Am Heart J.* 2014;167:133–40.

33. Testa L, Biondi Zoccai G, Tomai F, Ribichini F, Indolfi C, Tamburino C, Bartorelli A et al. Italian Diffuse/Multivessel Disease ABSORB Prospective Registry (IT-DISAPPEARS). Study design and rationale. *J Cardiovasc Med.* 2015;16:253–8.

34. Grundeken MJ, Hassell ME, Kraak RP, de Bruin DM, Koch KT, Henriques JP, van Leeuwen TG et al. Treatment of coronary bifurcation lesions with the Absorb bioresorbable vascular scaffold in combination with the Tryton dedicated coronary bifurcation stent: Evaluation using two- and three-dimensional optical coherence tomography. *EuroIntervention. Journal of EuroPCR in Collaboration with the Working Group on Interventional Cardiology of the European Society of Cardiology.* 2014.

35. Diletti R, Onuma Y, Farooq V, Gomez-Lara J, Brugaletta S, van Geuns RJ, Regar E et al. 6-month clinical outcomes following implantation of the bioresorbable everolimus-eluting vascular scaffold in vessels smaller or larger than 2.5 mm. *J Am Coll Cardiol.* 2011;58:258–64.

36. Wald DS, Morris JK, Wald NJ, Chase AJ, Edwards RJ, Hughes LO, Berry C et al. Randomized trial of preventive angioplasty in myocardial infarction. *New Engl J Med.* 2013;369:1115–23.

37. Gershlick AH, Khan JN, Kelly DJ, Greenwood JP, Sasikaran T, Curzen N, Blackman DJ et al. Randomized trial of complete versus lesion-only revascularization in patients undergoing primary percutaneous coronary intervention for STEMI and multivessel disease: The CvLPRIT trial. *J Am Coll Cardiol.* 2015;65:963–72.

# Bioresorbable coronary scaffolds in non-ST elevation acute coronary syndromes

CHARIS MAMILOU AND TOMMASO GORI

## INTRODUCTION

Acute coronary syndromes (ACSs) count to the most serious of acute cardiac disorders and are the leading cause of mortality in adults, being responsible for hundreds of thousands of deaths each year worldwide [1]. Importantly, the clinical spectrum of non-ST elevation ACSs is broad and ranges from patients free of symptoms at presentation (with an occasional finding of elevated myocardial biomarkers), to patients with crescendo angina, to those presenting with ongoing ischemia, electrical or hemodynamic instability (but no ST-elevation in the ECG). Additional to general clinical parameters such as age, diabetes, and kidney failure, the initial clinical presentation is obviously an important predictor of prognosis [2]. There is also a large spectrum of mechanisms that potentially underlie the non-ST ACSs. Building on the observation that differences in the underlying mechanisms also influence patient therapy and prognosis, the Universal Definition of Myocardial Infarction classifies myocardial ischemia into 5 types [3]. For the purpose of this chapter, however, we will focus only on the so-called "spontaneous myocardial infarction," or type 1, i.e., the form of ischemia that is related to atherosclerotic plaque rupture, ulceration, fissuring, erosion, or dissection with resulting intraluminal thrombus. Importantly, the instabilization of atherosclerosis leading to the above events is a systemic vascular pathology that often affects multiple vessels at the same time (up to 44–59% [4]), and the mechanical problem (i.e., thrombotic occlusion of the coronary) has to be seen as the result of more complex biological phenomena in which endothelial dysfunction plays a central role.

Central to the possible role of bioresorbable scaffolds in the therapy of non-ST elevation ACS (and acute coronary syndromes in general) is the consideration that although the acute manifestation of the disease results from a mechanical obstruction of the vessel, much more complex biological phenomena underlie this condition. As a corollary, the concept that a mechanical therapy (with a metal stent) might represent a definitive therapy to this disease appears overly simplistic (Figure 7.6.1).

Atherosclerosis is a chronic disease with generally prolonged quiescence periods and rapid progressions and phases of instabilization [5,6]. During these acute events, a dysfunctional endothelium/vascular wall leads to an increased expression of prothrombotic factors, chemokines, and proinflammatory mediators along with reduction of endothelial progenitor cells [7,8]. Furthermore, a reduced bioavailability of endothelial mediators is associated with the overexpression of intercellular adhesion molecules and increased binding of lymphocytes and monocytes, followed by their passage in the subendothelium and their transformation in foam cells [9,10]. Finally, the exposure of tissue factor in the setting of plaque erosion/rupture resulting from the thinning or rupture of the fibrous cap of the plaques is a potent stimulus to the activation of the coagulation cascade and of platelet aggregation. The resulting thrombus formation and lumen reduction leads to ischemia and (N)STEMI or unstable angina [11,12]. The plaques at higher risk to induce such phenomena, termed "thin cap fibroatheroma," are defined by the presence of a thin fibrous cap (<65 μm thickness) which overlays a hemorrhagic, necrotic, or necrotic-calcific core with thin-walled microvessels migrated from the adventitia (Figure 7.6.2) [13]. Finally, determinants of plaque rupture vulnerability include a core larger than 40% of the plaque volume and the collagen content/type of the cap [14,15] In sum, although they are caused by a mechanical phenomenon, acute coronary syndromes are biological entities, mediated by phenomena such as inflammation, endothelial dysfunction/activation, and oxidative stress.

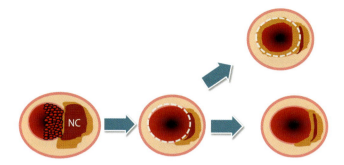

**Figure 7.6.1** Pathogenesis of acute coronary syndromes and fate after stenting: An acute coronary syndrome is caused mostly by plaque erosion/rupture which triggers the activation of the coagulation cascade and the aggregation of thrombi. The ensuing thrombus occludes the vessel lumen, causing ischemia. In the majority of the cases, these events are associated with thin fibrous cap fibroatheromas, with a necrotic core (NC) and a thin fibrotic layer (yellow). Stenting resolves only the mechanical problem. On long term, in the case of metal stents, only a concentric remodeling, causing lumen loss, is possible (upper right panel). This neointimal layer, however, biologically and mechanically stabilizes the plaque, and a stent is not necessary and rather harmful. The reabsorption of a BVS (mid-right panel) leaves the possibility of a remodeling of the now biologically stable vessel segment.

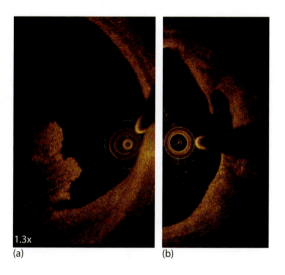

**Figure 7.6.2 (a)** intravascular thrombus likely caused by plaque erosion. **(b)** plaque dissection at the level of a plaque shoulder. Part of the plaque content has embolized into the lumen.

## THE POTENTIAL FOR BIORESORBABLE SCAFFOLDS IN NON-STEMI ACS

While they provide effective mechanical support, the drawback of traditional metallic stents is that they trigger immune/inflammatory and oxidative foreign-body-like reactions [16–22]. Such changes have been identified as a possible cause of in-stent restenosis and in-stent thrombosis, and

they surely lead to further worsening of endothelium-dependent vasomotor function [23]. In the setting of acute coronary syndromes, where the processes leading to the instabilization of a plaque appear to be based on inflammatory phenomena, the implantation of a permanent foreign body, as a possible continuous source of inflammation, appears particularly inadequate. As such, the introduction of bioresorbable scaffolds paves the way for a new paradigm in the therapy of ACS. The transient nature of the scaffold struts offers a number of theoretical advantages compared to metallic DES, including a lesser induction of inflammatory reactions, potentially resulting in a less prolonged endothelial dysfunction after stenting [24]. As well, acute coronary syndromes are in many cases caused by factors such as vasospasm, plaque erosion, or embolic events, which do not necessarily benefit from a permanent stent. In these cases, the resorption of the scaffold, together with plaque/media reduction and vessel lumen enlargement (as opposed to late luminal loss with permanent stents) may protect vascular geometry/biomechanics and restore important vascular functions such as pulsatility in response to changes in shear stress [25–28]. All these processes depend on the biology of the vessels and plaques, and appear to be particularly important for plaques that present the above characteristics of instability/vulnerability.

## CLINICAL OUTCOMES OF BVS IN NON-ST ELEVATION ACS

Despite the above advantages, the clinical outcomes of BVS implantation in the setting of acute coronary syndromes remain poorly explored. These can be classified into two major sections: anatomical and functional stabilization (preclinical evidence) and clinical evidence.

### Anatomical and functional stabilization

The concept of "plaque healing" or "plaque passivation" is central to the application of temporary scaffolds for the treatment of unstable/culprit plaques. In the months following the implantation of a stent, optical coherence tomography witnesses the formation of a fibrotic layer that covers the remnants of the plaque and protects from further erosion/rupture events (Figure 7.6.3). Such findings of a layer presenting OCT characteristics possibly compatible with those of a fibrous cap have been previously hypothesized to witness the transformation of vulnerable lesions to stable plaques [29–31]. Although the hypothesis of plaque passivation (and the existence of a threshold for a "stable" in-stent cap) remains speculative, evidence exists that in-stent thin caps are also markers of worse prognosis: in a report enrolling patients with stent failure, those presenting with relapsing unstable (vs. stable) angina also had a thinner fibrous cap and other OCT findings suggestive of instability, including TCFA-containing neointima [32]. Recent evidence suggests that the implantation of a BVS was systematically associated with the formation of a neointimal layer that transformed

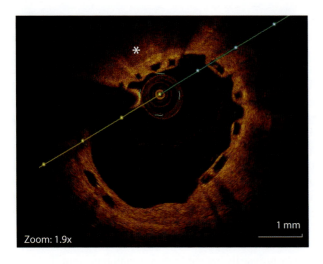

**Figure 7.6.3** Twelve months after BVS implantation for the treatment of a thrombotic plaque. The plaque (*) is now covered and stabilized by a neointimal layer.

the TCFA into thick-cap fibroatheromas; interestingly, while this neointima formation initially reduced luminal dimensions, the subsequent positive remodeling was associated with a lumen gain that compensated for this reduction [29,33,34]. This evidence from stable patients and type A lesions was further investigated by our group in the setting of acute coronary syndromes. In our recent paper, we investigated a series of 133 patients who underwent BVS implantation for the treatment of ACSs [35]. One year after implantation, OCT revealed that the remnants of the culprit plaque were covered in the large majority (95.7%) of cases by a homogeneous, signal-rich tissue thicker than 65 μm (Figure 7.6.4), witnessing the transformation of vulnerable lesions to stable plaques. In sum, the formation of a thick neointimal layer creates a *de novo* cap with functional

endothelium analogous to the original fibrous cap of the plaque [29,36,37]. Unique to BVS, due to late positive remodeling, this anatomical passivation is not associated with late lumen loss.

With regard to the composition of the underlying plaque, important evidence was recently published by Brugaletta et al. [38]. By analyzing with virtual histology the outcomes 12 months after implantation of bioresorbable scaffolds in patients from the cohort B trial, they demonstrate a mid-term increase in the size of the plaque located behind the polymeric struts of the scaffold, mostly due to an increase in its (stable) fibrous and fibrofatty content. Importantly, this finding was associated with a significant decrease in features of unstable necrotic core and dense calcium tissue. Any conclusions regarding the possible mechanisms of this "plaque passivation" remain speculative. A possible role could have been played by the drug eluted, since everolimus has been associated with reduction in intra-plaque macrophage content by triggering autophagy processes [39]. Alternatively, this improvement might result from the prolonged treatment with statins [40], or simply by the passing of time. Whatever the mechanism, this observation is important in the context of plaque stabilization, as the presence of macrophages and calcific core are hallmarks of plaque destabilization [21], and it correlates well with the return of endothelium-dependent vasodilator responses described below. Whether this effect is specific (or more pronounced) for scaffolds can also not be stated surely. However, the above evidence emphasizes the concept that a permanent stent, whatever its chemical nature, is not necessary as early as 12 months after treatment of a culprit lesion.

Vasomotion, mechanostransduction, adaptive shear stress, and the subsequent late luminal gain are all phenomena in which endothelial function is of paramount importance. From the functional perspective, the implantation

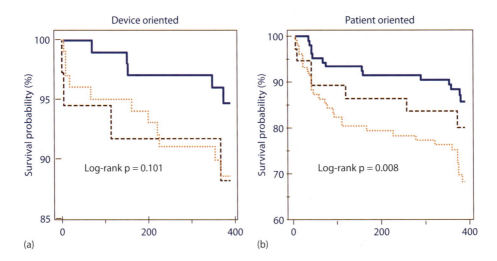

**Figure 7.6.4 (a)** Kaplan–Meier estimate of the incidence of a device-oriented endpoint following BVS implantation for the treatment of stable angina (blue), unstable angina (yellow), or NSTEMI (red). Although a trend is visible, there is no significant difference between groups. There is also absolutely no difference between unstable angina and NSTEMI. **(b)** Patient-oriented endpoint. Here a clear difference is visible, with a progressively worse prognosis for stable angina, unstable angina, and NSTEMI.

of a metal-stent significantly limits these functions. In a recent study from our group, we quantified the in-scaffold vasomotor in response to three different doses of acetylcholine, which allowed us to document both endothelium-dependent vasodilation and spasm phenomena, and to nitroglycerin, an endothelium-independent vasodilator [35]. While acetylcholine responses are an accepted diagnostic and risk stratification tool [41], data on the functional normalization of vessels previously treated in the setting of an acute event have not been reported before. In our population, endothelium-dependent vasodilation was observed in about 30% of the subjects. Nitroglycerin-induced vasodilation was observed in about half of the lesions. Of note, these figures might further improve after further withdrawal of the scaffolding function of the BVS. Collectively, these data demonstrate functional normalization in a large fraction of the segments treated with a BVS already after 1 year.

## Clinical evidence of bioresorbable scaffold in non-STEMI ACS

In terms of clinical outcomes, little data are available with regard specifically to non-STEMI ACS as the presence of thrombus-containing lesions was an exclusion criterion in the initial proof-of-concept trials. With regard to the acute procedural data, data from POLAR-ACS, the Polish National Registry (about 50% of the patients with ACS), the GHOST-EU (47% ACS), and AMC PCI registries (39% ACS) documented the safety of BVS implantation [28,42–44]. In line with this, target lesion failure rates at 6 months between 5 and 8% have been reported, similar to those in metals stents [27,28,43]. Interesting data were published in two important randomized-controlled trials: in the EVERBIO II, which compared ABSORB BVS with two types of metal stents, 9-month late lumen loss (the primary endpoint of the study) did not differ among treatment groups [45]. In this trial, subgroup analyses revealed an interaction between ACS and late loss, with a trend toward more neointima formation in the BVS group. The extent of neointima proliferation in this study, however, was larger than that reported by our group, and these observations remain to be confirmed [46]. With regard to more prolonged periods of observation, data are available from two large registries. In our recent paper [35], the rate of the composite endpoint of death, target lesion revascularization, and myocardial infarction was in the range of 13.5% at 1 year, higher than expected when compared to those previously observed in BVS-treated stable patients [30], but comparable with analogous figures in DES-treated patients [47–51]. In the GHOST-EU registry, a multicentric registry enrolling 1477 patients, ACSs were a predictor of both patient-oriented and device-oriented endpoints (unpublished data). In the first database of our group (n = 342), index presentation was a predictor of patient-oriented, but not of device-oriented endpoints (Figure 7.6.4). Of importance, both the GHOST-EU and our single center register provided evidence of a higher-than

expected incidence of in scaffold thrombosis, but the incidence of this event was not affected by the clinical presentation at index [46]. The recently published randomized trials with the ABSORB BVS included patients with stabilized ACSs along with patients with stable angina, but specific post-hoc analyses are not yet available. In the ABSORB III trial, 386 patients in the ABSORB group and 181 in the XIENCE group were treated for unstable angina or recent myocardial infarction. The incidence of the primary endpoint target lesion failure (cardiac death, target vessel myocardial infarction, and ischemia-driven target lesion failure) was 6.5 and 6.6 in the two groups, with an HR of 0.98 (050–1.90) [52].

Insufficient data are currently available with other scaffold platforms. Potential advantages of the DESolve platform include a larger range of expansion and a degree of "self-expansion," which might represent an advantage in thrombotic lesions [53,54]. However, no data on ACSs are currently available.

## CONCLUSIONS

Clinical experience of BVS implantation in non-STEMI ACSs remains limited, but insights from large registries and preliminary data from one randomized trial suggest that it is associated with good acute and midterm performance. While the importance of lesion preparation and adequate vessel sizing (particularly in the setting of spasm and intravascular thrombus) needs to be emphasized, the evidence supporting the biological rationale for use of scaffolds in ACS and the clinical literature available to date appear to suggest that this might remain one of the major indications for this novel technology.

## REFERENCES

1. American College of Emergency P, Society for Cardiovascular A, Interventions et al. 2013 ACCF/AHA guideline for the management of ST-elevation myocardial infarction: A report of the American College of Cardiology Foundation/American Heart Association Task Force on Practice Guidelines. *J Am Coll Cardiol.* 2013;61:e78–140.
2. Antman EM, Cohen M, Bernink PJ et al. The TIMI risk score for unstable angina/non-ST elevation MI: A method for prognostication and therapeutic decision making. *JAMA.* 2000;284:835–42.
3. Thygesen K, Alpert JS, Jaffe AS et al. Third universal definition of myocardial infarction. *Eur Heart J.* 2012;33:2551–67.
4. Rioufol G, Finet G, Ginon I et al. Multiple atherosclerotic plaque rupture in acute coronary syndrome: A three-vessel intravascular ultrasound study. *Circulation.* 2002;106:804–8.
5. Wang JC, Normand SL, Mauri L, Kuntz RE. Coronary artery spatial distribution of acute myocardial infarction occlusions. *Circulation.* 2004;110:278–84.

6. Davies MJ, Thomas AC. Plaque fissuring—The cause of acute myocardial infarction, sudden ischaemic death, and crescendo angina. *Br Heart J.* 1985;53:363–73.

7. Davies MJ, Woolf N, Rowles PM, Pepper J. Morphology of the endothelium over atherosclerotic plaques in human coronary arteries. *Br Heart J.* 1988;60:459–64.

8. Quyyumi AA. Prognostic value of endothelial function. *Am J Coll Cardiol.* 2003;91:19H–24H.

9. Khan BV, Harrison DG, Olbrych MT, Alexander RW, Medford RM. Nitric oxide regulates vascular cell adhesion molecule 1 gene expression and redox-sensitive transcriptional events in human vascular endothelial cells. *Proc Natl Acad Sci USA.* 1996;93:9114–9.

10. Hansson GK. Inflammation, atherosclerosis, and coronary artery disease. *New Engl J Med.* 2005;352:1685–95.

11. Ambrose JA, Singh M. Pathophysiology of coronary artery disease leading to acute coronary syndromes. F1000prime reports 2015;7:08.

12. Srikanth S, Ambrose JA. Pathophysiology of coronary thrombus formation and adverse consequences of thrombus during PCI. *Curr Cardiol Rev.* 2012;8:168–76.

13. Virmani R, Kolodgie FD, Burke AP, Farb A, Schwartz SM. Lessons from sudden coronary death: A comprehensive morphological classification scheme for atherosclerotic lesions. *Arterioscl Throm Vasc Biol.* 2000;20:1262–75.

14. Burke AP, Kolodgie FD, Farb A et al. Healed plaque ruptures and sudden coronary death: Evidence that subclinical rupture has a role in plaque progression. *Circulation.* 2001;103:934–40.

15. Glagov S, Weisenberg E, Zarins CK, Stankunavicius R, Kolettis GJ. Compensatory enlargement of human atherosclerotic coronary arteries. *New Engl J Med.* 1987;316:1371–5.

16. Bonz AW, Lengenfelder B, Strotmann J et al. Effect of additional temporary glycoprotein IIb/IIIa receptor inhibition on troponin release in elective percutaneous coronary interventions after pretreatment with aspirin and clopidogrel (TOPSTAR trial). *J Am Coll Cardiol.* 2002;40:662–8.

17. Goldberg A, Zinder O, Zdorovyak A et al. Diagnostic coronary angiography induces a systemic inflammatory response in patients with stable angina. *Am Heart J.* 2003;146:819–23.

18. Almagor M, Keren A, Banai S. Increased C-reactive protein level after coronary stent implantation in patients with stable coronary artery disease. *Am Heart J.* 2003;145:248–53.

19. Aggarwal A, Blum A, Schneider DJ, Sobel BE, Dauerman HL. Soluble CD40 ligand is an early initiator of inflammation after coronary intervention. *Coron Artery Dis.* 2004;15:471–5.

20. Aggarwal A, Schneider DJ, Sobel BE, Dauerman HL. Comparison of inflammatory markers in patients with diabetes mellitus versus those without before and after coronary arterial stenting. *Am J Coll Cardiol.* 2003;92:924–9.

21. Aggarwal A, Schneider DJ, Terrien EF, Gilbert KE, Dauerman HL. Increase in interleukin-6 in the first hour after coronary stenting: An early marker of the inflammatory response. *J Thromb Thrombolysis.* 2003;15:25–31.

22. Aggarwal A, Schneider DJ, Terrien EF, Terrien CM, Jr., Sobel BE, Dauerman HL. Comparison of effects of abciximab versus eptifibatide on C-reactive protein, interleukin-6, and interleukin-1 receptor antagonist after coronary arterial stenting. *Am J Cardiol.* 2003;91:1346–9.

23. Park DW, Yun SC, Lee JY et al. C-reactive protein and the risk of stent thrombosis and cardiovascular events after drug-eluting stent implantation. *Circulation.* 2009;120:1987–95.

24. Puricel S, Kallinikou Z, Espinola J et al. Comparison of endothelium-dependent and -independent vasomotor response after abluminal biodegradable polymer biolimus-eluting stent and persistent polymer everolimus-eluting stent implantation (COMPARE-IT). *Int J Cardiol.* 2016;202:525–31.

25. Onuma Y, Serruys PW. Bioresorbable scaffold: The advent of a new era in percutaneous coronary and peripheral revascularization? *Circulation.* 2011;123:779–97.

26. Iqbal J, Onuma Y, Ormiston J, Abizaid A, Waksman R, Serruys P. Bioresorbable scaffolds: Rationale, current status, challenges, and future. *Eur Heart J.* 2014;35:765–76.

27. Gori T, Schulz E, Hink U et al. Early outcome after implantation of Absorb bioresorbable drug-eluting scaffolds in patients with acute coronary syndromes. *EuroIntervention.* 2014;9:1036–41.

28. Capodanno D, Gori T, Nef H et al. Percutaneous coronary intervention with everolimus-eluting bioresorbable vascular scaffolds in routine clinical practice: Early and midterm outcomes from the European multicentre GHOST-EU registry. *EuroIntervention.* 2015;10:1144–53.

29. Brugaletta S, Radu MD, Garcia-Garcia HM et al. Circumferential evaluation of the neointima by optical coherence tomography after ABSORB bioresorbable vascular scaffold implantation: Can the scaffold cap the plaque? *Atherosclerosis.* 2012;221:106–12.

30. Serruys PW, Onuma Y, Dudek D et al. Evaluation of the second generation of a bioresorbable everolimus-eluting vascular scaffold for the treatment of de novo coronary artery stenosis: 12-month clinical and imaging outcomes. *J Am Coll Cardiol.* 2011;58:1578–88.

31. Brugaletta S, Gogas BD, Garcia-Garcia HM et al. Vascular compliance changes of the coronary vessel wall after bioresorbable vascular scaffold implantation in the treated and adjacent segments. *Circ J.* 2012;76:1616–23.

32. Park SJ, Kang SJ, Virmani R, Nakano M, Ueda Y. In-stent neoatherosclerosis: A final common pathway of late stent failure. *J Am Coll Cardiol.* 2012;59:2051–7.

33. Bourantas CV, Farooq V, Zhang Y et al. Circumferential distribution of the neointima at six-month and two-year follow-up after a bioresorbable vascular scaffold implantation: A substudy of the ABSORB Cohort B Clinical Trial. *EuroIntervention.* 2015;10:1299–306.

34. Bourantas CV, Serruys PW, Nakatani S et al. Bioresorbable vascular scaffold treatment induces the formation of neointimal cap that seals the underlying plaque without compromising the luminal dimensions: A concept based on serial optical coherence tomography data. *EuroIntervention.* 2015;11:746–56.

35. Gori T, Schulz E, Hink U et al. Clinical, angiographic, functional, and imaging outcomes 12 months after implantation of drug-eluting bioresorbable vascular scaffolds in acute coronary syndromes. *JACC Cardiovasc Interv.* 2015;8:770–7.

36. Onuma Y, Serruys PW, Perkins LE et al. Intracoronary optical coherence tomography and histology at 1 month and 2, 3, and 4 years after implantation of everolimus-eluting bioresorbable vascular scaffolds in a porcine coronary artery model: An attempt to decipher the human optical coherence tomography images in the ABSORB trial. *Circulation.* 2010;122:2288–300.

37. Serruys PW, Ormiston JA, Onuma Y et al. A bioabsorbable everolimus-eluting coronary stent system (ABSORB): 2-year outcomes and results from multiple imaging methods. *Lancet.* 2009;373:897–910.

38. Brugaletta S, Gomez-Lara J, Garcia-Garcia HM et al. Analysis of 1 year virtual histology changes in coronary plaque located behind the struts of the everolimus eluting bioresorbable vascular scaffold. *Int J Cardiovasc Imaging.* 2012;28:1307–14.

39. Martinet W, Verheye S, De Meyer GR. Everolimus-induced mTOR inhibition selectively depletes macrophages in atherosclerotic plaques by autophagy. *Autophagy.* 2007;3:241–4.

40. Hong MK, Park DW, Lee CW et al. Effects of statin treatments on coronary plaques assessed by volumetric virtual histology intravascular ultrasound analysis. *JACC Cardiovasc Interv.* 2009;2:679–88.

41. Montalescot G, Sechtem U, Achenbach S et al. 2013 ESC guidelines on the management of stable coronary artery disease: The Task Force on the management of stable coronary artery disease of the European Society of Cardiology. *Eur Heart J.* 2013;34:2949–3003.

42. Dudek D, Rzeszutko L, Zasada W et al. Bioresorbable vascular scaffolds in patients with acute coronary syndromes: The POLAR ACS study. *Pol Arch Med Wewm.* 2014;124:669–77.

43. Kraak RP, Hassell ME, Grundeken MJ et al. Initial experience and clinical evaluation of the Absorb bioresorbable vascular scaffold (BVS) in real-world practice: The AMC Single Centre Real World PCI Registry. *EuroIntervention.* 2015;10:1160–8.

44. Rzeszutko L, Siudak Z, Wlodarczak A et al. Use of bioresorbable vascular scaffolds in patients with stable angina and acute coronary syndromes. Polish National Registry. *Kardiol Pol.* 2014;72:1394–9.

45. Puricel S, Arroyo D, Corpataux N et al. Comparison of everolimus- and biolimus-eluting coronary stents with everolimus-eluting bioresorbable vascular scaffolds. *J Am Coll Cardiol.* 2015;65:791–801.

46. Puricel S, Cuculi F, Weissner M et al. Bioresorbable coronary scaffold thrombosis: Multicenter comprehensive analysis of clinical presentation, mechanisms, and predictors. *J Am Coll Cardiol.* 2016;67:921–31.

47. Raber L, Kelbaek H, Ostojic M et al. Effect of biolimus-eluting stents with biodegradable polymer vs bare-metal stents on cardiovascular events among patients with acute myocardial infarction: The COMFORTABLE AMI randomized trial. *JAMA.* 2012;308:777–87.

48. Kang WC, Ahn T, Lee K et al. Comparison of zotarolimus-eluting stents versus sirolimus-eluting stents versus paclitaxel-eluting stents for primary percutaneous coronary intervention in patients with ST-elevation myocardial infarction: Results from the Korean Multicentre Endeavor (KOMER) acute myocardial infarction (AMI) trial. *EuroIntervention.* 2011;7:936–43.

49. Palmerini T, Genereux P, Caixeta A et al. Prognostic value of the SYNTAX score in patients with acute coronary syndromes undergoing percutaneous coronary intervention: Analysis from the ACUITY (Acute Catheterization and Urgent Intervention Triage StrategY) trial. *J Am Coll Cardiol.* 2011;57:2389–97.

50. Dvir D, Barbash IM, Torguson R et al. Clinical outcomes after treating acute coronary syndrome patients with a drug-eluting stent: Results from REWARDS-EMI (Endeavor for Myocardial Infarction Registry). *Cardiovasc Revasc Med.* 2013;14:128–33.

51. Sabate M, Cequier A, Iniguez A et al. Everolimus-eluting stent versus bare-metal stent in ST-segment elevation myocardial infarction (EXAMINATION): 1 year results of a randomised controlled trial. *Lancet.* 2012;380:1482–90.

52. Ellis SG, Kereiakes DJ, Metzger DC et al. Everolimus-eluting bioresorbable scaffolds for coronary artery disease. *New Engl J Med.* 2015;373:1905–15.

53. Verheye S, Ormiston JA, Stewart J et al. A next-generation bioresorbable coronary scaffold system: From bench to first clinical evaluation: 6- and 12-month clinical and multimodality imaging results. *JACC Cardiovasc Interv.* 2014;7:89–99.

54. Wiebe J, Bauer T, Dorr O, Mollmann H, Hamm CW, Nef HM. Implantation of a novolimus-eluting bioresorbable scaffold with a strut thickness of 100 microm showing evidence of self-correction. *EuroIntervention.* 2015;11:204.

# Bioresorbable vascular scaffold in ST-segment elevation myocardial infarction: Clinical evidence, tips, and tricks

GIUSEPPE GIACCHI AND MANEL SABATÉ

## INTRODUCTION

Primary percutaneous coronary intervention (PCI) with drug eluting stent (DESs) is nowadays the gold standard treatment for patients presenting with ST-segment elevation myocardial infarction (STEMI) [1]. However, permanent delivery of metallic platform is affected by several drawbacks, such as caging and jailing of the vessels, impairment of vasomotion, and impossibility of lumen enlargement [2]. Furthermore, PCI in the context of STEMI portends a higher risk of acute and late acquired stent malapposition than that in stable patients, due to common presence of vasospasm and thrombus sequestration behind the struts [3,4]. For these reasons, bioresorbable vascular scaffold (BRSs) could be a good therapeutic option to overcome metallic stent drawbacks.

## BRSs: A NEW THERAPEUTIC TOOL FOR STEMI PATIENTS

Patients suffering from a STEMI are often young and therefore with long life expectancy. Ruptured plaques are usually soft in nature with relatively small plaque burden. Most of the current evidence by the use of BRSs resides in the experience of the ABSORB™ bioabsorbable scaffold (Abbott Vascular, Santa Clara, CA). The structure of the ABSORB BRSs with thick struts linked by straight bridges helps create a rough plane that promotes the formation of a thin layer of neointimal tissue which eventually may lead to a reduction in the risk of thrombosis [5,6]. Moreover, at long-term follow-up the implantation of an ABSORB BRSs is associated with lumen enlargement, side branch patency, struts reabsorption, and recovery of physiological reactivity to vasoactive stimuli [7,8]. Finally, the complete bioresorption of polymeric struts may also be associated with a reduction

in the incidence of angina during follow-up (REF ABSORB 2). Taken together, all these data support the concept of "plaque sealing." Theoretically then, STEMI patients may benefit more from temporary polymeric caging than from permanent stent implantation [9].

## BRSs IN STEMI: DATA FROM REGISTRIES AND CLINICAL TRIALS

Current available data are mostly limited to observational registries and a few ongoing randomized trials (Tables 7.7.1 and 7.7.2).

1. *Single-center registries:* Several registries reported a 1-month MACE rate ranging between 2.6% and 10.7% [10–12]. Besides, Gori et al. compared outcomes of BRSs patients with a control group of patients treated with XIENCE (Abbott, Abbott Park, IL), showing comparable results at 1- and 6-months follow-up [12]. Wiebe et al also evaluated in a single-center fashion the performance of BRSs in STEMI showing a MACE rate of 8.3% at 137 days [13]. Kochman et al in an optical coherence tomography study demonstrated a high strut apposition rate (>95%) immediately after implantation and only one instance of subacute scaffold thrombosis [14]. The POLAR-ACS Registry included patients with acute coronary syndrome (16% STEMI) showing a 2% MACE rate at 1-year follow-up [20].
2. *Multicenter registries:* Several multicenter registries also included patients with STEMI. The Polish National Registry (11% of STEMI) showed good acute clinical and angiographic outcomes (technical success 100%) [22]. The GHOST-EU (16% STEMI) and AMC PCI registry (13% STEMI) showed a target lesion failure rate at 6 months of 4.4% and 8.5%, respectively

369

**Table 7.7.1** Published registry and clinical trials

| Study title | Study type/design | Number of patients | STEMI (%) | Primary outcome | Reference number |
|---|---|---|---|---|---|
| AMC PCI Registry | Prospective, observational registry, open label patients who were enrolled according to operator's discretion | 135 | 13.0 | Angiographic success (residual stenosis <30% with TIMI 3 flow) = 96%<br>TVF (all-cause mortality, MI, TVR) at 6 months = 8.5% | [15] |
| ASSURE registry | Prospective, multi-center registry, that enrolled consecutive patients with lesion length <28 mm, vessel diameter between 2.0 and 3.3 mm | 183 | 27 | Procedural success = 100%<br>MACE (cardiovascular death, MI, ischemia driven TLR) at 1 year = 5% | [16] |
| BVS-EXAMINATION Study | Retrospective, multi-center trial, comparing a cluster of STEMI-BRSs consecutive patients with another two of STEMI-XIENCE/BMS patients (EXAMINATION population) | 290 | 100 | DOCE (cardiac death, TVre-MI, TLR) at 1 year – p BRSs/DESs = 0.994 (BRSs 4.1% – DESs 4.1%)<br>p BRSs/BMS = 0.306 (BRSs 4.1% – BMS 5.9%) | [17] |
| BVS STEMI first study | Non randomized, prospective, single arm study | 49 | 100 | – Device success (BRSs delivery with residual stenosis <30%) = 97.9%<br>– Procedural success (device success and no major periprocedural complications) = 97.9%<br>– Clinical success (procedural success and no in–hospital MACE) = 97.9%<br>– Device-oriented TLF (cardiac death, target-vessel MI, ischemia-driven TLR) at 30 days = 0%<br>– MACE (cardiac death, any re-MI, emergent CABG, or clinically driven TLR) at 30 days = 2.6%<br>– TVF (cardiac death, target-vessel MI, clinically driven TVR) at 30 days = 0% | [12] |
| EVERBIO II | Randomized, assessor-blinded, single center, all-comers study, comparing BRSs with DESs Promus Element and Biomatrix Flex (randomization ratio 1:1:1) | 240 | 10 | Late lumen loss at nine months – p BRSs/DESs = 0.30 (BRSs 0.28 ± 0.39 mm – DES 0.25 ± 0.36 mm) | [18] |
| GHOST-EU registry | Retrospective, multicenter registry, open label patients | 1189 | 16.1 | TLF (cardiac death, TV-MI, clinically driven TLR) at six months = 4.4% | [19] |
| Gori T et al. | Prospective, consecutive ACS-patients treated with BRSs. Control group of patients treated with XIENCE | 150 | 44 | MACE (death, non fatal MI, any PCI) at 30 days = $p > 0.8$ (BRSs 10.7%, DES 15.5%) | [11] |

(Continued)

**Table 7.7.1 (Continued)** Published registry and clinical trials

| Study title | Study type/design | Number of patients | STEMI (%) | Primary outcome | Reference number |
|---|---|---|---|---|---|
| Kochman J et al. | Single arm registry, open label patients with STEMI | 23 | 100 | – Device success = 100%<br>– Procedural success = 95.7%<br>– Clinical success = 95.7%<br>– OCT analysis: struts well apposed 95.4 ± 7.96% – struts malapposed 4.6 ± 5.71% – minimum lumen diameter 2.6 ± 0.35 mm – minimum scaffold area 6.9 ± 1.54 mm² – final residual stenosis 8.8 ± 24.37% – edge dissections 7.7%<br>– Clinical adverse events at follow-up: 1 MI at 229 (199–248) days | [14] |
| Kajiya T et al. | Registry, single group, STEMI patients who underwent PCI with intent of BRSs | 11 | 100 | MACE (cardiac death, MI, TVR) at 1 month = 9.1% | [10] |
| POLAR ACS Study | Prospective, single group registry with consecutive patients presenting ACS | 100 | 16 | MACE (death, MI, clinically driven TLR) at 1 year = 2% | [20] |
| Prague 19 | Prospective registry, consecutive STEMI patients with lesion length <24 mm, culprit vessel caliber between 2.3 and 3.7 mm | 41 | 100 | Device success (BRSs delivery with residual stenosis ≤20%) = 98%<br>MACE (death, MI, TVR) at 6 months = 5% | [21] |
| Polish National Registry | Retrospective, single group, open label patients who had a previous PCI with BRSs | 591 | 11 | Technical success (successful BRSs delivery) 100%, dissection 2.9%, slow-flow 0.5%, no-reflow 0.17%, side branch occlusion 0.33% | [22] |
| RAI registry | Prospective, single arm registry, open label lesions with 2.2 mm ≤RVD ≤3.7 mm, depending on operator's discretion | 74 | 100 | Procedural success (successful BRSs delivery, residual stenosis <30%, TIMI 3 flow without in-hospital MACE – cardiac death, MI, emergent revascularization) = 97.4%<br>MACE (cardiac death, MI, TLR, BRSs thrombosis) at 6 months = 8.1% | [23] |
| TROFI II study | Prospective, randomized (1 BRSs:1 XIENCE), single blinded, non-inferiority trial | 190 | 100 | HS lower in the BRSs arm vs. XIENCE arm (1.74 vs. 2.80; difference [90% CI] –1.06 [–1.96, –0.16]; $p_{\text{non-inferiority}}$, 0.001) | |
| Wiebe J et al. | Registry, single group, STEMI patients who underwent PCI with intent of BRSs | 25 | 100 | – Implant success (BRSs delivery with residual stenosis <30%) = 96.8%<br>– MACE (cardiac death, TV-MI, TVR) at 137.0 days (70.0 – 186.0) = 8.3% | [13] |

*Abbreviations:* ACS = acute coronary syndrome; BMS = bare metal stent; BRSs = bioresorbable vascular scaffold; CABG = coronary artery bypass graft; DESs = drug eluting stent; DOCE = device-oriented endpoint; MACE = major adverse cardiovascular event; MI = myocardial infarction; OCT = optical coherence tomography; PCI = percutaneous coronary intervention; RVD = reference vessel diameter; STEMI = ST-elevation myocardial infarction; TIMI = thrombolysis in myocardial infarction; TLF = target vessel failure; TLR = target lesion revascularization; TVF = target vessel failure; TV-MI = target vessel myocardial infarction; TVR = target vessel revascularization; TVre-MI = target vessel re-myocardial infarction.

**Table 7.7.2** Ongoing registry and randomized clinical trials

| Study title | Study type/design | Number of patients | STEMI (%) | Primary outcome | Status | ClinicalTrials.org number |
|---|---|---|---|---|---|---|
| ABSORB-ACS | Prospective registry, open label patients | 300 | Not provided | – MACE (death, MI, TLR, TVR and scaffold thrombosis) at 30 days and 1 year | Recruiting | NCT02071342 |
| ABSORB BVS | Prospective, multicenter registry, open label patients with de novo coronary artery lesions | 1801 | Not provided | Cardiac death, TV-MI, ischemia driven TLR at 1 year | Ongoing, not recruiting | NCT01759290 |
| ABSORB UK | Prospective, single arm, post-market registry | 1000 | Not provided | – Device success: BRSs delivery with residual stenosis <50%<br>– Procedural success: device success with no cardiac death, TV-MI, TLR within 3 days of index procedure<br>– MACE (cardiac death, MI, ischemia driven TLR) at 1 and 3 years | Recruiting | NCT01977534 |
| AIDA | Prospective, randomized (1 BRSs:1 XIENCE), single blinded, all-comers, non-inferiority trial | 2690 | Not provided | TVF (cardiac death, MI, TVR) at 2 years | Recruiting | NCT01858077 |
| Bioresorbable Vascular Scaffold in Patients With Myocardial Infarction | Prospective, randomized (BRSs vs. XIENCE), open label trial | 100 | 100 | Procedural (BRSs delivery with residual stenosis <20%, TIMI 2-3 flow without major complications) and clinical (deaths, re-MI, urgent revascularization, stroke, major bleedings) success for the duration of hospital stay (4–8 days) | Completed, but results pending | NCT02151929 |
| BVS in STEMI | Prospective, randomized (BRSs vs. XIENCE), non blinded, open label trial | 120 | 100 | Coronary Stent Healing Index at 1 year | Recruiting | NCT02067091 |
| BVS-RAI | Prospective registry, open label patients younger than 75-year old and successful delivery of at least 1 BRSs | 2000 | Not provided | Scaffold thrombosis and TLR at 1 year | Recruiting | NCT02298413 |

(Continued)

**Table 7.7.2 (Continued)** Ongoing registry and randomized clinical trials

| Study title | Study type/design | Number of patients | STEMI (%) | Primary outcome | Status | ClinicalTrials.org number |
|---|---|---|---|---|---|---|
| CSI-Ulm-BVS | Non randomized, single group, open label patients with planned delivery of at least 1 BRSs | 2000 | Not provided | MACE at 10 years | Recruiting | NCT02162056 |
| FRANCE-ABSORB | Prospective, single arm, open label with Frances patients in de novo coronary lesions | 2000 | Not provided | MACE (death, MI, ischemia driven TLR, CABG) at 1 year | Recruiting | NCT02238054 |
| ISAR-ABSORB MI | Prospective, randomized (BRSs vs. XIENCE), non-inferiority, open label patients with STEMI and planned stenting in vessels with 2.5 mm ≤RVD ≤3.9 mm | 260 | 100 | Percentage diameter stenosis at coronary angiography at 6–8 months follow-up | Recruiting | NCT01942070 |
| IT-Disappears | Non randomized, single group, open label patients with multivessel disease, or single lesions >24 mm | 1000 | Not provided | MACE (cardiac death, non-fatal MI, clinically driven TLR) at 1 year | Recruiting | NCT02004730 |
| PROSPECT II & PROSPECT ABSORB | Multicenter, prospective, randomized (BRSs treatment of vulnerable plaques vs. optical medical therapy) of patients with ACS and plaques prone to rupture and future clinical events | 900 | Not provided | – Patient level non-culprit lesion related MACE at 2 years (PROSPECT II)<br>– MLA in vessel with vulnerable plaques at 2 years (PROSPECT ABSORB) | Recruiting | NCT02171065 |
| REPARA study | Prospective registry, patients with lesion length <28 mm and 2.0 mm ≤RVD ≤3.8 mm | 1500 | Not provided | MACE (cardiac death, MI, ischemia driven TLR) at 1 year | Recruiting | NCT02256449 |

*Source:* All data from www-clinicaltrials.gov.
*Abbreviations:* ACS = acute coronary syndrome; BRSs = bioresorbable vascular scaffold; CABG = coronary artery bypass graft; MACE = major adverse cardiovascular event; MI = myocardial infarction; MLA = minimal lumen area; OCT = optical coherence tomography; RVD = reference vessel diameter; STEMI = ST-elevation myocardial infarction; TIMI = thrombolysis in myocardial infarction; TLR = target lesion revascularization; TVF = target vessel failure; TV-MI = target vessel myocardial infarction; TVR = target vessel revascularization.

[15,19]. Of note, the cumulative incidence of definite/probable scaffold thrombosis was rather high (2.1% in GHOST-EU registry and 3.0% in AMC PCI registry). The ASSURE Registry (27% STEMI) showed a rather low MACE rate at 1 year (5%) [16]. The Prague 19 and the RAI registries focused exclusively on STEMI [21,23]. Both registries reported encouraging midterm results. In the Prague 19, BRSs patients were compared with a control group (treated with metallic stent), showing similar outcomes.

3. *Propensity score matching comparison:* The BVS-EXAMINATION Study was designed to compare the 1-year outcome between the ABSORB BRSs and the everolimus-eluting metallic stent (EES) and bare metal stent (BMS) in STEMI [17]. A total of 290 consecutive STEMI treated by BRSs were matched with 290 STEMI subjects treated with EESs and 290 treated with BMS. Primary endpoint was device-oriented endpoint. Device thrombosis rate was also investigated. The three groups achieved a similar primary outcome rate at 1 year (4.1%, 4.1%, and 5%, respectively). Device thrombosis rate was numerically but not significantly higher by the use of BRSs (2.4% vs. 1.4% in the EES and 1.7% in the BMS arm) [17].

4. *Randomized-controlled trials:* EVERBIO II is a randomized trial containing STEMI treated with BRSs (10% of enrolled BRSs subjects) [18]. A total of 240 patients were randomly assigned 1:1:1 to BRSs or EES (Promus Element; Boston Scientific, Marlborough, MA) or biolimus-eluting stent (Biomatrix Flex, Biosensors Europe SA, Morges, Switzerland). Late lumen loss as primary endpoint did not differ between groups. The ABSORB STEMI TROFI II trial randomized 190 STEMI patients to either BRSs or EES.

Primary endpoint was arterial healing at 6-month follow-up as measured by optical coherence tomography. As a result, healing score in the BRSs arm was comparable with that of metallic EES at 6 months [24]. Among the ongoing randomized trials, the ISAR-ABSORB-MI trial (NCT01942070) with an angiographic outcome at 9 months will shed light on the safety and midterm efficacy of these devices as compared to second-generation DESs.

## PROCEDURAL ASPECTS: BRSs PITFALLS AND TECHNICAL TRICKS

Although preliminary clinical experience with BRSs in STEMI is promising, several concerns have arisen from initial registries.

Scaffold thrombosis appeared to be a non-negligible drawback of polymeric scaffolds [17–19,25] (Figure 7.7.1). Scaffold thrombosis can be linked to several factors. First, current generation BRSs present a rather bulky structure (strut thickness ≈150 μm) [26]. Acute and chronic inflammatory reaction following BRSs implantation could also play a role [27]. The presence of high thrombus burden in the context of STEMI and postprocedure enhanced platelet reactivity could facilitate the thrombosis [28]. Some procedure-related factors, such as acute incomplete apposition or inappropriate vessel sizing leading to scaffold infraexpansion, could also be taken into account [28,29]. Vasoconstriction of coronary arteries and the presence of thrombus are common features in the context of STEMI. These features should be taken into consideration to correctly select the scaffold size [30]. In this scenario, several thrombectomy passages and the use of

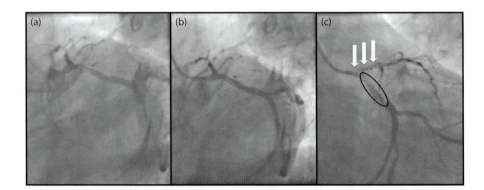

**Figure 7.7.1** Case of acute scaffold thrombosis. A 38-year-old man was admitted for STEMI secondary to thrombotic lesion of proximal left circumflex (LCx) **(a)**. After performing manual thrombectomy, a bioresorbable vascular scaffold 3.5/28 mm was delivered and postdilated with a 3.5 mm noncompliant balloon, inflated at high pressure. The patient was treated with prasugrel 60 mg bolus, aspirin 300 mg, and abciximab (bolus + infusion). Final result was good **(b)**. Twenty minutes later, the patient had a new episode of chest pain with ST-segment reelevation. Coronary angiography revealed thrombosis of the scaffold (black circle, **c**), which also involved left anterior descending and left main coronary arteries (white arrows, **c**). Despite an urgent procedure including new thrombectomy passages, postdilatation, and intra-aortic balloon pump, the patient suffered from a cardiac arrest, cardiogenic shock, electromechanical dissociation, and finally died.

intracoronary nitrates may be helpful. Although routine use of thombectomy has not demonstrated any clinical benefit in the overall population [1,31] we believe that when a BRSs is planned, the use of manual aspiration catheter may provide an additional value beyond thrombus removal and BRSs sizing; that is, the capacity to predict crossability of the lesion [30]. If predilatation is still needed after thrombectomy (i.e., residual high plaque burden), it has to be performed with a noncompliant balloon in a balloon-artery ratio 1:1 [30–32]. Postdilatation is currently advocated after BRSs implantation [33]. In the context of STEMI it is also advisable to use a noncompliant balloon and not to exceed 0.5 mm the size of the current generation BRSs. The use of intracoronary imaging is encouraged especially during the initial implants. Intravascular ultrasound imaging may facilitate correct balloon and scaffold sizing as well as evaluation of BRSs expansion. In turn, optical coherence tomography may obtain more accurate images of BRSs integrity, apposition, and presence of residual thrombus or edge dissections [30].

Antiplatelet regimen is another critical issue of BRSs in STEMI. Although no specific recommendations are given in guidelines [1], it is advisable to optimize the antithrombotic regimen in the acute phase (i.e., use of IIb/IIIa inhibitors) and to use the more potent oral agents available (prasugrel or ticagrelor). Regarding the duration of DAPT, the evidence is still lacking. However, in the event of complex procedures, with multiple overlapping scaffolds, it may be recommended to prolong DAPT up to the theoretical complete resorption of the scaffold [34].

## FUTURE BRSs DEVELOPMENTS IN STEMI

Current CE-approved BRSs (ABSORB, Abbott Vascular, Santa Clara, CA; DESolve™, Elixir Medical Corporation, Sunnyvale, CA) [35] are made of poly-lactic acid and have strut thickness of 150 μm. New BRSs platforms are currently under development (Table 7.7.3). Overall, new platforms will reduce strut thickness and improve distensibility. Besides, drug kinetics, materials, and bioresorption rate will also differ. Therefore, accurate knowledge of the new

Table 7.7.3 Bioresorbable scaffolds in clinical development

| | Scaffold | Strut thickness | Distensibility |
|---|---|---|---|
| Poly-lactic acid platform | | | |
| | ArterioSorb (Arterius, Breadford, UK) | <150 μm up to 3.5 mm size | No |
| | DESolve AMI (Elixir Medical Corporation, Sunnyvale, CA) | 100 μm | Self-correct to 0.25 mm above nominal diameter |
| | Fortitude (Amaranth Medical, Mountain View, CA) | 120 μm | Possible 1 mm overexpansion |
| | MeRes (Meril Lifescience, Vapi, Gujarat, India) | 100 μm | No |
| | Mirage Microfiber Scaffold (ManLi Cardiology, Singapore, Republic of Singapore) | 125 μm up to 3.0 mm size | No |
| Tyrosine polycarbonate alloy | | | |
| | REVA Fantom (Reva Medical Inc., San Diego, CA) | 125 μm | One of 3.0 mm caliber can be postdilated up to 4.87 mm |
| | REVA ReZolve (Reva Medical Inc., San Diego, CA) | 122 μm | Not reported |
| Magnesium structure | | | |
| | AMS series (Biotronik, Berlin, Germany) | No (165 μm) | Allowed > 2.0 mm postdilatation |
| | DREAMS series (Biotronik, Berlin, Germany) | 120 μm for DREAMS 1.0 | Allowed > 2.0 mm postdilatation |
| Nitride iron-based framework | | | |
| | Iron-based Biocorrodible Scaffold (Lifetech Scientific Corporation, Shenzhen, China) | 70 μm | Not reported |

Source: Data from TCTmd slide presentations, BRSs 2014 meeting: http://www.tctmd.com/list.aspx?fid=968379.

devices and future trials to test the safety and efficacy of second generation BRSs are warranted.

## CONCLUSIONS

Clinical experience of BRSs implantation in STEMI is currently limited. Available data suggest good acute and mid-term performance although acute scaffold thrombosis rate appears to be higher-than-expected in a few registries. In this regard, large-scale randomized trials with long-term follow-up will provide the potentials and limitations of current generation BRSs in this context. Finally, new generation BRSs may overcome most current technical pitfalls and may therefore improve clinical outcomes.

## CLINICAL CASES

**Case #1:** A 56-year-old male was admitted with an inferior STEMI. Coronary angiography revealed thrombotic lesion on the right coronary artery (black circle, Figure 7.7.2a). Lesion was predilated with a 2.5 mm semicompliant balloon and a BRSs ABSORB 3.5/28 mm was implanted. Final angiographic result was good with TIMI 3 flow (Figure 7.7.2b). Six months later, angiographic and OCT follow-up was performed. It showed good angiographic result with complete tissue coverage of scaffold and adequate BRSs expansion and apposition (Figure 7.7.2c and d; Video 7.7.1.).

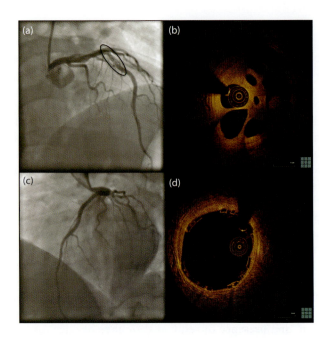

**Figure 7.7.3** Baseline angiography showing culprit lesion on LAD, with haziness and multiple filling defects (black rim, **a**). OCT imaging showed critical stenosis with a high thrombus burden, composed of multiple small channels divided by thin septa (**b**). Coronary angiography after scaffold implantation showed good results, without signs of edge dissections (**c**). OCT imaging showed good scaffold expansion and apposition (**d**).

**Case #2:** A 29-year-old male patient was emergently sent to the catheterization laboratory. Coronary angiography showed thrombotic lesion on the left anterior descending artery (black rim Figure 7.7.3a). OCT was performed, revealing a critical stenosis with high thrombus burden, composing multiple small channels (Figure 7.7.3b). An ABSORB 3.0/18 mm was delivered, with good scaffold expansion and apposition, no signs of edge dissection, and TIMI 3 flow (Figure 7.7.3c and d).

## VIDEO

**Video 7.7.1** Clinical Case #1: Optical coherence tomography at 6-month follow-up showing complete scaffold coverage, adequate expansion and apposition, without signs of edge dissections: https://youtu.be/ZKD_9QqlP0s.

## REFERENCES

1. Authors/Task Force members, Windecker S, Kolh P, Alfonso F, Collet JP, Cremer J, Falk V et al. 2014 ESC/EACTS guidelines on myocardial revascularization: The Task Force on Myocardial Revascularization of the European Society of Cardiology (ESC) and the European Association for Cardio-Thoracic Surgery (EACTS) Developed with the special contribution of the European Association of Percutaneous Cardiovascular Interventions (EAPCI). *Eur Heart J.* 2014;35:2541–619.

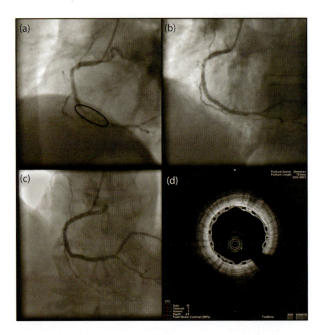

**Figure 7.7.2** Coronary angiography showed thrombotic lesion on right coronary artery (black circle, **a**). After BRSs 3.5/28 mm implantation, good angiographic result was obtained with TIMI 3 flow (**b**). Six-month angiographic follow-up revealed good result of previous procedure (**c**). Optical coherence tomography (OCT) showed complete tissue coverage of the BRSs with adequate scaffold expansion and apposition (**d**).

2. Serruys PW, Garcia-Garcia HM, Onuma Y. From metallic cages to transient bioresorbable scaffolds: Change in paradigm of coronary revascularization in the upcoming decade? *Eur Heart J.* 2012;33:16–25b.

3. Hong MK, Mintz GS, Lee CW, Kim YH, Lee SW, Song JM, Han KH et al. Incidence, mechanism, predictors, and long-term prognosis of late stent malapposition after bare-metal stent implantation. *Circulation.* 2004;109:881–6.

4. Hong MK, Mintz GS, Lee CW, Park DW, Park KM, Lee BK, Kim YH et al. Late stent malapposition after drug-eluting stent implantation: An intravascular ultrasound analysis with long-term follow-up. *Circulation.* 2006;113:414–9.

5. Scalone G, Brugaletta S, Gómez-Monterrosas O, Otsuki S, Sabaté M. Bioresorbable scaffolds: Focus on vascular response and long-term safety. *Panminerva Med.* 2015;57:1–13.

6. Brugaletta S, Radu MD, Garcia-Garcia HM, Heo JH, Farooq V, Girasis C, van Geuns RJ et al. Circumferential evaluation of the neointima by optical coherence tomography after ABSORB bioresorbable vascular scaffold implantation: Can the scaffold cap the plaque? *Atherosclerosis.* 2012;22:106–12.

7. Karanasos A, Simsek C, Gnanadesigan M, van Ditzhuijzen NS, Freire R, Dijkstra J, Tu S et al. OCT assessment of the long-term vascular healing response 5 years after everolimus-eluting bioresorbable vascular scaffold. *J Am Coll Cardiol.* 2014;64:2343–56.

8. Brugaletta S, Heo JH, Garcia-Garcia HM, Farooq V, van Geuns RJ, de Bruyne B, Dudek D et al. Endothelial-dependent vasomotion in a coronary segment treated by ABSORB everolimus-eluting bioresorbable vascular scaffold system is related to plaque composition at the time of bioresorption of the polymer: Indirect finding of vascular reparative therapy? *Eur Heart J.* 2012;33:1325–33.

9. Scalone G, Brugaletta S, Gómez-Monterrosas O, Otsuki S, Sabaté M. ST-segment elevation myocardial infarction—Ideal scenario for bioresorbable vascular scaffold implantation? *Circ J.* 2015;79(2):263–70.

10. Kajiya T, Liang M, Sharma RK, Lee CH, Chan MY, Tay E, Chan KH et al. Everolimus-eluting bioresorbable vascular scaffold (BVS) implantation in patients with ST-segment elevation myocardial infarction (STEMI). *EuroIntervention.* 2013;9:501–4.

11. Gori T, Schulz E, Hink U, Wenzel P, Post F, Jabs A, Münzel T. Early outcome after implantation of ABSORB bioresorbable drug-eluting scaffolds in patients with acute coronary syndromes. *EuroIntervention.* 2014;9:1036–41.

12. Diletti R, Karanasos A, Muramatsu T, Nakatani S, Van Mieghem NM, Onuma Y, Nauta ST et al. Everolimus-eluting bioresorbable vascular scaffolds for treatment of patients presenting with ST-segment elevation myocardial infarction: BVS STEMI first study. *Eur Heart J.* 2014;35:777–86.

13. Wiebe J, Möllmann H, Most A, Dörr O, Weipert K, Rixe J, Liebetrau C et al. Short-term outcome of patients with ST-segment elevation myocardial infarction (STEMI) treated with an everolimus-eluting bioresorbable vascular scaffold. *Clin Res Cardiol.* 2014;103:141–8.

14. Kochman J, Tomaniak M, Pietrasik A, Kołtowski L, Rdzanek A, Huczek Z, Mazurek T et al. Bioresorbable everolimus-eluting vascular scaffold in patients with ST-segment elevation myocardial infarction: Optical coherence tomography evaluation and clinical outcomes. *Cardiol J.* 2015;22(3):315–22.

15. Kraak RP, Hassell ME, Grundeken MJ, Koch KT, Henriques JP, Piek JJ, Baan J Jr et al. Initial experience and clinical evaluation of the ABSORB bioresorbable vascular scaffold (BVS) in real-world practice: The AMC Single Centre Real World PCI Registry. *EuroIntervention.* 2015;10(10):1160–8.

16. Wöhrle J, Naber C, Schmitz T, Schwencke C, Frey N, Butter C, Brachmann J et al. Beyond the early stages: Insights from the ASSURE registry on bioresorbable vascular scaffolds. *EuroIntervention.* 2015;11(2):149–56.

17. Brugaletta S, Gori T, Low AF, Tousek P, Pinar E, Gomez-Lara J, Scalone G et al. ABSORB bioresorbable vascular scaffold versus everolimus-eluting metallic stent in St-segment elevation myocardial infarction: 1-year results of a propensity score matching comparison: The BVS-EXAMINATION Study (Bioresorbable Vascular Scaffold-A Clinical Evaluation of Everolimus Eluting Coronary Stents in the Treatment of Patients With ST-segment Elevation Myocardial Infarction). *JACC Cardiovasc Interv.* 2015;8:189–97.

18. Puricel S, Arroyo D, Corpataux N, Baeriswyl G, Lehmann S, Kallinikou Z, Muller O et al. Comparison of everolimus- and biolimus-eluting coronary stents with everolimus-eluting bioresorbable vascular scaffolds. *J Am Coll Cardiol.* 2015;65:791–801.

19. Capodanno D, Gori T, Nef H, Latib A, Mehilli J, Lesiak M, Caramanno G et al. Percutaneous coronary intervention with everolimus-eluting bioresorbable vascular scaffolds in routine clinical practice: Early and midterm outcomes from the European multicentre GHOST-EU registry. *EuroIntervention.* 2015;10(10):1144–53

20. Dudek D, Rzeszutko Ł, Zasada W, Depukat R, Siudak Z, Ochała A, Wojakowski W et al. Bioresorbable vascular scaffolds in patients with acute coronary syndromes: The POLAR ACS study. *Pol Arch Med Wewn.* 2014;124:669–77.

21. Kočka V, Malý M, Toušek P, Buděšínský T, Lisa L, Prodanov P, Jarkovský J et al. Bioresorbable vascular scaffolds in acute ST-segment elevation myocardial infarction: A prospective multicentre study 'Prague 19'. *Eur Heart J.* 2014;35:787–94.

22. Rzeszutko Ł, Siudak Z, Włodarczak A, Lekston A, Depukat R, Ochała A, Gil RJ et al. Use of bioresorbable vascular scaffolds in patients with stable angina and acute coronary syndromes. Polish National Registry. *Kardiol Pol.* 2014;72:1394–9.

23. Ielasi A, Cortese B, Varricchio A, Tespili M, Sesana M, Pisano F, Loi B et al. Immediate and midterm outcomes following primary PCI with bioresorbable vascular scaffold implantation in patients with ST-segment myocardial infarction: Insights from the multicentre "Registro ABSORB Italiano" (RAI registry). *EuroIntervention.* 2015;11(2):157–62.

24. Sabaté M, Windecker S, Iñiguez A, Okkels-Jensen L, Cequier A, Brugaletta S, Hofma SH, Räber L, Christiansen EH, Suttorp M, Pilgrim T, Anne van Es G, Sotomi Y, García-García HM, Onuma Y, Serruys PW. Everolimus-eluting bioresorbable stent vs. durable polymer everolimus-eluting metallic stent in patients with ST-segment elevation myocardial infarction: Results of the randomized ABSORB ST-segment elevation myocardial infarction-TROFI II trial. *Eur Heart J.* 2016;37(3):229–40.

25. Fernández-Rodríguez D, Brugaletta S, Otsuki S, Sabaté M. Acute ABSORB bioresorbable vascular scaffold thrombosis in ST-segment elevation myocardial infarction: To stent or not to stent? *EuroIntervention.* 2014;10:600.

26. Kolandaivelu K, Swaminathan R, Gibson WJ, Kolachalama VB, Nguyen-Ehrenreich KL, Giddings VL, Coleman L et al. Stent thrombogenicity early in high-risk interventional settings is driven by stent design and deployment and protected by polymer-drug coatings. *Circulation.* 2011;123:1400–9.

27. Otsuka F, Pacheco E, Perkins LE, Lane JP, Wang Q, Kamberi M, Frie M et al. Long-term safety of an everolimus-eluting bioresorbable vascular scaffold and the cobalt-chromium XIENCE V stent in a porcine coronary artery model. *Circ Cardiovasc Interv.* 2014;7:330–42.

28. Kirtane AJ, Stone GW. How to minimize stent thrombosis. *Circulation.* 2011;124:1283–7.

29. Brown AJ, McCormick LM, Braganza DM, Bennett MR, Hoole SP, West NE. Expansion and malapposition characteristics after bioresorbable vascular scaffold implantation. *Cath Cardiovasc Interv.* 2014;84:37–45.

30. Tamburino C, Latib A, van Geuns RJ, Sabate M, Mehilli J, Gori T, Achenbach S et al. Contemporary practice and technical aspects in coronary intervention with bioresorbable scaffolds: A European perspective. *EuroIntervention.* 2015;11(1):45–52.

31. Jolly SS, Cairns JA, Yusuf S, Meeks B, Pogue J, Rokoss MJ, Kedev S et al. Randomized trial of primary PCI with or without routine manual thrombectomy. *N Engl J Med.* 2015;372:1389–1398.

32. Brown AJ, McCormick LM, Braganza DM, Bennett MR, Hoole SP, West NE. Expansion and malapposition characteristics after bioresorbable vascular scaffold implantation. *Cath Cardiovasc Interv.* 2014;84:37–45.

33. Mattesini A, Secco GG, Dall'Ara G, Ghione M, Rama-Merchan JC, Lupi A, Viceconte N et al. ABSORB biodegradable stents versus second-generation metal stents: A comparison study of 100 complex lesions treated under OCT guidance. *JACC Cardiovasc Interv.* 2014;7:741–50.

34. Ishibashi Y, Onuma Y, Muramatsu T, Nakatani S, Iqbal J, Garcia-Garcia HM, Bartorelli AL et al. Lessons learned from acute and late scaffold failures in the ABSORB EXTEND trial. *EuroIntervention.* 2014;10:449–57.

35. Wiebe J, Nef HM, Hamm CW. Current status of bioresorbable scaffolds in the treatment of coronary artery disease. *J Am Coll Cardiol.* 2014;64:2541–51.

# Bioresorbable scaffolds for treating coronary artery disease in patients with diabetes mellitus

AYYAZ SULTAN, TAKASHI MURAMATSU, AND JAVAID IQBAL

## INTRODUCTION

Coronary artery disease remains the most common cause of mortality and morbidity in the diabetic population due to accelerated atherosclerosis driven by complex pathophysiological effect of hyperglycemia, augmented serum levels of advanced glycation end-products, insulin resistance, and high free fatty acid levels. Advancements in percutaneous coronary intervention (PCI) and advent of newer generation drug eluting stents (DESs) have improved outcomes in patients with diabetes mellitus. However, diabetes is still a strong risk factor for adverse clinical outcomes after PCI due to higher rate of restenosis, stent thrombosis, and lower 1-year survival in diabetic compared to non-diabetic population. Bioresorbable scaffolds (BRSs) are novel devices for coronary revascularization and offer potential to improve long-term outcomes. It remains to be proven whether PCI with BRS may improve the outcomes in diabetic patients. This chapter reviews the revascularization strategy in patients with diabetes mellitus, with particular focus on the role of BRS in this patient group.

## REVASCULARIZATION IN PATIENTS WITH DIABETES

Diabetes is a major risk factor for development of coronary artery disease and for poor outcomes after revascularization with either coronary artery bypass grafting (CABG) or PCI [1]. Clinical trials comparing balloon angioplasty or bare metal stents with CABG are of limited relevance to contemporary practice. Similarly, registry data where the treating physicians made the decision on treatment modality cannot reliably compare the outcomes with two strategies. This may explain the divergent results in some studies; however, data from dedicated trials reports a clear advantage of CABG over PCI, especially in patients with multivessel coronary disease.

The FREEDOM trial is the largest ($n = 1900$) contemporary trial in patients with diabetes and multivessel coronary artery disease. Patients were randomized to receive either PCI using DES or CABG surgery and were followed-up for a median period of 3.8 years. The primary endpoint (composite of death from any cause, nonfatal myocardial infarction, or stroke) occurred more frequently in the PCI group (26.6% vs. 18.7%, $p = 0.005$) [2]. The benefit of CABG surgery was driven by differences in both rates of death from any cause ($p = 0.049$) and of myocardial infarction (MI) ($p < 0.001$) [2]. However, the incidence of stroke was more frequent in those undergoing CABG surgery (PCI 2.4% vs. CABG surgery 5.2%, $p = 0.03$) [2].

BARI 2D trial enrolled 2368 diabetic patients with coronary artery disease who underwent revascularization (PCI or CABG) with intensive medical therapy or intensive medical therapy alone. Primary endpoints were the rate of death and a composite of death, MI, or stroke. At 5-year follow-up, there was no significant difference in major adverse cardiac and cerebrovascular events (MACCEs) between the PCI group and the medical-therapy group. However, the MACCE rates were significantly lower in the CABG surgery group than in the medical-therapy group (22.4% vs. 30.5%, $p = 0.01$). Mortality, however, was not significantly different between the revascularization group and the medical-therapy group in either the CABG or the PCI stratum [3]. CARDia trial compared PCI with CABG surgery in patients with diabetes and multivessel disease. Although repeat revascularization was more frequent in those receiving PCI (9.9% vs. 2.0%, $p < 0.001$), even in the DES PCI group (7.3% vs. 2.0%, $p < 0.013$), the CARDia trial showed no significant difference in 1-year mortality (PCI 3.2% vs. CABG surgery 3.3%, $p = 0.83$) or 1-year MACCE events (PCI 10.2% vs. CABG surgery 11.8%) [4]. However, the trial was discontinued prematurely due to poor recruitment and was underpowered. A subgroup analysis of 452 patients with diabetes in the SYNTAX trial demonstrated a higher rate of MACCE for patients treated with PCI, but did not find any difference in mortality [1]. At 5-year follow-up, rates of MACCE (PCI 46.5% vs. CABG surgery 29.0%, $p < 0.001$) and repeat revascularization (PCI 35.3% vs. CABG surgery 14.6%, $p < 0.001$) were significantly higher for PCI compared with CABG surgery. No statistical difference was found for all-cause death (PCI 19.5% vs. CABG surgery 12.9%, $p = 0.065$), stroke (PCI 3.0% vs. CABG surgery 4.7%, $p = 0.34$), or MI (PCI 9.0% vs. CABG surgery 5.4%, $p = 0.20$) [5].

Based on these trials, it is recommended that patients with diabetes and multivessel disease should preferably be treated with CABG. However, diabetic patients with less extensive coronary disease (low Syntax score) can be treated with PCI.

# PCI IN PATIENTS WITH DIABETES

## Balloon angioplasty

Balloon angioplasty revolutionized the treatment of patients with symptomatic coronary artery disease. However, several studies have confirmed poor outcome in diabetic patients when compared to non-diabetic population who underwent balloon angioplasty. Stein et al. compared outcomes in 1133 diabetic and 9300 non-diabetic patients who underwent elective angioplasty from 1980 to 1990 [6]. They reported similar rates of procedural success and in-hospital complications in patients with or without diabetes mellitus. However, 5 years' survival and freedom from MI was considerably lower in diabetics. Kip et al. reported short- and long-term outcomes for diabetic ($n = 281$) and non-diabetic patients ($n = 1181$) from 1985 to 1986 in NHLBI PTCA registry and found that diabetics had three times higher in-hospital mortality and two times higher mortality at 9 years when compared with non-diabetics [7].

## Bare metal stents

Introduction of bare metal stents was a major breakthrough, which lead to substantial reduction in acute arterial closure and major adverse cardiac events even in diabetics. However, restenosis remained a major cause for repeat revascularization, MI, and death especially in the diabetic population. Carrozza et al. showed that diabetics had a significantly higher rate of restenosis (55% vs. 20%, $p = 0.001$) compared with non-diabetics due to greater late luminal loss ($1.66 \pm 1.28$ mm vs. $1.23 \pm 0.97$ mm, $p = 0.04$) [8]. Elize et al. compared outcome of 715 diabetic patients with 2839 non-diabetic patients. At 1 year, the diabetic population had significantly reduced MI free survival (89.9% vs. 94.4%, $p < 0.001$) and survival free of death, MI, and target lesion repeat revascularization (73.1% vs. 78.5%, $p < 0.001$) [9]. This was mainly driven by significantly higher rate of restenosis

(37.5% vs. 28.3%, $p < 0.001$) and target vessel occlusion in diabetics compared with non-diabetics (5.3% vs. 3.4%, $p = 0.037$).

## Drug eluting stents

The advent of drug eluting stents (DESs) improved the outcomes compared with bare metal stents by reducing restenosis rate and repeat target lesion revascularization, even in high-risk populations such as diabetics. However, with the DES came across a new problem, the late stent thrombosis.

### FIRST-GENERATION DES

Several clinical trials appraised the efficacy and safety of first-generation DES (CYPHER®—a sirolimus eluting stent [SES] and TAXUS®—a paclitaxel eluting stent [PES]) in diabetic population [10–14]. The subanalysis of diabetic patients from SIRIUS [15,16] and TAXUS IV [17,18] trials showed promising results with significant reduction in rates of target lesion revascularization (TLR) in patients who received DESs when compared to BMSs. DIABETES trial specifically compared 80 diabetics who received CYPHER with 80 diabetics who received BMS and showed significant reduction in late luminal loss, irrespective of type of diabetes [19]. DECODE [20], SCORPIUS [21], and DESSERT [22] trials further confirmed a significant reduction of late luminal loss at 6–9 months follow-up. A meta-analysis of 35 trials by Stettler et al. showed significant reduction in the rate of TLR in diabetics with the use of first-generation DES compared with BMS [23]. The number needed to treat with DES to prevent one event of TLR over 4 years is only 6 for diabetics (8 for non-diabetics). Five head-to-head studies found considerable reduction in late luminal loss with SES use compared to PES in the diabetic population [24–27].

First-generation DES undoubtedly reduced restenosis and TLR; however, several clinical trials and meta-analyses have indicated no significant improvement in hard clinical outcomes including mortality, MI, or stent thrombosis in diabetic population [28–33].

### NEWER GENERATION DES

Newer generation DES have improved design, material, polymer, and antiproliferative drugs [34]. However, outcomes in diabetic patients remain poor. In a pooled analysis of SPIRIT II to IV and COMPARE trials, patients with diabetes failed to gain significantly with everolimus-eluting stent (EES) compared to PES [35]. In SPIRIT-V DIABETIC trial, the composite endpoint of death, MI, and target vessel revascularization (TVR) was similar between EES and PES at 2 years (16.3 vs. 16.4%) [36]. ESSENCE-DIABETES demonstrated similar 1-year clinical outcomes of ischemia-driven TLR, death, and MI between EES and SES. SORT OUT IV found significantly high MACE in diabetics compared to non-diabetics (13.1 vs. 6.4%; HR: 2.08; 95% CI: 1.51–2.86; $p < 0.001$), irrespective of EES or SES implantation.

## Limitations of DES in diabetics

Several studies raised concern over the long-term safety of DES [37–40], largely due to late restenosis, neoatherosclerosis, and very late stent thrombosis. Numerous factors may contribute to stent thrombosis such as thrombus burden at the time of stent deployment, delayed healing due to localized inflammation, tissue necrosis, uncovered stent struts, stent underexpansion or malapposition and interruption of dual antiplatelet therapy [41–46]. Several clinical trials and registries have shown that diabetes mellitus is an independent predictor of stent thrombosis [47–52].

Permanent metal stents pose several limitations such as lifelong caging of the vessel, loss of restoration of coronary vasomotion [53,54], permanent jailing of side branch, lack of vessel remodeling [55,56], hindering noninvasive coronary imaging such as CT or MRI and barring the option for future surgical revascularization, especially in young diabetics.

## BIORESORBABLE SCAFFOLDS IN DIABETES

Bioresorbable scaffolds (BRSs), a two-decades old concept [57], may offer a solution for the above-mentioned limitations of permanent metallic stents. Several BRS are available currently, however, only two have been acknowledged by Conformité Européenne (CE) mark. These novel devices offer a promising future; however, initial studies were largely conducted in low risk populations and therefore the proportion of diabetic patients has been quite low (Table 7.8.1). We have summarized the available data on use of BRS in diabetic patients.

## ABSORB BVS

The first-in-human, nonrandomized, open-label, prospective ABSORB Cohort A trial showed promising safety and feasibility data over 6 months [58], 1 year [58], 2 years [59], and 5 years [60] in 30 patients, including one diabetic patient, with single *de novo* coronary lesions treated with first-generation BVS 1.0. The ABSORB Cohort B trial was a multicenter, nonrandomized, prospective, open-label trial, involving 101 patients in two groups B1 and B2 with clinical and multimodality imaging follow-up at 6/24 months [61–63] and 12/36 months [63,64], respectively, reinforced the safety and efficacy of second-generation BVS 1.1 [65, 66]. There were 17 diabetic patients in total (6/45 patients in B1 and 11/56 patients in B2). ABSORB EXTEND [67] is an ongoing, nonrandomized, prospective, single-arm, open-label trial which aims to recruit up to 800 patients at up to 100 international sites. It allows treatment of a maximum of two *de novo* native coronary artery lesions when each lesion is situated in a different coronary artery and patients with longer lesions (≤28 mm in length) and smaller reference vessel diameter (2.0–3.8 mm), as assessed by online QCA or IVUS, when compared with ABSORB Cohort B inclusion criteria. ABSORB EXTEND interim report by Abizaid [68] of the first 512 patients, including 128 diabetics enrolled in the study, at 1 year, showed the composite endpoints of ischemia-driven MACE, ischemia-driven target lesion failure, and ischemia-driven target vessel failure were 4.3%, 4.3%, and 4.9%, respectively. Definite and probable acute, subacute, and late scaffold thrombosis rates, as defined by Academic Research Consortium (ARC), were 0.0% (0/512), 0.4% (2/512), and 0.4% (2/512), respectively. Another report by Carrie in 2014 showed encouraging 24-months subanalysis of first 250 patients (including 25% diabetics) as suggested by the MACE and TVF rates of 7.3% and 8.1%, respectively.

The pooled analysis of the ABSORB Cohort B, ABSORB EXTEND, and SPIRIT FIRST through IV trials was the first report to evaluate the outcomes of BVS in diabetic patients compared to metallic drug eluting stent [69]. One hundred thirty-six diabetic patients were compared with 415 non-diabetic patients with 1 year follow-up from ABSORB Cohort B and ABSORB EXTEND trials. Furthermore, 102 diabetics who received BVS from the two ABSORB trials were compared with 1:2 propensity matched 172 diabetics, from SPIRIT trials, who received Everolimus eluting

**Table 7.8.1** Number of diabetic patients enrolled in different clinical studies evaluating brioresorbable scaffolds

| Scaffold | Study | Total patients | Diabetic n (%) | Outcome data in diabetics? |
|---|---|---|---|---|
| ABSORB BVS | Cohort A | 30 | 1 (3%) | No |
| | Cohort B | 101 | 17 (17%) | Yes |
| | ABSORB Extend | 512 | 128 (25%) | Yes |
| | ABSORB-II | 501 | 115 (23%) | No |
| | GHOST EU | 1187 | 295 (25%) | No |
| DESolve | DESolve FIM | 15 | 1 (7%) | No |
| | DESolve NX | 126 | 27 (21%) | No |
| AMS | PROGRESS AMS | 63 | 11 (18%) | No |
| DREAMS | BIOSOLVE-1 | 46 | 7 (15%) | No |
| RESOLVE | RESTORE | 25 | 9 (36%) | No |

coronary stent system. Incidence rate of device-oriented composite endpoint (DoCE = cardiac death, target vessel MI, or target lesion revascularization) in diabetics treated with BVS was reduced, though statistically nonsignificant, when compared to non-diabetics (3.7% vs. 5.1%, $p = 0.64$) and diabetics treated with EESs for non-complex coronary artery disease (3.9% for the BVS vs. 6.4% for EES, $p = 0.38$) in the propensity matched study group at 1 year follow-up. Similarly, patient-oriented composite endpoint (PoCE = all death, all MI, and all revascularizations) was similar in diabetics and non-diabetics treated with BVS (7.8% vs. 8.4%, $p = 0.86$). PoCE was nonsignificantly lower in BVS treated diabetics when compared to EES treated diabetics with noncomplex coronary artery disease in propensity matched study groups (7.8% vs. 11.0%, $p = 0.39$). There was no significant difference in 1-year rate of stent thrombosis when BVS treated diabetics were compared with non-diabetics (1% vs. 1%, $p = 1.0$) and EES treated diabetics (1% vs. 1.7%, $p = 1$) [69]. Further comparison at 2-year follow-up was presented by Iqbal et al., at TCT in 2014 [70]. They compared outcomes in 142 diabetic and 434 non-diabetic patients treated with BVS from ABSORB Cohort B and ABSORB EXTEND. Furthermore, BVS treated diabetic patients ($n = 103$) were compared with propensity matched diabetic patients ($n = 175$) treated with metallic XIENCE everolimus-eluting stents (EES) from SPIRIT First, II, III, and IV studies. BVS treated diabetic patients had similar baseline characteristics as BVS treated non-diabetics except for the presence of diabetes mellitus (100% vs. 0%) and hypertension (74% vs. 62%, $p = 0.008$). At 2-year follow-up, there were no significant differences in PoCE (diabetics 10.6% vs. non-diabetics 12.9%, $p = 0.46$) and DoCE (diabetics 4.2% vs. non-diabetics 7.6%, $p = 0.16$; Figure 7.8.1). There was also no difference in definite (diabetics 0.7% vs. non-diabetics 0.7%, $p = 1.0$) and definite/probable (diabetics 0.7% vs. non-diabetics 0.9%, $p = 1.0$) scaffold thrombosis between the two groups. BVS and EES treated diabetic patients were well matched for demographic, clinical, and procedural characteristics, except for longer duration of DAPT in the BVS group (BVS 89% vs. EES 63%, $p < 0.001$ at 2 years). PoCE (BVS 12.6% vs. EES 10.9%, $p = 0.66$), and DoCE (BVS 5.8% vs. EES 5.7%, $p = 0.97$; Figure 7.8.2) were similar in the diabetic patients treated with BVS or EES at 2-year follow-up. There was no difference in definite (BVS 1.0% vs. EES 0.6%, $p = 1.0$) and definite/probable (BVS 1.0% vs. EES 0.6%, $p = 1.0$) scaffold/stent thrombosis in the diabetic patients treated with BVS or EES at 2-year follow-up [70].

ABSORB II, a multicenter, single-blind randomized trial, enrolled 501 patients (23% diabetics and 6% insulin-dependent diabetics) with 1 or 2 *de novo* native coronary lesions in different epicardial vessels and evidence of myocardial ischemia, aimed to receive treatment with a BVS or treatment with an EES [71]. However, outcome of BVS as compared to EES in diabetic patients was not described in the results published.

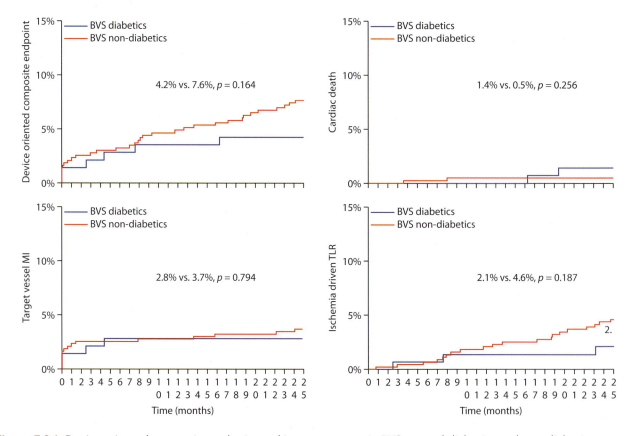

**Figure 7.8.1** Device oriented composite endpoint and its components in BVS treated diabetics and non-diabetics.

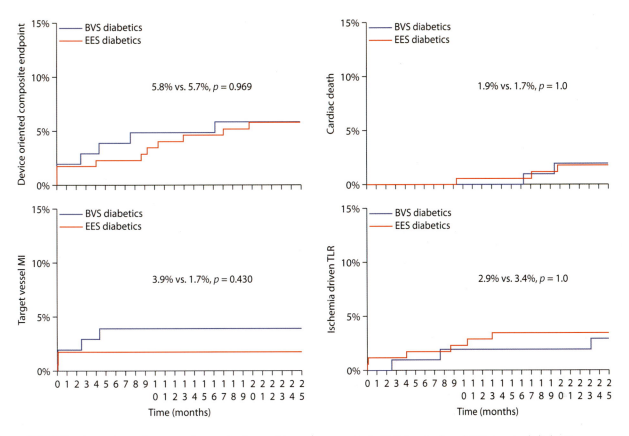

**Figure 7.8.2** Device oriented composite endpoint and its components in BVS treated and EES treated diabetics.

ABSORB III, a multi-center, single blind, randomized trial, enrolled 2008 patients with stable or unstable angina and up to two *de novo* coronary artery lesions in separate coronary arteries, in 2:1 fashion to the ABSORB BVS or XIENCE stents. Patients with myocardial infarction were excluded. Of the 1320 patients who received the ABSORB stent, 31.5% were diabetic compared to 32.7% of the 686 patients who received the XIENCE stent. At 1 year, the rate of device thrombosis (definite or probable) was 3.2% in diabetic patients with BVS compared to 1.4% in diabetic patients with EES (RR 2.34; 95% CI 0.23–2.78; *p* = 0.78) [72].

In the largest ever patient-level, propensity score-matched pooled analysis of ABSORB EXTEND and SPIRIT clinical trials, diabetic patients treated with the ABSORB BVS (*n* = 215) had similar rates of major adverse cardiac events (5.7% vs. 5.6%, respectively; HR 0.99; 0.44–2.20; *p* = 0.98) as compared with diabetics treated with EES (*n* = 882), after 393 days of follow-up [73].

In a recent prospective registry of 236 patients treated by BVS, diabetes mellitus and length of BVS were significant predictors for the occurrence of a device-oriented endpoint including cardiac death, target-vessel myocardial infarction, and target lesion revascularization, over mean follow-up period of 382 days [74].

The GHOST-EU [75] registry evaluated "real-world clinical practice" related early and mid-term clinical outcomes in 1189 patients treated with BVS; including patients with acute coronary syndromes, chronic total occlusions, and calcified

and bifurcation lesion. Two hundred ninety-five (24.8%) were diabetic patients and 106 were insulin-dependent. A total of 1731 BVSs were deployed with technical success attained in 99.7% of cases. The cumulative incidence of TLF (defined as the combination of cardiac death, target vessel myocardial infarction, or clinically driven TLR) was 2.2% at 30 days, 4.4% at 6 months, and the annualized rate of TLF and TVF were 10.1% and 11.9%, respectively. The cumulative incidence of definite/probable scaffold thrombosis was 1.5% at 30 days and 2.1% at 6 months. In multivariate analysis, diabetes mellitus was the only independent predictor of TLF (HR 2.41, 95% CI 1.28–4.53; *p* = 0.006). GHOST-EU registry revealed that, in unselected patients and lesions from routine clinical practice, BVS has acceptable safety and early/mid clinical outcomes comparable to contemporary second-generation EES. However, occurrence of early scaffold thrombosis (within 30 days) in 16/23 patients (43% diabetic patients), consistent with previously published results [71,76,77], points toward importance of patients and lesion selection and robust measure to ensure optimal deployment of BVS.

## Data for other BRSs

The DESolve® BRS (Elixir Medical, Sunnyvale, CA) is a novel PLLA-based bioresorbable scaffold, eluting antiproliferative metabolite of sirolimus, myolimus in earlier iterations, and novolimus in subsequent devices. The first-in-human trial

[78] demonstrated promising initial results for the efficacy and safety of the DESolve BRS in a multicenter, nonrandomized, prospective study of 15 patients (6.7% diabetics) [79]. This led to international enrolment of 126 patients (21% diabetics) for DESolve Nx trial, which showed significant increase in lumen area (5.9 vs. 6.43 mm²; 17%) and scaffold area (5.86 mm vs. 6.78 mm²; 16%) by IVUS examination and 99% coverage of the scaffold struts by OCT examination at 6 months. The MACE incidence was 3.25% including one cardiac death, one target vessel MI, and two TLRs [80]. However, the authors did not discuss outcome results specifically in diabetics.

PROGRESS-AMS [81] prospectively evaluated 63 patients for safety and efficacy of absorbable magnesium scaffold (AMS). There were 11 (18%) diabetics enrolled; however, the long-term follow up analysis [82] did not include any diabetic population. No data are available for the 7 diabetics enrolled in BIOSOLVE-1 [83], which showed satisfactory efficacy and safety profile based on clinical and angiographic outcomes up to 12 months for DREAMS, a paclitaxel-eluted AMS, in a total of 46 patients. Therefore, in summary, there are limited data on use of BRS in a diabetic population and further studies are needed.

## TIPS FOR USING BRSs IN DIABETIC PATIENTS

Diabetic patients frequently have small caliber vessels and diffuse coronary disease. They are prone to restenosis, neoatherosclerosis, and progression of disease in nonintervened arteries, which often require repeat PCI or CABG. Therefore, some special precautions are needed when using BRS in diabetic patients.

### Patient and lesion selection

Patient selection remains fundamental when considering implantation of BRSs to achieve safe long-term clinical outcomes. Patients who are likely to need further revascularization (e.g., young diabetics, diabetics with renal disease, history of restenosis, etc.) may benefit from use of BRSs, so that future revascularization option with either PCI or CBAG remains possible.

Suitable lesion selection, in diabetics, is pivotal to reduce incidence of late TLR and stent thombosis, as polymeric BRSs come with entirely different strut structure and biomechanical properties. This demands extreme caution due to challenges in deliverability [84] secondary to relatively larger crossing profile, stretchability/expansion, and radial strength of BVS and potential for strut fracture in complex lesions such as calcified lesions, tortuous lesions, bifurcations, vessel size 4.0 mm or more, vein grafts, small size vessels, and thrombotic lesions. Selection of relatively simple "ABSORB A/B or EXTEND" like lesions in native coronary arteries with diameter 2.5–3.75 and lesion length ≤24 mm would be appropriate.

### PSP technique

A simple "PSP" implantation technique has recently been recommend.

1. *P—Prepare the vessel*: Pre-dilate using a 1:1 balloon-to-artery ratio using a noncompliant balloon (it can also help accurately size the vessel). Use plaque-modification devices if needed. Confirm full expansion of balloon and residual stenosis of <40% in two orthogonal views.
2. *S—Size the vessel*: It is vital to appropriately size the vessel and select device accordingly. Use of IVUS or OCT is recommended to aid vessel sizing.
3. *P—Postdilatation*: Dilate to high pressure with a noncompliant balloon up to 0.5 mm above nominal scaffold diameter. Verify <10% final residual stenosis in two orthogonal views, and ensure full strut apposition.

### General considerations

The general recommendations for scaffold deployment advocate a gentle and deliberate expansion by 2 atm every 5 seconds up to the rated burst pressure. The stent-balloon inflation should be maintained for 30 seconds before complete deflation and cautious withdrawal of the balloon.

Particular attention is demanded when a second BRS is used to treat a long lesion in diabetics, while considering an overlap due to thicker struts (150 mm). Hence, at the overlap zone, a combined thickness of 300 mm can impact vessel lumen especially in relatively small caliber vessels in diabetics. The platinum markers in BVSs, each at the end of unexpanded balloons and within scaffold edges, should be laid side by side with an aim of overlap not more than 1–4 mm. It may also be appropriate to use adjacent positioning, instead of overlapping technique.

## CURRENT CHALLENGES AND FUTURE DIRECTIONS

PCI in the presence of diabetes is challenging due to relatively small caliber arteries, diffuse and long lesions, severity of calcification, multivessel involvement, and higher risk for stent thrombosis. Diabetic population has been under represented in most trials evaluating efficacy and safety of the BRS devices. BVS have a bulky profile relative to modern generation DES due to thicker stent struts which can compromise the deliverability of the device through the diabetic coronary anatomy. Optimal deployment without loss of radial strength is an additional challenge, as there is an inherent limitation to stretchability of the scaffold beyond which the risk of strut-fracture will potentially have a negative impact. This demands an accurate determination of the reference vessel size and selection of the correct scaffold diameter especially when dealing with high thrombus-laden lesions such as during STEMI.

There is a need for dedicated and adequately powered studies in the diabetic population to determine the short- and long-term success of BRS device, including clinical and angiographic outcomes, the need for repeat revascularization, and incidence of stent thrombosis.

## REFERENCES

1. Banning AP, Westaby S, Morice MC et al. Diabetic and nondiabetic patients with left main and/or 3-vessel coronary artery disease: Comparison of outcomes with cardiac surgery and paclitaxel-eluting stents. *J Am Coll Cardiol.* 2010;55:1067–75.

2. Farkouh ME, Domanski M, Sleeper LA et al. Strategies for multivessel revascularization in patients with diabetes. *New Engl J Med.* 2012;367:2375–84.

3. Bari 2D Study Group, Frye RL, August P et al. A randomized trial of therapies for type 2 diabetes and coronary artery disease. *New Engl J Med.* 2009;360:2503–15.

4. Kapur A, Hall RJ, Malik IS et al. Randomized comparison of percutaneous coronary intervention with coronary artery bypass grafting in diabetic patients. 1-year results of the CARDia (Coronary Artery Revascularization in Diabetes) trial. *J Am Coll Cardiol.* 2010;55:432–40.

5. Kappetein AP, Head SJ, Morice MC et al. Treatment of complex coronary artery disease in patients with diabetes: 5-year results comparing outcomes of bypass surgery and percutaneous coronary intervention in the SYNTAX trial. *Eur J Cardiothorac Surg. Official Journal of the Eur J Cardiothorac Surg.* 2013;43:1006–13.

6. Stein B, Weintraub WS, Gebhart SP et al. Influence of diabetes mellitus on early and late outcome after percutaneous transluminal coronary angioplasty. *Circulation.* 1995;91:979–89.

7. Kip KE, Faxon DP, Detre KM, Yeh W, Kelsey SF, Currier JW. Coronary angioplasty in diabetic patients. The National Heart, Lung, and Blood Institute Percutaneous Transluminal Coronary Angioplasty Registry. *Circulation.* 1996;94:1818–25.

8. Carrozza JP, Jr., Kuntz RE, Fishman RF, Baim DS. Restenosis after arterial injury caused by coronary stenting in patients with diabetes mellitus. *Ann Int Med.* 1993;118:344–9.

9. Elezi S, Kastrati A, Pache J et al. Diabetes mellitus and the clinical and angiographic outcome after coronary stent placement. *J Am Coll Cardiol.* 1998;32:1866–73.

10. Morice MC, Serruys PW, Sousa JE et al. A randomized comparison of a sirolimus-eluting stent with a standard stent for coronary revascularization. *New Engl J Med.* 2002;346:1773–80.

11. Serruys PW, Degertekin M, Tanabe K et al. Intravascular ultrasound findings in the multicenter, randomized, double-blind RAVEL (RAndomized study with the sirolimus-eluting VElocity balloon-expandable stent in the treatment of patients with de novo native coronary artery Lesions) trial. *Circulation.* 2002;106:798–803.

12. Morice MC, Serruys PW, Barragan P et al. Long-term clinical outcomes with sirolimus-eluting coronary stents: Five-year results of the RAVEL trial. *J Am Coll Cardiol.* 2007;50:1299–304.

13. Lemos PA, Serruys PW, van Domburg RT et al. Unrestricted utilization of sirolimus-eluting stents compared with conventional bare stent implantation in the "real world": The Rapamycin-Eluting Stent Evaluated At Rotterdam Cardiology Hospital (RESEARCH) registry. *Circulation.* 2004;109:190–5.

14. Kelbaek H, Klovgaard L, Helqvist S et al. Long-term outcome in patients treated with sirolimus-eluting stents in complex coronary artery lesions: 3-year results of the SCANDSTENT (Stenting Coronary Arteries in Non-Stress/Benestent Disease) trial. *J Am Coll Cardiol.* 2008;51:2011–6.

15. Moses JW, Leon MB, Popma JJ et al. Sirolimus-eluting stents versus standard stents in patients with stenosis in a native coronary artery. *New Engl J Med.* 2003;349:1315–23.

16. Moussa I, Leon MB, Baim DS et al. Impact of sirolimus-eluting stents on outcome in diabetic patients: A SIRIUS (SIRolImUS-coated Bx Velocity balloon-expandable stent in the treatment of patients with de novo coronary artery lesions) substudy. *Circulation.* 2004;109:2273–8.

17. Halkin A, Mehran R, Casey CW et al. Impact of moderate renal insufficiency on restenosis and adverse clinical events after paclitaxel-eluting and bare metal stent implantation: Results from the TAXUS-IV Trial. *Am Heart J.* 2005;150:1163–70.

18. Stone GW, Ellis SG, Cox DA et al. One-year clinical results with the slow-release, polymer-based, paclitaxel-eluting TAXUS stent: The TAXUS-IV trial. *Circulation.* 2004;109:1942–7.

19. Sabate M, Jimenez-Quevedo P, Angiolillo DJ et al. Randomized comparison of sirolimus-eluting stent versus standard stent for percutaneous coronary revascularization in diabetic patients: The diabetes and sirolimus-eluting stent (DIABETES) trial. *Circulation.* 2005;112:2175–83.

20. Chan C, Zambahari R, Kaul U et al. A randomized comparison of sirolimus-eluting versus bare metal stents in the treatment of diabetic patients with native coronary artery lesions: The DECODE study. *Catheter Cardiovasc Interv.* 2008;72:591–600.

21. Baumgart D, Klauss V, Baer F et al. One-year results of the SCORPIUS study: A German multicenter investigation on the effectiveness of sirolimus-eluting stents in diabetic patients. *J Am Coll Cardiol.* 2007;50:1627–34.

22. Maresta A, Varani E, Balducelli M et al. Comparison of effectiveness and safety of sirolimus-eluting stents versus bare-metal stents in patients with

diabetes mellitus (from the Italian Multicenter Randomized DESSERT Study). *Am J Cardiol.* 2008;101:1560–6.

23. Stettler C, Allemann S, Wandel S et al. Drug eluting and bare metal stents in people with and without diabetes: Collaborative network meta-analysis. *BMJ.* 2008;337:a1331.

24. Kim MH, Hong SJ, Cha KS et al. Effect of Paclitaxel-eluting versus sirolimus-eluting stents on coronary restenosis in Korean diabetic patients. *J Interv Cardiol.* 2008;21:225–31.

25. Maeng M, Jensen LO, Galloe AM et al. Comparison of the sirolimus-eluting versus paclitaxel-eluting coronary stent in patients with diabetes mellitus: The diabetes and drug-eluting stent (DiabeDES) randomized angiography trial. *Am J Cardiol.* 2009;103:345–9.

26. Lee SW, Park SW, Kim YH et al. A randomized comparison of sirolimus- versus Paclitaxel-eluting stent implantation in patients with diabetes mellitus. *J Am Coll Cardiol.* 2008;52:727–33.

27. Tomai F, Reimers B, De Luca L et al. Head-to-head comparison of sirolimus- and paclitaxel-eluting stent in the same diabetic patient with multiple coronary artery lesions: A prospective, randomized, multi-center study. *Diabetes Care.* 2008;31:15–9.

28. Spaulding C, Daemen J, Boersma E, Cutlip DE, Serruys PW. A pooled analysis of data comparing sirolimus-eluting stents with bare-metal stents. *New Engl J Med.* 2007;356:989–97.

29. Raber L, Wohlwend L, Wigger M et al. Five-year clinical and angiographic outcomes of a randomized comparison of sirolimus-eluting and paclitaxel-eluting stents: Results of the Sirolimus-Eluting Versus Paclitaxel-Eluting Stents for Coronary Revascularization LATE trial. *Circulation.* 2011;123:2819–28, 6 p following 28.

30. Lee SW, Park SW, Kim YH et al. A randomized comparison of sirolimus- versus paclitaxel-eluting stent implantation in patients with diabetes mellitus: 4-year clinical outcomes of DES-DIABETES (drug-eluting stent in patients with DIABETES mellitus) trial. *JACC Cardiovasc Interv.* 2011;4:310–6.

31. de Waha A, Dibra A, Kufner S et al. Long-term outcome after sirolimus-eluting stents versus bare metal stents in patients with diabetes mellitus: A patient-level meta-analysis of randomized trials. *Clin Res Cardiol. Official Journal of the German Cardiac Society* 2011;100:561–70.

32. Kirtane AJ, Ellis SG, Dawkins KD et al. Paclitaxel-eluting coronary stents in patients with diabetes mellitus: Pooled analysis from 5 randomized trials. *J Am Coll Cardiol.* 2008;51:708–15.

33. Kufner S, de Waha A, Tomai F et al. A meta-analysis of specifically designed randomized trials of sirolimus-eluting versus paclitaxel-eluting stents in diabetic patients with coronary artery disease. *Am Heart J.* 2011;162:740–7.

34. Iqbal J, Gunn J, Serruys PW. Coronary stents: Historical development, current status and future directions. *Br Med Bull.* 2013;106:193–211.

35. Stone GW, Rizvi A, Sudhir K et al. Randomized comparison of everolimus- and paclitaxel-eluting stents. 2-year follow-up from the SPIRIT (Clinical Evaluation of the XIENCE V Everolimus Eluting Coronary Stent System) IV trial. *J Am Coll Cardiol.* 2011;58:19–25.

36. Grube E, Chevalier B, Guagliumi G et al. The SPIRIT V diabetic study: A randomized clinical evaluation of the XIENCE V everolimus-eluting stent vs the TAXUS Liberte paclitaxel-eluting stent in diabetic patients with de novo coronary artery lesions. *Am Heart J.* 2012;163:867–75 e1.

37. Camenzind E, Steg PG, Wijns W. Stent thrombosis late after implantation of first-generation drug-eluting stents: A cause for concern. *Circulation.* 2007;115:1440–55; discussion 55.

38. Farb A, Boam AB. Stent thrombosis redux—The FDA perspective. *New Engl J Med.* 2007;356:984–7.

39. McFadden EP, Stabile E, Regar E et al. Late thrombosis in drug-eluting coronary stents after discontinuation of antiplatelet therapy. *Lancet.* 2004;364:1519–21.

40. Finn AV, Joner M, Nakazawa G et al. Pathological correlates of late drug-eluting stent thrombosis: Strut coverage as a marker of endothelialization. *Circulation.* 2007;115:2435–41.

41. Joner M, Finn AV, Farb A et al. Pathology of drug-eluting stents in humans: Delayed healing and late thrombotic risk. *J Am Coll Cardiol.* 2006;48:193–202.

42. Daemen J, Wenaweser P, Tsuchida K et al. Early and late coronary stent thrombosis of sirolimus-eluting and paclitaxel-eluting stents in routine clinical practice: Data from a large two-institutional cohort study. *Lancet.* 2007;369:667–78.

43. Finn AV, Nakazawa G, Joner M et al. Vascular responses to drug eluting stents: Importance of delayed healing. *Arterioscler Thromb Vasc Biol.* 2007;27:1500–10.

44. Virmani R, Kolodgie FD, Burke AP, Farb A, Schwartz SM. Lessons from sudden coronary death: A comprehensive morphological classification scheme for atherosclerotic lesions. *Arterioscler Thromb Vasc Biol.* 2000;20:1262–75.

45. Hwang CW, Levin AD, Jonas M, Li PH, Edelman ER. Thrombosis modulates arterial drug distribution for drug-eluting stents. *Circulation.* 2005;111:1619–26.

46. Cook S, Wenaweser P, Togni M et al. Incomplete stent apposition and very late stent thrombosis after drug-eluting stent implantation. *Circulation.* 2007;115:2426–34.

47. Wiviott SD, Braunwald E, Angiolillo DJ et al. Greater clinical benefit of more intensive oral antiplatelet therapy with prasugrel in patients with diabetes mellitus in the trial to assess improvement in therapeutic

outcomes by optimizing platelet inhibition with prasugrel-thrombolysis in myocardial infarction 38. *Circulation.* 2008;118:1626–36.

48. Aoki J, Lansky AJ, Mehran R et al. Early stent thrombosis in patients with acute coronary syndromes treated with drug-eluting and bare metal stents: The Acute Catheterization and Urgent Intervention Triage Strategy trial. *Circulation.* 2009;119:687–98.

49. Lagerqvist B, Carlsson J, Frobert O et al. Stent thrombosis in Sweden: A report from the Swedish Coronary Angiography and Angioplasty Registry. *Circ Cardiovasc Interv.* 2009;2:401–8.

50. Urban P, Gershlick AH, Guagliumi G et al. Safety of coronary sirolimus-eluting stents in daily clinical practice: One-year follow-up of the e-Cypher registry. *Circulation.* 2006;113:1434–41.

51. Machecourt J, Danchin N, Lablanche JM et al. Risk factors for stent thrombosis after implantation of sirolimus-eluting stents in diabetic and nondiabetic patients: The EVASTENT Matched-Cohort Registry. *J Am Coll Cardiol.* 2007;50:501–8.

52. Iqbal J, Sumaya W, Tatman V et al. Incidence and predictors of stent thrombosis: A single-centre study of 5,833 consecutive patients undergoing coronary artery stenting. *EuroIntervention. Journal of EuroPCR in Collaboration with the Working Group on Interventional Cardiology of the European Society of Cardiology* 2013;9:62–9.

53. Plass CA, Sabdyusheva-Litschauer I, Bernhart A et al. Time course of endothelium-dependent and -independent coronary vasomotor response to coronary balloons and stents. Comparison of plain and drug-eluting balloons and stents. *JACC Cardiovasc Interv.* 2012;5:741–51.

54. Maier W, Windecker S, Kung A et al. Exercise-induced coronary artery vasodilation is not impaired by stent placement. *Circulation.* 2002;105:2373–7.

55. Mintz GS, Popma JJ, Pichard AD et al. Arterial remodeling after coronary angioplasty: A serial intravascular ultrasound study. *Circulation.* 1996;94:35–43.

56. Kimura T, Kaburagi S, Tamura T et al. Remodeling of human coronary arteries undergoing coronary angioplasty or atherectomy. *Circulation.* 1997;96:475–83.

57. van der Giessen WJ, Slager CJ, van Beusekom HM et al. Development of a polymer endovascular prosthesis and its implantation in porcine arteries. *J Interv Cardiol.* 1992;5:175–85.

58. Ormiston JA, Serruys PW, Regar E et al. A bioabsorbable everolimus-eluting coronary stent system for patients with single de-novo coronary artery lesions (ABSORB): A prospective open-label trial. *Lancet.* 2008;371:899–907.

59. Serruys PW, Ormiston JA, Onuma Y et al. A bioabsorbable everolimus-eluting coronary stent system (ABSORB): 2-year outcomes and results from multiple imaging methods. *Lancet.* 2009;373:897–910.

60. Onuma Y, Dudek D, Thuesen L et al. Five-year clinical and functional multislice computed tomography angiographic results after coronary implantation of the fully resorbable polymeric everolimus-eluting scaffold in patients with de novo coronary artery disease: The ABSORB cohort A trial. *JACC Cardiovasc Interv.* 2013;6:999–1009.

61. Serruys PW, Onuma Y, Ormiston JA et al. Evaluation of the second generation of a bioresorbable everolimus drug-eluting vascular scaffold for treatment of de novo coronary artery stenosis: Six-month clinical and imaging outcomes. *Circulation.* 2010;122:2301–12.

62. Ormiston JA, Serruys PW, Onuma Y et al. First serial assessment at 6 months and 2 years of the second generation of absorb everolimus-eluting bioresorbable vascular scaffold: A multi-imaging modality study. *Circ Cardiovasc Interv.* 2012;5:620–32.

63. Serruys PW, Onuma Y, Garcia-Garcia HM et al. Dynamics of vessel wall changes following the implantation of the absorb everolimus-eluting bioresorbable vascular scaffold: A multi-imaging modality study at 6, 12, 24 and 36 months. *EuroIntervention. Journal of EuroPCR in Collaboration with the Working Group on Interventional Cardiology of the European Society of Cardiology* 2014;9:1271–84.

64. Serruys PW, Onuma Y, Dudek D et al. Evaluation of the second generation of a bioresorbable everolimus-eluting vascular scaffold for the treatment of de novo coronary artery stenosis: 12-month clinical and imaging outcomes. *J Am Coll Cardiol.* 2011;58:1578–88.

65. Diletti R, Farooq V, Girasis C et al. Clinical and intravascular imaging outcomes at 1 and 2 years after implantation of absorb everolimus eluting bioresorbable vascular scaffolds in small vessels. Late lumen enlargement: Does bioresorption matter with small vessel size? Insight from the ABSORB cohort B trial. *Heart.* 2013;99:98–105.

66. Onuma Y, Serruys PW, Muramatsu T et al. Incidence and imaging outcomes of acute scaffold disruption and late structural discontinuity after implantation of the absorb Everolimus-eluting fully bioresorbable vascular scaffold: Optical coherence tomography assessment in the ABSORB cohort B Trial (A Clinical Evaluation of the Bioabsorbable Everolimus Eluting Coronary Stent System in the Treatment of Patients With De Novo Native Coronary Artery Lesions). *JACC Cardiovasc Interv.* 2014;7:1400–11.

67. Ishibashi Y, Onuma Y, Muramatsu T et al. Lessons learned from acute and late scaffold failures in the ABSORB EXTEND trial. *EuroIntervention.* 2014;10:449–57.

68. Abizaid A, Costa JR, Jr., Bartorelli AL et al. The ABSORB EXTEND study: Preliminary report of the twelve-month clinical outcomes in the first 512 patients enrolled. *EuroIntervention.* 2014.

69. Muramatsu T, Onuma Y, van Geuns RJ et al. 1-year clinical outcomes of diabetic patients treated with everolimus-eluting bioresorbable vascular scaffolds: A pooled analysis of the ABSORB and the SPIRIT trials. *JACC Cardiovasc Interv.* 2014;7:482–93.

70. Iqbal J, Onuma Y, Van Geuns RJ et al. TCT-245 Diabetic patients treated with bioresorbable vascular scaffolds show good clinical outcomes at two-year follow-up: A pooled analysis from the ABSORB and SPIRIT trials. *J Am Coll Cardiol.* 2014;64.

71. Serruys PW, Chevalier B, Dudek D et al. A bioresorbable everolimus-eluting scaffold versus a metallic everolimus-eluting stent for ischaemic heart disease caused by de-novo native coronary artery lesions (ABSORB II): An interim 1-year analysis of clinical and procedural secondary outcomes from a randomised controlled trial. *Lancet.* 2015;385:43–54.

72. Ellis SG, Kereiakes DJ, Metzger DC et al. Everolimus-eluting bioresorbable scaffolds for coronary artery disease. *New Engl J Med.* 2015;373:1905–15.

73. Campos CM, Abizaid A, Caixeta A, Bartorelli AL, Whitbourn RJ, Perin MA. TCT-600 short and mid-term outcomes of diabetic patients treated with everolimus-eluting bioresorbable scaffolds versus second-generation drug eluting stents: A propensity score-matched analysis of ABSORB EXTEND and SPIRIT clinical trials. *J Am Coll Cardiol.* 2015;66.

74. Seeger J, Marcovic S, Gonska B, Walcher D, Rottbauer W, Wöhrle J. TCT-509 Clinical follow-up after implantation of bioresorbable drug-eluting scaffolds—A prospective single center experience up to 3 years. *J Am Coll Cardiol.* 2015;66.

75. Capodanno D, Gori T, Nef H et al. Percutaneous coronary intervention with everolimus-eluting bioresorbable vascular scaffolds in routine clinical practice: Early and midterm outcomes from the European multicentre GHOST-EU registry. *EuroIntervention.* 2015;10:1144–53.

76. Kraak RP, Hassell ME, Grundeken MJ et al. Initial experience and clinical evaluation of the Absorb bioresorbable vascular scaffold (BVS) in real-world practice: The AMC Single Centre Real World PCI Registry. *EuroIntervention. Journal of EuroPCR in Collaboration with the Working Group on Interventional Cardiology of the European Society of Cardiology* 2015;10:1160–8.

77. Jaguszewski M, Ghadri JR, Zipponi M et al. Feasibility of second-generation bioresorbable vascular scaffold implantation in complex anatomical and clinical scenarios. *Clin Res Cardiol. Official Journal of the German Cardiac Society* 2015;104:124–35.

78. Ormiston J, Webster M, Stewart J et al. First-in-human evaluation of a bioabsorbable polymer-coated sirolimus-eluting stent: Imaging and clinical results of the DESSOLVE I Trial (DES with sirolimus and a bioabsorbable polymer for the treatment of patients with de novo lesion in the native coronary arteries). *JACC Cardiovasc Interv.* 2013;6:1026–34.

79. Verheye S, Ormiston JA, Stewart J et al. A next-generation bioresorbable coronary scaffold system: From bench to first clinical evaluation: 6- and 12-month clinical and multimodality imaging results. *JACC Cardiovasc Interv.* 2014;7:89–99.

80. Abizaid A, Schofer J, Maeng M et al. TCT-37 Prospective, multi-center evaluation of the DESolve Nx novolimus-eluting bioresorbable coronary scaffold: First report of one year clinical and imaging outcomes. *J Am Coll Cardiol.* 2013;62:B13–B.

81. Erbel R, Di Mario C, Bartunek J et al. Temporary scaffolding of coronary arteries with bioabsorbable magnesium stents: A prospective, non-randomised multicentre trial. *Lancet.* 2007;369:1869–75.

82. Waksman R, Erbel R, Di Mario C et al. Early- and long-term intravascular ultrasound and angiographic findings after bioabsorbable magnesium stent implantation in human coronary arteries. *JACC Cardiovasc Interv.* 2009;2:312–20.

83. Haude M, Erbel R, Erne P et al. Safety and performance of the drug-eluting absorbable metal scaffold (DREAMS) in patients with de-novo coronary lesions: 12 month results of the prospective, multicentre, first-in-man BIOSOLVE-I trial. *Lancet.* 2013;381:836–44.

84. Iqbal J, Onuma Y, Ormiston J, Abizaid A, Waksman R, Serruys P. Bioresorbable scaffolds: Rationale, current status, challenges, and future. *Eur Heart J.* 2014;35:765–76.

# 7.9

# BRSs in calcified lesions

ASHOK SETH AND BABU EZHUMALAI

The bioresorbable scaffolds (BRSs) is being increasingly used for the treatment of significant coronary artery disease since the commercial launch of the ABSORB BVS (A-BVS) (Abbott Vascular, Santa Clara, CA) in 2012. The A-BVS has been demonstrated to be as safe and effective in the short term as the "best in class" metallic drug eluting stent (mDES) at least in noncomplex patient and lesion subsets [1]. However, the probable long-term benefits of a "temporary stent" remain to be proven as we eagerly await the results of ongoing longer-term studies. Its natural extended application to more complex "real world" cases has been limited by the fact that A-BVS is a thick strut bulky device that is "plastic" in nature and has unique physical and expansion characteristics. Hence, it does not behave like a third-generation thin strut mDES, with which the interventional cardiology community is more confident, comfortable, and familiar. A new set of "tricks and tips" is necessary for its safe and effective implantation in complex lesion subsets. Additionally, there is apprehension regarding its results in the "real world" patients, as presently only small registries outlining short-term outcomes are available [2].

Calcified vessels and lesions form a very challenging subgroup of complex lesions faced in the real world practice. Calcified vessels account for nearly 35–40% of percutaneous coronary intervention (PCI) in most busy cath labs [3] of which 15–20% may be moderate to severely calcified, and often represent more extensive and diffuse atherosclerotic burden.

Calcified lesions are more likely to have stent thrombosis and restenosis. Severe calcification is also an independent predictor of death, MI, and repeat revascularization at follow-up even with a good second-generation mDES [4]. They present a technical nightmare for the operator creating problems in stent delivery, difficulties in lesion dilatation, higher chances of dissections and perforations, and often require the use of adjunctive devices like rotational atherectomy (RA) and cutting/scoring balloons to decalcify the lesion to enable optimal stent expansion and apposition. The procedure takes greater time, radiation exposure, and contrast load. Because of the above reasons, patients with calcified vessels often undergo incomplete revascularization.

## CONCERNS AND CHALLENGES OF BRS IN CALCIFIED LESIONS

The concerns of BRSs in calcified coronary anatomy relate both to the procedural challenges as well as uncertain outcomes.

A-BVS is a high profile, 156 micron thick strut device and behaves like a first-generation mDES. It is poorly deliverable through calcified arteries especially with tortuosities. There are additional concerns about the lack of adequate radial strength of this "plastic stent" in calcified lesions and that incomplete expansion, poor apposition, recoil, and residual stenosis could all lead to higher scaffold thrombosis in the short term and higher restenosis and target vessel failure in the intermediate term. Uncertainty also exists as to whether the potential long-term benefits of BRSs, i.e., return of vasomotor tone, late lumen enlargement and positive remodeling, ability to use CT imaging, etc. will have any relevant advantages in rigid calcified coronary arteries.

On the other hand, the natural concern that the plastic scaffold lacks the radial strength to support calcified arteries may be unjustified. On bench testing the radial strength of the A-BVS is equivalent to XIENCE Vision (Abbott Vascular, Santa Clara, CA) [5]. Also, calcified arteries have stiffer mechanical properties and low elasticity and once the calcium ring is disrupted by adjunctive tools, the radial compression and recoil factor is low [6]. Mild to moderately calcified vessels could also exhibit positive remodeling, return of vasomotor tone at follow-up and the same long-term benefits could be possible even for severely calcified lesions if they were decalcified with rotational atherectomy prior to BRS implantation. There are other obvious long-term benefits of the lack of a permanent implant like discontinuation of dual antiplatelet therapy at will if needed and absence of neoatherosclerosis. One could also argue that BRS could be ideal for the treatment of long and diffusely diseased vessels which are often calcified. It is conceivable that a strategy of decalcifying long diffuse calcified lesions by RA followed by multiple BRS implantations could improve outcomes in this difficult subgroup of patients.

Hence, it may be reasonable to treat select cases of moderate to severely calcified vessels with BRSs.

## TECHNICAL CONSIDERATIONS OF BRS IMPLANTATION IN CALCIFIED LESIONS

Experience has taught us that the meticulous attention to the tips, tricks, and implantation techniques can achieve a high degree of success in calcified lesions with low complication rates and favorable short-term outcomes.

The following are the procedural principles of techniques of PCI using BRS for calcified lesion [7] that need emphasis to achieve the best results:

1. **A firm guide catheter support;** hence, preferably 7F guide should be used.

2. **Pre-assessment of vessel up to the lesion** should be performed for tortuosity, calcification at curves, and the extent of calcification at the lesion by careful angiographic evaluation or use of IVUS/OCT. Calcification at curves and tortuosity at the lesion site are the most common reasons for inability to deliver BRS in the first go.

3. **For mild to moderate calcification,** high pressure predilatation (≥18–20 atm) with a near optimal size noncompliant (NC) balloon and occasionally with scoring/cutting balloon should be performed to break the lesion completely and achieve less than 20% residual stenosis.

   **For severe calcification,** RA as per standard technique [8] followed by NC balloon high pressure predilatation should be performed (Cases 1–3).

4. **All efforts should be made to deliver the scaffold in the first attempt as withdrawal of A-BVS is to be avoided**. Routine use of support wires (like Balance Heavy Weight and All Star [Abbott Vascular, Santa Clara, CA]) to deliver the device to the lesion through the calcified artery and on occasions upfront use of buddy wire help to achieve delivery success in the first go (Case 4).

5. **If the BRS is unable to traverse a calcified curve,** then sustained and firm pressure would gradually slip the BRS though calcified curves; "dottering" as done with mDES should not be done with BRS (Case 5).

6. **Mother and child catheters like Guideliner** (Vascular Solutions Inc., Minneapolis, MN) can be used to deliver BRS through difficult tortuous calcified anatomy but familiarity with practice points is required [9] (see Figure 7.9.1, Cases 6 and 7).

7. **Proper sizing of the BRS to the vessel** is very important as the BRS should not be expanded to more than 0.5 mm beyond its original diameter.

8. **High pressure postdilatation (despite a good angiographic result after deployment) with a 0.25–0.5 mm higher NC balloon to ≥20 atm** (but keeping within the recommended expansion limit of the BRS) is necessary to achieve optimization especially if imaging is not used. It has been shown that within the vessel, the A-BVS does not necessarily achieve the dimension as listed in the compliance chart and expansion is impaired mostly by calcification [10]. This can be optimized by high pressure postdilatation, which should be performed routinely in all calcified lesions [11].

9. **Final imaging with IVUS/OCT** is recommended to assess adequate expansion and full strut apposition.

10. **Meticulous attention to antiplatelet regimen** postprocedure is essential to avoid scaffold thrombosis.

**A) 7F "Guideliner" (6F guideliner for 7F Guide Catheter), ID: 0.062"**
    a. All sizes of A-BVS can be delivered through a 7F Guideliner.
    b. The 3.5 mm BVS is tight fit and needs to be preloaded.

**B) 6F GL (5F GL in 6F Guide Catheter), ID: 0.056"**
    a. The 2.5 mm and 3.0 mm A-BVS are tight fit and should be preloaded into the GL and then advanced into the guide catheter.
    b. The 3.5 mm A-BVS cannot be preloaded into a 6F GL.

    NB: This information is important for radial intervention where predominantly 6F guide catheters are used.

**C) Entry of A-BVS through the proximal metallic collar of GL**
    a. Is much improved in GL version 3.
    b. Occasionally there is a intertwining of wire with the shaft of GL, hence entry of A-BVS into the GL extension tube through proximal collar should be under direction vision and extremely gentle.
    c. If difficulty in advancing A-BVS through proximal collar of the extension tube
        i. Withdraw GL back into thoracic aorta so entry of A-BVS more coaxial
        ii. Intubate the GL deeply into the vessel and withdraw the guide catheter by 4–5 cm to alter the alignment of A-BRS to the entry collar and remove Guidewire bias.

**Figure 7.9.1** Tips and tricks of using Guideliner (GL) (Vascular Solutions Inc., Minneapolis, MN) for delivering A-BVS. (From Seth A, Ravisekar V, Kaul U. *Indian Heart* 2014;66:453–458.)

## ILLUSTRATIVE CASES

### CASE 1: Severe calcified lesion pretreated with rotational atherectomy and long A-BVS implanted under OCT guidance

- **Clinical history:**
  - 53-year-old male
  - Hypertension for 1 year
  - Diabetes mellitus for 9 years
  - Strong positive family history of coronary artery disease
  - Presented with chronic stable angina (CCS class III) and positive treadmill test
  - Attempt at PCI failed at another center as even a 1.25 mm balloon could not cross the lesion
  - LVEF 60%
- **Angiographic finding:** Severely calcified mid-RCA 95% lesion.
- **Cine 1:** Coronary angiogram performed in LAO projection with 7F JR 3.5 guiding catheter demonstrated severely calcified mid-RCA 95% lesion.
- **Cine 2:** Rotational atherectomy was performed with 1.5 mm burr.
- **Cine 3:** Wire exchanged for All Star wire (Abbott Vascular, Santa Clara, CA); OCT was performed. Predilatation performed with 3 × 15 mm noncompliant balloon at 17 atm.
- **Cine 4:** A-BVS 3 × 28 mm positioned across the lesion and gradually deployed at 8 atm. Postdilatation was performed with 3.25 × 15 mm noncompliant balloon at 24 atm.
- **Cine 5:** Angiogram performed after postdilatation of A-BVS. OCT was performed.
- **Cine 6:** Again postdilatation was performed using 3.5 × 12 mm noncompliant balloon at 22 atm. OCT was performed.
- **Cine 7:** Final angiogram in LAO projection demonstrating no residual stenosis with TIMI III flow.
- **OCT findings:**
  - OCT Clip 1: OCT performed at baseline demonstrated tight stenosis with calcification seen in mid-RCA.
  - OCT clip 2: OCT performed after first postdilatation with 2.5 × 15 mm noncompliant balloon at 24 atm demonstrated underexpanded malapposed scaffolds.
  - OCT clip 3: OCT performed after second postdilatation with 3.25 × 15 mm noncompliant balloon at 26 atm, demonstrated well-embedded, well-apposed, and well-expanded scaffolds.
- **Follow up:**
  - Patient doing well and asymptomatic at 6 weeks follow-up.

### CASE 2: Severe calcified lesion pretreated with rotational atherectomy followed by implantation of A-BVS with bifurcation T-stenting

- **Clinical History:**
  - 56-year-old male
  - No family history of coronary artery disease
  - Non-smoker
  - Dyslipidemia
  - Presented with atypical chest pain
  - Stress echo demonstrated fresh exercise-induced ischemia with distal septal hypokinesia
  - LVEF 60%
- **Angiographic finding:** 80% calcified bifurcation lesion of distal LAD/diagonal.
- **Cine 1 and 2:** Angiogram performed in AP cranial and LAO cranial projections with 7F XB 3.5 guiding catheter demonstrated 80% calcified bifurcation lesion of distal LAD/diagonal (Medina 1,1,1).
- **Cine 3:** Rotational atherectomy was performed with 1.5 mm burr.
- **Cine 4:** Rotawire was exchanged to All Star wire (Abbott Vascular, Santa Clara, CA) in LAD and Sion blue wire (Asahi Intecc, Aichi, Japan) was passed into the second diagonal branch. Predilatation of LAD was performed using 2.75 × 12 mm noncompliant balloon at 18 atm, following which the large second diagonal branch was pinched.

- **Cine 5:** The second diagonal was also dilated using 2.75 × 12 mm balloon at 14 atm.
- **Cine 6:** A-BVS 2.5 × 18 mm was positioned into the second diagonal in a manner that the proximal balloon marker lies just proximal to the side branch ostium. A 3.0 × 8 mm noncompliant balloon was placed in LAD and the side branch scaffold was deployed at 10 atm and then dilated with 2.75 x 12 mm noncompliant balloon to 20 atm. The proximal scaffold marker lies just beyond the ostium of the side branch with minimal protrusion of the scaffold into the main branch.
- **Cine 7:** Then wire in diagonal was removed. A 3 × 18 mm A-BVS was then deployed at 12 atm in the LAD across the second diagonal to perform T stenting.
- **Cine 8:** The LAD A-BVS was postdilated with a 3.5 × 8 mm noncompliant balloon to 16 atm distally and then 20 atm proximally.
- **Cine 9:** The struts of the LAD A-BVS were crossed with Sion blue wire into the second diagonal through the side branch scaffold. The struts of the main branch scaffold were dilated with a 2 mm noncompliant balloon followed by a 2.5 mm noncompliant balloon. A final snuggle balloon dilatation was performed as shown using a 3.25 × 15 mm noncompliant balloon in main branch and a 2.75 × 12 mm noncompliant balloon in side branch.
- **Cine 10 and 11:** Final result of a bifurcation T stenting using A-BVS in a calcified lesion demonstrated in LAO cranial and AP cranial projections.
- **Follow-up:**
  - Stress echo done at 12 months post-index procedure was negative for inducible ischemia.
  - CT coronary angiogram at 12 months post-index procedure demonstrated patent scaffolds and no restenosis.

## CASE 3: Long severe calcified lesion pretreated with rotational atherectomy followed by multiple A-BVS implantation with 18-months CT coronary angiography follow-up

- **Clinical History:**
  - 74-year-old female
  - Hypertension for 20 years
  - Dyslipidemia
  - Atypical chest pain
  - LVEF 60%
  - Stress thallium demonstrates anterior wall ischemia
- **Angiographic finding:** Long severely calcified lesion 80% in proximal to mid-LAD lesion also involving a large first diagonal branch.
- **Cine 1 and 2:** Coronary angiography with 7F XB 3.0 guiding catheter in RAO caudal and AP cranial projections demonstrating a long severely calcified lesion 80% in proximal to mid-LAD lesion also involving a large first diagonal branch (Medina 1,1,0).
- **Cine 3:** Rotational atherectomy was performed using 1.5 mm burr.
- **Cine 4:** Following rotational atherectomy, All Star wire (Abbott Vascular, Santa Clara, CA) was placed in LAD; BMW wire (Abbott Vascular, Santa Clara, CA) was placed in the first diagonal; predilatation was performed with 2.5 × 12 mm noncompliant balloon to 22 atm. A-BVS 2.5 × 28 mm was positioned distally and deployed at 12 atm. Then postdilatation was performed with 2.75 × 15 mm noncompliant balloon to 22 atm.
- **Cine 5:** A second A-BVS 3 × 28 mm was positioned proximally with the distal balloon marker of this scaffold abutting the proximal marker of the distal scaffold. It was deployed at 12 atm and then postdilated with 3 × 15 mm noncompliant balloon to 24 atm.
- **Cine 6:** The side branch wire was removed. Then a third A-BVS 3.5 × 12 mm was positioned in proximal LAD, so that the distal balloon maker of this scaffold abuts the proximal marker of the second scaffold. Then this scaffold was deployed at 10 atm and postdilated with 3.75 × 8 mm noncompliant balloon to 18 atm.
- **Cine 7:** AP cranial projection demonstrating the overlapped scaffolds in LAD with scaffold markers side by side.
- **Cine 8 and 9:** Final angiogram in AP cranial and RAO caudal projections demonstrating very good result with TIMI 3 flow and maintained patency of first diagonal with moderate stenosis at its origin.
- **Follow-up:**
  - Stress thallium scan done at 6 months post-index procedure was negative for inducible ischemia.
  - CT coronary angiogram at 18 months post-index procedure demonstrated maintained patency of scaffolds and no restenosis.

## CASE 4: Long severe calcified lesion pretreated with rotational atherectomy and multiple A-BVS delivered under OCT guidance and 1 year CT coronary angiography follow-up

- **Clinical history:**
  - 63-year-old male
  - Dyslipidemia for 10 years
  - Ex-smoker, stopped smoking 25 years ago
  - With history of breathlessness, sweating, chest pain, 1 year back
  - Treadmill test positive for reversible myocardial ischemia
- **Angiographic finding:** Triple vessel coronary artery disease.
  - Proximal LAD 60–70% lesion (FFR = 0.83)
  - Proximal OM1 shows 50% lesion
  - Long severely calcified lesion 95% in proximal and mid-RCA
- **Cine 1 and 2:** Coronary angiogram performed in LAO and RAO projections with 7F JR 3.5 guiding catheter demonstrated long severely calcified lesion 95% in mid-RCA.
- **Cine 3:** Lesion crossed with Fielder FC wire (Asahi Intecc, Aichi, Japan), predilated with 1.2 × 06 mm balloon at 16 atm and then using a microcatheter, this wire was exchanged to rotawire.
- **Cine 4 and 5:** Rotational atherectomy along the lesion was performed with 1.25 mm burr and then followed by 1.5 mm burr.
- **Cine 6:** Angiogram performed after rotablation.
- **Cine 7:** The rotawire wire exchanged for All Star wire was passed into PLB, another upfront buddy wire Sion blue (Asahi Intecc, Aichi, Japan) was passed into PDA. The length of the lesion was predilated with 2.5 × 12 mm noncompliant balloon at 16 atm. A-BVS 2.5 × 28 mm was passed over the buddy wire deployed at 11 atm and then postdilated with 2.5 × 12 mm noncompliant balloon at 28 atm and then with 2.75 × 15 mm noncompliant balloon at 22 atm.
- **Cine 8:** A-BVS 3 × 28 mm had difficulty in being delivered through the proximal scaffold and calcified lesion.
- **Cine 9:** This scaffold was placed in mid-RCA with the distal balloon marker of this scaffold abutting the proximal scaffold marker of the distal scaffold. This second scaffold was deployed at 10 atm and then postdilated with 3 × 12 mm noncompliant balloon at 22 atm.
- **Cine 10:** Then A-BVS 3.5 × 18 mm was positioned in proximal RCA minimally overlapping the second scaffold, so that the distal balloon marker of this scaffold abutting the proximal scaffold marker of the second scaffold. This third scaffold was gradually deployed at 10 atm.
- **Cine 11:** Postdilation of the third scaffold was performed with 3.5 × 15 mm noncompliant balloon at 24 atm.
- **Cine 12 and 13:** Final angiogram performed in LAO and RAO projections demonstrated no residual stenosis with TIMI III flow.
- **OCT findings:**
  - OCT clip 1: OCT performed after postdilatation of the lesion with high pressure noncompliant balloons demonstrated well-apposed, well-expanded, and well-embedded struts of scaffolds.
- **Follow-up:**
  - Exercise thallium scan performed at 12 months post-index procedure was negative for inducible ischemia.
  - CT coronary angiography performed at 12 months post-index procedure demonstrated patent scaffolds.

## CASE 5: Sustained and firm pressure to deliver A-BVS through calcified tortuous OM artery

- **Clinical history:**
  - 46-year-old male
  - Hypertension for 10 years
  - Dyslipidemia
  - Hypothyroidism
  - No family history of coronary artery disease
  - Presented with non-ST elevation MI; ECG showing ST depression in V4-V6, elevated blood levels of cardiac biomarkers
  - Normal LV function

- **Angiographic finding:**
  - Triple vessel coronary artery disease
  - Calcified 80% lesion in proximal LAD—treated with 3.5 × 18 mm A-BVS
  - Calcified tortuous proximal OM1 with 90% lesion
  - 50% lesion in mid-RCA
- **Cine 1:** Coronary angiogram performed in AP cranial projection with 7F XB 3.5 guiding catheter demonstrated calcified 80% lesion in proximal LAD and calcified tortuous proximal OM1 with 90% lesion.
- **Cine 2:** All Star wire (Abbott Vascular, Santa Clara, CA) was passed into OM1. Another buddy wire BMW (Abbott Vascular, Santa Clara, CA) also passed into OM1. Lesion was predilated with 2.5 × 15 mm noncompliant balloon at 12 atm.
- **Cine 3:** With sustained and firm pressure 2.5 × 28 mm A-BVS gradually slipped through the calcified curve. It was positioned across the lesion and deployed at 10 atm. Postdilated with 2.75 × 15 mm noncompliant balloon at 22 atm. Dissection occurred in proximal stent edge. So this was covered with 2.75 × 8 mm XIENCE Xpedition stent (Abbott Vascular, Santa Clara, CA) deployed at 18 atm.
- **Cine 4:** Final result in RAO caudal projection demonstrating no residual stenosis with TIMI 3 flow.
- **Follow-up:**
  - Patient doing well at 6 weeks post-index procedure.

## CASE 6: Guideliner use for delivering A-BVS in tortuous calcified LAD after failed attempts

- **Clinical history:**
  - 60 years old
  - Hypertension
  - PCI with Cypher 2.75 × 28 mm stent to proximal LAD 11 years ago
  - Presented with unstable angina
  - ECG showing T-wave inversion in Lead III and aVF
  - Normal blood levels of cardiac biomarkers
  - LVEF 55%
- **Angiographic finding:** Tortuous calcified proximal LAD with patent stent in mid-LAD and a long 80–90% tortuous lesion in distal LAD. Proximal LAD shows tortuosity with moderate to severe calcification while distal LAD lesion shows moderate calcification.
- **Cine 1:** Angiogram performed in RAO cranial projection with 7F XB 3.5 catheter demonstrated tortuous calcified proximal LAD with patent stent in mid-LAD and a long 80–90% tortuous lesion in distal LAD. Proximal LAD showed tortuosity with moderate to severe calcification while distal LAD lesion demonstrated moderate calcification.
- **Cine 2:** All Star wire (Abbott Vascular, Santa Clara, CA) was passed into LAD. There was difficulty in crossing the distal lesion with 2.25 × 12 mm balloon with the guiding catheter backing out.
- **Cine 3:** Lesion was predilated with a 1.5 mm balloon followed by a 2.25 × 12 mm with noncompliant balloon at 20 atm. Various maneuvers to get a 2.5 × 28 mm A-BVS across proximal tortuous LAD failed.
- **Cine 4:** A-BVS was withdrawn and 7F guideliner was passed across the proximal LAD tracking up to mid-LAD.
- **Cine 5:** A-BVS 2.5 × 28 mm was passed through the guideliner and positioned across the lesion in distal LAD.
- **Cine 6:** Guideliner was removed and A-BVS 2.5 × 28 mm was gradually deployed at 10 atm at the lesion site. Then this scafflold was postdilated with 2.5 × 15 mm noncompliant balloon at 24 atm.
- **Cine 7:** Final result in RAO cranial projection showing no residual stenosis with TIMI 3 flow.
- **Follow-up:**
  - Patient continues to do well with negative stress echo at 5 months post-index procedure.

CASE 7: Guideliner preloaded with A-BVS for delivering the scaffold across a calcified angulated RCA after failed attempts

- **Clinical history:**
  - 65 years old
  - Hypertension
  - Diabetes mellitus
  - Chronic stable angina (CCS class III)
  - LVEF 60%
  - Renal dysfunction
- **Angiographic finding:** Double vessel coronary artery disease; 95% calcified angulated in proximal RCA and 80–90% long lesion in LAD. In view of renal dysfunction, staged procedure was done to reduce contrast load. LAD was lesion treated with 2.5 × 28 mm A-BVS and 2.75 × 8 mm XIENCE V stent in another sitting.
- **Cine 1:** Coronary angiogram performed in LAO projection with 7F guiding catheter demonstrated 95% calcified lesion in angulated proximal RCA.
- **Cine 2:** Lesion was crossed with All Star wire (Abbott Vascular, Santa Clara, CA); predilated with 3 × 12 mm noncompliant balloon at 20 atm.
- **Cine 3:** Inability to deliver a 3.5 × 18 mm A-BVS across the tortuous calcified lesion despite various maneuvers including deep throttling of guide catheter.
- **Cine 4:** A-BVS was withdrawn because of failed attempts in delivering it to the lesion site.
- **Cine 5:** Further dilatation was performed with a 3.5 × 12 mm noncompliant balloon at 20 atm.
- **Cine 6:** Buddy wire BMW (Abbott Vascular, Santa Clara, CA) was passed into PDA. There was inability to deliver the scaffold despite various guide catheter maneuvers.
- **Cine 7:** Scaffold and buddy wire were withdrawn and 7F guideliner was placed across the calcified proximal RCA angulation. There was inability to get A-BVS through the proximal metal collar of guideliner into the extension tube.
- **Cine 8:** The guideliner was preloaded with 3.5 × 18 mm A-BVS and brought to the tip of guide catheter.
- **Cine 9:** The guideliner was then advanced into the lesion using a guide catheter backup and the 3.5 × 18 mm A-BVS was being delivered across the lesion.
- **Cine 10:** A-BVS 3.5 × 18 mm was deployed at 12 atm and then postdilated with 3.5 × 12 mm noncompliant balloon at 24 atm.
- **Cine 11:** Final result in LAO projection demonstrated no residual stenosis and no dissection with TIMI 3 flow.
- **Follow-up:**
  - Exercise thallium scan performed at 24 months post-index procedure demonstrated no inducible ischemia.

## RESULTS AND OUTCOMES

Sparse data exist presently regarding the procedural outcomes of BRS in calcified lesions. These lesions were excluded from the initial studies of BRS but with increasing experience most of the real world registries have included calcified lesions.

The ABSORB Extend Registry excluded severely calcified lesions [12]. The Ghost EU Registry does not mention the incidence of calcified lesions or whether they had any relationship to adverse outcomes [13]. The ABSORB First Worldwide Registry [14], the ASSURE German Registry [15], and the AMC Netherlands Registry [16] had 18.8%, 15.7%, and 11% moderate to heavily calcified lesions. Though the numbers of severely calcified lesions in the registries are small and the procedural and short-term outcomes of this specific subgroup are unclear, yet in none of these registries were any adverse outcomes in the immediate and short-term related to the calcified lesions. In B-Search Registry [17], inability to deliver this device did relate to calcified vessels. Hence, based on the present data no strong

recommendation can be made regarding the appropriateness of BRS in severely calcified lesions [18].

Panoulas et al. [19] published their initial experience of use of A-BVS in calcified lesions in 163 real world patients 62 (38%) of whom had moderate to heavy calcification and compared them to the remainder 101 patients who had noncalcified lesions. The calcified lesion group had a higher prevalence of diabetes, chronic kidney disease, more complex lesions, and longer lesions. Predilatation with NC balloon and scoring balloon was significantly higher in calcified lesions versus the noncalcified group. RA was used in nearly 11.8% calcified lesion versus none in noncalcified lesions and cutting/scoring balloons in 26.3% versus 6.9%. IVUS was used in 96% of the calcified lesions for lesion assessment and result optimization. Post-BRS implantation, the acute gain and the minimal scaffold area were no different in the two groups. While the angiographic success was similar in both groups, there was a higher rate of periprocedural MI in the calcified lesion subgroup (13.1% vs. 5.0%,

$p = .067$). It is unclear from the article whether this difference was primarily related to just CPK rise alone, which could occur from distal embolization due to RA, longer length of lesion coverage with occlusion of very small side branches by thick scaffold struts, and high pressure postdilatation along the long length of the scaffolds. At a median follow-up at 14 months, no difference in MACE was observed between the two groups for death, MI, TLR, or stent thrombosis.

In our own experience in the first 200 real world cases performed between January 2013 and August 2013, our device delivery success rate was 96%. All eight delivery failures related to calcified lesions. Of these 8 patients, 6 (6%) occurred in the first 100 patients and 2 (2%) in the next 100, thereby outlining the learning curve. The device was withdrawn once in 4 patients, twice in 2 patients, and three times in 2 patients. In all patients, the device was finally delivered (procedural success rate 100%) by using a combination of buddy wire with a support wire (3 patients) and/or more aggressive lesion and vessel preparation by further high pressure predilatation with a larger NC balloon (3 patients), RA (1 patient), and Guideliner

use (3 patients). Our early experience has taught us to carefully evaluate the vessel and lesion, and use these strategies upfront to achieve successful delivery in the first go.

To date in our experience, 100 patients with angiographic calcification (142 lesions) have been treated between January 2013 and December 2014 using 192 A-BVS (1.9 BVS per patient). Thirty-three of these patients (33%) underwent RA for severe calcification prior to A-BVS implantation (Figures 7.9.2 and 7.9.3). Over a median follow-up of 15 months, clinical follow-up is available in 30 of the 31 patients (94%). CT coronary angiography (7 patients) and stress echocardiogram (14 patients) have been performed at 1 year in 21 of these 31 patients (68%), 8 of the 31 patients remain event-free at a median follow up of 15 months. Two patients developed restenosis treated with further stent implantation and one patient had progression of another lesion in the target vessel needing further stent implantation. Most importantly, there was no acute, subacute, or late scaffold thrombosis or acute MI. Thus, our experience of RA followed by A-BVS implantation for heavily calcified lesions is associated with low complication rates and favorable intermediate-term outcomes. However, BVS in calcified vessels <2.75 mm should be avoided due to increased risk for thrombosis.

## CONCLUSION

BRS can be safely used to treat calcified coronary arteries with favorable immediate and short-term outcomes. This requires understanding the procedural tips and tricks to achieve delivery success, and it requires aggressive and adequate lesion preparation using high pressure predilatation with NC balloons/scoring or cutting balloons. Use of RA especially in long severely calcified lesions is important to achieve successful implantation of long, multiple BRS. High pressure postdilatation with a NC balloon is a must for all cases and regular use of imaging modalities helps to optimize the final results. Meticulous attention to technical details including antiplatelet

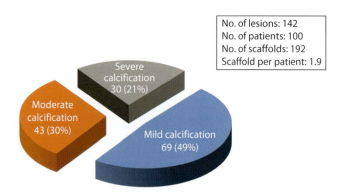

No. of lesions: 142
No. of patients: 100
No. of scaffolds: 192
Scaffold per patient: 1.9

Severe calcification 30 (21%)

Moderate calcification 43 (30%)

Mild calcification 69 (49%)

**Figure 7.9.2** Severity of calcification in 100 patients (142 lesions) with angiographic calcification undergoing A-BVS implantation between January 2013 and December 2014 at Fortis Escorts Heart Institute.

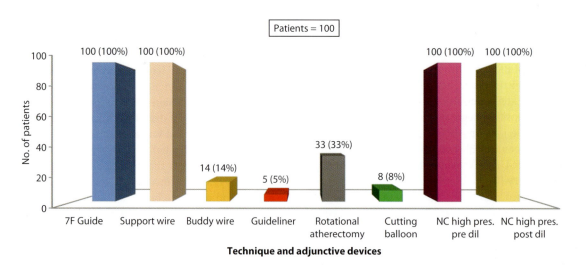

**Figure 7.9.3** Technical considerations for implantation of A-BVS in 100 calcified vessels (Fortis Escorts Heart Institute Experience).

regimens in this complex subgroup of patients ensures low scaffold thrombosis rates and favorable long-term outcomes, comparable to those of BRS in noncalcified lesions or mDES. At this stage, the routine use of BRS in mild to moderate calcified lesion is acceptable, but in heavily calcified lesion is not recommended. The potential advantage of BRS for long diffuse calcified disease would need to be proven. It could have potential advantages especially for long and diffuse calcific disease. Thus, we await the results of more dedicated and larger studies with long-term follow-up especially with angiography and intravascular imaging to define its definitive role in the treatment of this difficult lesion subgroup.

## REFERENCES

1. Felix C, Everaert B, Diletti R, Van Mieghem N, Daemen J, Valgimigli M, de Jaegere PP et al. Current status of clinically available bioresorbable scaffolds in percutaneous coronary interventions. *Neth Heart J.* 2015 Mar;23(3):153–60.

2. Seth A, Kumar V. Bioresorbable scaffold: "Looking at the 'real world' through a plastic tube." *Cathet Cardiovasc Interv.* 2014;84:53–54.

3. Mintz GS, Popma JJ, Pichard AD, Kent KM, Satler LF, Chuang YC, Ditrano CJ, Leon MB. Patterns of calcification in coronary artery disease. A statistical analysis of intravascular ultrasound and coronary angiography in 1155 lesions. *Circulation.* 1995;91:1959–65.

4. Bourantas CV, Zhang YJ, Garg S, Iqbal J, Valgimigli M, Windecker S, Mohr FW et al. Prognostic implications of coronary calcification in patients with obstructive coronary artery disease treated by percutaneous coronary intervention: A patient-level pooled analysis of 7 contemporary stent trials. *Heart.* 2014 Aug;100(15):1158–64.

5. Oberhauser JP, Hossainy S, Rapoza RJ. Design principles and performance of bioresorbable polymeric vascular scaffolds. *EuroIntervention.* 2009 Dec 15;5 Suppl F:F15–22.

6. Tanimoto S, Bruining N, van Domburg RT, Rotger D, Radeva P, Ligthart JM, Serruys PW. Late stent recoil of the bioabsorbable everolimus-eluting coronary stent and its relationship with plaque morphology. *J Am Coll Cardiol.* 2008 Nov 11;52(20):1616–20.

7. Costopoulos C, Naganuma T, Colombo A. Tools and techniques clinical: Percutaneous intervention of calcific coronary lesions. *EuroIntervention.* 2014;9:1–10.

8. Tomey MI, Kini AS, Sharma SK. Current status of rotational atherectomy. *JACC Cardiovasc Interv.* 2014 Apr;7(4):345–53.

9. Seth A, Ravisekar V, Kaul U. Use of 'Guideliner' catheter to overcome failure of delivery of Absorb™ bioresorbable vascular scaffold in calcified tortuous coronary lesions: Technical considerations in 'real world patients'. *Indian Heart J.* 2014;66:453–458.

10. Attizzani GF, Ohno Y, Capodanno D, Francaviglia B, Grasso C, Sgroi C, Wang W et al. New insights on acute expansion and longitudinal elongation of bioresorbable vascular scaffolds in vivo and at bench test: A note of caution on reliance to compliance charts and nominal length. *Cathet Cardiovasc Interv.* 2015;85(4):E99–E107.

11. Seth A, Kumar V, Rastogi V. BRS in complex lesions: Massaging (and messaging) the right pressure points. *EuroIntervention.* 2015;11:131–135.

12. Abizaid A, Costa Jr. JR, Bartorelli AL, Whitbourn R, Jan van Geuns R, Chevalier B, Patel T et al. The ABSORB EXTEND study: Preliminary report of the twelve-month clinical outcomes in the first 512 patients enrolled. *EuroIntervention.* 2015;10:1396–1401.

13. Capodanno D, Gori T, Nef H, Latib A, Mehilli J, Lesiak M, Caramanno G et al. Percutaneous coronary intervention with everolimus-eluting bioresorbable vascular scaffolds in routine clinical practice: Early and midterm outcomes from the European multi-centre GHOST-EU registry. *EuroIntervention.* 2015 Feb;10(10):1144–53.

14. Eeckhout E, Naber CK, Mao VW, Miquel-Hebert K, Gao Y, Cheong W-F, Staehr P et al. ABSORB FIRST real-world registry: One-year clinical outcomes on 958 patients. Presented at EuroPCR 2015.

15. Wöhrle J, Naber C, Schmitz T, Schwencke C, Frey N, Butter C, Brachmann J et al. Beyond the early stages: Insights from the ASSURE registry on bioresorbable vascular scaffolds. *EuroIntervention.* 2015 Jun;11(2):149–56.

16. Kraak RP, Hassell ME, Grundeken MJ, Koch KT, Henriques JP, Piek JJ, Baan J Jr et al. Initial experience and clinical evaluation of the Absorb bioresorbable vascular scaffold (BVS) in real-world practice: The AMC Single Centre Real World PCI Registry. *EuroIntervention.* 2015 Feb;10(10):1160–8.

17. Simsek C, Magro M, Onuma Y, Boersma E, Smits P, Dorange C, Veldhof S et al. Procedural and clinical outcomes of the Absorb everolimus-eluting bioresorbable vascular scaffold: One-month results of the Bioresorbable vascular Scaffold Evaluated At Rotterdam Cardiology Hospitals (B-SEARCH). *EuroIntervention.* 2014 Jun;10(2):236–40.

18. Everaert B, Felix C, Koolen J, den Heijer P, Henriques J, Wykrzykowska JJ, van der Schaaf R et al. Appropriate use of bioresorbable vascular scaffolds in percutaneous coronary interventions: A recommendation from experienced users: A position statement on the use of bioresorbable vascular scaffolds in the Netherlands. *Neth Heart J.* (2015) 23:161–165.

19. Panoulas VF, Miyazaki T, Sato K, Naganuma T, Sticchi A, Kawamoto H, Figini F et al. Procedural outcomes of patients with calcified lesions treated with bioresorbable vascular scaffolds. *EuroIntervention.* 2016 Mar;11(12):1355–62.

# Invasive sealing of vulnerable, high-risk lesions

CHRISTOS V. BOURANTAS, RYO TORRI, NICOLAS FOIN, AJAY SURI, ERHAN TENEKECIOGLU,
VIKAS THONDAPU, TOM CRAKE, PETER BARLIS, AND PATRICK W.J.C. SERRUYS

## THE CONCEPT OF THE VULNERABLE PLAQUE

Pioneering histology-based studies performed at the beginning of the last century have demonstrated that the culprit lesions responsible for sudden death have specific morphological characteristics [1–4]. More recently, Davies and Thomas have shown that plaque disruption was the main cause of coronary thrombosis and is associated with crescendo angina, myocardial infarction, and sudden death [5,6]. These landmark studies have attracted attention and efforts were made to identify features associated with plaque vulnerability. Today it is known that the high-risk lesions have a specific phenotype called thin cap fibroatheroma (TCFA) that exhibits an increased plaque burden, with a necrotic core that is covered by a thin fibrous cap and is rich in macrophages [7–10]. More recent evidence has shown that vulnerable lesions also have micro-calcifications and are rich in neo-vessels and cholesterol crystals [11–13].

## IN VIVO DETECTION OF VULNERABLE LESIONS: CURRENT EVIDENCE

The advent of intravascular imaging and the introduction of intravascular ultrasound (IVUS) in the clinical arena in the early 1990s enabled for the first time in vivo assessment of coronary plaque morphology and evaluation of its vulnerability [14,15]. Small-scale imaging studies have shown that lesions that progressed to cause events have a different morphology than those that remained dormant creating hope that intravascular imaging can detect these high-risk plaques [16]. The PROSPECT and the VIVA studies were the first prospective large-scale studies of coronary atherosclerosis [17,18]. The PROSPECT study included 697 patients admitted with an acute coronary syndrome that had complete revascularization and IVUS-virtual histology (VH) imaging in the nonculprit vessels. At 3-year follow-up, 104 new lesions developed in the nonculprit vessels, of which only 55 were studied by IVUS-VH. It was shown that an increased plaque burden (>70%), a minimum lumen area <4 mm$^2$ and a TCFA phenotype were all independent predictors of lesions that progressed and caused events. Of note the positive predictive value of IVUS-VH in detecting these high-risk lesions was only 18.2%. Similar were the results of the VIVA study that included 170 patients admitted with stable angina or an acute coronary syndrome that were treated with percutaneous coronary intervention (PCI) and had IVUS-VH in the nonculprit vessels. At 1-year follow-up there were 13 nonculprit lesion-related events, and as for the PROSPECT study, a lumen area (<4 mm$^2$), plaque burden (>70%), and a TCFA phenotype were associated future events.

Finally, the PREDICTION study was the only prospective study that investigated the prognostic implications of the local hemodynamic forces. In this study, 506 patients admitted with an acute coronary event had IVUS imaging in the non-culprit vessels at baseline and at 6–10 months follow-up. The IVUS data at baseline were fused with the angiographic data to reconstruct coronary anatomy and in the obtained models blood flow simulation was performed. Low endothelial shear stress (ESS) at baseline appeared to associate with a lumen reduction and an increase in plaque burden at follow-up. An increased plaque burden and low ESS were the only predictors of lesions that progressed and required revascularization at follow-up (positive predictive value: 41%) [19]. A recent meta-analysis of the PREDICTION study that included information about the composition of the plaque, which was provided by the radiofrequency analysis of the IVUS backscatter signal, has demonstrated that the addition of plaque component to the ESS and plaque burden increased considerably the positive predictive value of the developed model from 41% to 53% [20].

## EMERGING INVASIVE AND NONINVASIVE IMAGING MODALITIES

The first invasive imaging-based studies of coronary atherosclerosis have provided robust evidence that intravascular imaging is able to identify vulnerable, high-risk lesions but also revealed significant limitations of the existing techniques [21]. The low accuracy of the available modalities in detecting these lesions and assessing accurately the composition of the plaque [22–25], the fact that they do not enable assessment of the entire coronary tree, and the risk of complications (i.e., in the PROSPECT study the complication rate was 1.6% and in the PREDICTION 0.6%) are significant drawbacks that cannot justify their use in the clinical arena. To overcome these limitations, efforts were made over the last years to develop advanced intravascular imaging techniques that would enable more accurate assessment of plaque pathobiology. Therefore, apart from IVUS, optical coherence tomography (OCT), and near infrared spectroscopy (NIRS) that have already applications in the clinical arena, several other invasive imaging techniques have recently emerged including: near infrared fluorescence (NIRF) imaging [26], intravascular photoacoustic imaging (IVPA) [27], time resolved fluorescence spectroscopy (TRFS) [28], and Raman spectroscopy [29]. These techniques appear able to provide complementary information about plaque composition, biology, and vulnerability. In parallel efforts are currently underway to develop dual-probe catheters that combine two imaging modalities with complementary strengths and allow complete assessment of plaque pathobiology [30]. Several prototypes are available today and include the combined NIRS-IVUS catheter, the IVUS-OCT [31,32], the OCT-NIRF [33], the IVUS-NIRF [34], the OCT-NIRS [35], the IVUS-IVPA [36,37], and the combined IVUS-TRFS [38,39]. Two of these devices—the NIRS-IVUS and the OCT-NIRF catheters—already have applications in the clinical arena. Histology-based studies have shown that combined NIRS and IVUS imaging allows more accurate detection of high-risk plaques than standalone IVUS [40], while small-scale clinical studies have demonstrated that NIRS-IVUS-derived plaque characteristics can differentiate with high accuracy culprit from nonculprit lesions in patients admitted with ST-elevation myocardial infarction (STEMI) [41] or non-STEMI and unstable angina [42]. These findings created hope that NIRS-IVUS imaging would be able to accurately identify vulnerable lesions and two prospective studies (the PROSPECT II, NCT02171065 and the LRP study, NCT02033694) are currently underway to investigate the value of NIRS-IVUS in detecting lesions that are prone to progress and cause events.

Recently Ughi et al. have demonstrated the feasibility of OCT-NIRF imaging in humans [43]. Experimental studies have provided evidence that combined OCT-NIRF imaging can assess plaque morphology, detect the presence of inflammation, and evaluate vessel wall healing and fibrin deposition in stented segments [33,44]. Therefore, this catheter is expected to provide unique insights about the role of plaque biology on atherosclerotic evolution and stent failure.

In parallel, advances in computed tomographic coronary angiography (CTCA, e.g., the use of dual X-ray sources, the increased number of detectors, the decreased slice thickness and the faster rotation gantry) have permitted assessment of coronary artery anatomy and morphology with reduced radiation dose. Numerous studies in patients without established coronary artery disease have demonstrated that CTCA can detect the lumen, outer vessel wall, and plaque dimensions, and provide information about the composition of the plaque [45–48] while histology-based studies have shown that CTCA can also detect the phenotype of the plaque: a napkin-ring sign in CTCA constitutes a typical signature of high-risk atherosclerotic lesions with an increased lipid core component [49–51]. In a study that included 895 patients, CTCA-derived plaque characteristics (i.e., positive remodeling, low attenuated plaques, and napkin-ring sign) appeared to enable identification of lesions that are prone to progress and cause adverse cardiovascular events [52], while a larger retrospective analysis which included 1650 patients has shown that the culprit lesions that cause events at 2-year follow-up had different morphological characteristics at baseline CTCA (i.e., an increased plaque burden, lower attenuation, and a smaller lumen area) from those that remained silent [53].

Recent advances in nuclear medicine have enabled the identification of new positron emission tomographic tracers that are able to detect noninvasively vascular inflammation. $^{18}$F-fluoride and $^{68}$Ga-DOTATATE have been used to study plaque biology and today there is evidence to support their value in detecting inflamed plaques and vulnerable lesions [54–57]. Currently, the PREFFIR (NCT02278211) study is underway and aims to investigate the prognostic value of $^{18}$F-fluoride positron emission tomography-CTCA imaging in 700 patients admitted with an acute coronary syndrome, and examine its value in detecting lesions that will progress and cause events.

## ROLE OF BIORESORBABLE VASCULAR SCAFFOLDS IN SEALING HIGH-RISK VULNERABLE LESIONS

The aforementioned advances in intravascular and more importantly noninvasive imaging modalities have created hope that in the future we will be able to more accurately detect vulnerable lesions and treat them more aggressively. However, an invasive sealing of high-risk vulnerable lesions can be justified only if the endovascular devices used for this purpose are effective and safe. Initial reports demonstrated an unacceptable high risk of complications in nonflow limiting lesions treated with balloon angioplasty or bare metal stents (BMSs), while new developments in stent design and the introduction of drug eluting stents (DESs) may have reduced the risk of complications but have not eradicated them [58]. The risk of neo-atherosclerosis and stent thrombosis as well as the distortion of vessel physiology and the permanent caging of the treated vessel are considerable drawbacks of the metallic stents [59]. Bioresorbable scaffolds (BRSs) were introduced to overcome these limitations and have revolutionized the treatment of coronary artery disease. These devices have the ability to provide temporary scaffolding, safeguard the patency of the vessel, and then gradually resolve liberating the vessel from its cage allowing restoration of vessel integrity and physiology. The ABSORB bioresorbable vascular scaffold (ABSORB BVSs, Abbott Vascular, Santa Clara, CA) is the most well-studied BRSs and has received CE Mark approval for the treatment of coronary artery disease. Histology-based studies in animal models and imaging data from the first-in-human studies have shown that ABSORB BVSs have the ability to seal the underlying plaques providing a unique potential for the invasive passivation of high-risk lesions. The evidence supporting the role of ABSORB BVSs in sealing high-risk plaques is discussed in the following sections.

## Implications of ABSORB BVSs implantation of the phenotype of the plaque: Histological data

Histology-based studies in porcine arteries have allowed detailed assessment of the vessel wall response following ABSORB BVSs implantation. In a seminal study Onuma et al. [60] examined the scaffold resorption and the vessel healing process following ABSORB BVSs implantation. Thirty-five scaffolds (3.0 × 12.0 mm) were implanted in the coronary arteries of 17 pigs. OCT imaging was performed and the studied models were euthanized immediately ($n = 2$), at 28 days ($n = 2$), at 2 years ($n = 3$), at 3 years ($n = 5$), and at 4 years ($n = 5$) follow-up. All of the studied vessels were histologically evaluated and were correlated with OCT. At 28-days follow-up, a thin fibromuscular layer had developed over the struts that maintained their structural integrity (Figure 7.10.1). At 2-years follow-up, the polymeric struts had discrete borders consisting of hyaline material that was stained positive by Alcian Blue, indicating that it is rich in proteoglycans. Minor calcification was noted around the struts but there was no evidence of inflammation. At 3 years, 43% of the struts were replaced by connective tissue, while at 4 years all the struts were fully resorbed. Movat pentachrome staining at this time point showed that the developed neointima tissue was rich in smooth muscle cells and connective tissue but had limited inflammation, while von Kossa staining suggested minimal calcification.

Similar were the results of a histological analysis performed during the autopsy study of two patients treated with Igaki–Tamai stents (a BRSs with similar composition to the ABSORB BVSs) 3.5 and 10 years before their death. There was no evidence of inflammation in both cases. At 3.5-years follow-up, the struts of the scaffold were replaced by proteoglycan while at 10 years, these spaces have completely disappeared and there was only intimal thickening in the treated lesion that was rich in smooth muscle cells and fibrotic tissue [61,62].

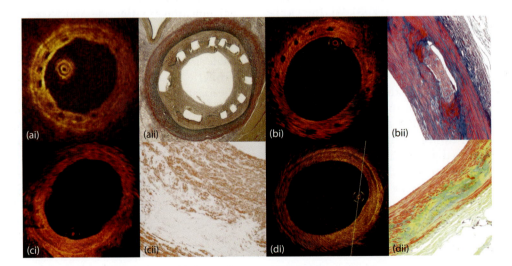

**Figure 7.10.1** OCT and the corresponding histological images portraying scaffold resorption and vessel wall healing process following ABSORB BVSs implantation in porcine models. At 28 days neointima tissue has been developed **(ai)** that is rich in connective tissue as shown in elastin staining **(aii)** and covered the polymeric struts. At 2 years the ABSORB BVSs struts can be seen in OCT **(bi)** but histology indicates that these have been replaced by proteoglycans which are surrounded by connective tissue and smooth muscle cells as shown by trichrome staining **(bii)**. At 3 years, only a very few struts are discernible by OCT **(ci)**. Actin immunohistochemistry staining confirms the presence of smooth muscle cells in the neointima tissue **(cii)**. At 4 years, the ABSORB BVSs is no longer visible **(di)**. Movat's pentachrome staining indicates that the developed tissue is rich in smooth muscle cells, collagen, and proteoglycans **(dii)**.

The findings from these studies indicate that scaffold implantation promotes the development of a thick layer of fibromuscular neo-tissue that has features associated with plaque stability while at long-term follow-up the deployed scaffold is fully resorbed liberating the vessel from its cage.

## Implications of ABSORB BVSs implantation of the phenotype of the plaque: Imaging data

Several intravascular imaging studies have examined the vessel wall healing response following ABSORB BVS implantation [63–65]. Brugaletta et al. were the first to examine the distribution of neointima proliferation in patients implanted with an ABSORB BVS [63]. They analyzed OCT data from patients recruited in the ABSORB Cohort B study (A Clinical Evaluation of the Everolimus Eluting Bioresorbable Vascular Scaffold System in the Treatment of Patients with de Novo Native Coronary Artery Lesions, NCT00856856). This study was a prospective multicenter single-arm trial that examined the safety and efficacy of the ABSORB BVS in 101 patients with single or two-vessel *de novo* lesions [66]. In brief, the recruited patients were divided in two groups of which the first group (Cohort B1) underwent repeat coronary angiography, grayscale IVUS, IVUS-VH, and OCT evaluation at baseline postprocedure, at 6-months, and at 2-year follow-up; while the second group (Cohort B2) had these invasive investigations at baseline, 1-year, and 3-year follow-up. In the analysis of Brugaletta et al., 58 patients (59 lesions) who had OCT at 6 months ($n = 28$ patients/lesions) or 12 months follow-up ($n = 30$ patients/31 lesions) were included. The authors reported a reduction in the lumen area at 12 months compared to 6-months follow-up ($5.64 \pm 1.41$ mm$^2$ vs. $6.42 \pm 1.40$ mm$^2$, $p = 0.05$), while the neointima thickness was increased at this time point [80 (40–120) μm vs. 50 (30–80) μm, $p = 0.071$] and had a more symmetric distribution.

Similar were the findings of the analysis performed by Bourantas et al. [64]. The authors analyzed OCT data acquired at baseline, 6-months, and 2-years follow-up in 23 patients recruited in the ABSORB Cohort B1 substudy. They reported a statistically significant decrease in the lumen area at 6-months follow-up comparing to baseline, but no further change at 2-years follow-up [7.49 (6.13–8.00) mm$^2$ at baseline vs. 6.31 (4.75–7.06) mm$^2$ at 6 months, $p < 0.0001$; vs. 6.01 (4.67–7.11) mm$^2$ at 2 years, $p = 0.373$]. On the other hand, the neointima area continued to increase [mean neointima: 189 (173–229) mm$^2$ at 6 months vs. 258 (222–283) mm$^2$ at 2 years, $p < 0.0001$] and had a more symmetrical distribution at 2-years follow-up. This paradox, i.e., the increase in neointima and preservation of luminal dimensions, was attributed to the fact that the scaffold tended to expand at 2-year follow-up [7.62 (6.49–8.23) mm$^2$ at baseline vs. 7.86 (6.57–8.68) mm$^2$ at 6 months, $p = 0.057$; vs. 8.31 (6.96–9.41) mm$^2$ at 2 years, $p = 0.373$] and was statistically increased at this time point comparing to baseline ($p = 0.027$). It appears that the expanded scaffold was able to accommodate the

developed neointima that covered the underlying plaques (in 76% of the analyzed frames the minimum neointima thickness was >65 μm at 2 years), maintaining the luminal dimensions.

The implications of this process on the phenotype of the plaque were evaluated in detail in a recent study conducted by the same research group [65]. The authors analyzed OCT data from 46 patients treated with an ABSORB BVS that had OCT at baseline, at short-term (6–12 months), and mid-term (24–36 months) follow-up and from 20 patients treated with a BMS that underwent OCT imaging at baseline and at 6-months follow-up. The TCFA and the calcific tissue were identified in the treated segments and in the adjacent native segments at baseline, and the neointima thickness was measured over these tissues at follow-up. Spread-out plots of the studied segments were created that allowed visualization of the detected tissues (lipid in red, fibrotic tissue in green and calcific tissue in white, Figure 7.10.2) and assessment of their burden in the superficial plaque. At short-term follow-up, only 8% of the TCFA detected at baseline were present in the ABSORB BVS and 27% in the BMS implantation segment ($p = 0.231$) while at mid-term follow-up all the TCFA in the ABSORB BVS were fully covered. On the other hand, 60% of the TCFA in the native segments did not change their phenotype at follow-up. The lumen area was considerably reduced at short-term follow-up in both BMS and ABSORB BVS group; however, the lumen reduction was higher in the BMS group ($-2.11 \pm 1.97$ mm$^2$ vs. $-1.34 \pm 0.99$ mm$^2$, $p = 0.026$). In ABSORB BVS the neointima tissue continued to develop at mid-term follow-up ($2.17 \pm 048$ mm$^2$ vs. $1.38 \pm 0.52$ mm$^2$, $p < 0.0001$) and covered the underlying tissues without compromising the luminal dimensions ($5.93 \pm 1.49$ mm$^2$ vs. $6.14 \pm 1.49$ mm$^2$, $p = 0.571$) as it was accommodated by the expanded scaffold ($8.28 \pm 1.74$ mm$^2$ vs. $7.67 \pm 1.28$ mm$^2$, $p < 0.0001$). Mixed model analysis (including the underlying tissue, follow-up time, and stent type) for the mean neointima thickness showed a significant effect for follow-up time (lower at short-term, $p = 0.040$) and stent type (lower in ABSORB BVS, $p = 0.006$) but not for the plaque type. These findings indicate that ABSORB BVS implantation promotes the development of a thick layer of fibromuscular tissue that covers all the underlying plaques irrespective of their composition leading to their passivation. The changes in the phenotype of the plaque appear to have an effect on its mechanical properties resulting in a reduced vessel wall strain [67] that indicates plaque stability [68,69].

Karanasos et al. has recently reported the long-term implications of ABSORB BVS implantation on the composition of the plaque [70]. They analyzed the OCT data acquired at 5-year follow-up in 8 patients implanted with the first-generation ABSORB BVS. The lumen area gradually increased with time ($4.89 \pm 1.29$ mm$^2$ at 6-months to $5.03 \pm 1.24$ mm$^2$ at 2-years and $6.39 \pm 1.18$ mm$^2$ at 5-years follow-up). At 5 years, all the struts were fully resorbed and there was a thin layer of fibromuscular tissue with

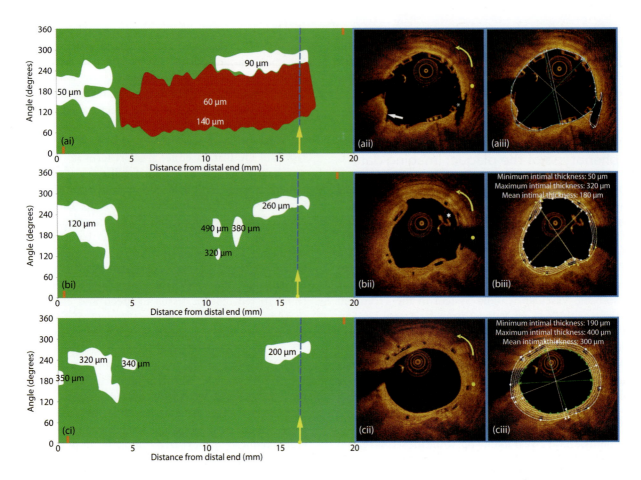

**Figure 7.10.2** Spread-out plots of a scaffolded coronary segment at baseline **(ai)**, at 6 months **(bi)**, and at 2 years follow-up **(ci)**. The X axis represents the distance from the distal end of the scaffold while the Y axis the circumferential segment (angle) where the different plaque components are located. The axial position of the metallic nontranslucent to light markers seen at the borders of the scaffold is shown with orange markers. The red color corresponds to TCFA, the white to calcific, and the green to fibrous tissue. The minimum thickness of the tissue that covers the detected calcific spots and the TCFA is also provided. A mixed lipid/calcific plaque is detected [in the middle of the spread-out scaffold plot in panel **(ai)**] and the calcific tissue is portrayed in a semitransparent fashion. The blue dashed lines indicate the location of the frames portrayed at panels **(aii)**, **(bii)**, and **(cii)**. The yellow spot in panels **(aii)**, **(bii)**, and **(cii)** denotes the 0 degree location in the spread-out scaffold plot while the yellow arrow the counterclockwise direction followed to evaluate the circumferential location of the detected tissues. The minimum thickness of the cap in panel aii was measured using the Sheehy's method 60 µm (white arrow) [71]. The intimal dissection seen at baseline is healed at follow-up (*) examination while the strut discontinuity (*) detected at 6-months follow-up disappears at 2 years. As is shown in panels **(aiii)**, **(biii)**, and **(ciii)**, neointima tissue gradually develops which covers the lipid tissue. The developed neointima covers the whole circumference of the vessel wall at 6 months and it has a more uniform distribution at 2 years.

a mean thickness of 310 ± 113 µm (minimum thickness: 155 ± 90 µm) that covered the necrotic cores and calcific component (Figure 7.10.3 [72]). Of note, IVUS imaging confirmed an increase in the lumen area between 2- and 5-years follow-up (6.17 ± 0.74 mm² at 6 months, 6.56 ± 1.16 mm² at 2 years and 6.96 ± 1.13 mm² at 5 years) but also a reduction in plaque area (9.17 ± 1.86 mm² at 6 months, 7.54 ± 1.24 mm² at 2 years, and 7.57 ± 1.63 mm² at 5 years) [73].

Summarizing the evidence from the abovementioned studies, it appears that ABSORB BVS implantation alters the morphological characteristics of the plaque that have been associated with plaque vulnerability in

the PROSPECT and VIVA studies (i.e., TCFA phenotype, reduced lumen area <4 mm², and plaque burden >70%), as it promotes the formation of a thick layer of neointima tissue that seals the underlying—potentially high-risk—plaques while at long-term follow-up there is also a reduction in plaque burden accompanied by lumen enlargement.

## Implications of ABSORB BVSs implantation of the local hemodynamic forces

Several studies in the past have assessed the implications of local hemodynamic forces on neointima tissue formation

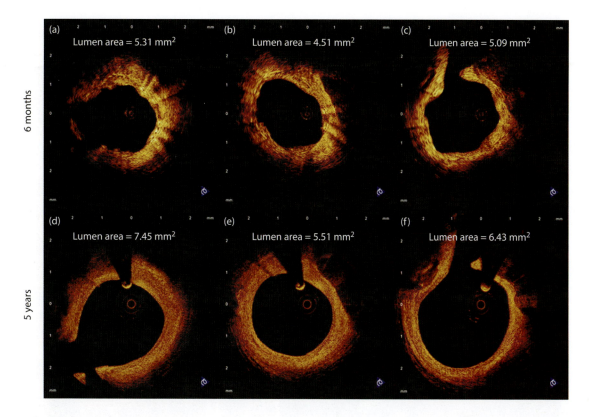

**Figure 7.10.3** Corresponding OCT images at 6-months (**a** and **c**) and 5-years follow-up (**d** and **f**) following ABSORB BVS implantation. Panel (**b**) shows the minimum lumen areas at 6 months (4.51 mm²) whereas (**e**) the minimum lumen area at 5 years (5.51 mm²). It is apparent that the lumen area has increased in all matched sites [5.31 mm² vs. 7.45 mm² in panels (**a, d**), and 5.09 mm² vs. 6.43 mm² in panels (**c, f**)]. (Image obtained with permission from Karanasos A et al. *Circulation*. Aug 14 2012;126(7):e89–91.)

and demonstrated that low ESS promotes neointima proliferation in BMS while in DESs the association between ESS and neointima thickness is weak and appears to be affected by the mechanisms of action and probably by the release kinetics of the eluted drug [74–76]. However, these studies used IVUS imaging to reconstruct coronary artery anatomy, an imaging technique with low resolution (65–150 μm) that does not allow detailed assessment of the luminal morphology in stented/scaffolded segments and evaluation of the effect of the protruding struts on the local hemodynamic forces.

These limitations were addressed with the introduction of advanced reconstruction methodologies that enable three-dimensional (3D) reconstruction of coronary anatomy from OCT and X-ray angiography [77–79]. These technical developments permitted detailed reconstruction and evaluation of the local hemodynamic micro-environment in segments implanted with ABSORB BVS [80,81]. In a recent study, Bourantas et al. were the first who assessed the association between ESS and neointima proliferation in OCT-based reconstructions [82]. They analyzed data from 12 patients who recruited in the ABSORB Cohort B2 study that had OCT imaging at baseline and 1-year follow-up. The OCT data

acquired at 1 year were used to reconstruct coronary anatomy and blood flow simulation was performed in the scaffold surface which was assumed that represented the lumen surface at baseline. It was shown that the protruding struts created flow disturbances and disruptions resulting in recirculation zones in the areas between the struts. This created a low ESS environment (61% of the estimated ESS was <1 Pa) that promoted neointima proliferation at 1-year follow-up. The neointima thickness was increased in the segments between the struts, where the ESS was low and minimal on the top of the struts where high ESS was noted. A strong negative correlation was found between ESS and neointima thickness at 1-year follow-up (average correlation coefficient: −0.385, $p < 0.0001$).

The long-term implications of ABSORB BVS implantation on the local hemodynamic micro-environment has been assessed in a case report published by the same research group [83]. They used the OCT data to reconstruct coronary anatomy at baseline immediately after device implantation and at 2-years follow-up and performed blood flow simulation (Figure 7.10.4). At baseline the rugged luminal surfaces in the scaffolded segment obstructed flow, and created flow disturbances and recirculation zones resulting in a low

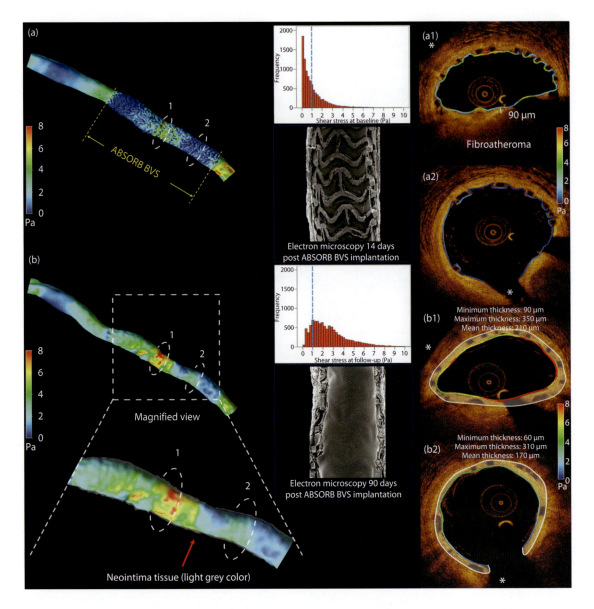

**Figure 7.10.4** Three-dimensional reconstruction of a left anterior descending coronary artery from X-ray angiographic and OCT data at baseline, immediately after implantation of an ABSORB BVS. Blood flow simulation was performed in the reconstructed models and the local ESS are color-coded displayed (blue indicates low and red high ESS) **(a)**. The distribution of the ESS in the scaffolded segment is portrayed at the top right side of the panel, and below there is an electron microscopy image acquired 14 days after ABSORB BVS implantation in a rabbit model showing the rugged luminal surface created by the deployed device. Panels **(a1, a2)** illustrate the baseline ESS distribution around the circumference of the vessel wall in two OCT cross-sectional images. Normal-to-high ESS noted over a fibroatheroma with a minimum cap thickness of 90 μm in panel **(a1)**, whereas in panel **(a2)** the ESS is low over the vessel wall and normal over the struts. The asterisk (*) in both frames indicates the origin of a side branch. At follow-up, the ESS is higher compared to baseline **(b)**. The magnified view shows the thin layer of neointima that has been developed and is portrayed with light gray. The ESS is high over the fibroatheroma detected at baseline, but the neointima tissue has sealed the plaque **(b1)**, while the low ESS estimated at baseline across the circumference of the vessel wall in **(a2)** is normalized at follow-up **(b2)**. (Reprinted with permission from Bourantas CV et al. *JACC Cardiovasc Interv.* Jan 2014;7(1):100–101.)

ESS environment (62% of the measured ESS was <1 Pa). At 2-years follow-up, neointima tissue had been developed in the areas between the struts and smoothed the luminal surface which was exposed to a homogenous athero-protective high ESS environment (16.5% of the measured ESS was <1 Pa). It appears that the low ESS noted immediately after scaffold implantation promoted neointima proliferation that sealed the underlying high-risk plaque and filled in the gaps between the protruding struts resulting in a smooth luminal surface and an athero-protective ESS environment that is anticipated to inhibit the development of vulnerable lesions.

# RANDOMIZED CONTROL STUDIES INVESTIGATING THE POTENTIAL OF BIORESORBABLE SCAFFOLD IMPLANTATION IN TREATING VULNERABLE LESIONS

The evidence from these studies has attracted attention and currently two prospective randomized control trials are underway and investigate the potential value of ABSORB BVS in sealing vulnerable lesions. The first is PROSPECT II and PROSPECT-ABSORB study (NCT02171065) which has two components: PROSPECT II aims to recruit 600 patients and investigate the value of NIRS-IVUS imaging in detecting plaques that are prone to rupture and cause clinical events; while PROSPECT-ABSORB aims to randomize 300 patients with vulnerable high-risk plaques—detected by NIRS-IVUS and defined as lesions with a plaque burden ≥70%—to treatment with either an ABSORB BVS or conservative management in order to investigate whether ABSORB BVS implantation safely increases the lumen area at 2-years follow-up. The study is expected to be completed by the end of 2018.

The second study is the PREVENT study (NCT02316886), which commenced in 2015, aims to recruit 1600 patients with established coronary artery disease, and investigate whether ABSORB BVS implantation in nonflow limiting high-risk vulnerable plaques—defined as lesions with a fractional flow reserve <0.80 which meet two of the following criteria: (1) minimum lumen area <4 mm$^2$, (2) plaque burden >70%, (3) lipid-rich plaque on NIRS, and (4) TCFA phenotype in OCT—reduces major adverse cardiovascular events. The study endpoint is death, myocardial infarction, or unplanned rehospitalization due to unstable angina at 2-year follow-up; the study is anticipated to be completed by the end of 2019.

## CONCLUSIONS—FUTURE TRENDS

Evidence from invasive imaging-based studies of coronary atherosclerosis demonstrated that intravascular imaging enables identification of lesions that are prone to progress and cause future cardiovascular events. Recent developments in intravascular imaging have permitted more accurate assessment of plaque vulnerability, while advances in CTCA have allowed noninvasive assessment of plaque morphology and identification of high-risk plaques. These advances combined with the new developments in stent technology and the introduction of BRSs, challenge the current practice [84,85]. These devices, in contrast to the traditional metallic stents, have the ability to provide at short-term temporal scaffolding that safeguards the patency of the vessel and create a rugged luminal surface that causes flow disruption and a low ESS environment which promotes the development of a neointima that seals the underlying plaques; while at long term, the device disappears allowing restoration of vessel wall physiologic function and structural integrity, resulting in plaque regression, and normalization of the ESS that act athero-protectively. These unique effects have attracted the attention of the scientific community and currently randomized control trials are exploring for the first time the safety, efficacy, and clinical benefit of an invasive sealing of vulnerable high-risk lesions. A decade ago, the potential to rescind these high-risk plaques was once regarded a fantasy, but with current advances, we tantalizingly move closer toward this becoming a reality.

## REFERENCES

1. Friedman M, Van den Bovenkamp GJ. The pathogenesis of a coronary thrombus. *Am J Pathol.* Jan 1966;48(1):19–44.
2. Clark E, Graef I, Chasis H. Thrombosis of the aorta and coronary arteries with specific reference to the "fibrinoid" lesions. *Arch Pathol.* 1936;22:183–212.
3. Constantinides P. Plaque fissures in human coronary thrombosis. *J Atheroscler Res.* 1966;6:1–17.
4. Wartman WB. Occlusion of the coronary arteries by hemorrhage into their walls. *Am Heart J.* 1938;15:459–470.
5. Davies MJ, Thomas A. Thrombosis and acute coronary-artery lesions in sudden cardiac ischemic death. *N Engl J Med.* May 3 1984;310(18):1137–1140.
6. Davies MJ, Thomas AC. Plaque fissuring—The cause of acute myocardial infarction, sudden ischaemic death, and crescendo angina. *Br Heart J.* Apr 1985;53(4):363–373.
7. Varnava AM, Mills PG, Davies MJ. Relationship between coronary artery remodeling and plaque vulnerability. *Circulation.* Feb 26 2002;105(8):939–943.
8. Burke AP, Farb A, Malcom GT, Liang YH, Smialek J, Virmani R. Coronary risk factors and plaque morphology in men with coronary disease who died suddenly. *N Engl J Med.* May 1 1997;336(18):1276–1282.
9. Moreno PR, Bernardi VH, Lopez-Cuellar J et al. Macrophages, smooth muscle cells, and tissue factor in unstable angina. Implications for cell-mediated thrombogenicity in acute coronary syndromes. *Circulation.* Dec 15 1996;94(12):3090–3097.
10. Falk E. Plaque rupture with severe pre-existing stenosis precipitating coronary thrombosis. Characteristics of coronary atherosclerotic plaques underlying fatal occlusive thrombi. *Br Heart J.* Aug 1983;50(2):127–134.
11. Ehara S, Kobayashi Y, Yoshiyama M, Ueda M, Yoshikawa J. Coronary artery calcification revisited. *J Atheroscler Thromb.* Feb 2006;13(1):31–37.
12. Virmani R, Kolodgie FD, Burke AP et al. Atherosclerotic plaque progression and vulnerability to rupture: Angiogenesis as a source of intraplaque hemorrhage. *Arterioscler Thromb Vasc Biol.* Oct 2005;25(10):2054–2061.

13. Duewell P, Kono H, Rayner KJ et al. NLRP3 inflammasomes are required for atherogenesis and activated by cholesterol crystals. *Nature*. Apr 29 2010;464(7293):1357–1361.

14. Nishimura RA, Edwards WD, Warnes CA et al. Intravascular ultrasound imaging: In vitro validation and pathologic correlation. *J Am Coll Cardiol*. Jul 1990;16(1):145–154.

15. Gussenhoven EJ, Essed CE, Lancee CT et al. Arterial wall characteristics determined by intravascular ultrasound imaging: An in vitro study. *J Am Coll Cardiol*. Oct 1989;14(4):947–952.

16. Sano K, Kawasaki M, Ishihara Y et al. Assessment of vulnerable plaques causing acute coronary syndrome using integrated backscatter intravascular ultrasound. *J Am Coll Cardiol*. Feb 21 2006;47(4):734–741.

17. Stone GW, Maehara A, Lansky AJ et al. A prospective natural-history study of coronary atherosclerosis. *N Engl J Med*. Jan 20 2011;364(3):226–235.

18. Calvert PA, Obaid DR, O'Sullivan M et al. Association between IVUS findings and adverse outcomes in patients with coronary artery disease: The VIVA (VH-IVUS in Vulnerable Atherosclerosis) Study. *JACC Cardiovasc Imaging*. Aug 2011;4(8):894–901.

19. Stone PH, Saito S, Takahashi S et al. Prediction of progression of coronary artery disease and clinical outcomes using vascular profiling of endothelial shear stress and arterial plaque characteristics: The PREDICTION Study. *Circulation*. Jul 10 2012;126(2):172–181.

20. Papafaklis MI, Mizuno S, Takahashi S et al. Incremental predictive value of combined endothelial shear stress, plaque necrotic core, and plaque burden for future cardiac events: A post-hoc analysis of the PREDICTION study. *Int J Cardiol*. Jan 1 2016;202:64–66.

21. Bourantas CV, Garcia-Garcia HM, Torii R et al. Vulnerable plaque detection: An unrealistic quest or a feasible objective with a clinical value? *Heart*. Jan 18 2016.

22. Murray SW, Palmer ND. What is behind the calcium? The relationship between calcium and necrotic core on virtual histology analyses. *Eur Heart J*. Jan 2009;30(1):125; author reply 125–126.

23. Sales FJ, Falcao BA, Falcao JL et al. Evaluation of plaque composition by intravascular ultrasound "virtual histology": The impact of dense calcium on the measurement of necrotic tissue. *EuroIntervention*. Aug;6(3):394–399.

24. Thim T, Hagensen MK, Wallace-Bradley D et al. Unreliable assessment of necrotic core by virtual histology intravascular ultrasound in porcine coronary artery disease. *Circ Cardiovasc Imaging*. Jul;3(4):384–391.

25. Kawasaki M, Bouma BE, Bressner J et al. Diagnostic accuracy of optical coherence tomography and integrated backscatter intravascular ultrasound images for tissue characterization of human coronary plaques. *J Am Coll Cardiol*. Jul 4 2006;48(1):81–88.

26. Jaffer FA, Calfon MA, Rosenthal A et al. Two-dimensional intravascular near-infrared fluorescence molecular imaging of inflammation in atherosclerosis and stent-induced vascular injury. *J Am Coll Cardiol*. Jun 21 2011;57(25):2516–2526.

27. Jansen K, van Soest G, van der Steen AF. Intravascular photoacoustic imaging: A new tool for vulnerable plaque identification. *Ultrasound Med Biol*. Jun 2014;40(6):1037–1048.

28. Marcu L. Fluorescence lifetime in cardiovascular diagnostics. *J Biomed Opt*. Jan–Feb 2010;15(1):011106.

29. Brennan JF, 3rd, Nazemi J, Motz J, Ramcharitar S. The vPredict Optical Catheter System: Intravascular Raman Spectroscopy. *EuroIntervention*. Mar 2008;3(5):635–638.

30. Bourantas CV, Garcia-Garcia HM, Naka KK et al. Hybrid intravascular imaging: Current applications and prospective potential in the study of coronary atherosclerosis. *J Am Coll Cardiol*. Apr 2 2013;61(13):1369–1378.

31. Li J, Ma T, Jing J et al. Miniature optical coherence tomography-ultrasound probe for automatically coregistered three-dimensional intracoronary imaging with real-time display. *J Biomed Opt*. Oct 2013;18(10):100502.

32. Yin J, Li X, Jing J et al. Novel combined miniature optical coherence tomography ultrasound probe for in vivo intravascular imaging. *J Biomed Opt*. Jun 2011;16(6):060505.

33. Yoo H, Kim JW, Shishkov M et al. Intra-arterial catheter for simultaneous microstructural and molecular imaging in vivo. *Nat Med*. Dec 2011;17(12):1680–1684.

34. Dixon AJ, Hossack JA. Intravascular near-infrared fluorescence catheter with ultrasound guidance and blood attenuation correction. *J Biomed Opt*. May 2013;18(5):56009.

35. Fard AM, Vacas-Jacques P, Hamidi E et al. Optical coherence tomography—near infrared spectroscopy system and catheter for intravascular imaging. *Opt Express*. Dec 16 2013;21(25):30849–30858.

36. Li X, Wei W, Zhou Q, Shung KK, Chen Z. Intravascular photoacoustic imaging at 35 and 80 MHz. *J Biomed Opt*. Oct 2012;17(10):106005.

37. Li Y, Gong X, Liu C et al. High-speed intravascular spectroscopic photoacoustic imaging at 1000 A-lines per second with a 0.9-mm diameter catheter. *J Biomed Opt*. Jun 2015;20(6):065006.

38. Bec J, Ma DM, Yankelevich DR et al. Multispectral fluorescence lifetime imaging system for intravascular diagnostics with ultrasound guidance: In vivo validation in swine arteries. *J Biophotonics.* May 2014;7(5):281–285.

39. Ma D, Bec J, Yankelevich DR, Gorpas D, Fatakdawala H, Marcu L. Rotational multispectral fluorescence lifetime imaging and intravascular ultrasound: Bimodal system for intravascular applications. *J Biomed Opt.* Jun 2014;19(6):066004.

40. Kang SJ, Mintz GS, Pu J et al. Combined IVUS and NIRS detection of fibroatheromas: Histopathological validation in human coronary arteries. *JACC Cardiovasc Imaging.* Feb 2015;8(2):184–194.

41. Madder RD, Goldstein JA, Madden SP et al. Detection by near-infrared spectroscopy of large lipid core plaques at culprit sites in patients with acute ST-segment elevation myocardial infarction. *JACC Cardiovasc Interv.* Aug 2013;6(8):838–846.

42. Madder RD, Husaini M, Davis AT et al. Detection by near-infrared spectroscopy of large lipid cores at culprit sites in patients with non-ST-segment elevation myocardial infarction and unstable angina. *Catheter Cardiovasc Interv.* Nov 15 2015;86(6):1014–1021.

43. Ungi GJ. Next-generation intravascular imaging: Dual-modality OCT and near-infrared autofluorescence (NIRAF) for the simultaneous acquisition of microstructural and molecular/chemical information within the coronary vasculature: Early human clinical experience. *Transcatheter Cardiovascular Therapeutics.* Washington, October, 2014.

44. Hara T, Ughi GJ, McCarthy JR et al. Intravascular fibrin molecular imaging improves the detection of unhealed stents assessed by optical coherence tomography in vivo. *Eur Heart J.* Dec 18 2015.

45. Boogers MJ, Broersen A, van Velzen JE et al. Automated quantification of coronary plaque with computed tomography: Comparison with intravascular ultrasound using a dedicated registration algorithm for fusion-based quantification. *Eur Heart J.* Apr 2012;33(8):1007–1016.

46. Schlett CL, Maurovich-Horvat P, Ferencik M et al. Histogram analysis of lipid-core plaques in coronary computed tomographic angiography: Ex vivo validation against histology. *Invest Radiol.* Sep 2013;48(9):646–653.

47. Schlett CL, Ferencik M, Celeng C et al. How to assess non-calcified plaque in CT angiography: Delineation methods affect diagnostic accuracy of low-attenuation plaque by CT for lipid-core plaque in histology. *Eur Heart J Cardiovasc Imaging.* Nov 2013;14(11):1099–1105.

48. Papadopoulou SL, Neefjes LA, Schaap M et al. Detection and quantification of coronary atherosclerotic plaque by 64-slice multidetector CT: A systematic head-to-head comparison with intravascular ultrasound. *Atherosclerosis.* Nov 2011;219(1):163–170.

49. Maurovich-Horvat P, Hoffmann U, Vorpahl M, Nakano M, Virmani R, Alkadhi H. The napkin-ring sign: CT signature of high-risk coronary plaques? *JACC Cardiovasc Imaging.* Apr 2010;3(4):440–444.

50. Maurovich-Horvat P, Schlett CL, Alkadhi H et al. The napkin-ring sign indicates advanced atherosclerotic lesions in coronary CT angiography. *JACC Cardiovasc Imaging.* Dec 2012;5(12):1243–1252.

51. Seifarth H, Schlett CL, Nakano M et al. Histopathological correlates of the napkin-ring sign plaque in coronary CT angiography. *Atherosclerosis.* Sep 2012;224(1):90–96.

52. Otsuka K, Fukuda S, Tanaka A et al. Napkin-ring sign on coronary CT angiography for the prediction of acute coronary syndrome. *JACC Cardiovasc Imaging.* Apr 2013;6(4):448–457.

53. Versteylen MO, Kietselaer BL, Dagnelie PC et al. Additive value of semiautomated quantification of coronary artery disease using cardiac computed tomographic angiography to predict future acute coronary syndrome. *J Am Coll Cardiol.* Jun 4 2013;61(22):2296–2305.

54. Li X, Bauer W, Kreissl MC et al. Specific somatostatin receptor II expression in arterial plaque: (68) Ga-DOTATATE autoradiographic, immunohistochemical and flow cytometric studies in apoE-deficient mice. *Atherosclerosis.* Sep 2013;230(1):33–39.

55. Rominger A, Saam T, Vogl E et al. In vivo imaging of macrophage activity in the coronary arteries using 68Ga-DOTATATE PET/CT: Correlation with coronary calcium burden and risk factors. *J Nucl Med.* Feb 2010;51(2):193–197.

56. Dweck MR, Chow MW, Joshi NV et al. Coronary arterial 18F-sodium fluoride uptake: A novel marker of plaque biology. *J Am Coll Cardiol.* Apr 24 2012;59(17):1539–1548.

57. Joshi NV, Vesey AT, Williams MC et al. 18F-fluoride positron emission tomography for identification of ruptured and high-risk coronary atherosclerotic plaques: A prospective clinical trial. *Lancet.* Feb 22 2014;383(9918):705–713.

58. Mercado N, Maier W, Boersma E et al. Clinical and angiographic outcome of patients with mild coronary lesions treated with balloon angioplasty or coronary stenting. Implications for mechanical plaque sealing. *Eur Heart J.* Mar 2003;24(6):541–551.

59. Serruys PW, Garcia-Garcia HM, Onuma Y. From metallic cages to transient bioresorbable scaffolds: Change in paradigm of coronary revascularization in the upcoming decade? *Eur Heart J.* Jan 2012;33(1):16–25b.

60. Onuma Y, Serruys PW, Perkins LE et al. Intracoronary optical coherence tomography and histology at 1 month and 2, 3, and 4 years after implantation of everolimus-eluting bioresorbable vascular scaffolds

in a porcine coronary artery model: An attempt to decipher the human optical coherence tomography images in the ABSORB trial. *Circulation*. Nov 30 2010;122(22):2288–2300.

61. Nishio S, Kosuga K, Igaki K et al. Long-term (>10 years) clinical outcomes of first-in-human biodegradable poly-l-lactic acid coronary stents: Igaki–Tamai stents. *Circulation*. May 15 2012;125(19):2343–2353.

62. Nishio S. Igaki–Tamai stent. *PCR Focus Group on Bioresorbable Scaffolds*. 2012; Rotterdam, Netherlands, 2012.

63. Brugaletta S, Radu MD, Garcia-Garcia HM et al. Circumferential evaluation of the neointima by optical coherence tomography after ABSORB bioresorbable vascular scaffold implantation: Can the scaffold cap the plaque? *Atherosclerosis*. Mar 2012;221(1):106–112.

64. Bourantas CV, Farooq V, Zhang Y et al. Circumferential distribution of the neointima at six-month and two-year follow-up after a bioresorbable vascular scaffold implantation: A substudy of the ABSORB Cohort B Clinical Trial. *EuroIntervention*. Mar 2015;10(11):1299–1306.

65. Bourantas CV, Serruys PW, Nakatani S et al. Bioresorbable vascular scaffold treatment induces the formation of neointimal cap that seals the underlying plaque without compromising the luminal dimensions: A concept based on serial optical coherence tomography data. *EuroIntervention*. Nov 22 2015;11(8):746–756.

66. Serruys PW, Onuma Y, Ormiston JA et al. Evaluation of the second generation of a bioresorbable everolimus drug-eluting vascular scaffold for treatment of de novo coronary artery stenosis: Six-month clinical and imaging outcomes. *Circulation*. Nov 30 2010;122(22):2301–2312.

67. Bourantas CV, Garcia-Garcia HM, Campos CA et al. Implications of a bioresorbable vascular scaffold implantation on vessel wall strain of the treated and the adjacent segments. *Int J Cardiovasc Imaging*. Mar 2014;30(3):477–484.

68. de Korte CL, Sierevogel MJ, Mastik F et al. Identification of atherosclerotic plaque components with intravascular ultrasound elastography in vivo: A Yucatan pig study. *Circulation*. Apr 9 2002;105(14):1627–1630.

69. Schaar JA, Regar E, Mastik F et al. Incidence of high-strain patterns in human coronary arteries: Assessment with three-dimensional intravascular palpography and correlation with clinical presentation. *Circulation*. Jun 8 2004;109(22):2716–2719.

70. Karanasos A, Simsek C, Gnanadesigan M et al. OCT assessment of the long-term vascular healing response 5 years after everolimus-eluting bioresorbable vascular scaffold. *J Am Coll Cardiol*. Dec 9 2014;64(22):2343–2356.

71. Sheehy A, Gutierrez-Chico JL, Diletti R et al. In vivo characterisation of bioresorbable vascular scaffold strut interfaces using optical coherence tomography with Gaussian line spread function analysis. *EuroIntervention*. Feb 2012;7(10):1227–1235.

72. Karanasos A, Simsek C, Serruys P et al. Five-year optical coherence tomography follow-up of an everolimus-eluting bioresorbable vascular scaffold: Changing the paradigm of coronary stenting? *Circulation*. Aug 14 2012;126(7):e89–91.

73. Simsek C, Karanasos A, Magro M et al. Long-term invasive follow-up of the everolimus-eluting bioresorbable vascular scaffold: Five-year results of multiple invasive imaging modalities. *EuroIntervention*. Jan 22 2016;11(9):996–1003.

74. Papafaklis MI, Bourantas CV, Theodorakis PE et al. The effect of shear stress on neointimal response following sirolimus- and paclitaxel-eluting stent implantation compared with bare-metal stents in humans. *JACC Cardiovasc Interv*. Nov 2010;3(11):1181–1189.

75. Wentzel JJ, Krams R, Schuurbiers JC et al. Relationship between neointimal thickness and shear stress after Wallstent implantation in human coronary arteries. *Circulation*. Apr 3 2001;103(13):1740–1745.

76. Cheng C, Tempel D, Oostlander A et al. Rapamycin modulates the eNOS vs. shear stress relationship. *Cardiovasc Res*. Apr 1 2008;78(1):123–129.

77. Papafaklis MI, Bourantas CV, Yonetsu T et al. Anatomically correct three-dimensional coronary artery reconstruction using frequency domain optical coherence tomographic and angiographic data: Head-to-head comparison with intravascular ultrasound for endothelial shear stress assessment in humans. *EuroIntervention*. Aug 2015;11(4): 407–415.

78. Toutouzas K, Chatzizisis YS, Riga M et al. Accurate and reproducible reconstruction of coronary arteries and endothelial shear stress calculation using 3D OCT: Comparative study to 3D IVUS and 3D QCA. *Atherosclerosis*. Jun 2015;240(2):510–519.

79. Li Y, Gutierrez-Chico JL, Holm NR et al. Impact of Side Branch Modeling on Computation of Endothelial Shear Stress in Coronary Artery Disease: Coronary Tree Reconstruction by Fusion of 3D Angiography and OCT. *J Am Coll Cardiol*. Jul 14 2015;66(2):125–135.

80. Bourantas CV, Papafaklis MI, Lakkas L et al. Fusion of optical coherence tomographic and angiographic data for more accurate evaluation of the endothelial shear stress patterns and neointimal distribution after bioresorbable scaffold implantation: Comparison with intravascular ultrasound-derived reconstructions. *Int J Cardiovasc Imaging*. Mar 2014;30(3):485–494.

81. Papafaklis MI, Bourantas CV, Farooq V et al. In vivo assessment of the three-dimensional haemodynamic micro-environment following drug-eluting bioresorbable vascular scaffold implantation in a human coronary artery: Fusion of frequency domain optical coherence tomography and angiography. *EuroIntervention*. Nov 2013;9(7):890.

82. Bourantas CV, Papafaklis MI, Kotsia A et al. Effect of the endothelial shear stress patterns on neointimal proliferation following drug-eluting bioresorbable vascular scaffold implantation: An optical coherence tomography study. *JACC Cardiovasc Interv*. Mar 2014;7(3):315–324.

83. Bourantas CV, Papafaklis MI, Garcia-Garcia HM et al. Short- and long-term implications of a bioresorbable vascular scaffold implantation on the local endothelial shear stress patterns. *JACC Cardiovasc Interv*. Jan 2014;7(1):100–101.

84. Bourantas CV, Garcia-Garcia HM, Diletti R, Muramatsu T, Serruys PW. Early detection and invasive passivation of future culprit lesions: A future potential or an unrealistic pursuit of chimeras? *Am Heart J*. Jun 2013;165(6):869–881 e864.

85. Serruys PW, Garcia-Garcia HM, Regar E. From post-mortem characterization to the in vivo detection of thin-capped fibroatheromas: The missing link toward percutaneous treatment: What if Diogenes would have found what he was looking for? *J Am Coll Cardiol*. Sep 4 2007;50(10):950–952.

# PART 8

# Complications (incidence, diagnosis, potential mechanisms and treatment)

# Acute and subacute scaffold thrombosis

DAVIDE CAPODANNO

## INTRODUCTION

Evolution in stent platforms, polymers, and drug load may contribute to explaining the low rate of stent thrombosis observed with current-generation drug-eluting stents (DESs) as compared with earlier generation DESs and even bare metal stents [1]. However, stent thrombosis still results in death or myocardial infarction in the vast majority of cases, which justifies enduring research efforts to additionally minimize its incidence rate. It has been hypothesized that the lack of any residual foreign material and restoration of functional endothelial coverage after disappearance of bioresorbable scaffolds (BRSs) might result in reduced thrombosis [2]. Still, since the bioresorption process of BRSs takes months to years, their putative (yet unproven) advantage in reducing thrombotic complications is necessarily confined to late events. In the early term, the presence of the scaffold may still exert a theoretical prothrombotic stimulus, and cases of acute and subacute thrombosis have already been reported in the BRSs literature [3]. This chapter provides an overview on acute and subacute BRSs thrombosis, with a focus on incidence rates, putative mechanisms, prevention, and management strategies.

## INCIDENCE

### Randomized clinical trials

Six studies have thus far reported randomized comparative data of BRSs versus DESs. In the ABSORB II trial, the Absorb BRSs (Abbott Vascular, Santa Clara, CA) was 2:1 compared to everolimus-eluting stents (EESs) in 501 patients with mostly B lesions according to the classification system of the American College of Cardiology/American Heart Association (ACC/AHA). Two definite scaffold thrombosis (0.6%) leading to myocardial infarction were documented in an interim 1-year report of the trial, one acute (0.3%) and another subacute (0.3%) on day 2 [4]. The two thrombotic events involved in one case two overlapping scaffolds and in the other case bifurcation scaffolding, a protocol deviation. No stent thrombosis was observed in the DESs group, corresponding to 0.3% differences for acute and subacute definite thrombosis between the ABSORB BRSs and the EESs, although large 95% confidence intervals were observed for these difference estimates (–1.98% to 1.67% and –1.98% to 1.68% for acute and subacute definite thrombosis, respectively), reflecting the low statistical power of the trial for assessing relatively infrequent clinical endpoints. Another trial, named EVERBIO II, randomly assigned 240 patients with about 30% of ACC/AHA $B_2$/C lesions in a 1:1:1 fashion to EESs, biolimus-eluting stents or the ABSORB BRSs [5]. The authors reported no definite or probable thrombosis in any of the groups at 30 days. In TROFI II, a small trial that included only patients with ST-segment elevation myocardial infarction (STEMI), one case of definite subacute stent thrombosis occurred in the ABSORB BRSs arm (1.1% vs. 0% EESs; $p$ = NS) [6]. Again, these studies do not inform meaningfully on the incidence rate of early scaffold thrombosis and the comparative efficacy versus DESs due to the small number of patients randomized.

Recently, three regulatory trials conducted in broader PCI populations have been almost simultaneously published from China, Japan, and the United States. In ABSORB-CHINA ($n$ = 480), only one case of probable subacute thrombosis was reported, in the ABSORB BRSs arm (0.4% vs. 0% EESs; $p$ = 1.00) [7]. In ABSORB-JAPAN ($n$ = 400), there were no cases of acute scaffold thrombosis, whereas three definite subacute cases occurred in the ABSORB BRSs arm versus one case in the EESs arm (1.1% vs. 0.8%; $p$ = 1.00) [8]. In ABSORB III, the largest randomized study conducted so far ($n$ = 2008), acute definite or probable thrombosis was reported acutely in 0.2% and 0.6% of patients in the ABSORB BRSs and EESs groups, respectively ($p$ = 0.19), and subacutely in 0.9% and 0.1%, respectively ($p$ = 0.04) [9].

## Observational data

Registries are useful complements to randomized clinical trials in that they generally enroll more complex populations and better capture low frequency events. However, currently published observational studies of BRSs are typically small sized, have short follow-up, document site-reported events, and/or lack a control group [10–29] (Table 8.1.1). In the GHOST-EU registry, a pioneering, multicenter ($n = 1189$) all-comers BRSs study, Kaplan–Meier estimates of definite or probable scaffold thrombosis were 1.5% at 30 days and 2.1% at 6 months [29]. Most episodes occurred early (5 in the first 24 hours), were in patients on dual antiplatelet therapy, and led to death or myocardial infarction. As with DESs, the clinical context in which BRSs are implanted might play an important role in the likelihood of scaffold thrombosis. Indeed, in published series, early scaffold thrombosis ranged between 0.0% and 0.4% in patients with stable coronary artery disease [10–14], between 0.0% and 1.4% in patients with acute coronary syndromes [16,17], between 0.0% and 4.3% in patients with ST-elevation myocardial infarction (STEMI) [18–22], and between 0.0% and 2.2% in all-comers patients undergoing percutaneous coronary intervention [23–29].

## Meta-analyses

A meta-analysis from Ishibashi and colleagues, lumping 4309 patients from published and unpublished observational studies, weighted an early scaffold thrombosis average of 0.8% (0.2% acute, 0.6% subacute), with total scaffold thrombosis estimates of 0.9% in stable CAD and 2.2% in acute coronary syndromes, at an average follow-up of 10 months [30]. Several meta-analyses have been published after the reporting of most recent trials and registries of ABSORB BRSs versus EESs. A study-level meta-analysis of six trials from Cassese et al. [31] showed that compared with metallic DESs patients treated with the ABSORB BRSs had a significant time-dependent risk of early definite or probable thrombosis (acute, OR 0.36 [95% CI 0.07–1.71]; $p = 0.21$; subacute, OR 3.11 [95% CI 1.24–7.82]; $p = 0.02$, $p$ for interaction <0.0001). In contrast, a patient-level meta-analysis of ABSORB II, ABSORB III, ABSORB-CHINA, and ABSORB-JAPAN reported nonsignificantly different cumulative rates of early thrombosis in patients treated with ABSORB BRSs and patients treated with EESs (0.9% vs. 0.5% $p = 0.22$) [32]. Lipinski et al. performed a focused meta-analysis of scaffold thrombosis including over 10,000 patients from trials and registries of the ABSORB BRSs, with a mean follow-up of 6.4 months. In patients who received the ABSORB BRSs, acute scaffold thrombosis was reported in 0.27% and subacute scaffold thrombosis in 0.57%. The ORs for early scaffold thrombosis with the ABSORB BRSs versus the DESs were 2.51 (95% CI 0.12–52.61) in a meta-analysis that only included ABSORB II and EVERBIO II, and 2.10 (95% CI 0.57–7.73) in a meta-analysis of five comparative registries reporting on this outcome (overall OR 2.02, 95%

CI 0.69–5.93; $p = 0.20$), with large confidence intervals suggesting inconclusive results for this endpoint [33].

In aggregate, current data suggest that acute and subacute scaffold thrombosis is <1% in selected patients from the early trials experience, but its incidence could be sensibly higher in less selected real-world all-comers and acute coronary syndrome patients undergoing percutaneous coronary intervention. Compared with metallic DESs, ABSORB BRSs seem to be associated with more thrombosis within the first 30 days after implant.

## MECHANISMS

Meaningful predictors of scaffold thrombosis have not yet been identified and unlikely will be so in the near future, due to the young age of the BRSs technology. Indeed, to identify statistically significant predictors of scaffold thrombosis, very large BRSs datasets with a proper number of events are needed. In fact, multivariable methods render incorrect results if an insufficient number of outcome events are available relative to the number of variables analyzed in the model (i.e., <10 events per variable) [34]. Therefore, for example, if 10 variables are tested in a multivariable model to identify independent predictors of 30-day scaffold thrombosis (with a putative incidence rate of 1%), then 100 events are needed, corresponding to approximately 10,000 patients. The above-mentioned meta-analysis of Stone et al., encompassing about 35 definite or probable device thrombosis events in about 3300 patients, identified diabetes, small vessel disease, and ACC/AHA B2/C lesions as independent predictors [32]. However, this analysis also included patients who received DESs; therefore, the specific predictors of BRSs thrombosis remain uncertain. Anyway, some lessons still can be drawn from prior experiences with DESs, and multiple potential mechanisms for scaffold thrombosis advocated (Figure 8.1.1).

### Patient-related mechanisms

Patients with acute coronary syndromes are at higher risk of early stent thrombosis regardless of the stent implanted [35]. This can be partly ascribed to the prothrombotic milieu itself, along with potential mechanical factors specific to acute coronary syndromes, including stent underexpansion (i.e., due to vasospasm resolution) and incomplete apposition (i.e., due to thrombus eventually disappearing and leaving a gap between the stent and the vessel wall). Other individual predisposing conditions have been advocated as responsible for thrombosis of DESs, including smoking, diabetes mellitus, chronic kidney disease, and impaired left ventricular ejection fraction [3]. Whether these factors also play a role in scaffold thrombosis remains hypothetical but unproven at this stage. Similar to DESs, it is also highly expected that platelet-specific risk factors can also trigger scaffold thrombosis. These include thrombocytosis, high on-treatment platelet reactivity (an occurrence that has been mitigated but not abolished by prasugrel and ticagrelor

**Table 8.1.1** Rates of definite or definite/probable scaffold thrombosis in published registries

| Study/first author | Year | Sample size | Device | Population | Follow up | Acute ST | Subacute ST | Early ST | Total ST |
|---|---|---|---|---|---|---|---|---|---|
| ABSORB Cohort A [10] | 2013 | 30 | ABSORB BVS | Stable CAD | 60 months | 0.0% | 0.0% | 0.0% | 0.0% |
| ABSORB Cohort B [11] | 2014 | 101 | ABSORB BVS | Stable CAD | 36 months | 0.0% | 0.0% | 0.0% | 0.0% |
| ABSORB EXTEND [12] | 2014 | 512 | ABSORB BVS | Stable CAD | 12 months | 0.0% | 0.4% | 0.4% | 0.8% |
| CTO-ABSORB [13] | 2014 | 35 | ABSORB BVS | Stable CAD | 6 months | 0.0% | 0.0% | 0.0% | 0.0% |
| DESolve FIM [14] | 2014 | 16 | Elixir DESolve | Stable CAD | 12 months | 0.0% | 0.0% | 0.0% | 0.0% |
| ASSURE [15] | 2014 | 183 | ABSORB BVS | Stable CAD/UA | 12 months | 0.0% | 0.0% | 0.0% | 0.0% |
| POLAR ACS [16] | 2014 | 100 | ABSORB BVS | ACS | 12 months | 0.0% | 0.0% | 0.0% | 1.0% |
| Gori et al. [17] | 2015 | 133 | ABSORB BVS | ACS | 12 months | 0.7% | 0.7% | 1.4% | 3.1% |
| Kajiya et al. [18] | 2013 | 11 | ABSORB BVS | STEMI | 3 months | 0.0% | 0.0% | 0.0% | 0.0% |
| BVS STEMI First [19] | 2014 | 49 | ABSORB BVS | STEMI | 30 days | 0.0% | 0.0% | 0.0% | 0.0% |
| PRAGUE 19 [20] | 2014 | 41 | ABSORB BVS | STEMI | 4 months | 0.0% | 2.4% | 2.4% | 2.4% |
| Kochman et al. [21] | 2014 | 23 | ABSORB BVS | STEMI | 8 months | 0.0% | 4.3% | 4.3% | 4.3% |
| RAI [22] | 2014 | 74 | ABSORB BVS | STEMI | 6 months | 0.0% | 1.4% | 1.4% | 1.4% |
| BVS-EXAMINATION | 2015 | 290 | ABSORB BVS | STEMI | 12 months | 0.7% | 0.7% | 1.4% | 1.7% |
| AMC [23] | 2014 | 135 | ABSORB BVS | All comers | 6 months | 0.0% | 2.2% | 2.2% | 3.0% |
| Mattesini et al. [24] | 2014 | 73 | ABSORB BVS | All comers | 8 months | 0.0% | 0.0% | 0.0% | 0.0% |
| Azzalini et al. [25] | 2015 | 339 | ABSORB BVS | All comers | 30 days | 0.0% | 1.2% | 1.2% | 1.2% |
| Sato et al. [26] | 2015 | 96 | ABSORB BVS | All comers | 12 months | 1.0% | 0.0% | 1.0% | 1.0% |
| Jaguszewski [27] | 2015 | 106 | ABSORB BVS | All comers | 5 months | 0.0% | 0.0% | 0.0% | 0.0% |
| Robaei et al. [28] | 2015 | 100 | ABSORB BVS | All comers | 30 days | 0.0% | 0.0% | 0.0% | 0.0% |
| GHOST-EU [29] | 2015 | 1189 | ABSORB BVS | All comers | 6 months | 0.4% | 0.9% | 1.5% | 2.1% |

*Note:* In case of multiple overlapping publications from the same registry, the most updated is reported. Incidences of scaffold thrombosis are reported as crude rates or Kaplan–Meier estimates.

*Abbreviations:* ACS = acute coronary syndromes; CAD = coronary artery disease; CTO = chronic total occlusions; ST = stent thrombosis; STEMI = ST-elevation myocardial infarction; UA = unstable angina.

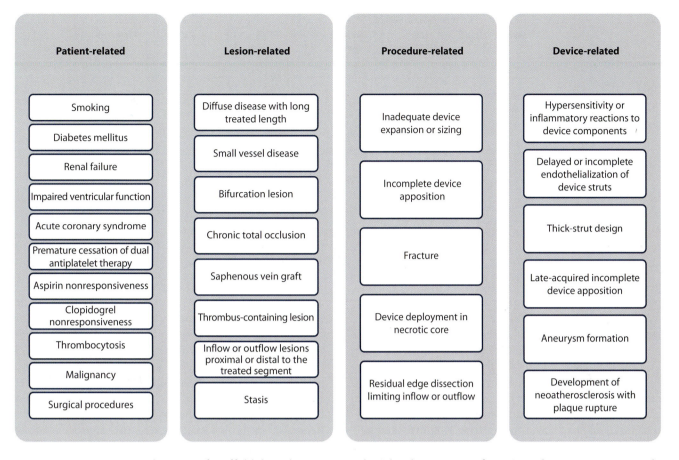

**Figure 8.1.1** Putative mechanisms of scaffold thrombosis. (Reproduced with permission from Capodanno D, Joner M and Zimarino M. *EuroIntervention.* 2015;11 Suppl V:V181–4.)

[36]) and premature dual antiplatelet therapy (DAPT) discontinuation [37].

## Lesion-related mechanisms

Intuitively, both DESs and BRSs thrombosis are statistically more likely to occur in a patient if multiple or long coronary segments are treated, a circumstance that is typically associated with diffuse or multivessel coronary artery disease. For the reasons detailed above, thrombus-containing lesions could also be associated with an increased risk of scaffold thrombosis. It is also reasonable to assume that the increased risk of early DESs thrombosis observed in complex angiographic subsets such as small vessel disease, chronic total occlusions, bifurcation lesions, and saphenous vein grafts cannot be abolished by current-generation BRSs, or could be even amplified due to technical limitations of current generation thick-strut devices.

## Procedure-related mechanisms

In the GHOST-EU registry, the observed clustering of thrombotic events during the first 30 days of follow-up suggested a specific role for procedure-related factors [29]. Due

to its material construct, placement of BRSs typically require more dedication and time than corresponding placement of a metallic stent, with multiple steps necessarily involved to avert the risk of fracture, acute incomplete apposition, underexpansion, and flow-limiting dissection [38]. All these procedural complications may theoretically trigger scaffold thrombosis. Acute scaffold fracture was a relatively rare iatrogenic phenomenon, possibly related to overexpansion, observed in 2 of 51 (3.9%) patients of the ABSORB Cohort B study who had postimplantation optical coherence tomography (OCT) imaging [39]. Incomplete scaffold apposition was reported at 6.2% in another small OCT study, being more frequently demonstrated in fibro-calcific plaques [40]. Importantly, incomplete scaffold apposition has been linked to BRSs strut uncoverage and the presence of intraluminal masses by OCT at 6 months [41]. Also, a notable delay in strut coverage has been documented at the site of BRSs overlaps in animal models [42].

## Device-related mechanisms

Strut thickness of the ABSORB BRSs—the most used BRSs in the market—is about 150 μm, resembling that of a first-generation DESs and almost doubling that of a second-generation DESs (Figure 8.1.2). Bulky struts are known to

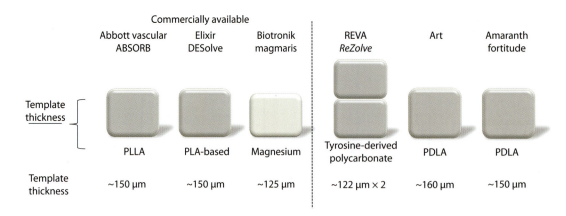

**Figure 8.1.2** Strut thickness of currently available and investigational bioresorbable scaffolds.

generate flow disturbances and activate the coagulation pathway, as shown by seminal studies conducted with bare metal stents [43]. Extrapolating results from previous stent studies, the greater strut dimension of the BRSs might also be theoretically responsible for delayed endothelialization [44]. Also notably, due to the nonmetallic nature of the BRSs, plaque composition and morphology may significantly impact on important features such as expansion and eccentricity [45,46]. Acute and chronic vascular inflammatory reactions may play a role in triggering early and late thrombotic events in patients who receive DESs [47]. In preclinical models, mild to moderate inflammatory reactions have been observed acutely after implantation and chronically during the biodegradation phase of the BRSs, which exceeded those observed with the second generation DESs [48].

## PREVENTION AND MANAGEMENT

### Prevention of scaffold thrombosis

A general rule of common sense to prevent early thrombotic events is to avoid implanting a BRSs in lesions where suboptimal results and loss of scaffold integrity can be anticipated. The instructions of the manufacturer should be followed thoroughly, and special care should be devoted in vessel sizing, lesion preparation, scaffold implantation, and optimization. Overlaps, when necessary, should be as short as possible.

Intravascular imaging is intuitively effective to detect potential mechanical causes of early scaffold thrombosis and guide further interventions, although its clinical impact remains difficult to demonstrate [38]. Intravascular ultrasound allows optimization of scaffold size while reducing the risk of disruption with oversized balloons. With its higher resolution, OCT provides precise assessment of scaffold integrity, apposition to the underlying wall, edge dissections, and presence of thrombus [24].

Dual antiplatelet therapy is the cornerstone of thrombosis preventions in patients undergoing percutaneous coronary intervention. Prasugrel or ticagrelor, when they are noncontraindicated, are recommended in patients who present with an acute coronary syndrome [49]. To limit the incidence of early BRSs thrombosis in patients undergoing elective PCI in the context of stable coronary artery disease, some centers adopt a strategy of de-escalation with newer $P2Y_{12}$ inhibitors during the first month after implantation, and switch to clopidogrel thereafter, on a background of aspirin therapy [38]. Due to lacking evidences of safety and effectiveness, this approach cannot be presently recommended, but it is the object of ongoing investigations. The length of DAPT after implantation of BRSs is another matter of debate. Current European guidelines advocate a 6-month DAPT period after implantation of DESs, but prolonging DAPT beyond 6 months may still be considered in patients at high thrombotic risk and low bleeding risk [49]. None of the several recent trials of DAPT duration included patients who received BRSs [50]. Notably, the vast majority of patients in the ABSORB II trial and GHOST-EU registry were still on DAPT at 12 months [4,29]. Indisputably, compliance to DAPT should be regularly assessed in patients who receive BRSs, particularly in the early period.

### Management of acute and subacute scaffold thrombosis

When scaffold thrombosis occurs early, a fundamental step is to exclude one of two factors to be responsible: mechanical causes and suboptimal antithrombotic therapy. OCT is key to identify (or to rule out) underlying mechanical reasons including edge dissection, fractures, incomplete apposition, and underexpansion (Figure 8.1.3). In case of thrombosis arising from an uncovered dissection, another stent or scaffold should be positioned. In case of fracture, placement of a DESs is advisable [38]. In case of incomplete scaffold apposition, one should consider the desired final vessel diameter and the nominal diameter of the scaffold: if the scaffold is too small, then placement of a DESs should be considered, otherwise postdilatation with a properly sized

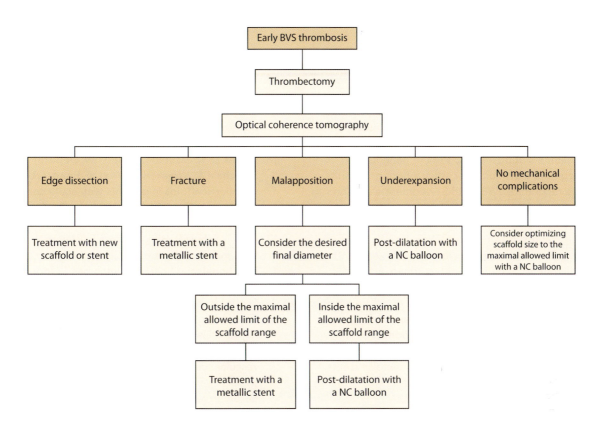

**Figure 8.1.3** Algorithm for the treatment of early scaffold thrombosis. (Reproduced with permission from Tamburino C, Latib A, van Geuns RJ, Sabate M, Mehilli J, Gori T, Achenbach S et al. *EuroIntervention*. 2015;10.)

noncompliant balloon may help the scaffold to reach the final dimension and avoid multiple strut layering. Use of noncompliant balloons should also be advocated in cases of thrombosis sustained by scaffold underexpansion. Finally, if BRSs thrombosis occurs in patients on clopidogrel therapy, switch to more potent antiplatelet agents (i.e., prasugrel or ticagrelor) is recommended.

## CONCLUSIONS

Disappearance of a BRSs with recovery of functional endothelial lining represents a paradigm shift in percutaneous coronary intervention, with the potential to reduce late thrombotic events. However, in the early term after implantation, scaffold thrombosis can be triggered by the unfavorable rheology of current thick-strut devices and the potential procedural shortcomings of BRSs implantation in complex clinical and lesions subsets. Next-generation devices with thinner struts (~100–120 µm) may contribute to ameliorate these issues. Determining the true incidence of early scaffold thrombosis is challenged by the paucity of data, which are mostly site-reported and collected in small and selected populations. Mechanisms of scaffold thrombosis are likely multifactorial, stemming from patient- to lesion-specific considerations, along with procedural- and device-related factors that may play a prominent role in the incidence of acute and subacute events. Prevention of procedural causes with extensive use of best implantation

practice, intravascular imaging and adoption of optimal antithrombotic therapies remains essential. When early scaffold thrombosis occurs, understanding and removing the underlying mechanism is the principal condition to avoid recurrences.

## REFERENCES

1. Palmerini T, Biondi-Zoccai G, Della Riva D, Mariani A, Genereux P, Branzi A and Stone GW. Stent thrombosis with drug-eluting stents: Is the paradigm shifting? *J Am Coll Cardiol*. 2013;62:1915–21.
2. Iqbal J, Onuma Y, Ormiston J, Abizaid A, Waksman R and Serruys P. Bioresorbable scaffolds: Rationale, current status, challenges, and future. *Eur Heart J*. 2014;35:765–76.
3. Capodanno D, Joner M and Zimarino M. What about the risk of scaffold thrombosis with BRSs? *EuroIntervention*. 2015;11 Suppl V:V181–4.
4. Serruys PW, Chevalier B, Dudek D, Cequier A, Carrie D, Iniguez A, Dominici M et al. A bioresorbable everolimus-eluting scaffold versus a metallic everolimus-eluting stent for ischaemic heart disease caused by de-novo native coronary artery lesions (ABSORB II): An interim 1-year analysis of clinical and procedural secondary outcomes from a randomised controlled trial. *Lancet*. 2015;385:43–54.

5. Puricel S, Arroyo D, Corpataux N, Baeriswyl G, Lehmann S, Kallinikou Z, Muller O et al. Comparison of everolimus- and biolimus-eluting coronary stents with everolimus-eluting bioresorbable vascular scaffolds. *J Am Coll Cardiol.* 2015;65:791–801.

6. Sabate M, Windecker S, Iniguez A, Okkels-Jensen L, Cequier A, Brugaletta S, Hofma SH et al. Everolimus-eluting bioresorbable stent vs. durable polymer everolimus-eluting metallic stent in patients with ST-segment elevation myocardial infarction: Results of the randomized ABSORB ST-segment elevation myocardial infarction-TROFI II trial. *Eur Heart J.* 2016;37:229–40.

7. Gao R, Yang Y, Han Y, Huo Y, Chen J, Yu B, Su X et al. Bioresorbable vascular scaffolds versus metallic stents in patients with coronary artery disease: ABSORB China Trial. *J Am Coll Cardiol.* 2015;66:2298–309.

8. Kimura T, Kozuma K, Tanabe K, Nakamura S, Yamane M, Muramatsu T, Saito S et al. A randomized trial evaluating everolimus-eluting Absorb bioresorbable scaffolds vs. everolimus-eluting metallic stents in patients with coronary artery disease: ABSORB Japan. *Eur Heart J.* 2015;36:3332–42.

9. Ellis SG, Kereiakes DJ, Metzger DC, Caputo RP, Rizik DG, Teirstein PS, Litt MR et al. Everolimus-eluting bioresorbable scaffolds for coronary artery disease. *N Engl J Med.* 2015;373:1905–15.

10. Onuma Y, Dudek D, Thuesen L, Webster M, Nieman K, Garcia-Garcia HM, Ormiston JA et al. Five-year clinical and functional multislice computed tomography angiographic results after coronary implantation of the fully resorbable polymeric everolimus-eluting scaffold in patients with de novo coronary artery disease: The ABSORB cohort A trial. *JACC Cardiovasc Interv.* 2013;6:999–1009.

11. Serruys PW, Onuma Y, Garcia-Garcia HM, Muramatsu T, van Geuns RJ, de Bruyne B, Dudek D et al. Dynamics of vessel wall changes following the implantation of the ABSORB everolimus-eluting bioresorbable vascular scaffold: A multi-imaging modality study at 6, 12, 24 and 36 months. *EuroIntervention.* 2014;9:1271–84.

12. Abizaid A, Costa JR, Jr., Bartorelli AL, Whitbourn R, van Geuns RJ, Chevalier B, Patel T et al. The ABSORB EXTEND study: Preliminary report of the twelve-month clinical outcomes in the first 512 patients enrolled. *EuroIntervention.* 2015;10(12):1396–401.

13. Vaquerizo B, Barros A, Pujadas S, Bajo E, Estrada D, Miranda-Guardiola F, Rigla J et al. Bioresorbable everolimus-eluting vascular scaffold for the treatment of chronic total occlusions: CTO-ABSORB pilot study. *EuroIntervention.* 2015;11(5):555–63.

14. Verheye S, Ormiston JA, Stewart J, Webster M, Sanidas E, Costa R, Costa JR, Jr. et al. A next-generation bioresorbable coronary scaffold system: From bench to first clinical evaluation: 6- and 12-month clinical and multimodality imaging results. *JACC Cardiovasc Interv.* 2014;7:89–99.

15. Wohrle J, Naber C, Schmitz T, Schwencke C, Frey N, Butter C, Brachmann J et al. Beyond the early stages: Insights from the ASSURE registry on bioresorbable vascular scaffolds. *EuroIntervention.* 2015;11:149–56.

16. Dudek D, Rzeszutko L, Zasada W, Depukat R, Siudak Z, Ochala A, Wojakowski W et al. Bioresorbable vascular scaffolds in patients with acute coronary syndromes: The POLAR ACS study. *Pol Arch Med Wewn.* 2014;124:669–77.

17. Gori T, Schulz E, Hink U, Kress E, Weiers N, Weissner M, Jabs A et al. Clinical, Angiographic, Functional, and Imaging Outcomes 12 Months After Implantation of Drug-Eluting Bioresorbable Vascular Scaffolds in Acute Coronary Syndromes. *JACC Cardiovasc Interv.* 2015;8:770–7.

18. Kajiya T, Liang M, Sharma RK, Lee CH, Chan MY, Tay E, Chan KH et al. Everolimus-eluting bioresorbable vascular scaffold (BVS) implantation in patients with ST-segment elevation myocardial infarction (STEMI). *EuroIntervention.* 2013;9:501–4.

19. Diletti R, Karanasos A, Muramatsu T, Nakatani S, Van Mieghem NM, Onuma Y, Nauta ST et al. Everolimus-eluting bioresorbable vascular scaffolds for treatment of patients presenting with ST-segment elevation myocardial infarction: BVS STEMI first study. *Eur Heart J.* 2014;35:777–86.

20. Kocka V, Maly M, Tousek P, Budesinsky T, Lisa L, Prodanov P, Jarkovsky J et al. Bioresorbable vascular scaffolds in acute ST-segment elevation myocardial infarction: A prospective multicentre study 'Prague 19'. *Eur Heart J.* 2014;35:787–94.

21. Kochman J, Tomaniak M, Pietrasik A, Koltowski L, Rdzanek A, Huczek Z, Mazurek T et al. Bioresorbable everolimus-eluting vascular scaffold in patients with ST-segment elevation myocardial infarction: Optical coherence tomography evaluation and clinical outcomes. *Cardiol J.* 2015;22(3):315–22.

22. Ielasi A, Cortese B, Varricchio A, Tespili M, Sesana M, Pisano F, Loi B et al. Immediate and midterm outcomes following primary PCI with bioresorbable vascular scaffold implantation in patients with ST-segment myocardial infarction: Insights from the multicentre 'Registro ABSORB Italiano' (RAI registry). *EuroIntervention.* 2015;11:157–62.

23. Kraak RP, Hassell ME, Grundeken MJ, Koch KT, Henriques JP, Piek JJ, Baan J, Jr. et al. Initial experience and clinical evaluation of the ABSORB bioresorbable vascular scaffold (BVS) in real-world practice: The AMC Single Centre Real World PCI Registry. *EuroIntervention.* 2015;10:1160–8.

24. Mattesini A, Secco GG, Dall'Ara G, Ghione M, Rama-Merchan JC, Lupi A, Viceconte N et al. ABSORB biodegradable stents versus second-generation

metal stents: A comparison study of 100 complex lesions treated under OCT guidance. *JACC Cardiovasc Interv.* 2014;7:741–50.

25. Azzalini L and L'Allier PL. Bioresorbable vascular scaffold thrombosis in an all-comer patient population: Single-center experience. *J Invasive Cardiol.* 2015;27:85–92.

26. Sato K, Latib A, Panoulas VF, Kawamoto H, Naganuma T, Miyazaki T and Colombo A. Procedural feasibility and clinical outcomes in propensity-matched patients treated with bioresorbable scaffolds vs new-generation drug-eluting stents. *Can J Cardiol.* 2015;31:328–34.

27. Jaguszewski M, Ghadri JR, Zipponi M, Bataiosu DR, Diekmann J, Geyer V, Neumann CA et al. Feasibility of second-generation bioresorbable vascular scaffold implantation in complex anatomical and clinical scenarios. *Clin Res Cardiol.* 2015;104:124–35.

28. Robaei D, Back LM, Ooi SY, Pitney MR and Jepson N. Everolimus-eluting bioresorbable vascular scaffold implantation in real world and complex coronary disease: Procedural and 30-day outcomes at two Australian Centres. *Heart Lung Circ.* 2015;24:854–9.

29. Capodanno D, Gori T, Nef H, Latib A, Mehilli J, Lesiak M, Caramanno G et al. Percutaneous coronary intervention with everolimus-eluting bioresorbable vascular scaffolds in routine clinical practice: Early and midterm outcomes from the European multicentre GHOST-EU registry. *EuroIntervention.* 2015;10:1144–53.

30. Ishibashi Y, Nakatani S and Onuma Y. Definite and probable bioresorbable scaffold thrombosis in stable and ACS patients. *EuroIntervention.* 2015;11:e1–2.

31. Cassese S, Byrne RA, Ndrepepa G, Kufner S, Wiebe J, Repp J, Schunkert H et al. Everolimus-eluting bioresorbable vascular scaffolds versus everolimus-eluting metallic stents: A meta-analysis of randomised controlled trials. *Lancet.* 2016;387:537–44.

32. Stone GW, Gao R, Kimura T, Kereiakes DJ, Ellis SG, Onuma Y, Cheong WF et al. 1-year outcomes with the ABSORB bioresorbable scaffold in patients with coronary artery disease: A patient-level, pooled meta-analysis. *Lancet.* 2016;387:1277–89.

33. Lipinski MJ, Escarcega RO, Baker NC, Benn HA, Gaglia MA Jr, Torguson R and Waksman R. Scaffold thrombosis after percutaneous coronary intervention with ABSORB bioresorbable vascular scaffold: A systematic review and meta-analysis. *JACC Cardiovasc Interv.* 2016;9:12–24.

34. van Domburg R, Hoeks S, Kardys I, Lenzen M and Boersma E. Tools and techniques—Statistics: How many variables are allowed in the logistic and Cox regression models? *EuroIntervention.* 2014;9:1472–3.

35. Kukreja N, Onuma Y, Garcia-Garcia HM, Daemen J, van Domburg R and Serruys PW. The risk of stent thrombosis in patients with acute coronary syndromes treated with bare-metal and drug-eluting stents. *JACC Cardiovasc Interv.* 2009;2:534–41.

36. Lemesle G, Schurtz G, Bauters C and Hamon M. High on-treatment platelet reactivity with Ticagrelor versus Prasugrel: A systematic review and meta-analysis. *J Thromb Haemost.* 2015;13:931–42.

37. Mehran R, Baber U, Steg PG, Ariti C, Weisz G, Witzenbichler B, Henry TD et al. Cessation of dual antiplatelet treatment and cardiac events after percutaneous coronary intervention (PARIS): 2 year results from a prospective observational study. *Lancet.* 2013;382:1714–22.

38. Tamburino C, Latib A, van Geuns RJ, Sabate M, Mehilli J, Gori T, Achenbach S et al. Contemporary practice and technical aspects in coronary intervention with bioresorbable scaffolds: A European perspective. *EuroIntervention.* 2015;10.

39. Onuma Y, Serruys PW, Muramatsu T, Nakatani S, van Geuns RJ, de Bruyne B, Dudek D et al. Incidence and imaging outcomes of acute scaffold disruption and late structural discontinuity after implantation of the absorb Everolimus-Eluting fully bioresorbable vascular scaffold: Optical coherence tomography assessment in the ABSORB cohort B Trial (A Clinical Evaluation of the Bioabsorbable Everolimus Eluting Coronary Stent System in the Treatment of Patients With De Novo Native Coronary Artery Lesions). *JACC Cardiovasc Interv.* 2014;7:1400–11.

40. Brown AJ, McCormick LM, Braganza DM, Bennett MR, Hoole SP and West NE. Expansion and malapposition characteristics after bioresorbable vascular scaffold implantation. *Catheter Cardiovasc Interv.* 2014;84:37–45.

41. Gomez-Lara J, Radu M, Brugaletta S, Farooq V, Diletti R, Onuma Y, Windecker S et al. Serial analysis of the malapposed and uncovered struts of the new generation of everolimus-eluting bioresorbable scaffold with optical coherence tomography. *JACC Cardiovasc Interv.* 2011;4:992–1001.

42. Farooq V, Serruys PW, Heo JH, Gogas BD, Onuma Y, Perkins LE, Diletti R et al. Intracoronary optical coherence tomography and histology of overlapping everolimus-eluting bioresorbable vascular scaffolds in a porcine coronary artery model: The potential implications for clinical practice. *JACC Cardiovasc Interv.* 2013;6:523–32.

43. Kolandaivelu K, Swaminathan R, Gibson WJ, Kolachalama VB, Nguyen-Ehrenreich KL, Giddings VL, Coleman L et al. Stent thrombogenicity early in high-risk interventional settings is driven by stent design and deployment and protected by polymer-drug coatings. *Circulation.* 2011;123:1400–9.

44. Pache J, Kastrati A, Mehilli J, Schuhlen H, Dotzer F, Hausleiter J, Fleckenstein M et al. Intracoronary stenting and angiographic results: Strut thickness effect on restenosis outcome (ISAR-STEREO-2) trial. *J Am Coll Cardiol.* 2003;41:1283–8.

45. Shaw E, Allahwala UK, Cockburn JA, Hansen TC, Mazhar J, Figtree GA, Hansen PS et al. The effect of coronary artery plaque composition, morphology and burden on Absorb bioresorbable vascular scaffold expansion and eccentricity—A detailed analysis with optical coherence tomography. *Int J Cardiol.* 2015;184c:230–236.

46. Attizzani GF, Ohno Y, Capodanno D, Francaviglia B, Grasso C, Sgroi C, Wang W et al. New insights on acute expansion and longitudinal elongation of bioresorbable vascular scaffolds in vivo and at bench test: A note of caution on reliance to compliance charts and nominal length. *Catheter Cardiovasc Interv.* 2015;85:E99–e107.

47. Inoue T, Croce K, Morooka T, Sakuma M, Node K and Simon DI. Vascular inflammation and repair: Implications for re-endothelialization, restenosis, and stent thrombosis. *JACC Cardiovasc Interv.* 2011;4:1057–66.

48. Otsuka F, Pacheco E, Perkins LE, Lane JP, Wang Q, Kamberi M, Frie M et al. Long-term safety of an everolimus-eluting bioresorbable vascular scaffold and the cobalt-chromium XIENCE V stent in a porcine coronary artery model. *Circ Cardiovasc Interv.* 2014;7:330–42.

49. Windecker S, Kolh P, Alfonso F, Collet JP, Cremer J, Falk V, Filippatos G et al. 2014 ESC/EACTS Guidelines on myocardial revascularization: The Task Force on Myocardial Revascularization of the European Society of Cardiology (ESC) and the European Association for Cardio-Thoracic Surgery (EACTS) Developed with the special contribution of the European Association of Percutaneous Cardiovascular Interventions (EAPCI). *Eur Heart J.* 2014;35:2541–619.

50. Palmerini T, Benedetto U, Bacchi-Reggiani L, Riva DD, Biondi-Zoccai G, Feres F, Abizaid A et al. Mortality in patients treated with extended duration dual antiplatelet therapy after drug-eluting stent implantation: A pairwise and Bayesian network meta-analysis of randomised trials. *Lancet.* 2015;385(9985):2371–82.

# Late and very late scaffold thrombosis

ANTONIOS KARANASOS, BU-CHUN ZHANG, JORS VAN DER SIJDE, JIANG MING FAM,
ROBERT-JAN M. VAN GEUNS, AND EVELYN REGAR

Bioresorbable scaffolds (BRSs) are a new treatment for coronary artery disease. As these devices are expected to resorb after providing the mechanical support required the first months after percutaneous coronary intervention (PCI), they could potentially be associated with several long-term advantages over the metallic stents, such as a lack of permanent vessel caging that enables restoration of the vessel vasomotor tone, adaptive shear stress, late luminal enlargement with late expansive remodeling, preservation of long-term side-branch patency, and allowing future revascularization options, while free of complications observed with metallic stents such as neoatherosclerosis and late failure [1]. First-in-human studies of BRSs have shown promising results demonstrating a favorable healing response at long-term with complete scaffold resorption, late lumen enlargement, recovery of vasomotion, and a potentially favorable plaque modification [2,3]. Furthermore, initial clinical results were also promising showing a low rate of adverse events and a complete absence of late and very late thrombotic events. Utilization of BRSs in more complex lesions and populations was associated with a higher event rate, while several cases of late and very late scaffold thrombosis were reported. In this chapter, we aim to briefly summarize current insights from late and very late metallic stent thrombosis, give basic insights into BVSs healing, review current experience on BRSs thrombosis, and suggest potential mechanisms and preventive measures for this complication.

## LATE AND VERY LATE THROMBOSIS IN METALLIC STENTS

Late thrombosis, defined as the occurrence of stent thrombosis beyond 1 month after baseline implantation, had not received much attention from the interventional community during the first years of metallic stents. However, the report of several angiographically confirmed cases of first-generation metallic drug-eluting stent (DESs) thrombosis related to antiplatelet therapy discontinuation brought this issue in the spotlight [4], and intracoronary devices have

ever since been scrutinized for the occurrence of this complication. First-generation DESs had been considered the main devices associated with this complication, with an annual incidence rate of late and very late (defined as stent thrombosis occurring beyond 1 year since initial implantation) stent thrombosis of 0.6% per year in a large two-center registry [5]. However, accumulating experience has shown that an ongoing thrombotic risk is present with all devices, including bare metal stents (BMS) with cases of thrombosis reported up to 15–20 years postimplantation [6,7]. Similarly, although second-generation drug-eluting stents have been associated with an improved long-term safety profile with lower risk of stent thrombosis in meta-analyses [8], it appears that late thrombosis remains an issue with these devices as well, with an annual incidence rate of definite very late stent thrombosis of 0.2% [9]. It is therefore evident that late and very late stent thrombosis is consistently observed with all metallic stents, although the incidence might vary depending on stent type.

Several factors have been implicated in the pathogenesis of stent thrombosis, including patient-related factors (acute coronary syndrome, diabetes, renal failure, impaired left ventricular function, prior brachytherapy, malignancy), lesion factors (lesion/stent length, vessel/stent diameter, bifurcation, total occlusion, saphenous venous graft lesions), procedural factors (inadequate stent expansion or sizing, malapposition, stent deployment in necrotic core, residual edge dissections), antithrombotic and antiplatelet therapy (premature dual antiplatelet therapy discontinuation, aspirin or clopidogrel nonresponsiveness), and device-related factors (hypersensitivity to stent polymer or drug, incomplete endothelialization, stent design, covered stents) [10,11].

Pathologic studies were the first to assess the pathomechanisms of metallic stent thrombosis [12,13]. These observations hinted to the underlying plaque as an important substrate in BMS thrombosis, whereas with DESs an impaired healing response with high incidence of incomplete strut coverage and stent malapposition was identified as the main mechanism [13]. Namely in first-generation

DESs, this pattern of healing response has been associated with vessel wall toxicity either due to the released drug or to the polymer [14]. These initial pathologic observations were expanded by *in vivo* optical coherence tomography (OCT) studies which tried to evaluate imaging findings in patients with late and very late metallic stent thrombosis (Figure 8.2.1). As the high resolution of OCT allows for the detection of tissue with ~10 μm resolution, strut coverage by OCT has been used to assess strut endothelialization. Although numerous studies have assessed OCT coverage as a surrogate for healing, the percentage of uncovered struts has not been prospectively associated with stent thrombosis thus far [15]. Nevertheless, studies focusing on patients with events have shown a high incidence of incomplete coverage in patients with late and very late metallic DESs thrombosis [16–24]. Similarly, stent malapposition has also been suggested to play a role in metallic stent thrombosis. As with incomplete coverage, acute malapposition has not been prospectively associated with stent thrombosis [25]; however, metallic stents with late thrombosis have a very high incidence of malapposition [16–24], while late malapposition has been associated with the presence of local inflammation in first-generation metallic DESs and prospectively linked to very late adverse outcome [26]. Importantly, findings of incomplete coverage and malapposition are exaggerated within the stent in segments with thrombus versus segments without thrombus [24].

Overall in these studies, this impaired healing response accounts for approximately half of the very late thrombotic events in metallic DESs. In the rest of the cases with very late DESs thrombosis and also in the vast majority of very late bare metal stent (BMS) thrombosis, another mechanism, consisting of *de novo* development of atherosclerosis within the stented segment and called neoatherosclerosis, seems to prevail [27–30]. Indeed, several reports have linked neoatherosclerosis to in-stent plaque rupture and subsequent thrombosis within the stent [6], while neoatherosclerotic plaque rupture has been associated with acute coronary syndrome presentation, although it can be also encountered in asymptomatic or stable patients [27]. Finally, a third more rare mechanism is identified in some cases, consisting of a native plaque rupture at the edges of a stent triggering thrombosis within the stented segment [16,21].

It becomes thus apparent that late and very late metallic stent thrombosis is to some extent triggered by the permanent metallic structure of the implanted devices which might be a source of vascular toxicity, while it massively limits the vessel's ability for remodeling, plaque regression, and lumen enlargement, thus leading inevitably to lumen narrowing with or without neoatherosclerosis over time. Conceptually, bioresorbable scaffolds could allow for a different healing response with recovery of the native vessel morphology over time [2] (Figure 8.2.2).

## HEALING RESPONSE IN BIORESORBABLE SCAFFOLDS

First-in-human bioresorbable scaffold studies have employed multimodality imaging for evaluating the vascular healing response after BRSs implantation [31–34]. Therefore, the healing response of several bioresorbable scaffolds has been well documented. The more extensively studied bioresorbable scaffold is the ABSORB BVSs (Abbott Vascular, Santa Clara, CA) with two generations: ABSORB BVSs 1.0 evaluated in the ABSORB A study, and ABSORB BVSs 1.1, which was evaluated in the ABSORB B study. Invasive imaging follow-up of ABSORB A has documented a favorable healing response of the ABSORB BVSs 1.0 with strut integration within the vessel wall and resolution of acute malapposition by 6 months, although accompanied by moderate acute and chronic recoil [35]. Longer-term follow-up, namely 5 years postimplantation, has demonstrated complete strut resorption, recovery of vasomotion at the scaffolded segment, late luminal enlargement due to plaque regression, increased luminal symmetry, side-branch patency, and development of a signal-rich and low-attenuating by OCT tissue layer covering potentially thrombogenic plaque components [2,3]. Similarly, ABSORB BVSs 1.1 has exhibited a favorable

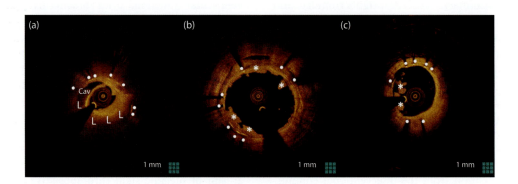

**Figure 8.2.1** Different mechanisms of very late stent thrombosis in metallic stents. **(a)** Neointimal rupture with in-stent cavity formation. **(b)** Thrombus attached to malapposed struts. **(c)** Thrombus attached to an uncovered strut. Annotations: L = necrotic core, white bullets = stent struts, white asterisk = white thrombus, Cav = cavity.

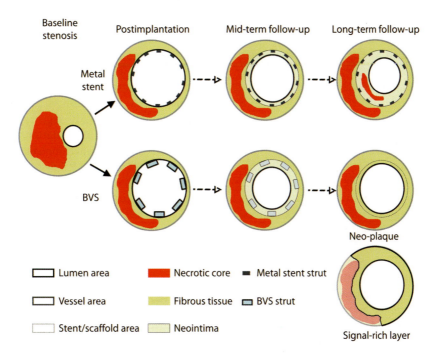

**Figure 8.2.2** Long-term vascular healing response in metal stents and bioresorbable scaffolds. After metal stent implantation, struts are preserved and the neointimal area is clearly delineated between stent and lumen contour even at long-term follow-up, with possible development of neoatherosclerosis within the neointima. Conversely, in long-term follow-up of bioresorbable scaffolds, neointimal boundaries are unclear after bioresorption (dotted line), and the intima resembles a native plaque, defined as neoplaque. The signal-rich layer is the layer that separates the underlying plaque components from the lumen. BVS = bioresorbable vascular scaffold. (Adapted from Karanasos et al., *J Am Coll Cardiol* 2014;64:2343–56.)

healing response with an incidence of ~3% of uncovered struts at 6 months, decreasing to ~1.5% over 3 years, while scaffold-level malapposition decreased from 81% postimplantation to 16% at 3 years [32].

The DESolve BCS (Elixir Medical, Sunnyvale, CA) has also demonstrated a good healing response with 1.32% uncovered struts and 0.04% malapposed struts at 6 months [33], and ongoing bioresorption with 14% reduction in the number of discernible struts by OCT. Likewise, the magnesium bioresorbable platform (DREAMS; Biotronik, Bülach, Switzerland) has demonstrated excellent healing with 100% strut coverage at 6 months and 2.8% malapposed struts at 6 months that diminished to 0.2% at 1 year [34].

## CURRENT EXPERIENCE WITH LATE SCAFFOLD THROMBOSIS

These imaging observations suggest a good healing response for bioresorbable scaffolds. However, the main limitation of these imaging studies is that they have mainly focused on relatively simple patient and lesion subsets. As a result, the complication rate was low and no cases of late or very late stent thrombosis have been reported in these first-in-human studies. Nevertheless, vascular healing and also complication rate could differ in more complex lesions. Implantation

of overlapping ABSORB BVSs in animal models has demonstrated a delayed coverage of segments with strut overlap compared to segments without strut overlap [36]. Similarly, it is known from metallic stents that implantation in myocardial infarction is associated with higher rates of uncovered and malapposed struts compared to implantation in stable patients [37,38].

Recently, the ABSORB BVSs and the DESolve BCS have received approval for commercial use in several countries. Consequently, these scaffolds were also implanted in patients and lesions not usually encountered in the context of clinical trials and several registries recording the outcomes in patients treated with bioresorbable scaffolds—mainly with ABSORB BVSs—have been published [39–48]. As these registries tend to include more complex patient and lesion subsets, outcome in these registries could differ from the ones reported in the first-in-human studies. Indeed, scaffold thrombosis has been reported, with an incidence that varies across the different series, and comprises mainly cases with acute or subacute thrombosis. In these registries, the reported rate of 6-month definite scaffold thrombosis has ranged from 0% to 2.7% [49]. Additionally to (sub)acute thrombosis, several cases of late thrombosis have also been reported in these studies.

Due to the limited number of patients included in these registries and the limited available follow-up—as most registries have reported outcomes up to 6 months—it is difficult to make firm estimations for the incidence of a relatively rare complication such as late scaffold thrombosis. Next to the first-in-human studies, only a limited number of studies with follow-up up to 1 year have been reported: ABSORB EXTEND, ABSORB II, ASSURE, POLAR-ACS, and BVSs EXAMINATION [42–44,50,51] (Table 8.2.1). The reported 1-year incidence of late scaffold thrombosis in these registries has ranged from 0 to 0.4%.

Thus far, a total of 12 cases of late scaffold thrombosis has been reported in the literature. For the majority of these cases, the etiology was not completely elucidated; however, early discontinuation of antiplatelet therapy has been implicated in some of them. The majority of these cases come from the multicenter GHOST registry. In this registry of 1189 patients at a median follow-up of 184 days, seven cases of definite or probable late scaffold thrombosis occurring from 34 to 239 days since implantation have been reported [41]. A detailed description of the mechanism for the majority of these cases was not provided. High-risk characteristics in this series include baseline implantation performed due to acute coronary syndrome in three out of seven cases, while two of the implantations had been performed in type C lesions. In two of the cases (34 and 149 days postimplantation), DAPT had been discontinued prematurely at the time of the event. Two additional cases have been reported in ABSORB EXTEND registry [52]. One of them occurred three months after implantation in a bifurcation lesion, and in this case platelet function tests revealed a normal ADP-induced platelet aggregation, potentially due to resistance to clopidogrel. The second case occurred 239 days postimplantation without clear identification of the pathomechanism; however, the close temporal correlation

of the acute coronary syndrome with a bee sting has raised speculation by the authors regarding a possible participation of spasm in the pathogenesis of this case. One case of probable late scaffold thrombosis at 335 days has also been documented at the 1-year follow-up report of ABSORB II, a randomized comparison of ABSORB BVSs with metallic stents [51]. In the AMC registry with 6-month follow-up after ABSORB BVSs implantation, one case of late scaffold thrombosis 3 months after implantation was reported, which was associated with DAPT discontinuation due to gastrointestinal bleeding [46]. Finally, one more case of late scaffold thrombosis occurring at 96 days postimplantation has been reported in the BVSs EXAMINATION registry, a registry investigating the 1-year outcomes following ABSORB BVSs implantation in 290 STEMI patients; however, more details were not available [42].

## CURRENT EXPERIENCE WITH VERY LATE SCAFFOLD THROMBOSIS

In line with expectations of a very low incidence of very late scaffold thrombosis with BRSs, considering that a significant fraction of the scaffold mass is expected to have been resorbed after 1 year, only four cases of very late scaffold thrombosis have been reported in the literature. In one case from our center, scaffold thrombosis occurred almost 2 years post-initial implantation, soon after dual antiplatelet therapy discontinuation [54] (Figures 8.2.3 and 8.2.4). Imaging findings in this case included extensive scaffold discontinuity with struts protruding into the lumen and thrombus formation. This observed scaffold deformation was possibly caused by a repeat procedure where the scaffolded segment had been subjected to postdilation, performed 1 year after the baseline implantation. As by that time point, the scaffold is expected to have lost a large part of its mechanical support, intervention or catheter manipulation at the scaffolded segment could have resulted in scaffold disruption, which in turn triggered thrombosis soon after antiplatelet therapy discontinuation. Another case of very late scaffold thrombosis which occurred 16 months after implantation, after scheduled dual antiplatelet therapy at 12 months was recently reported [55]. Imaging by intravascular ultrasound revealed the presence of scaffold underexpansion. The underexpansion was attributed to late recoil, although this diagnosis was not supported by intravascular ultrasound measurements at baseline and event demonstrating a reduction in scaffold area. Finally, two more cases of very late scaffold thrombosis have been reported; however, OCT imaging findings have not provided further insight into the mechanisms [56,57]; interestingly, the common link between these two cases is that both these patients were not receiving any antiplatelet therapy at the time of thrombosis.

In our center, we have witnessed two additional cases of very late scaffold thrombosis [58]. The first occurred on day 371 after implantation, 6 days after discontinuation of

Table 8.2.1 Studies of bioresorbable scaffolds reporting on 1-year scaffold thrombosis rates

| Study | Population size, n | Definite/probable late scaffold thrombosis, n (%) |
| --- | --- | --- |
| ABSORB BVS | | |
| ABSORB A [31] | 30 | 0 (0) |
| ABSORB B [32] | 101 | 0 (0) |
| ABSORB EXTEND [50] | 512 | 2 (0.4) |
| ABSORB II [51] | 335 | 1 (0.3) |
| ASSURE [44] | 180 | 0 (0) |
| POLAR ACS [43] | 98 | 0 (0) |
| BVS EXAMINATION [42] | 290 | 1 (0.3) |
| | | |
| DESolve BCS | | |
| DESolve First-in-Man [33] | 16 | 0 (0) |
| | | |
| DREAMS | | |
| BIOSOLVE-I [53] | 43 | 0 (0) |

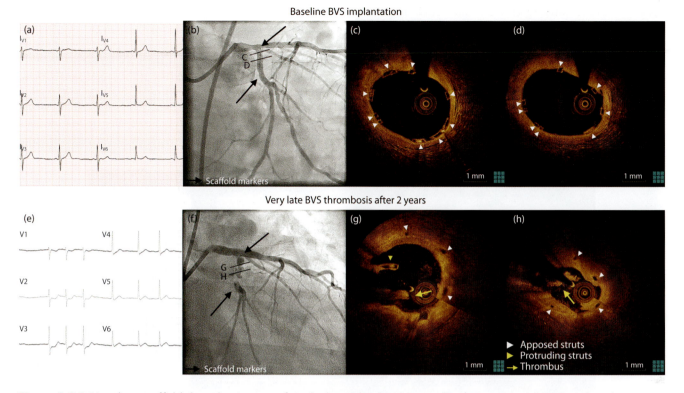

**Figure 8.2.3** Very late scaffold thrombosis soon after dual antiplatelet therapy discontinuation. **(a)** ECG prebaseline implantation. **(b–d)** Angiogram and OCT images post-ABSORB BVS implantation in the ostial left circumflex artery (LCx). **(e)** ECG at event 2 years after implantation. **(f)** Coronary angiogram at event showed a filling defect in the scaffolded segment. **(g, h)** OCT at event showing intracoronary thrombus and scaffold discontinuity. (Adapted with permission from Karanasos et al., *Eur Heart J* 2014;35:1781.)

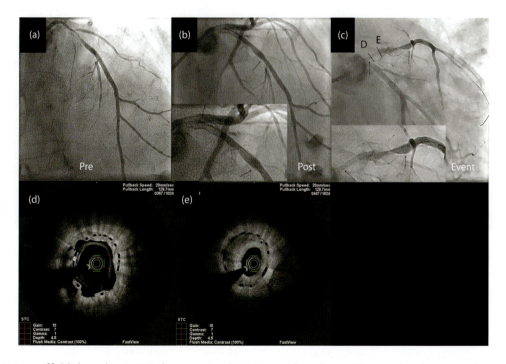

**Figure 8.2.4** Late scaffold thrombosis 112 days postimplantation with malapposition and underexpansion. Implantation of a 3.5 × 28 mm ABSORB BVS in an ostial LAD lesion **(a)** with suspected underexpansion by angiography **(b)**. **(c)** Angiogram at event after thrombus aspiration. OCT reveals sites with malapposed struts with thrombus **(d)** and focal restenosis in underexpanded segments (minimal scaffold diameter: 2.71 mm) **(e)**.

both aspirin and clopidogrel, which the patient had been consistently taking since implantation. This patient had a complex BVSs implantation for non-ST myocardial infarction in a vessel with heavy calcification by OCT, proximally overlapping a first-generation metallic DESs, with extensive malapposition due to intra-scaffold dissections. The other case occurred 478 days after implantation, while the patient was on aspirin alone. The imaging findings included thrombus arising from a site with possible minor late discontinuity and malapposition, and several adjacent uncovered struts.

## IMAGING OBSERVATIONS IN LATE AND VERY LATE SCAFFOLD THROMBOSIS

Overall, eight cases with late or very late scaffold thrombosis have been documented in our center up to June 2014 [58]. OCT was performed at the time of the event in seven

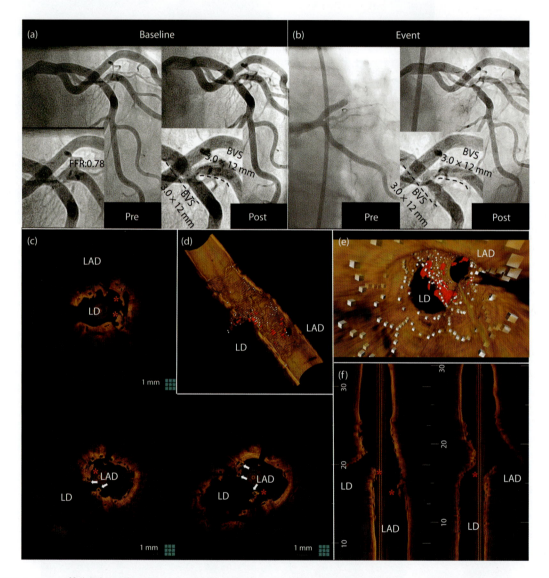

**Figure 8.2.5** Late scaffold thrombosis in a patient with complex bifurcation intervention and antiplatelet therapy discontinuation. **(a)** Implantation of two 3.0 × 12 mm ABSORB BVSs with T-stenting in a LAD-diagonal bifurcation due to stable angina with fractional flow reserve <0.80. **(b)** The patient had discontinued both antiplatelet agents after an atrial fibrillation-related embolic ischemic cerebrovascular accident and suffered a late scaffold thrombosis 129 days postimplantation, while on oral anticoagulants alone, treated with balloon dilation, rheolytic thrombectomy, and eptifibatide infusion. **(c)** OCT performed after treatment demonstrated reasonable expansion and apposition, but with uncovered struts (arrows) protruding at the bifurcation, and thrombus (asterisks) mainly located at the site of the bifurcation. **(d)** Three-dimensional longitudinal cut-away view demonstrating the localization of the thrombus (red). **(e)** The three-dimensional downstream fly-through view reveals the patency of both vessel ostia, but with the presence of multiple protruding struts proximal to the carina covered with thrombus. The presence of these multiple struts could affect local hemodynamics and comprise a focus for platelet aggregation in the absence of platelet inhibition. **(f)** L-mode OCT images demonstrating the location of the thrombus. Three-dimensional rendering performed with QAngioOCT 1.0 (Medis specials bv, Leiden, the Netherlands). Abbreviations: LAD = left anterior descending artery; LD = diagonal branch.

of them. In most patients, (very) late BVSs thrombosis was observed in the presence of regional suboptimal flow conditions, such as underexpansion and strut protrusion into the lumen due to strut malapposition, scaffold fracture, or bifurcation intervention (Figures 8.2.4 and 8.2.5). In BVSs thrombosis, expansion was better in nonthrombosed versus thrombosed sites within the scaffolds. In these patients with (very) late scaffold thrombosis, the incidence of malapposed struts was 1.9 ± 2.2% not differing significantly from a control group of patients undergoing OCT during late metallic stent thrombosis. This range was higher than the range reported in follow-up of asymptomatic patients treated with second-generation metallic DESs [59]. Likewise, malapposition distance (486 ± 225 μm) was similar to that of the metallic stent control group, and at the range of previously reported values in metallic DESs thrombosis (mean value of 350 μm) [19]. These observations suggest a potential involvement of large-scale malapposition that can potentially affect flow conditions, in the mechanism of (very) late scaffold thrombosis. Similarly, in complex bifurcation interventions the presence of struts protruding into the lumen at the level of the bifurcation could be a cause of suboptimal flow conditions [60,61] (Figure 8.2.5). Such flow conditions could also be instigated by strut discontinuity associated with scaffold protrusion into the lumen, a finding observed in two patients in our series.

Importantly, among the eight patients in our series, two of the patients, concomitantly with these potentially impaired flow conditions, were not receiving any antiplatelet therapy at the time of the event, while on oral anticoagulants. This suggests a potential synergistic effect of lack of platelet inhibition with suboptimal flow conditions in the pathogenesis of late scaffold thrombosis.

## POTENTIAL MECHANISMS—PREVENTIVE MEASURES

Due to the small number of observations, the mechanisms underlying late and very late BRSs thrombosis are poorly understood at this moment. In the case of the ABSORB BVSs, its increased strut thickness (150 μm) has been suggested as a potential factor associated with increased thrombogenicity. This hypothesis has been derived from bench observations of increased thrombogenicity of thick struts, which might become exaggerated in the presence of factors potentially affecting flow conditions such as malapposition or overlap [62]. Therefore, the presence of underexpansion or excessive strut protrusion into the lumen, which are factors that potentially affect flow conditions, could comprise an adverse environment associated with higher risk for scaffold thrombosis. Hence, a meticulous implantation technique, possibly including imaging guidance, could help ensure an optimal implantation result without adverse effects on regional flow conditions. In cases where optimal flow conditions are not achieved, as in suboptimal implantation or complex interventions, absence of adequate antiplatelet inhibition could act synergistically in the pathogenesis of scaffold thrombosis. This might dictate the use of platelet reactivity testing, or of more potent antiplatelet therapy in such cases.

Furthermore, the observation that several reported cases of very late scaffold thrombosis have occurred in patients not receiving any antiplatelet therapy supports the notion that patients treated with BRSs should receive at least one antiplatelet agent at a minimum until confirmed scaffold resorption and possibly for life.

Finally, as the scaffold loses a part of its mechanical support over time, reintervention in the same vessel several months after initial implantation should be performed with caution in view of a potential scaffold disruption while recrossing with wires or catheters.

## CONCLUSIONS

The introduction of bioresorbable scaffolds has held promise for a reduction of late and very late scaffold thrombosis, as these devices are associated with a favorable healing response, while the vascular morphology can be restored after resorption with elimination of the permanent vessel caging. However, use of bioresorbable scaffolds in more complex patient and lesion subsets has given rise to a limited number of late and very late scaffold thrombosis cases. Although the mechanisms of this complication in bioresorbable scaffolds are not completely understood, we speculate based on preliminary observations on a possible role of suboptimal flow conditions in the pathogenesis, while appropriate antiplatelet therapy administration seems to be important in avoiding this complication. The increasing utilization of BRSs in clinical practice might enable the elucidation of the mechanisms of this complication, while properly sized prospective studies will help to define the optimal procedural strategy and optimal antiplatelet regimen that can help diminish the risk of late and very late bioresorbable scaffold thrombosis.

## REFERENCES

1. Serruys PW, Garcia-Garcia HM, Onuma Y. From metallic cages to transient bioresorbable scaffolds: Change in paradigm of coronary revascularization in the upcoming decade? *Eur Heart J.* 2012;33:16–25b.

2. Karanasos A, Simsek C, Gnanadesigan M, van Ditzhuijzen NS, Freire R, Dijkstra J, Tu S et al. OCT assessment of the long-term vascular healing response 5 years after everolimus-eluting bioresorbable vascular scaffold. *J Am Coll Cardiol.* 2014;64:2343–2356.

3. Simsek C, Karanasos A, Magro M, Garcia-Garcia HM, Onuma Y, Regar E, Boersma E et al. Long-term invasive follow-up of the everolimus-eluting bioresorbable vascular scaffold: Five-year results of multiple invasive imaging modalities. *EuroIntervention.* 2016;11(9):996–1003.

4. McFadden EP, Stabile E, Regar E, Cheneau E, Ong AT, Kinnaird T, Suddath WO et al. Late thrombosis in drug-eluting coronary stents after discontinuation of antiplatelet therapy. *Lancet.* 2004;364:1519–1521.

5. Daemen J, Wenaweser P, Tsuchida K, Abrecht L, Vaina S, Morger C, Kukreja N et al. Early and late coronary stent thrombosis of sirolimus-eluting and paclitaxel-eluting stents in routine clinical practice: Data from a large two-institutional cohort study. *Lancet.* 2007;369:667–678.

6. Karanasos A, Ligthart JM, Regar E. In-stent neoatherosclerosis: A cause of late stent thrombosis in a patient with "full metal jacket" 15 years after implantation: Insights from optical coherence tomography. *JACC Cardiovasc Interv.* 2012;5:799–800.

7. Yamaji K, Kimura T, Morimoto T, Nakagawa Y, Inoue K, Soga Y, Arita T et al. Very long-term (15 to 20 years) clinical and angiographic outcome after coronary bare metal stent implantation. *Circ Cardiovasc Interv.* 2010;3:468–475.

8. Palmerini T, Biondi-Zoccai G, Riva DD, Stettler C, Sangiorgi D, D'Ascenzo F, Kimura T et al. Stent thrombosis with drug-eluting and bare-metal stents: Evidence from a comprehensive network meta-analysis. *Lancet.* 2012;379:1393–1402.

9. Räber L, Magro M, Stefanini GG, Kalesan B, Domburg RT, Onuma Y, Wenaweser P et al. Very late coronary stent thrombosis of a newer-generation everolimus-eluting stent compared with early-generation drug-eluting stents a prospective cohort study. *Circulation.* 2012;125:1110–1121.

10. Holmes Jr DR, Kereiakes DJ, Garg S, Serruys PW, Dehmer GJ, Ellis SG, Williams DO et al. Stent thrombosis. *J Am Coll Cardiol.* 2010;56:1357–1365.

11. Windecker S, Meier B. Late coronary stent thrombosis. *Circulation.* 2007;116:1952–1965.

12. Farb A, Burke AP, Kolodgie FD, Virmani R. Pathological mechanisms of fatal late coronary stent thrombosis in humans. *Circulation.* 2003;108:1701–1706.

13. Finn AV, Joner M, Nakazawa G, Kolodgie F, Newell J, John MC, Gold HK et al. Pathological correlates of late drug-eluting stent thrombosis: Strut coverage as a marker of endothelialization. *Circulation.* 2007;115:2435–2441.

14. Nakazawa G, Finn AV, Vorpahl M, Ladich ER, Kolodgie FD, Virmani R. Coronary responses and differential mechanisms of late stent thrombosis attributed to first-generation sirolimus- and paclitaxel-eluting stents. *J Am Coll Cardiol.* 2011;57:390–398.

15. Gutierrez-Chico JL, Alegria-Barrero E, Teijeiro-Mestre R, Chan PH, Tsujioka H, de Silva R, Viceconte N et al. Optical coherence tomography: From research to practice. *Eur Heart J Cardiovasc Imaging.* 2012;13(5):370–84.

16. Alfonso F, Dutary J, Paulo M, Gonzalo N, Perez-Vizcayno MJ, Jimenez-Quevedo P, Escaned J et al. Combined use of optical coherence tomography and intravascular ultrasound imaging in patients undergoing coronary interventions for stent thrombosis. *Heart.* 2012;98:1213–1220.

17. Amabile N, Souteyrand G, Ghostine S, Combaret N, Slama MS, Barber-Chamoux N, Motreff P et al. Very late stent thrombosis related to incomplete neointimal coverage or neoatherosclerotic plaque rupture identified by optical coherence tomography imaging. *Eur Heart J Cardiovasc Imaging.* 2014;15:24–31.

18. Davlouros PA, Karantalis V, Xanthopoulou I, Mavronasiou E, Tsigkas G, Toutouzas K, Alexopoulos D. Mechanisms of non-fatal stent-related myocardial infarction late following coronary stenting with drug-eluting stents and bare metal stents. Insights from optical coherence tomography. *Circ J.* 2011;75:2789–2797.

19. Guagliumi G, Sirbu V, Musumeci G, Gerber R, Biondi-Zoccai G, Ikejima H, Ladich E et al. Examination of the in vivo mechanisms of late drug-eluting stent thrombosis: Findings from optical coherence tomography and intravascular ultrasound imaging. *JACC Cardiovasc Interv.* 2012;5:12–20.

20. Kang S-J, Lee CW, Song H, Ahn J-M, Kim W-J, Lee J-Y, Park D-W et al. OCT analysis in patients with very late stent thrombosis. *JACC Cardiovasc Interv.* 2013;6:695–703.

21. Karanasos A, Witberg K, Van Geuns RJ, Schultz C, Van Mieghem N De Jaegere P, Bruining N et al. Morphological characteristics by optical coherence tomography of ruptured neoatherosclerotic plaques in patients with very late stent thrombosis. *Eur Heart J.* 2012;33:176.

22. Ko Y-G, Kim D-M, Cho JM, Choi SY, Yoon JH, Kim J-S, Kim B-K et al. Optical coherence tomography findings of very late stent thrombosis after drug-eluting stent implantation. *Int J Cardiovasc Imaging.* 2012;28:715–723.

23. Miyazaki S, Hiasa Y, Takahashi T, Yano Y, Minami T, Murakami N, Mizobe M et al. In vivo optical coherence tomography of very late drug-eluting stent thrombosis compared with late in-stent restenosis. *Circ J.* 2012;76:390–398.

24. Parodi G, La Manna A, Di Vito L, Valgimigli M, Fineschi M, Bellandi B, Niccoli G et al. Stent-related defects in patients presenting with stent thrombosis: Differences at optical coherence tomography between subacute and late/very late thrombosis in the Mechanism Of Stent Thrombosis (MOST) study. *EuroIntervention.* 2013;9:936–944.

25. Karanasos A, Regar E. Standing on solid ground?: Reassessing the role of incomplete strut apposition in drug-eluting stents. *Circ Cardiovasc Interv.* 2014;7:6–8.

26. Cook S, Eshtehardi P, Kalesan B, Raber L, Wenaweser P, Togni M, Moschovitis A et al. Impact of incomplete stent apposition on long-term clinical outcome after drug-eluting stent implantation. *Eur Heart J.* 2012;33:1334–1343.

27. Karanasos A, Ligthart J, Witberg K, Toutouzas K, Daemen J, Van Soest G, Gnanadesigan M et al. Association of neointimal morphology by optical coherence tomography with rupture of neo-atherosclerotic plaque very late after coronary stent implantation. *Proc SPIE Progr Biomed Opt Imaging.* 2013;8565:856542.

28. Karanasos A, Witberg K, Ligthart J, Toutouzas K, Daemen J, Van Soest G, Gnanadesigan M et al. In-stent neoatherosclerosis: Are first generation drug eluting stents different than bare metal stents? An optical coherence tomography study. *Proc SPIE Progr Biomed Opt Imaging.* 2013;8565:856543.

29. Nakazawa G, Otsuka F, Nakano M, Vorpahl M, Yazdani SK, Ladich E, Kolodgie FD et al. The pathology of neoatherosclerosis in human coronary implants bare-metal and drug-eluting stents. *J Am Coll Cardiol.* 2011;57:1314–1322.

30. Otsuka F, Vorpahl M, Nakano M, Foerst J, Newell JB, Sakakura K, Kutys R et al. Pathology of second-generation everolimus-eluting stents versus first-generation sirolimus- and paclitaxel-eluting stents in humans. *Circulation.* 2014;129:211–223.

31. Onuma Y, Dudek D, Thuesen L, Webster M, Nieman K, Garcia-Garcia HM, Ormiston JA et al. Five-year clinical and functional multislice computed tomography angiographic results after coronary implantation of the fully resorbable polymeric everolimus-eluting scaffold in patients with de novo coronary artery disease: The ABSORB Cohort A Trial. *JACC Cardiovasc Interv.* 2013;6:999–1009.

32. Serruys PW, Onuma Y, Garcia-Garcia HM, Muramatsu T, van Geuns RJ, de Bruyne B, Dudek D et al. Dynamics of vessel wall changes following the implantation of the ABSORB everolimus-eluting bioresorbable vascular scaffold: A multi-imaging modality study at 6, 12, 24 and 36 months. *EuroIntervention.* 2014;9:1271–1284.

33. Verheye S, Ormiston JA, Stewart J, Webster M, Sanidas E, Costa R, Costa Jr JR et al. A next-generation bioresorbable coronary scaffold system—From bench to first clinical evaluation: Six- and 12-month clinical and multimodality imaging results. *JACC Cardiovasc Interv.* 2014;7:89–99.

34. Waksman R, Prati F, Bruining N, Haude M, Bose D, Kitabata H, Erne P et al. Serial observation of drug-eluting absorbable metal scaffold: Multi-imaging modality assessment. *Circ Cardiovasc Interv.* 2013;6:644–653.

35. Ormiston JA, Serruys PW, Regar E, Dudek D, Thuesen L, Webster MW, Onuma Y et al. A bioabsorbable everolimus-eluting coronary stent system for patients with single de-novo coronary artery lesions (ABSORB): A prospective open-label trial. *Lancet.* 2008;371:899–907.

36. Farooq V, Serruys PW, Heo JH, Gogas BD, Onuma Y, Perkins LE, Diletti R et al. Intracoronary optical coherence tomography and histology of overlapping everolimus-eluting bioresorbable vascular scaffolds in a porcine coronary artery model: The potential implications for clinical practice. *JACC Cardiovasc Interv.* 2013;6:523–532.

37. Gonzalo N, Barlis P, Serruys PW, Garcia-Garcia HM, Onuma Y, Ligthart J, Regar E. Incomplete stent apposition and delayed tissue coverage are more frequent in drug-eluting stents implanted during primary percutaneous coronary intervention for ST-segment elevation myocardial infarction than in drug-eluting stents implanted for stable/unstable angina: Insights from optical coherence tomography. *JACC Cardiovasc Interv.* 2009;2:445–452.

38. Diletti R, Karanasos A, Muramatsu T, Nakatani S, Van Mieghem NM, Onuma Y, Nauta ST et al. Everolimus-eluting bioresorbable vascular scaffolds for treatment of patients presenting with ST-segment elevation myocardial infarction: BVS STEMI first study. *Eur Heart J.* 2014;35:777–786.

39. Azzalini L, L'Allier PL. Bioresorbable vascular scaffold thrombosis in an all-comer patient population: Single-center experience. *J Invasive Cardiol.* 2015;27:85–92.

40. Costopoulos C, Latib A, Naganuma T, Miyazaki T, Sato K, Figini F, Sticchi A et al. Comparison of early clinical outcomes between ABSORB bioresorbable vascular scaffold and everolimus-eluting stent implantation in a real-world population. *Catheter Cardiovasc Interv.* 2015;85:E10–E15.

41. Capodanno D, Gori T, Nef H, Latib A, Mehilli J, Lesiak M, Caramanno G. Percutaneous coronary intervention with everolimus-eluting bioresorbable vascular scaffolds in routine clinical practice: Early and midterm outcomes from the European multicentre GHOST-EU registry. *EuroIntervention.* 2015;10:1144–1153.

42. Brugaletta S, Gori T, Low AF, Tousek P, Pinar E, Gomez-Lara J, Scalone G et al. ABSORB bioresorbable vascular scaffold versus everolimus-eluting metallic stent in ST-segment elevation myocardial infarction: 1-year results of a propensity score matching comparison: The BVS-EXAMINATION Study (Bioresorbable Vascular Scaffold-A Clinical Evaluation of Everolimus Eluting Coronary Stents in the Treatment of Patients With ST-segment Elevation Myocardial Infarction). *JACC Cardiovasc Interv.* 2015;8:189–197.

43. Dudek D, Rzeszutko Ł, Zasada W, Depukat R, Siudak Z, Ochała A, Wojakowski W et al. Bioresorbable vascular scaffolds in patients with acute coronary syndromes: The POLAR ACS study. *Pol Arch Med Wewn.* 2014;124:669–677.

44. Wohrle J, Naber C, Schmitz T, Schwencke C, Frey N, Butter C, Brachmann J et al. Beyond the early stages: Insights from the ASSURE registry on bioresorbable vascular scaffolds. *EuroIntervention.* 2015;11(2):149–56.

45. Sato K, Latib A, Panoulas VF, Kawamoto H, Naganuma T, Miyazaki T, Colombo A. Procedural feasibility and clinical outcomes in propensity-matched patients treated with bioresorbable scaffolds vs new-generation drug-eluting stents. *Can J Cardiol.* 2015;31:328–334.

46. Kraak RP, Hassell ME, Grundeken MJ, Koch KT, Henriques JP, Piek JJ, Baan J, Jr. et al. Initial experience and clinical evaluation of the ABSORB bioresorbable vascular scaffold (BVS) in real-world practice: The AMC Single Centre Real World PCI Registry. *EuroIntervention.* 2015;10:1160–1168.

47. Van Geuns RJ, De Jaegere P, Diletti R, Karanasos A, Muramatsu T, Nauta ST, Onuma Y et al. Short- and intermediate- term clinical outcomes after implantation of everolimus-eluting bioresorbable scaffold in complex lesions: A prospective single-arm study—ABSORB Expand trial. *J Am Coll Cardiol.* 2013;62:B133–B133.

48. Ielasi A, Cortese B, Varricchio A, Tespili M, Sesana M, Pisano F, Loi B et al. Immediate and mid-term outcomes following primary PCI with bioresorbable vascular scaffold implantation in patients with ST-segment myocardial infarction: Insights from the multicentre "Registro ABSORB Italiano" (RAI registry). *EuroIntervention.* 2015;11(2):157–62.

49. Ishibashi Y, Nakatani S, Onuma Y. Definite and probable bioresorbable scaffold thrombosis in stable and ACS patients. *EuroIntervention.* 2015;11(3):e1–2.

50. Abizaid A, Costa JR, Jr., Bartorelli AL, Whitbourn R, van Geuns RJ, Chevalier B, Patel T et al. The ABSORB EXTEND study: Preliminary report of the twelve-month clinical outcomes in the first 512 patients enrolled. *EuroIntervention.* 2014;10:1396–1401.

51. Serruys PW, Chevalier B, Dudek D, Cequier A, Carrié D, Iniguez A, Dominici M et al. A bioresorbable everolimus-eluting scaffold versus a metallic everolimus-eluting stent for ischaemic heart disease caused by de-novo native coronary artery lesions (ABSORB II): An interim 1-year analysis of clinical and procedural secondary outcomes from a randomised controlled trial. *Lancet.* 2015;385:43–54.

52. Ishibashi Y, Onuma Y, Muramatsu T, Nakatani S, Iqbal J, Garcia-Garcia HM, Bartorelli AL et al. Lessons learned from acute and late scaffold failures in the ABSORB EXTEND trial. *EuroIntervention.* 2014;10:449–457.

53. Haude M, Erbel R, Erne P, Verheye S, Degen H, Böse D, Vermeersch P et al. Safety and performance of the drug-eluting absorbable metal scaffold (DREAMS) in patients with de-novo coronary lesions: 12 month results of the prospective, multicentre, first-in-man BIOSOLVE-I trial. *Lancet.* 2013;381:836–844.

54. Karanasos A, van Geuns RJ, Zijlstra F, Regar E. Very late bioresorbable scaffold thrombosis after discontinuation of dual antiplatelet therapy. *Eur Heart J.* 2014;35:1781.

55. Cortese B, Piraino D, Ielasi A, Steffenino G, Orrego PS. Very late bioresorbable vascular scaffold thrombosis due to late device recoil. *Int J Cardiol.* 2015;189:132–133.

56. Sato T, Abdel-Wahab M, Richardt G. Very late thrombosis observed on optical coherence tomography 22 months after the implantation of a polymer-based bioresorbable vascular scaffold. *Eur Heart J.* 2015;36(20):1273.

57. Timmers L, Stella PR, Agostoni P. Very late bioresorbable vascular scaffold thrombosis following discontinuation of antiplatelet therapy. *Eur Heart J.* 2015;36:393–393.

58. Karanasos A, Van Mieghem N, Van Ditzhuijzen NS, Felix C, Daemen J, Autar A, Onuma Y et al. Angiographic and optical coherence tomography insights into bioresorbable scaffold thrombosis. A single-center experience. *Circ Cardiovasc Interv.* 2015; 8(5). pii: e002369.

59. Papayannis AC, Cipher D, Banerjee S, Brilakis ES. Optical coherence tomography evaluation of drug-eluting stents: A systematic review. *Catheter Cardiovasc Interv.* 2013;81:481–487.

60. Capranzano P, Francaviglia B, Tamburino CI, Gargiulo G, Longo G, Capodanno D, Tamburino C. One-year coverage by optical coherence tomography of a bioresorbable scaffold neocarina: Is it safe to discontinue dual antiplatelet therapy? *Can J Cardiol.* 2015 Sep;31(9):1205. e5–6.

61. Karanasos A, Li Y, Tu S, Wentzel JJ, Reiber JHC, van Geuns R-J, Regar E. Is it safe to implant bioresorbable scaffolds in ostial side-branch lesions? Impact of 'neo-carina' formation on main-branch flow pattern. Longitudinal clinical observations. *Atherosclerosis.* 2015;238:22–25.

62. Kolandaivelu K, Swaminathan R, Gibson WJ, Kolachalama VB, Nguyen-Ehrenreich KL, Giddings VL, Coleman L et al. Stent thrombogenicity early in high-risk interventional settings is driven by stent design and deployment and protected by polymer-drug coatings. *Circulation.* 2011;123:1400–1409.

# Treatment of bioresorbable scaffold failure

CORDULA M. FELIX, BERT EVERAERT, NIGEL JEPSON, CORRADO TAMBURINO, AND ROBERT-JAN M. VAN GEUNS

## INTRODUCTION

Bioresorbable scaffolds (BRSs) are a promising new interventional treatment strategy for coronary artery disease (CAD). They were developed to overcome some of the limitations of metal drug-eluting stents (DESs), mainly the late reinterventions that occur at a consistent rate after 1 year and have not been reduced by use of local drug-elution. Initial experience in noncomplex lesions established the efficacy in opening the vessel and the concept of bioresorption. However, with the use of BRSs in more complex lesions, also the incidence of BRSs failure, including both scaffold restenosis and thrombosis (ScT), has increased. Therefore, understanding of both the pathophysiology and of the available treatment options of scaffold failure remain important issues in ensuring procedural and long-term clinical success.

Over recent years, BRSs have evolved as a new treatment strategy for CAD with the ABSORB BVSs (BVSs, Abbott Vascular, Santa Clara, CA) being the device most intensively studied. Animal studies on the BVSs demonstrated that the length of the polymers are consistently reduced in the first 2 years with final resorption usually one year later [1]. In this way, BRSs offer transient vessel support to prevent acute vessel recoil during angioplasty while eluting an antiproliferative drug to minimize neointima hyperplasia during the healing process. The ABSORB Extend study and multiple randomized controlled trials (ABSORB II, ABSORB III, ABSORB China, and ABSORB Japan) in noncomplex patients showed comparable 1 year results to cobalt-chromium based everolimus eluting XIENCE V metal stent (CoCr-EESs; Abbott Vascular, Santa Clara, CA) [2–6]. It should be underlined that only lesions of moderate complexity were included in these trials. In more real world lesion registries [7–14] BVS failure (including both scaffold thrombosis [ScT] and scaffold restenosis [Figure 8.3.1]) occurs unfortunately more frequently, and implantation of BVSs in more complex patients seems to be associated with a higher rate of adverse events.

A different CE marked scaffold, the DESolve myolimus-eluting bioresorbable coronary scaffold system (Elixir Medical Corporation, Sunnyvale, CA), was introduced recently after successful preliminary clinical studies [15,16]. Although the DESolve platform is also PLLA based, the degradation and drug-elution profile is faster and different timings for failure strategies may apply. Recently, the Magmaris scaffold (previously known as DREAMS, Biotronik AG, Bülach, Switzerland), a sirolimus-eluting and magnesium-based scaffold, received the CE mark after its safety was tested in the BIOSOLVE-II first-in-human trial [17]. Resorption is faster than in PLLA-based scaffolds. For both scaffolds, very little is known about the performance in real-world patients.

In this chapter we will provide a short overview of the pathophysiology and the treatment options in the case of BRSs failure with a focus on the most frequently used BVSs and some remarks for the other faster resorbing scaffolds.

## RISK FACTORS FOR STENT AND SCAFFOLD RESTENOSIS

The mechanism for BMSs or DESs restenosis is multifactorial and consists of stent recoil, formation of neointima, organization of thrombus, geographical miss, and impaired endothelial function. The pivotal factor in the process of ISR is neointimal formation, due to migration and proliferation of smooth muscle cells and myofibroblasts. In the longer-term, metallic DESs might fracture at hinging points in the coronary artery inducing an inflammatory reaction. Occasionally, some patients seem to be "limus" resistant and develop early restenosis [18,19]. Finally, ongoing atherosclerosis contributes to the negative remodeling within the caged vessel wall [20]. In addition, hypersensitivity reaction to the DESs polymer is another important mechanism contributing to stent failure.

The rates of BMSs-ISR have been described to be as high as 60%, depending on several risk factors such as lesion

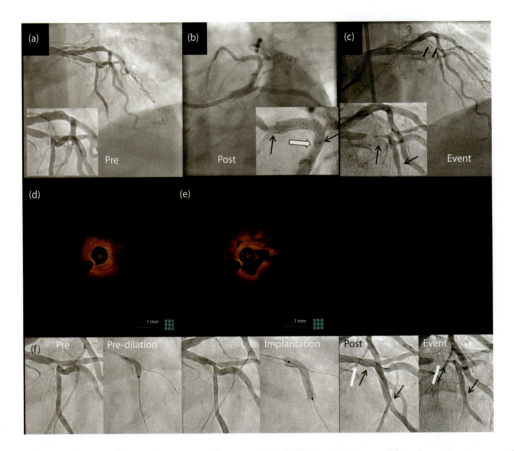

**Figure 8.3.1** BVSs failure due to edge. Edge restenosis treated with BVSs. A 65-year-old male patient presenting with an NSTEMI was treated with a 3.5 × 28 BVSs for a trifurcation lesion of the LAD and two diagonals **(a** and **b)**. One hundred forty-two days later he returned for unstable angina due to a subtotal occlusion of the LAD with slow flow distal to the scaffold (TIMI 1) **(c)**. OCT imaging revealed edge restenosis as the underlying mechanism for BRSs failure **(d)** and restenosis within the scaffold with a layered pattern **(e)** but no luminal thrombus. The patient was treated with thrombus aspiration and a 3.5 × 38 mm DESs (Promus). Retrospective review of the postprocedural angiogram at baseline showed proximal edge dissection **(b)** and incomplete lesion coverage with geographic miss as the reason for restenosis [**(f)** series]. Black arrows indicate the scaffold markers and white arrows the uncovered edge segment. (Reprinted from *EuroIntervention* 2015;11:Supplement V, Felix C, Everaert B, Jepson N, Tamburino C, van Geuns R-J, Treatment of bioresorbable scaffold failure, V175–V180, Copyright 2015, with permission from Europa Digital & Publishing.)

complexity, patient co-morbidities and vessel size [21–24]. The use of DESs has significantly reduced the rate of ISR, although DESs-ISR rates at 1 year have been observed to occur in 3–20% of the patients, depending on DESs generation and patient, lesion, and procedural characteristics [25].

Multiple patient, lesion, and procedure-related risk factors for ISR in BMSs and DESs have been reported, including diabetes mellitus, multivessel disease, stent length, bifurcation lesions, small caliber vessels, chronic total occlusion (CTO), strut thickness, usage of multiple stents, and stent underexpansion. ISR by itself is also a predictor for future ISR [25–30]. Also the stent type plays an important role which can be related to strut thickness, drug dosage, and drug release profile. In general, thicker stent struts cause more flow disturbances with reduced endothelial shear stress [31], which does enhance the process of neointimal hyperplasia.

It seems likely that most risk factors for ISR with BRSs are the same as for ISR with BMSs or DESs albeit that all current BRSs have biodegradable coatings for drug elution

eliminating a hypersensitivity reaction to the coatings of most current DESs. With the restoration of endothelial function potentially the triggers for accelerated atherosclerosis are eliminated. Recently, a case series reported on geographical miss and scaffold underexpansion as being the most frequent causes of BRSs failure [32].

## RISK FACTORS FOR STENT AND SCAFFOLD THROMBOSIS

Several risk factors for ST exist. Many of them are also predictive for stent restenosis. These risk factors can be categorized as lesion, patient, and procedure-related factors. Procedure-related factors are stent malapposition, stent undersizing, dissection, placement of multiple stents, stent overlap, and stent length. Lesion-related factors include coronary bifurcations, heavily calcified lesions, long lesion length, small vessel size, and CTO. Finally, there are the patient-related factors such as diabetes mellitus, advanced age, renal failure, low ejection fraction, smoking, prior

CABG, acute coronary syndromes (ACS) at presentation, (early) discontinuation of DAPT, or resistance to clopidogrel [33,34].

A meta-analysis, including 10,510 patients (BVSs: 8351 and DESs: 2159), revealed that patients with a BVSs were at higher risk of myocardial infarction (MI) and definite/probable ScT compared to DESs patients with a definite/probable ScT rate of 1.2% at 1 month [35].

Probably, consistent with DESs, the rate of ScT varies depending on lesion, patient, and procedure-related characteristics. The most remarkable difference between BVSs and current DESs is the increased strut thickness and width (comparable to old stainless steel BMSs and first generation DESs). This will increase the early uncovered surface significantly. Also, strut thickness induces convective flow patterns, triggering platelet deposition [36]. Susceptibility to platelet aggregation might be further aggravated by conditions such as scaffold underexpansion, treatment of thrombotic lesions, e.g., during ACS, and DAPT interruption.

Scaffold underexpansion is an important issue in BVSs [37] and is an important contributor to BRSs failure. It occurs less frequently if lesions are treated using an optimal implantation strategy. Specially, with the use of a noncompliant balloon with the same size as RVD for predilation, full expansion of the scaffold by high pressure postdilatation with a noncompliant balloon up to a maximum of 0.5 mm larger [38,39]. Discontinuation of DAPT and edge dissections have also been described as causes of ScT [40]. Currently ongoing and future all-comer, randomized controlled trials will indicate whether BRSs have more favorable rates of late ScT compared to the current generation DESs.

## SCAFFOLD DISLODGEMENT

In severely calcified or tortuous lesions, successful delivery of BRSs can be difficult and the scaffold could be potentially dislodged [41] in the same way as metallic stents. If dislodged BRSs cannot be retrieved and have to be secured in the coronary artery by additional DESs, a local asymmetric intracoronary lesion of approximately 400 µm remains with a potential trigger for a restenosis. However, after an early publication, no further cases of scaffold dislodgement have been reported and BVSs failure due to this mechanism has not been described.

For the recently introduced alternatives to the BVSs, insufficient experience exists to guarantee their retention in complex cases.

## HOW TO TREAT BRSs FAILURE

Multiple treatment options for treating BRSs failure exist: thrombus aspiration, balloon angioplasty (POBA), BMSs, DESs, BRSs, drug-eluting balloons (DEB), or medical treatment (e.g., with a thrombolytic agent or a glycoprotein IIbIIIa inhibitor [GPI]). Deciding which is most suitable

depends on the triggering mechanism and not infrequently multiple underlying factors are present. Understanding the fundamental pathophysiological mechanism underlying the TLF is of key importance to direct subsequent management. Invasive imaging modalities, such as optical coherence tomography (OCT) are of paramount importance to achieve treatment success. OCT enables the operator to determine the mechanism for BRSs-TLF including scaffold underexpansion, scaffold malapposition or undersizing, geographic miss (edge dissection, edge restenosis), neointimal hyperplasia, or scaffold strut fracture.

BRSs thrombosis after DAPT interruption, whether acute (<24 hours), subacute (<1 month), or late, can be managed with the use of thrombectomy, GPI, and/or POBA. In patients on clopidogrel that present with an occlusion of the target vessel due to a thrombus, platelet function testing and switching to more potent P2Y12 inhibitor has to be considered.

Early underexpansion and malapposition can be treated with POBA with noncompliant balloons in a 1:1 balloon–vessel ratio and with sufficient diameter and pressure, although the maximum overexpansion limit of 0.5 mm always has to be respected for BVSs, especially in the situation of undersizing (Figure 8.3.2). If the vessel is above 4 mm in diameter and there is serious malapposition, large metallic stents are indicated. Preferably a DESs is used, although potentially a BMS could be sufficient for treatment of acute or subacute (<30 days) scaffold failure. However, the negative effects of an additional dose of antiproliferative drugs when DESs are used seem only theoretical and hence not of clinical importance. If underexpansion cannot be managed by POBA alone, a BMSs or DESs is indicated to ensure additional radial support (Figure 8.3.3). To minimize stent overlap, only the insufficiently apposed areas need be covered with the new stent. After 30 days we strongly recommend DESs (or even a second BVSs in larger vessels) as the remaining dose of everolimus on the BVSs might not be sufficient to effectively reduce neointimal hyperplasia (Figure 8.3.3). For undersizing, POBA could be sufficient up to 6 months as the goal is ensuring optimal apposition without further vessel dilatation (low pressure) activating a new healing process.

After approximately 6 months the tie chains between the crystal polylactide lamellae in the BVSs become increasingly hydrolyzed and the radial strength and subsequent vessel support gradually decreases (Figure 8.3.4) [42]. BRSs failure after 6 months due to mechanical problems will need placement of an additional stent or scaffold. For the two new BRSs (Desolve and Magmaris), the resorption process is much faster and additional stents and scaffolds might be necessary as of 3 months after initial implant.

In the setting of a geographical miss leading to a clinically relevant acute or subacute edge dissection, a BRSs bailout strategy could be used. In the case of a geographical miss with apparent edge restenosis, placement of an additional BRSs is possible although converting to a DESs with a minimal risk of repeat ISR is more prudent. ISR due to intimal hyperplasia can be treated by a DEB (<6 months) but

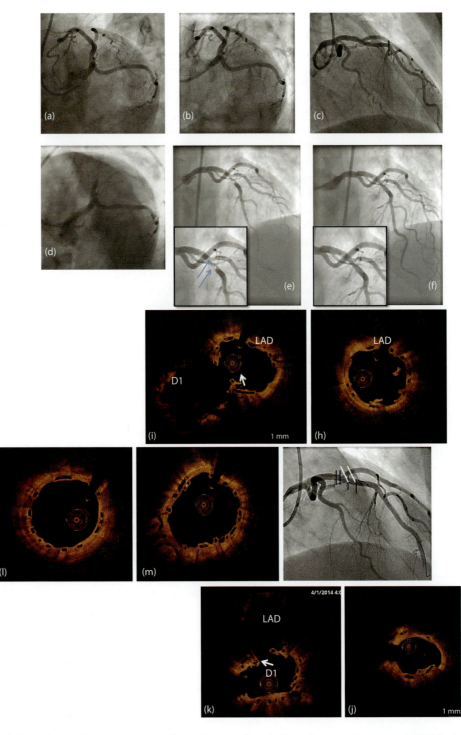

**Figure 8.3.2** BRSs failure due to discontinuation of DAPT treated with thrombus aspiration and POBA. A 60-year-old male patient with a history of smoking, hypertension, and heart failure presented with stable angina. There was one vessel disease and a LAD–first diagonal lesion (Medina 0, 0, 1) on angiography. Two 3.0 × 12 mm BRSs were placed in the LAD and first diagonal, using a T- and protrusion technique with good results in the spider **(b)** and RAO **(c)** projections. After 129 days the patient developed a STEMI due to an occluded LAD **(d)** potentially due to ascal and prasugrel discontinuation for CVA. POBA with a 3.0 mm balloon was then performed. After three Angiojet runs, the angiographic result was acceptable **(e)** and eptifibatide was continued for 24 hours. The treatment of BRSs failure was reviewed four days later using OCT **(f–m)**. Pullback from de LAD (lower row) showed some remaining thrombus **(h)**, and signs of fractures or double layer of uncovered struts **(i,** arrow). Pullback from the diagonal branch showed some undersizing distal **(j)** and same double layer and loss struts **(k,** arrow). Proximal to the bifurcation the struts were mainly well covered **(l** and **m)**. (Reprinted from *EuroIntervention* 2015;11:Supplement V, Felix C, Everaert B, Jepson N, Tamburino C, van Geuns R-J, Treatment of bioresorbable scaffold failure, V175–V180, Copyright 2015, with permission from Europa Digital & Publishing.)

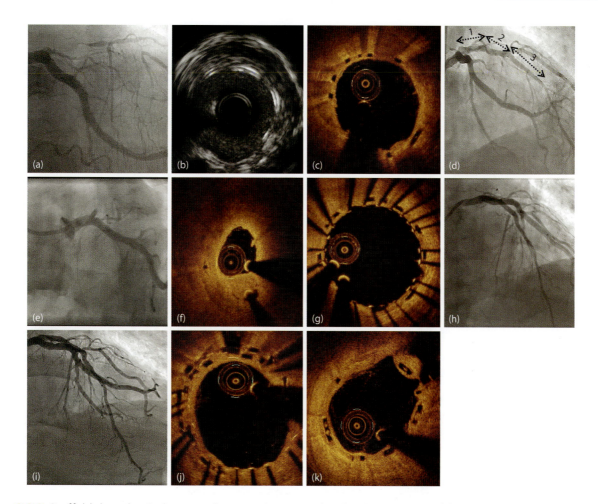

**Figure 8.3.3** Scaffold thrombosis due to underexpansion treated with DES. A 69-year-old male patient presented with an NSTEMI. Angiography showed one-vessel disease with long narrowing of the proximal and mid-LAD and collateral filling **(a)**. Three BVSs (3.0 × 28 mm, 3.5 × 18 mm, 3.5 × 18 mm) were implanted **(d)**. After placement of the first two scaffolds there was compression and thrombus in the first diagonal. Invasive imaging postprocedure revealed organized thrombus behind the struts of the proximal scaffold [**(b)** IVUS, and thrombus protrusion and **(c)** OCT] at the overlapping scaffolds. After 47 days the patient presented with a non-Q-wave myocardial infarction due to a full occlusion in the proximal LAD **(e)**. There was some underexpansion, but a large thrombus on OCT **(f)**. He was treated with thrombectomy, eptifibatide, and PCI with a 3.5 × 38 mm DESs (XIENCE) covering the proximal BVSs with good angiographic and OCT result **(g and h)**. The control diagnostic angiography made 110 days later **(i)** displayed good scaffold and stent apposition on OCT with good coverage of the struts of the new DESs **(j)** and the untreated original distal BVSs **(k)**. (Reprinted from *EuroIntervention* 2015;11:Supplement V, Felix C, Everaert B, Jepson N, Tamburino C, van Geuns R-J, Treatment of bioresorbable scaffold failure, V175–V180, Copyright 2015, with permission from Europa Digital & Publishing.)

after 6 months, additional vessel support is indicated (with a preference for a DESs) (Figure 8.3.1).

Last, in the case of limited scaffold strut fracture, POBA should be able to correct the malapposed segments [43]. For more extensive fractures or large diameter vessels, a new stent (BMSs or DESs) would be the treatment of choice. Again, after 6 months disintegration of the scaffold is in progress and additional radial strength is necessary. Implanting a DESs would be the most obvious treatment option; however, a case report described the metal-in-polymer (MIP) technique where late malapposition of the metal DESs occurred, probably due to vessel enlargement. Treatment of scaffold failure with a second scaffold should also be considered [44].

In the case of both fracture and underexpansion, lesion dilatation is necessary and we recommend an additional DESs from 30 days after the initial BRSs placement. Treatment options for BRSs failure are summarized in Table 8.3.1.

However, we reiterate that the bulk of clinical experience with BRSs failure is gained from the experience with the ABSORB BVSs platform, and that, given the paucity of trial numbers, very limited data are available for other BRSs subtypes such as the DESolve novolimus-eluting bioresorbable coronary scaffold system (Elixir) or metal-based (magnesium) resorbable devices. As such, these recommendations for the treatment of BRSs failure are only applicable to the ABSORB BVSs.

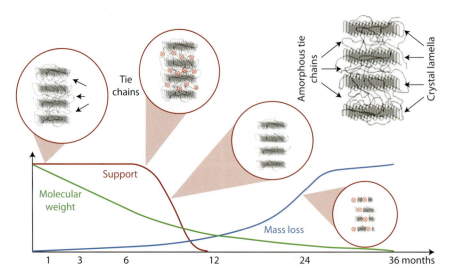

**Figure 8.3.4** Bioresorption of BVSs. Initially cleavage of polylactactes results in minimal molecular weight loss with remaining full support until 6 months. After 6 months degradation significant impact on tie chains between crystal lamella occurs rapidly, reducing radial support when the material starts to become brittle and implantation of additional vessel supportive therapy is indicated to successfully treat lumen reduction. (Reprinted from *EuroIntervention* 2015;11:Supplement V, Felix C, Everaert B, Jepson N, Tamburino C, van Geuns R-J, Treatment of bioresorbable scaffold failure, V175–V180, Copyright 2015, with permission from Europa Digital & Publishing.)

**Table 8.3.1** Treatment options for BRSs failure

| | Acute (<24 h) | Subacute (<30 days) | Late (<6 months)[a] | Very late (>6 months) |
|---|---|---|---|---|
| DAPT interruption | GPI/thrombectomy/POBA | | | |
| Underexpansion | POBA | | DES/BVSs | |
| Undersizing/malapposition | POBA: max 0.5 mm > nominal > 4 mm: DESs/BMSs[b] | | | DES/BVSs |
| Geographical miss | Dissection: BVSs bailout | | Edge stenosis: DESs/BVSs | |
| Neointimalhyperplasia | – | | DEBs | DESs/BVSs |
| Strut fracture | POBA: max 0.5 > nominal > 4 mm: DESs/BMSs[b] | | | DESs |

*Source:* Updated from Felix, C. et al. *EuroIntervention*, II Suppl V:V175–80, 2015. doi:10.4244/EIJV11SVA42. Review.
[a] For Magmaris and Desolve, additional vascular support might be needed already 3 months after implantation.
[b] In the first period, as drug release is still ongoing, BMS theoretically should be sufficient.

## SUMMARY

All BRSs are foreign bodies to the vessel and bloodstream before coverage and initial resorption. In this regard 1 year TLR rate is at least similar to current DESs and due to the increased strut thickness potentially even higher. Reintervention of the treated segment will be a common phenomenon for current DES. Treatment of scaffold failure should target any suboptimal result. After thrombus aspiration and aggressive medical treatment, intravascular imaging is advised to reveal any scaffold abnormalities. A wide range of strategies can be applied to correct suboptimal scaffold results. The major difference between BRSs and DESs in the treatment of target lesion failure is the more frequent need for additional vessel support (using a second BVSs or a DES). The timing when this additional support is needed is dependent on the construction of the specific BRSs targeted.

## ACKNOWLEDGMENTS

The authors thank EuroIntervention for the permission to reproduce the images.

## REFERENCES

1. Onuma Y, Serruys PW, Perkins LE et al. Intracoronary optical coherence tomography and histology at 1 month and 2, 3, and 4 years after implantation of everolimus-eluting bioresorbable vascular scaffolds in a porcine coronary artery model: An attempt to decipher the human optical coherence tomography images in the ABSORB trial. *Circulation.* 2010;122:2288–300.
2. Serruys PW, Chevalier B, Dudek D et al. A bioresorbable everolimus-eluting scaffold versus a metallic

everolimus-eluting stent for ischaemic heart disease caused by de-novo native coronary artery lesions (ABSORB II): An interim 1-year analysis of clinical and procedural secondary outcomes from a randomised controlled trial. *Lancet.* 2015;385(9962):43–54.

3. Abizaid A, Costa JR, Jr., Bartorelli AL et al. The ABSORB EXTEND study: Preliminary report of the twelve-month clinical outcomes in the first 512 patients enrolled. *EuroIntervention.* 2015;10(12):1396–401.

4. Ellis SG, Kereiakes DJ, Metzger DC et al. Everolimus-eluting bioresorbable scaffolds for coronary artery disease. *N Engl J Med.* 373:1905–1915.

5. Gao R, Yang Y, Han Y et al. Bioresorbable vascular scaffolds versus metallic stents in patients with coronary artery disease: ABSORB China trial. *J Am Coll Cardiol.* 2015;66(21):2298–309.

6. Kimura T, Kozuma K, Tanabe K et al. A randomized trial evaluating everolimus-eluting Absorb bioresorbable scaffolds vs. everolimus-eluting metallic stents in patients with coronary artery disease: ABSORB Japan. *Eur Heart J.* 2015;36:3332–42.

7. Capodanno D, Gori T, Nef H et al. Percutaneous coronary intervention with everolimus-eluting bioresorbable vascular scaffolds in routine clinical practice: Early and midterm outcomes from the European multicentre GHOST-EU registry. *EuroIntervention.* 2015;10(10):1144–53.

8. Wohrle J, Naber C, Schmitz T et al. Beyond the early stages: Insights from the ASSURE registry on bioresorbable vascular scaffolds. *EuroIntervention.* 2015;11(2):149–56.

9. Felix CM, Fam JM, Diletti R et al. Mid- to long-term clinical outcomes of patients treated with the everolimus-eluting bioresorbable vascular scaffold: The BVS Expand Registry. *JACC Cardiovasc Interv.* 2016;9(16):1652–63.

10. Fam JM, Felix C, van Geuns RJ et al. Initial experience with everolimus-eluting bioresorbable vascular scaffolds for treatment of patients presenting with acute myocardial infarction: A propensity-matched comparison to metallic drug eluting stents 18-month follow-up of the BVS STEMI first study. *EuroIntervention.* 2016;12:30–7.

11. Miyazaki T, Ruparelia N, Kawamoto H, Figini F, Latib A, Colombo A. Clinical outcomes following "off-label" versus "established" indications of bioresorbable scaffolds for the treatment of coronary artery disease in a real-world population. *EuroIntervention.* 2016;11:1475–8.

12. Felix CM, Onuma Y, Fam JM et al. Are BVS suitable for ACS patients? Support from a large single center real live registry. *Int J Cardiol.* 2016;218:89–97.

13. Kraak RP, Grundeken MJ, Hassell ME et al. Two-year clinical outcomes of Absorb bioresorbable vascular scaffold implantation in complex coronary artery disease patients stratified by SYNTAX score and ABSORB II study enrolment criteria. *EuroIntervention.* 2016;12:e557–65.

14. Capranzano P, Longo G, Tamburino CI et al. One-year outcomes after Absorb bioresorbable vascular scaffold implantation in routine clinical practice. *EuroIntervention.* 2016;12:e152–9.

15. Verheye S, Ormiston JA, Stewart J et al. A next-generation bioresorbable coronary scaffold system: From bench to first clinical evaluation: 6- and 12-month clinical and multimodality imaging results. *JACC Cardiovasc Interv.* 2014;7:89–99.

16. Abizaid A, Costa RA, Schofer J et al. Serial multi-modality imaging and 2-year clinical outcomes of the novel DESolve novolimus-eluting bioresorbable coronary scaffold system for the treatment of single de novo coronary lesions. *JACC Cardiovasc Interv.* 2016;9:565–74.

17. Haude M, Ince H, Abizaid A et al. Sustained safety and performance of the second-generation drug-eluting absorbable metal scaffold in patients with de novo coronary lesions: 12-month clinical results and angiographic findings of the BIOSOLVE-II first-in-man trial. *Eur Heart J.* 2016 37(35):2701–9.

18. Lemos PA, Saia F, Ligthart JM et al. Coronary restenosis after sirolimus-eluting stent implantation: Morphological description and mechanistic analysis from a consecutive series of cases. *Circulation.* 2003;108:257–60.

19. Felix C, Everaert B, Jepson N, Tamburino C, van Geuns RJ. Treatment of bioresorbable scaffold failure. *EuroIntervention.* 2015;11 Suppl V:V175–80.

20. Kibos A, Campeanu A, Tintoiu I. Pathophysiology of coronary artery in-stent restenosis. *Acute Card Care.* 2007;9:111–9.

21. Serruys PW, de Jaegere P, Kiemeneij F et al. A comparison of balloon-expandable-stent implantation with balloon angioplasty in patients with coronary artery disease. Benestent Study Group. *N Engl J Med.* 1994;331:489–95.

22. Babapulle MN, Eisenberg MJ. Coated stents for the prevention of restenosis: Part I. *Circulation.* 2002;106:2734–40.

23. Fischman DL, Leon MB, Baim DS et al. A randomized comparison of coronary-stent placement and balloon angioplasty in the treatment of coronary artery disease. Stent Restenosis Study Investigators. *N Engl J Med.* 1994;331:496–501.

24. Greenberg D, Bakhai A, Cohen DJ. Can we afford to eliminate restenosis? Can we afford not to? *J Am Coll Cardiol.* 2004;43:513–8.

25. Dangas GD, Claessen BE, Caixeta A, Sanidas EA, Mintz GS, Mehran R. In-stent restenosis in the drug-eluting stent era. *J Am Coll Cardiol.* 2010;56:1897–907.

26. Hoffmann R, Mintz GS, Dussaillant GR et al. Patterns and mechanisms of in-stent restenosis. A serial intravascular ultrasound study. *Circulation*. 1996;94:1247–54.

27. Hoffmann R, Mintz GS. Coronary in-stent restenosis—Predictors, treatment and prevention. *Eur Heart J*. 2000;21:1739–49.

28. Farooq V, Gogas BD, Serruys PW. Restenosis: Delineating the numerous causes of drug-eluting stent restenosis. *Circ Cardiovasc Interv*. 2011;4:195–205.

29. Weintraub WS. The pathophysiology and burden of restenosis. *Am J Cardiol*. 2007;100:3K–9K.

30. Kimura T, Morimoto T, Nakagawa Y et al. Very late stent thrombosis and late target lesion revascularization after sirolimus-eluting stent implantation: Five-year outcome of the j-Cypher Registry. *Circulation*. 2012;125:584–91.

31. Bourantas CV, Papafaklis MI, Kotsia A et al. Effect of the endothelial shear stress patterns on neointimal proliferation following drug-eluting bioresorbable vascular scaffold implantation: An optical coherence tomography study. *JACC Cardiovasc Interv*. 2014;7:315–24.

32. Longo G, Granata F, Capodanno D et al. Anatomical features and management of bioresorbable vascular scaffolds failure: A case series from the GHOST Registry. *Catheter Cardiovasc Interv*. 2015;85(7):1150–61.

33. Iakovou I, Schmidt T, Bonizzoni E et al. Incidence, predictors, and outcome of thrombosis after successful implantation of drug-eluting stents. *JAMA*. 2005;293:2126–30.

34. Machecourt J, Danchin N, Lablanche JM et al. Risk factors for stent thrombosis after implantation of sirolimus-eluting stents in diabetic and nondiabetic patients: The EVASTENT Matched-Cohort Registry. *J Am Coll Cardiol*. 2007;50:501–8.

35. Lipinski MJ, Escarcega RO, Baker NC et al. Scaffold thrombosis after percutaneous coronary intervention with ABSORB bioresorbable vascular scaffold: A systematic review and meta-analysis. *JACC Cardiovasc Interv*. 2016;9:12–24.

36. Duraiswamy N, Cesar JM, Schoephoerster RT, Moore JE, Jr. Effects of stent geometry on local flow dynamics and resulting platelet deposition in an in vitro model. *Biorheology*. 2008;45:547–61.

37. Karanasos A, Van Mieghem N, van Ditzhuijzen N et al. Angiographic and optical coherence tomography insights into bioresorbable scaffold thrombosis: Single-center experience. *Circ Cardiovasc Interv*. 2015;8(5). pii: e002369.

38. Brown AJ, McCormick LM, Braganza DM, Bennett MR, Hoole SP, West NE. Expansion and malapposition characteristics after bioresorbable vascular scaffold implantation. *Cathet Cardiovasc Interv*. 2014;84:37–45.

39. Puricel S, Cuculi F, Weissner M et al. Bioresorbable coronary scaffold thrombosis: Multicenter comprehensive analysis of clinical presentation, mechanisms, and predictors. *J Am Coll Cardiol*. 2016;67:921–31.

40. Azzalini L, L'Allier PL. Bioresorbable vascular scaffold thrombosis in an all-comer patient population: Single-center experience. *J Invasive Cardiol*. 2015;27:85–92.

41. Ishibashi Y, Onuma Y, Muramatsu T et al. Lessons learned from acute and late scaffold failures in the ABSORB EXTEND trial. *EuroIntervention*. 2014;10:449–57.

42. Serruys PW, Onuma Y, Dudek D et al. Evaluation of the second generation of a bioresorbable everolimus-eluting vascular scaffold for the treatment of de novo coronary artery stenosis: 12-month clinical and imaging outcomes. *J Am Coll Cardiol*. 2011;58:1578–88.

43. Pan M RM, Ojeda S, Suarez De Lezo Jr J, Segura J, Mazuelos F, Lopez J, Martin P et al. Rupture of bioresorbable vascular scaffold after side-branch dilation in bifurcation lesion. *Eur Heart J*. 2014;35 (Abstract Supplement).

44. Capranzano P, Francaviglia B, Capodanno D et al. Is the metallic stent a safe treatment for bioresorbable scaffold failure?: Insights from optical coherence tomography. *JACC Cardiovasc Interv*. 2016;9:976–7.

45. Serruys PW, Onuma Y, Garcia-Garcia HM et al. Dynamics of vessel wall changes following the implantation of the Absorb everolimus-eluting bioresorbable vascular scaffold: A multi-imaging modality study at 6, 12, 24 and 36 months. *EuroIntervention*. 2014;9:1271–84.

# Recoil and bioresorbable scaffolds

JOHN A. ORMISTON, BRUCE WEBBER, JANARTHANAN SATHANANTHAN, AND MARK W.I. WEBSTER

## MEASUREMENT OF STENT/SCAFFOLD RECOIL

### Bench measurements

**Durable metallic stents.** The ASTM (American Society for Testing Materials) F2079 (www.astm.org) defines recoil for the purposes of bench testing as the percentage stent diameter decrease from that measured on the inflated balloon at nominal pressure to that after balloon deflation. The test may be performed in air at room temperature unless there is a known temperature dependence of the material (such as with polymeric scaffolds).

**Polymeric scaffolds.** To measure polymeric scaffold recoil on the bench, the ASTM F2079-09 recommends expanding the scaffolds at nominal pressure while immersed unconstrained in a water bath that has heating and recirculation instruments to maintain the bath at 37°C. The expanded scaffold on the balloon may be removed briefly from the bath, measured, and returned to the bath for balloon deflation. After deflation, the scaffold may be briefly removed from the bath and photographed again [1].

## CLINICAL ASSESSMENT

Recoil has been assessed clinically by quantitative angiography and defined as the difference between mean diameter of the last inflated balloon at the highest pressure (X) and mean lumen diameter of the stent immediately after the last balloon deflation (Y). Acute percent recoil was defined as (X − Y)/X and expressed as a percentage [2,3]. Recoil can also been assessed by measurement of cross-sectional area using intravascular imaging with intravascular ultrasound (IVUS) and optical coherence tomography (OCT). With the area postprocedure (X) and stent area at follow-up (Y), late stent area recoil is defined as (X − Y)/X expressed as a percentage [4]. For the same recoiled stent or scaffold, the percentage recoil calculated from areas will be a larger number than the percentage calculated from diameter change.

## CONTRIBUTORS TO RECOIL

### Stent/scaffold design

Stent or scaffold design is an important factor for recoil. While both the Palmaz Schatz stent (Johnson & Johnson, New Brunswick, NJ) and the Gianturco-Roubin stent (Cook Medical, Bloomington, IN) were constructed from stainless steel, the diameter recoil of the former was measured as 6.9% and the latter 17.8% [5]. The "slide and lock" design of early REVA polymeric scaffolds (REVA Medical, San Diego, CA) was associated with 0% recoil in contrast to polymeric scaffolds with conventional designs [6].

### Vessel wall

Recoil is also dependent on characteristics of the vessel wall. The elastic properties of the arterial wall are affected by the plaque characteristics of the stented segment. Cross-sectional area recoil of an ABSORB scaffold (Abbott Vascular, Santa Clara, CA) was significantly less in calcified plaques (1.97 ± 22.2%) than when implanted in fibronecrotic plaques (12.4 ± 28.0%, $p \pm S0.001$) [4].

### Strut dimensions

To counter the lesser radial strength and greater recoil of polymeric construction materials, polymeric scaffolds are designed with thicker, wider struts than metallic durable stents (Table 8.4.1) [7]. There are advantages to thin struts and conversely disadvantages to thick, wide struts. Reduction in stent strut thickness has been associated with improved stent deliverability, improved procedural outcome, and lower rates of subsequent restenosis and

**Table 8.4.1** Strut thickness, strut width, recoil, and radial strength for a 3.0 mm diameter durable metallic DESs and two polymeric BRSs

|  | XIENCE expedition | | ABSORB | | DESolve | |
| --- | --- | --- | --- | --- | --- | --- |
| Strut thickness including polymer coat, (μm) | 89 | | 157 | | 120 | |
| Strut width including polymer coat, (μm) | 89–112 | | Connector | 140 | Connector | 100 |
|  |  |  | Hoop | 191 | Hoop | 165 |
| Diameter recoil, % | 1 min | 2.7% | 1 min | 3.4% | 1 min | 3.5% |
|  | 1 hour | 2.9% | 1 hour | 5.5% | 1 hour | −0.4% |
| Radial strength[a] | 1.64 ± 0.19 atm | | 1.37 ± 0.17 atm | | | |

*Source:* Ormiston JA, Webber B, Ben Ubod B, Darremont O and Webster MWI. *EuroIntervention*. 2015;11:60–67.
*Note:* The strut thickness and width for the BRSs are greater than those for the metallic durable stents to provide sufficient radial strength and limit recoil measured.
[a] Pressure to reduce stent scaffold cross-sectional area by 25%.

thrombosis [8–10]. Greater strut width has been associated with higher rates of periprocedural myocardial infarction than with narrower struts [11].

## Construction material

Construction material has a marked influence on stent scaffold recoil with stents constructed from stainless steel recoiling less than those from cobalt chromium which recoil less than those from nickel chromium (Figure 8.4.1). Scaffolds constructed from polylactic acid have recoil similar to those made from nickel chromium (Figure 8.4.1). Those constructed from a polylactide-derived polymer (DESolve, Elixir Medical, Sunnyvale, CA) had the least recoil at 1 hour after deployment [1].

## CLINICAL ANGIOGRAPHIC MEASUREMENTS OF IMMEDIATE DIAMETER RECOIL FOR BRSs

Immediate recoil was compared for bioresorbable scaffolds from the ABSORB Cohort B trial ($n$ = 88), and from the ABSORB Cohort A trial ($n$ = 27) with matched patients who received durable metallic XIENCE V stents in the Spirit I trial ($n$ = 27). Percentage diameter recoil of ABSORB scaffolds from Cohort B (6.7% ± 6.4%) was numerically larger than for the metallic XIENCE V stent (4.3% ± 7.1%) and similar to ABSORB Cohort A 6.9% ± 7.0%, but the differences were not statistically significant ($p$ = 0.22) [5]. Angiographic immediate diameter recoil in patients for the Elixir polymeric BRSs

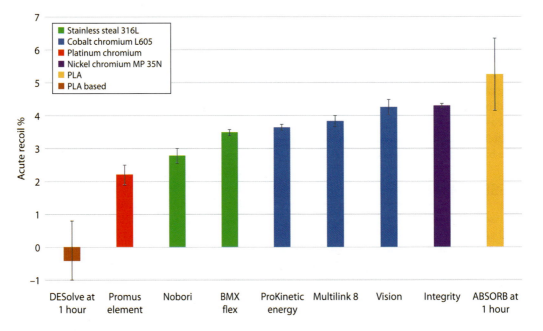

**Figure 8.4.1** Construction material influences recoil. Bench measurements of immediate diameter recoil for metallic stents compared with ABSORB and DESolve BRSs at 1 hour. All were 3.0 mm devices deployed at nominal pressure. The polymeric scaffolds were deployed in a water bath at 37°C and the stents were deployed in air. Stents constructed from stainless steel recoiled less than those constructed from cobalt chromium or cobalt nickel. Recoil at 1 hour of current ABSORB was greater than for most durable metallic stents. The DESolve scaffold at 1 hour was very similar in diameter to its diameter at baseline.

was similar to ABSORB (6.4 ± 4.6%) [12]. In the first-in-human trial (PROGRESS AMS) of a resorbable magnesium-based scaffold, immediate diameter recoil was similar to the polymeric BRSs at 7 ± 15% [13].

## COMPARISON OF BENCH DIAMETER RECOIL OVER ONE HOUR FOR TWO RESORBABLE POLYMERIC SCAFFOLD DESIGNS COMPARED WITH A DURABLE METALLIC STENT DESIGN

Because recoil measurements for different polymers may show time dependency (ASTM F2079-09), we compared diameter measurements of two bioresorbable scaffolds (ABSORB and DESolve) with the durable metallic Multilink 8 stent (Abbott Vascular) over an hour following deployment. The polymeric scaffolds were deployed in a water bath at 37°C (Figure 8.4.2). The external diameters of the ABSORB and DESolve scaffolds at deployment were greater than that of the ML8 stent because of their thicker struts (Figure 8.4.2). By 1 minute after deployment, all three devices had recoiled by approximately 0.1 mm. Between 1 minute and 10 minutes there was not much change in diameter. Between 10 minutes and 1 hour, the ABSORB scaffolds and ML8 stents showed little change but the DESolve scaffold increased in diameter to baseline dimensions ("self correction"), so that its diameter was larger than that of ML8 stent and ABSORB scaffold (Figure 8.4.2). This unique feature may correct strut malapposition and is being exploited in the design of the "Amity" scaffold (Elixir Medical) where there is at least 0.5 mm of self correction above nominal diameter which

may correct scaffold malapposition after resolution of thrombus and spasm following treatment of acute myocardial infarction or chronic total occlusion. Clearly it is important to state the time after deployment that recoil measurements are made because for different polymeric scaffolds the results at 1 minute may be very different from those at, for instance, 1 hour (Figure 8.4.2).

## SCAFFOLD RESORPTION AND RECOIL AFTER MONTHS

While current BRSs generally have adequate radial strength when deployed, this strength reduces over time as the scaffold is resorbed. The timing of scaffold strength reduction is important to limit recoil months after implantation. If a scaffold resorbs too quickly and before the process of arterial negative remodeling associated with percutaneous coronary intervention is completed, then the scaffold may be weakened and unable to counter these forces and hence may narrow [14]. With the first-generation magnesium BRSs [13], there was negative remodeling with a 42% reduction in volume enclosed by the external elastic lamina which the scaffold had failed to oppose. The scaffold failure accounts for some of the angiographic late loss seen. Similarly, in Cohort A of the ABSORB trial, IVUS showed scaffold area reduction from 6.08 mm$^2$ to 5.37 mm$^2$ ($p < 0.001$) between deployment and 6-months follow-up. In Cohort B there was no recoil with mean scaffold area at implantation by OCT of 7.53 ± 1.16 mm$^2$ and at 6 months of 7.74 ± 1.34 mm$^2$ ($p = 0.10$) [15]. Scaffolds may be damaged on deployment (Figure 8.4.3) and this may reduce radial strength and permit recoil especially if the resorption time is short.

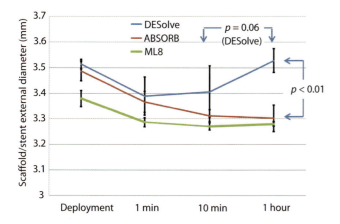

Figure 8.4.2 Recoil. Scaffold (or stent) external diameter immediately after deployment, at 1 minute, 10 minutes, and 1 hour after deployment. Durable metallic stents recoil immediately after deployment and then do not change much subsequently over time. This is very different from polymeric resorbable scaffolds. The ABSORB BRSs continues to recoil somewhat out to 1 hour in contrast to the DESolve where there is "self-correction" or enlargement between 10 minutes and 1 hour. (Ormiston JA, Webber B, Ben Ubod B, Darremont O and Webster MWI. *EuroIntervention*. 2015;11:60–67.)

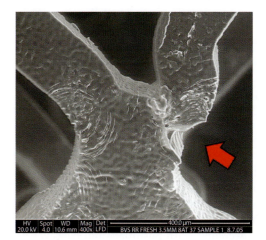

Figure 8.4.3 A first-generation 3.0 mm ABSORB scaffold as used in Cohort A that was damaged by postdilatation with a 3.5 mm semicompliant balloon inflated to 8 atm. Strut damage (arrow) may weaken a scaffold reducing radial strength and increasing recoil and potentially allow restenosis. In contrast to a complete strut fracture, this damage may not be detectable with OCT.

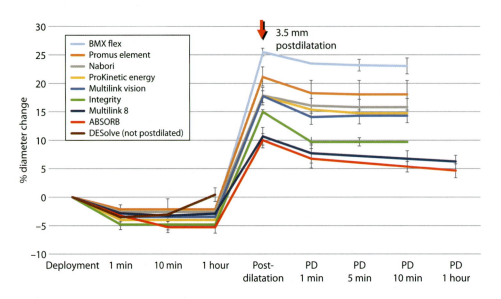

**Figure 8.4.4** Percentage diameter change for 3 mm stents/scaffolds from deployment to 1 hour then after postdilatation with a 3.5 mm balloon. Postdilatation improves stent/scaffold size and overcomes diameter loss due to recoil. Polymeric scaffold deployments were in a water bath at 3°C.

## TREATMENT OF RECOILED BRSs

Recoil can be overcome by careful postdilatation. We measured percentage diameter recoil of 3.0 mm stents and scaffolds immediately after deployment at nominal pressure then after postdilatation in the water bath for scaffolds and in air for the durable metallic stents (Figure 8.4.4). The diameter gain achieved after postdilatation was much greater than that lost by recoil. For safe postdilatation of polymeric scaffolds, it is important to recognize the safe postdilatation diameters to avoid strut fracture [1]. If there is strut fracture causing recoil, then the usual treatment has been stenting with a metallic DES [16]. The best treatment for BRSs restenosis is not established but could be a metallic DESs or a repeat BRSs rather than a drug-eluting balloon.

## SUMMARY

Stent recoil, which affects both metallic stents and bioresorbable scaffolds, differs between BRSs and durable stents and between different BRSs. Both bench testing and clinical trial data have shown that BRSs are at risk of immediate and late recoil. This can lead to adverse long-term clinical outcomes with increased restenosis and thrombosis. At the time of device deployment, recoil can be overcome with postdilatation. However postdilatation balloons must be appropriately sized, as oversized balloons can lead to scaffold fracture [1,16]. As interest in the field of BRSs evolves and with the introduction of new scaffolds, recoil must continue to be assessed on the bench and clinically.

## REFERENCES

1. Ormiston J, Webber B, Ubod B, Darremont O and Webster M. An independent bench comparison of two bioresorbable drug-eluting coronary scaffolds (ABSORB and DESolve) with a durable metallic drug-eluting stent (ML8/Expedition). *EuroIntervention.* 2015;11:60–67.
2. Tanimoto S, Serruys P, Thuesen L, Dudek D, de Bruyne B, Chevalier B and Ormiston J. Comparison of in vivo acute stent recoil between the bioabsorbable everolimus-eluting coronary stent and the everolimus-eluting cobalt chromium coronary stent: Insights from the ABSORB and SPIRIT trials. *Cathet Cardiovasc Interv.* 2007;70:515–523.
3. Onuma Y, Serruys P, Gomez J, de Bruyne B, Dudek D, Thuesen L, Smits P et al. Comparison of in vivo acute stent recoil between bioresorbable everolimus-eluting coronary scaffolds (revision 1.0 and 1.1) and the metallic everolimus-eluting stent. *Cathet Cardiovasc Interv.* 2011;78:3–12.
4. Tanimoto S, Bruining N, van Domburg R, Rotger D, Radeva P, Ligthart J and Serruys P. Late stent recoil of bioresorbable everolimus-eluting coronary stent and its relationship with plaque morphology. *J Am Coll Cardiol.* 2008;52:1616–1620.
5. Carrozza J, Hosley S, Cohen D and Bairn D. In vivo assessment of stent expansion and recoil in normal porcine coronary arteries. *Circulation.* 1999;100:756–760.
6. Pollman M. Engineering a bioresorbable stent: REVA programme update. *EuroIntervention Supplement.* 2009;5:F54–F57.

7. Ormiston JA, Webber B, Ben Ubod B, Darremont O and Webster MWI. An independent bench comparison of two bioresorbable drug-eluting coronary scaffolds (ABSORB and DESolve) with a durable metallic drug-eluting stent (ML8/Xpedition). *EuroIntervention*. 2015;11:60–67.

8. Kastrati A, Mehilli J, Dirschinger J, Dotzer F, Schuhlen H, Neuman F-J, Fleckenstein M et al. Strut thickness effect on restenosis outcome (JSAR STEREO) trial. *Circulation*. 2001;103:2816–2821.

9. Menown I, Noad R, Garcia E and Meredith I. The platinum chromium element stent platform: From alloy, to design, to clinical practice. *Adv Ther*. 2010;27:129–141.

10. Yamamoto Y, Brown D, Ischinger T, Arbab-Zadeh A and Penny W. Effect of stent design on reduction of elastic recoil: A comparison via quatitative intravascular ultrsound. *Cathet Cardiovasc Interv*. 1999;47:251–257.

11. Kawamoto H, Panoulas V, Sato K, Miyazaki S, Naganuma T, Sticchi A, Figini F et al. Impact of strut width in periprocedural myocardial infarction. A propensity-matched comparison between bioresorbable scaffolds and the first-generation sirolimus-eluting stent. *J Am Coll Cardiol Interv*. 2015;8:900–909.

12. Verheye S, Ormiston J, Stewart J, Webster M, Sanidas E, Costa R, Costa J et al. The next-generation bioresorbable coronary scaffold system: From bench to first clinical evaluation. *J Am Coll Cardiol Interv*. 2014;7:89–99.

13. Erbel R, Di Mario C, Bartunek J, Bonnier J, de Bruyne B, Erbeli FR, Erne P et al. Temporary scaffolding of coronary arteries with bioabsorbable magnesium stents: A prospective, non-randomized multicentre trial. *Lancet*. 2007;369:1869–1875.

14. Ormiston J and Serruys PW. Bioresorbable coronary stents. *Circ Cardiovasc Interv*. 2009;2:255–260.

15. Serruys P, Onuma Y, Ormiston J, de Bruyne B, Regar E, Dudek D, Thuesen L et al. Evaluation of the second generation of a bioresorbable everolimus drug-eluting vascular scaffold for treatment of de novo coronary artery stenosis: Six-month clinical and imaging outcomes. *Circulation*. 2010;122: 2301–12.

16. Ormiston J, De Vroey F, Serruys PW and Webster M. Bioresorbable polymeric vascular scaffolds: A cautionary tale. *Circ Cardiovasc Interv*. 2011;4:535–538.

# Acute scaffold disruption and late discontinuities

YOSHINOBU ONUMA, YOHEI SOTOMI, TAKESHI KIMURA, ROBERT-JAN M. VAN GEUNS, AND PATRICK W.J.C. SERRUYS

## INTRODUCTION

The current BRSs are composed of either a polymer or bioresorbable metal alloy. The key mechanical traits for candidate material in coronary indications include high elastic moduli to impart radial stiffness, large break strains to impart the ability to withstand deformations from the crimped to expanded states, and low yield strains to reduce the amount of recoil and overinflation necessary to achieve a target deployment. Primarily due to the mechanical properties of the selected materials, however, the functionality of the bioresorbable scaffold is somewhat limited (Table 8.5.1).

Numerous different polymers are available, whereas the most frequently used polymer in the current generation of BRSs is poly-L-lactic acid (PLLA). A potential drawback of the PLLA technology is its mechanical fragility related to the individual polymeric strut as exemplified by the disruption of the strut network when overexpanded. The elongation at break of raw PLLA is 2–5% so that raw material could break if it exceeds the limits. On the other hand, this acute mechanical disruption has to be distinguished from the structural discontinuity of the polymeric struts at a late stage, a biologically programmed fate during the course of bioresorption [1].

Taking into account the availability of the ex vivo, preclinical and clinical data, in this chapter, acute disruption and late discontinuities of the ABSORB everolimus-eluting PLLA scaffold are discussed.

## ACUTE DISRUPTION

### Phantom study

To define the OCT image findings associated with acute disruption, a phantom study was performed to intentionally create overexpansion and acute disruption of polymeric device. A BVSs (3.0 × 18 mm) was broken with an oversized balloon (4.0 mm) in a silicon phantom (left panel, Figure 8.5.1) [2]. After withdrawal of the balloon, OCT pullback was performed. OCT showed isolated struts in the middle of lumen or multiple struts overhanging in the same angular sector. In the proximal part of the scaffold, broken struts appeared as a double row of overhung struts malapposed to the phantom wall (Figure 8.5.1).

## Definition of strut disruption or late discontinuities on optical coherence tomography findings

Based on the phantom study, the acute (periprocedural) structural strut rupture was defined by the presence of at least one of the following in at least one cross-section: (1) if two struts overhang each other in the same angular sector of the lumen perimeter, with malapposition (overhang strut) or without malapposition (stacked strut) or (2) if there was an isolated strut located without obvious connection with other surrounding struts in 2-D OCT [2]. Isolated strut is defined as a strut located at a distance from the vessel wall (>1/3 of span between the center of gravity and the luminal border) [3,4]. Late discontinuity was judged when the above-mentioned findings were absent postprocedure but present at follow-up. If such findings were persistently observed at second follow-up, the case was classified as persistent late discontinuity. If late discontinuity observed at first follow-up became absent at second follow-up, the case was classified as resolved late discontinuity. Classification of OCT findings for acute disruption and late discontinuities is summarized in Table 8.5.2.

Table 8.5.1 Mechanical properties of biostable and bioresorbable material

| Polymer composition | Tensile modulus of elasticity (Gpa) | Tensile strength (Mpa) | Elongation at break (%) | Degradation time (months) |
|---|---|---|---|---|
| Poly (L-lactide) | 3.1–3.7 | 60–70 | 2–6 | >24 |
| Poly (DL-lactide) | 3.1–3.7 | 45–55 | 2–6 | 6–12 |
| Poly (glycolide) | 6.5–7.0 | 90–110 | 1–2 | 6–12 |
| 50/50 DL-lactide/glycolide | 3.4–3.8 | 40–50 | 1–4 | 1–2 |
| 82/18 L-lactide/glycolide | 3.3–3.5 | 60–70 | 2–6 | 12–18 |
| 70/30 L-Lactide/å-caprolactone | 0.02–0.04 | 18–22 | >100 | 12–24 |
| Cobalt chromium | 210–235 | 1449 | ~40 | Biostable |
| Stainless steel 316L | 193 | 668 | 40+ | Biostable |
| Nitinol | 45 | 700–1100 | 10–20 | Biostable |
| Magnesium alloy | 40–45 | 220–330 | 2–20 | 1–3 |

*Source:* Reproduced from Onuma Y, Serruys PW, *Circulation.* 2011;123(7):779–97.

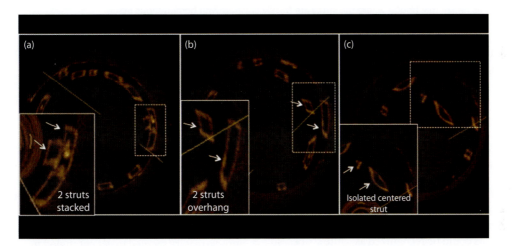

Figure 8.5.1 OCT criteria to diagnose acute scaffold disruption (phantom assessment). In a silicon phantom, a 3.0 mm ABSORB BVSs scaffold was disrupted through inflation of a semicompliant balloon up to 4.3 mm in diameter. OCT showed the following: more than 2 struts in the same angular sector with close contact (2 struts stacked; **a**) or without any contact (overhung struts; **b**). The other presentation of disrupted scaffold is the detection of an isolated malapposed strut located at the center of the lumen with loss of circularity of the scaffold **(c)**. The distance from the abluminal side of the strut to the luminal border should be more than a third of the distance from the center of gravity to the lumen border in the corresponding angular sector. (Illustrations reproduced from Onuma Y et al., *JACC Cardiovasc Interv.* 2014;7(12):1400–11. With permission.)

To visualize comprehensively in three dimensions the connections and disconnections of the struts inside the global structure of the scaffold, 3-D OCT analysis could be also used [3,4]. First, image sequences were generated from the OCT image files. Every single strut was detected in each OCT cross-section. After segmentation of scaffold struts, three-dimensional images were reconstructed using a volume rendering software (e.g., OSIRIX, version 3.8.1). X and Y axis pixel resolution were calculated in each image sequence using the image software, while the slice interval was set as 0.2 mm, according to the pull-back speed of 2.0 mm/s and the frame rate of 100 frames/second.

A spread-out-vessel graphic is also useful to summarize changes in the spatial distribution of the struts along the scaffold from postprocedure to late follow-up (Figure 8.5.2). The graphic is created by correlating the longitudinal distance from the distal edge of the scaffold to the strut (abscissa) with the angle where the struts were located in the circular cross-section with respect to the center of gravity of

Table 8.5.2 Classification of OCT findings

| | Etiology | Time of OCT observation | |
| --- | --- | --- | --- |
| | | Postprocedure | Late |
| Scaffold disruption | Procedure related | • Stacked struts | Late persistent[a]/Late procedural[b]<br>• Stacked struts with/without coverage, with/without malapposition |
| | | • Overhung struts | • Overhung struts with/without coverage, with/without malapposition |
| | | • Isolated intraluminal strut(s) | • Isolated malapposed struts with[c]/without coverage |
| Scaffold discontinuities | Resorption related | NA | Late acquired[a]<br>• Stacked/overhung/isolated or intraluminal strut(s) w/ or w/o coverage or malapposition |

Source: Reproduced from Onuma Y et al., JACC Cardiovasc Interv. 2014;7(12):1400–11. With permission.

Note: Artifacts such as non-uniform rotational deformation (NURD) and non-coaxial positioning of the catheter should be excluded with caution.

[a] Late persistent or late acquired can be only diagnosed when serial OCT is available (baseline/follow-up). If serial imaging cannot determine the etiology, the absence of a circular strut configuration at a late imaging time point may support a procedural disruption etiology whereas the presence of a circular strut configuration may support the etiology of a resorption-related discontinuity.

[b] Late procedural is related to the diagnostic procedure at follow-up, which either aggravates or creates the disruption.

[c] Can be detected as neointimal bridge where the struts are thickly covered with homogenous tissue.

the vessel (ordinates). The resultant graphic represents the scaffolded vessel, as if it had been cut longitudinally along the reference angle and spread out on a flat surface.

## Which imaging modality should be used to detect acute disruption and/or late discontinuities: angiography, OCT, or IVUS?

Considering the radio-lucency of the polymeric scaffold, angiography is not capable to detect any structural abnormality protruding into the lumen (Figure 8.5.3). On IVUS, the polymeric struts could be recognized as white stripes, so that in principle IVUS could detect structural abnormality of the scaffold. However, given the relatively low resolution, IVUS is less sensitive than OCT in the detection of acute strut disruption or late strut discontinuity. IVUS was able to detect major disruptions or discontinuities, but overlooked some disruptions or could not differentiate them from malapposition. OCT might be recommended as an additional diagnostic technique when the scaffolded vessel angiographically appears patent and oversizing and/or overexpansion is suspected.

## ACUTE DISRUPTION IN HUMANS

### ABSORB Cohort A

In humans, acute disruption was documented for the first time in an anecdotal case from the ABSORB Cohort A, where the prototype of ABSORB scaffold (ABSORB 1.0) was tested. At index procedure, a BVSs scaffold (3.0 × 12 mm) was implanted in the middle right coronary artery, followed by

postdilatation with 3.5 × 9 mm compliant balloon (Voyager) inflated at a pressure of 18 atm (nominal diameter at that level of inflation 3.84 mm). The overexpansion with a postdilatation balloon resulted in strut fracture as documented by OCT [5]. Of note, during this first-in-human trial, there was no instruction about the size of postdilatation balloon, since at that time the limit of expansion was not well established.

At 40 days, the patient experienced a single episode of angina at rest without electrographic evidence of ischemia. Repeat angiography showed a 42% of diameter stenosis in the BVSs by quantitative analysis (Figure 8.5.4) [5]. An attempt to cross the stenotic lesion with the pressure wire failed: the pressure wire seemed to get entangled in the scaffold strut at the site of the stenosis. Subsequent OCT image acquisition using a Helios catheter disclosed the following: (1) unhealed distal edge dissection, (2) two rows of overhung and malapposed struts, suggesting strut fracture, (3) minimal luminal area of 2.7 mm², due to reduction of treated area by 33% in comparison with baseline measurement, (4) late acquired struts malapposition, and (5) irregular intraluminal defects attached to the vessel wall. Although there was no evidence of ECG ischemia at rest, for a perceived safety reason the polymeric scaffold was covered by a drug-eluting metallic stent (non-ID TLR). After this repeat revascularization procedure, the patient had a slight rise in cardiac enzymes (peak troponin 2.21 ng/mL, CK-MB 87.7 µg/L), which was adjudicated as a non-Q wave MI [5].

At the time of event, the interpretation of the strange OCT image was not complete, since no data exists about the acute disruption either in clinical data or preclinical data. It was only after the subsequent phantom study that this clinical case was retrospectively diagnosed as "acute disruption" almost 3 years after this clinical event. It remained elusive what was the causal

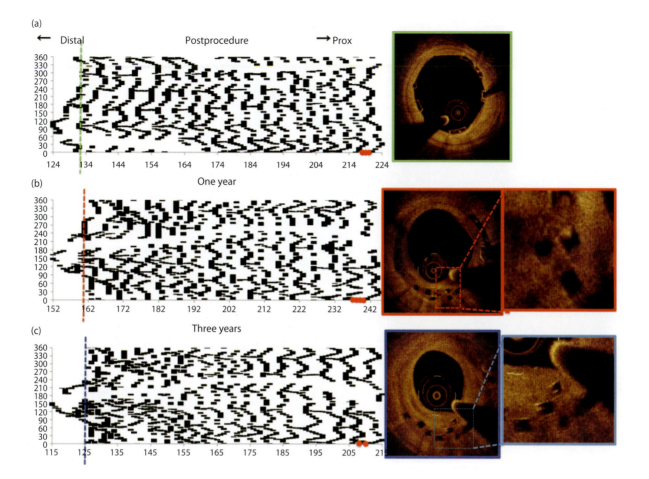

**Figure 8.5.2** Examples of spread-out view. The panels on the left in this figure represent spread-out-vessel graphics created by correlating the longitudinal distance from the distal scaffold edge to the individual struts detected in a single cross-section (abscissa) on the ordinate of the angle where the individual strut was located in the circular cross-section with respect to the center of gravity of the vessel (ordinates). In each cross-section (axial resolution of 200 micron), the circumferential length of each individual strut was depicted in an angular fashion. The resultant graphic represented the scaffolded vessel, as if it had been cut longitudinally along the reference angle and spread out on a flat surface. The spread-out view postprocedure **(a)** showed that the scaffold consisted of 19 rings interconnected by 3 links. At 1 year **(b)** and 3 years **(c)**, mechanical integrity has gradually subsided and the distal part of the scaffold was starting to show signs of dismantling, along which late discontinuities were observed. At baseline, in the distal edge of the scaffold (green dotted line in the foldout view), 2-dimensional OCT (with green frame) revealed well-apposed struts. At 1 year, in the distal edge (red dotted line in the foldout view), 2-dimensional OCT (with red frame) showed overhung and apposed struts. At 3 years, these struts remained overhung (blue line in the foldout view, corresponding to 2-D OCT with a blue frame). The phenomenon is considered benign since the struts are mostly covered at 1 and 3 years. Red dots in the figure represent the proximal metallic markers. (Illustrations reproduced from Onuma Y et al., *JACC Cardiovasc Interv.* 2014;7(12):1400–11. With permission.)

relationship between the scaffold disruption and the recurrence of rest angina, either with the collapsed lumen causing an ischemia or thrombotic formation of disrupted struts.

## ABSORB Cohort B

The frequency of acute disruption was systematically investigated in the ABSORB Cohort B, in 52 patients with OCT postprocedure. OCT was optionally performed postprocedure, at 6, 12, 24, and 36 months in a serial and nonserial manner [2]. Out of 50 patients with OCT imaging postprocedure, acute

strut fracture was observed in 2 (4%). The acute strut disruption at baselines was detectable on IVUS in 1 of the 2 cases.

One patient had a target lesion revascularization presumably associated with the acute fracture and its worsening at 1 month. In this case (Figure 8.5.3), an ABSORB 3.0 mm scaffold was implanted in an obtuse marginal branch with a reference diameter of 3.26 mm [6]. After postdilatation by a 3.25-mm noncompliant balloon at 24 atm, there remained malapposition at the proximal part of the scaffold on OCT. To correct the malapposition, an additional postdilatation was performed with a compliant 3.5 mm balloon at 16 atm

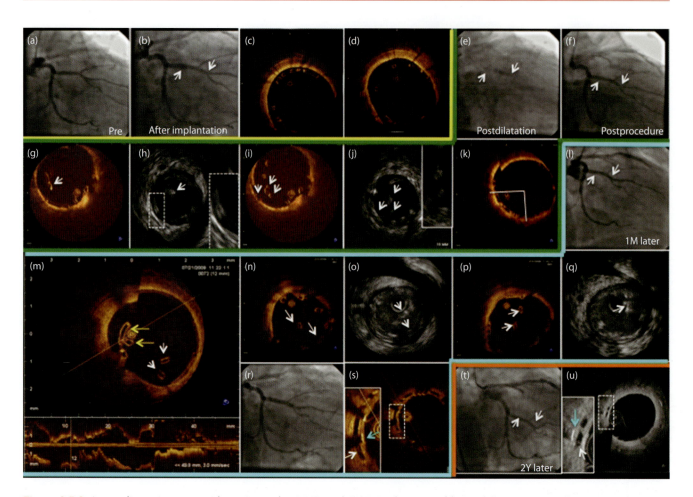

Figure 8.5.3 Acute disruption case with angiography, IVUS, and OCT. Each series of framed illustrations (yellow, green, blue, and orange) represents the observation at different time points (before postdilatation, after postdilatation, at 1 month, and at 2 years). An ABSORB BVSs 3.0 × 18 mm scaffold was implanted in an obtuse marginal branch (a: preprocedural angiography) with a reference diameter of 3.26 mm. After the first postdilatation by a 3.25-mm noncompliant balloon at 24 atm (panel b), malap-position remained at the proximal part of the scaffold on OCT (panel c and d). To correct the malapposition, an additional post-dilatation was performed with a compliant 3.5 mm balloon at 16 atm (expected diameter, approximately 4.0 mm, panel e). The angiographic result was successful (panel f) but the postprocedural OCT (panel g and i) and IVUS demonstrated acute strut dis-ruption (panel h and j) in the scaffolded segment. On both OCT and IVUS, isolated intraluminal struts (white arrow, OCT: g and IVUS: h) and overhung struts (white arrow, OCT: i and IVUS: j) were observed. At 1 month, the patient had 5 episodes of recur-rent angina at rest. The angiography (panel l) revealed a patent scaffold segment with a TIMI III flow, however, OCT (panel m and n) showed a deterioration of strut discontinuity (white arrows: isolated intraluminal or overhung struts). In the correspond-ing IVUS frames (o and q), the disrupted struts were also visible. A metallic XIENCE V stent was placed inside the ABSORB BVSs scaffold (panel r). Post-TLR OCT (panel s) showed the metallic struts, with shadows behind (blue arrows), are located inside of a polymeric strut (white arrow). At 2 years, the planned repeat angiography showed a patent stented segment (t), while OCT (u) showed in some cross-sections the presence of covered polymeric struts inside the metallic struts. (Illustrations reproduced from Onuma Y et al., JACC Cardiovasc Interv. 2014;7(12):1400–11. With permission.)

(expected diameter, approximately 4.0 mm). The repeat OCT and IVUS demonstrated acute strut fracture in the scaffolded segment. At 1 month, the patient had 5 episodes of recurrent angina at rest. Despite the fact that an exercise tolerance test was negative, the patient underwent recath-eterization because of persisting symptoms. The angiogra-phy revealed a patent scaffold segment with a TIMI III flow; however, OCT showed a deterioration of strut discontinuity. A metallic XIENCE V stent was placed inside the ABSORB scaffold, which eliminated his symptoms. After the nonisch-emic TLR procedure, there was a rise in troponin (0.09 uL/g

with an upper limit of normal of 0.03 uL/g), which was adju-dicated as a non-q-wave MI.

In the second case, overhang struts were observed on OCT at baselines in 5 cross-sections (Figure 8.5.5). According to the protocol, the asymptomatic patient under-went repeat angiography at 6 months with an IVUS and OCT imaging. After IVUS, the operator experienced dif-ficulty to cross the OCT in the scaffolded segment. After recrossing the wire, OCT was successfully acquired, which demonstrated an extremely malapposed strut close to the OCT catheter. The irregularity of the strut structure might

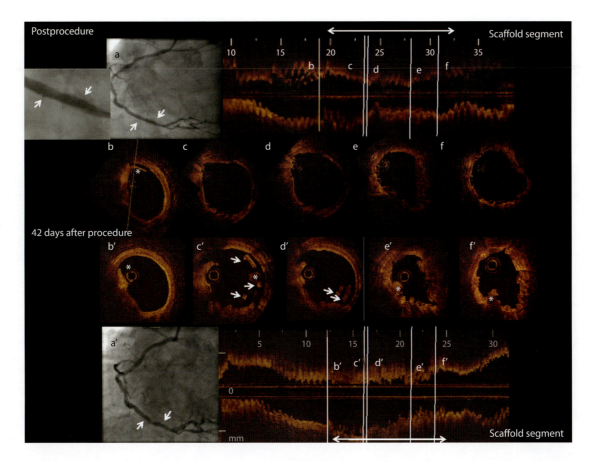

**Figure 8.5.4** Postprocedure, the final angiography showed a patent study stent identified with two metallic markers (panel **a**, white arrow) free from residual stenosis. The OCT images were acquired poststenting but before postdilatation. Distal to the BVSs, a small dissection was detected (panel **b**). In the middle portion, the scaffold was well expanded with a circular shape and struts were well apposed (panel **c**, **d**, **f**). At the site of the minimal luminal area (**e**), the lumen shape was triangular. Forty-two days after the procedure, the patient underwent repeat angiography due to recurrent angina, which revealed a moderate stenosis in the previously implanted BVSs (arrow indicates metallic markers, panel **a'**). The OCT cross-sections (**b'–f'**) were matched to the postprocedural OCT images (**b–f**). At the distal edge, the small dissection remained partially unhealed (asterisk, panel **b'**). In the middle of the scaffold (**c'**), struts are detached from the vessel wall (arrow), with an irregular intraluminal defect attached to the strut (asterisk). Two strut rows (**d'**, arrows) are overhung and malapposed in parallel, which suggests a disruption of scaffold structure. At the previous site of minimal luminal area, the lumen was deformed into a triangular shape (**e'**), due to late recoil of the scaffold. Occasionally, irregular intraluminal defects attached to the vessel wall were observed with attenuation (6–7 o'clock, asterisk, **f'**). (Illustration reproduced from Onuma Y et al., *EuroIntervention*. 2010;6(4):447–53. With permission.)

be induced by advancement of the wire to outside of the scaffold and pushing the OCT catheter under the abluminal side of struts. At 2-year imaging follow-up, OCT revealed the detached struts densely encapsulated with homogeneous tissues, as an arch extending from the proximal to the distal. On IVUS it was documented as a healed dissection in a scaffold segment. Despite the abnormal imaging findings, the patient remained asymptomatic up to 3 years.

## ABSORB Japan

The acute disruption was for the first time evaluated in a subgroup of the randomized ABSORB Japan trial comparing the ABSORB and XIENCE. In 125 patients subrandomized to OCT-1 group, postprocedural OCT was performed and was repeated at 2 years. In this series, no acute disruption was observed [7].

Compared to the Cohort B study, several technical differences are noted at the time of implantation. The sizing was based on angiography, and the clear instruction was given to the investigator to respect the limit of expansion. Postdilatation of BVSs was not mandatory but was allowed, using a low profile, high-pressure, noncompliant balloon with diameter ≤0.5 mm larger than the nominal BVSs size. Postdilatation of CoCr-EES was per standard of care. The careful sizing and avoidance of overexpansion with a too large postdilatation balloon could prevent the occurrence of acute disruption.

## LATE DISCONTINUITIES

### Definitions of late discontinuities

Late discontinuity is a programed phenomenon in the bioresorption process of the polymeric device. Six months after

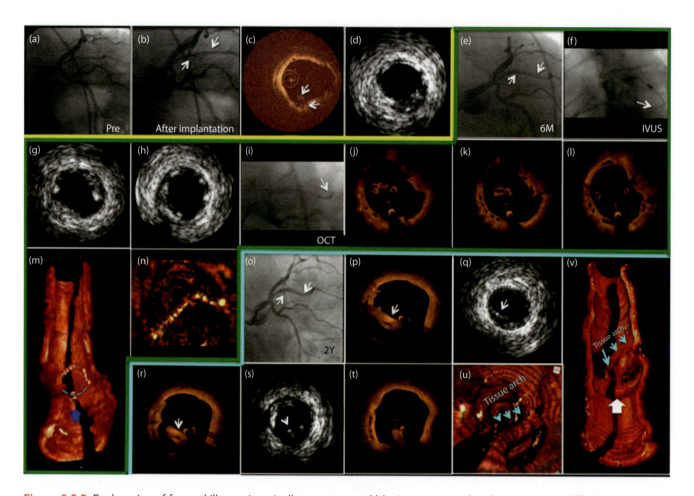

**Figure 8.5.5** Each series of framed illustrations (yellow, green, and blue) represents the observation at different time points (postprocedure, at 6 months, and at 2 years). An ABSORB BVSs scaffold was implanted in a small circumflex (reference vessel diameter 2.42 mm, **a**) followed by postdilatation with a 3.0 mm noncompliant balloon at a maximal pressure of 24 atm (**b**). Postprocedural OCT detected overhung struts or isolated struts in 5 cross-sections (**c**), which was not detected by IVUS (**d**). At 6-month follow-up, the patient underwent repeat angiography which revealed low angiographic late loss of 0.10 mm (**e**). According to the protocol, IVUS and OCT were performed. IVUS did not detect any abnormality (**g, h**). After IVUS, the operator experienced difficulty to cross the scaffolded segment with the OCT catheter (**i**). After rewiring the scaffolded segment, OCT was successfully acquired, and showed isolated struts close to the OCT catheter with loss of circularity of the scaffold (**j, k, l**: corresponding frames with **g** and **h**). On 3D-OCT, it was evident that one ring of scaffold was detached from the vessel wall (**m**) and divided the coronary flow (**n**; endoscopic view). The late disruption of the scaffold might have been induced by advancing the wire outside of the scaffold, pushing the OCT catheter under the abluminal side of the struts during the first crossing attempt. Despite the abnormal OCT findings, the patient remained asymptomatic up to 2 years. At 2-year angiographic follow-up (**o**), OCT revealed detached struts (**p, r, t**), which were fully covered by thick homogeneous tissue extending as an endoluminal arch connected proximally and distally to the vessel wall (3D: **u** and **v**). On IVUS it was documented as a "dissection" in a scaffold segment (**q** and **s**). (**p, r** and **q, s**) are the corresponding frames on OCT and IVUS, respectively. (Illustrations reproduced from Onuma Y et al., *JACC Cardiovasc Interv.* 2014;7(12):1400–11. With permission.)

device implantation, the polymeric scaffold starts losing its mechanical integrity and subsequent mass loss can lead to expected late discontinuity (Figure 8.5.6 [2]). This is theoretically a benign change during the bioresorption process and does not cause any problems if struts are well covered.

## ABSORB Cohort B

In the first-in-human ABSORB Cohort B trial, out of 50 patients (51 lesions), the OCT image was obtained in all but two patients at any follow-up (at 6 months, 1 year,

2 years or 3 years). Overall late structural discontinuity was observed in 21 patients (43%) [2]. The details of the case are presented in Figures 8.5.7 and 8.5.8.

In the series with 6- and 24-month follow-up, late discontinuities were observed in 3 cases at 6 months, which was persistently observed at second follow-up at 24 months. In 9 cases, late continuities were observed only at 2 years.

In the series with 1- and 3-year follow-up, late structural discontinuities were observed at 1 year in 7 cases. In 3 cases, no follow-up was performed at 3 years, so the fate

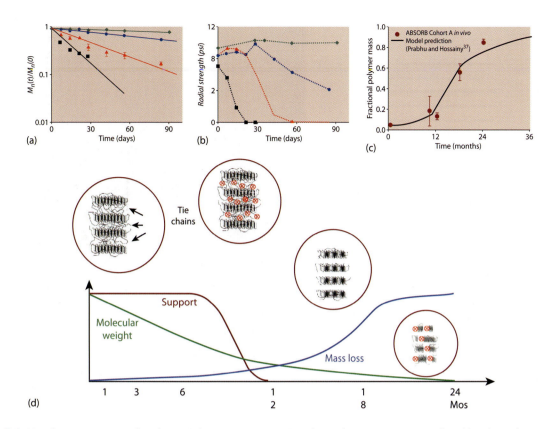

**Figure 8.5.6** Number-average molecular weight at various *in vitro* degradation times normalized by the value at $t = 0$ [$M_n$t/$M_n(0)$] for ABSORB Cohort B scaffolds with varying hydrolytic degradation rates (panel **a**). Data for $M_n$ were obtained using gel permeation chromatography with refractive index detection (panel **b**). Radial strength as a function of *in vitro* degradation time for the same lots of scaffolds as in panel **a**. (Panel **c**) Fractional polymer mass loss data versus time in the porcine animal model is shown in 2c. The curve represents the model of Prabhu and Hossainy [9]. The cartoon **(d)** described the initial reduction in molecular weight, the decrease in radial support around 6 months, and finally the loss in mass starting at 12 months, subsequently being completed at 24 months. The encircled graphical cartoons describe the progressive change in amorphous tie chains of PLLA and the progressive fragmentation of the crystal lamella. (Adapted from Oberhauser JP, Hossainy S and Rapoza RJ. *EuroIntervention*. 2009;5:F15–F22.)

of these discontinuities was unknown. Two discontinuities were persistently observed in serial OCT images at 3 years, while in 2 cases discontinuities were resolved at 3 years. In 2 cases, late structural discontinuities were observed only at 3 years.

There have been no events associated with these observations observed on OCT at follow-up except for one patient who underwent a nonischemia driven repeat revascularization (Figure 8.5.9). The 45-year-old male patient received a 3 × 18 mm ABSORB scaffold in the mid-LAD. At 1 year, the patient underwent a planned repeat angiography, which showed an enlargement of lumen. OCT showed late acquired discontinuity with malapposed overhanging struts over a length of 4 mm. Due to the pronounced malapposition, clopidogrel treatment was continued after 1 year. The patient had a stable angina of CCS class of 2–3 and underwent a repeat angiography on day 722. On angiography, the lumen became ectatic (QCA max diameter: 3.6 mm) without any significant stenosis in the scaffolded segment while on OCT one ring of scaffold showed a persistent discontinuity with malapposition. Despite the absence

of evidence of ischemia, it was thought that the anginal symptoms were somewhat related to the malappostion. A 3.0 × 28 mm metallic XIENCE Prime stent was placed in the scaffolded segment. After postdilatation with a 3.5 mm balloon, retention of angiographic contrast medium was observed within the new stent, diagnosed as malapposed struts on OCT. The segment was further dilated with a 4.5 mm balloon.

## ABSORB Japan

In the subpopulation of randomized study ($n = 77$), the serial OCT of the scaffold segment allowed the assessment of strut discontinuities, whether they were persistent or late acquired. The overhang or stacked struts were found at 2 years in approximately a quarter of the BVSs arm (19/77), although there was no acute strut disruption at postprocedure OCT [7]. However, the majority of such struts were well covered and apposed. In only 3 cases, such struts were uncovered and malapposed (Figure 8.5.10). There were no adverse events associated with these findings.

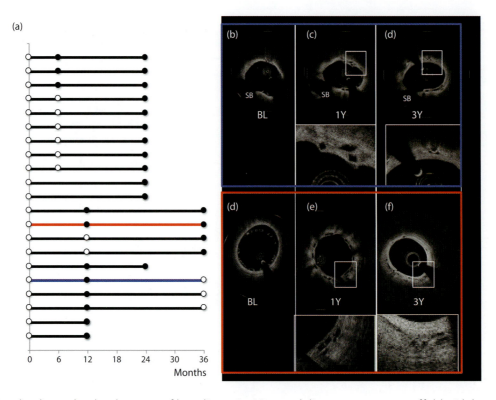

Figure 8.5.7  Panel **a** shows the development of late discontinuities, each line represents a scaffold with late discontinuities at various time points of follow-up (postprocedure, 6, 12, 24, and 36 months). White circle indicates OCT investigation without late strut discontinuities while the black circle represents OCT observation with late discontinuities at that time point. Framed illustrations in blue (**b**, **c**, and **d**) correspond to scaffolds with resolution at 36 months of late acquired discontinuity originally detected at 12 months. Framed illustrations in red (**d**, **e**, and **f**) correspond to a scaffold with persistent (at 36 months) late discontinuities detected at 12 months. In both cases, the stacked struts were already covered at 12 months. BL = baselines, 1Y = at 1-year follow-up, 3Y = at 3-year follow-up, SB = side-branch. (Illustrations reproduced from Onuma Y et al., *JACC Cardiovasc Interv.* 2014;7(12):1400–11. With permission.)

## PATHOLOGICAL RELATIONSHIP BETWEEN LATE DISCONTINUITIES AND LATE/VERY LATE SCAFFOLD THROMBOSIS

The current clinical data of ABSORB bioresorbable vascular scaffolds have generated concerns about scaffold thrombosis (ScT) both in early and late phases [8–15]. Recently published meta-analyses revealed that patients treated with the BVSs had a higher risk of definite or probable ScT than those treated with a metallic EES (odds ratio: 1.99–2.09) [16–18]. However, the causes of ScT both in early and late phases have yet to be fully elucidated.

In the current literatures [19], 100 case reports of definite ScT (acute and subacute ScT, *n* = 63; late and very late ScT, *n* = 37) were identified [8,11,12,20–39]. Out of these cases, imaging insights with IVUS and OCT were available in 5 and 38 cases, respectively. The other 57 cases did not undergo the intracoronary imaging assessment at the time of ScT event. Tables 8.5.3 and 8.5.4 and Figure 8.5.11 summarize the imaging findings of the 17 early ScT cases and 26 late ScT cases assessed by IVUS and OCT [19]. Representative examples of ScT underlying possible

mechanisms explored by OCT are summarized in Figure 8.5.12 [19].

In the 4 VLST cases of ABSORB Japan, the scaffolds were widely patent at 1-year angiographic follow-up, suggesting that the occurrence of VLST could relate to the structural abnormalities undetectable on angiography. In 3 cases, OCT at the time of or shortly after VLST demonstrated strut discontinuities, malapposition, and/or uncovered struts. These findings are in line with the previous reports by Karanosos et al. and Räber et al., demonstrating that incomplete lesion coverage, malapposition, strut discontinuities, and underexpansion of the scaffold were frequently observed by OCT in patients presenting with definite BVSs VLST [22,27]. The causal relationship of such OCT abnormalities and VLST, however, still remains undetermined. First, after the mechanical integrity of the scaffold disappears at 6 months after implantation, the scaffold structure becomes malleable so that wiring, thrombus aspiration, ballooning, or imaging procedure could induce strut discontinuities or malapposition [2]. Second, single OCT imaging only at the time of event could not differentiate the persistent acute disruption/malapposition and late acquired discontinuities. In general,

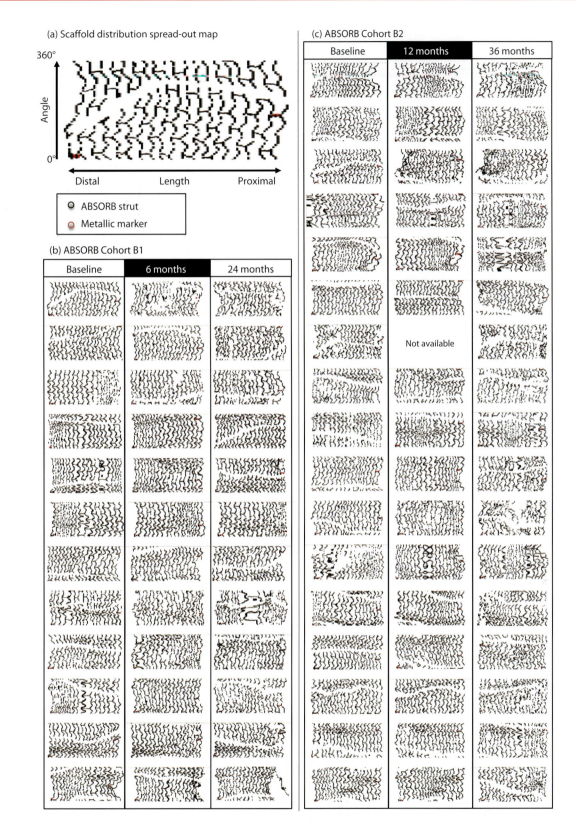

**Figure 8.5.8** Sequential changes of the spatial distribution of ABSORB struts in ABSORB Cohort B trial. Representative spread-out map is indicated in panel **a**. Horizontal axis indicates the distance from the distal edge of the devices. Vertical axis indicates the angle where the strut is located in the circular cross-section with respect to the center of gravity of the vessel (0° to 360°). Black dot indicates individual struts while the red dot indicates the location of metallic markers. Sequential changes of strut distribution in ABSORB Cohorts B1 and B2 are presented in panel **b** and **c**, respectively. Each row represents an individual lesion. Each column indicates the time point of the observation (baseline, 6, and 24 months in ABSORB Cohort B1; baseline, 12, and 36 months in ABSORB Cohort B2).

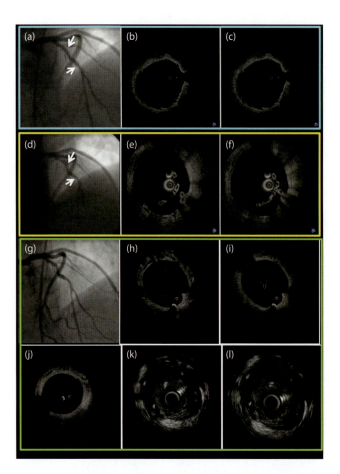

Figure 8.5.9 Each series of framed illustrations (light blue, yellow, and light green) represents the observation at different time points (postprocedure, at 1 year, and at 2 years). The figure shows a case with nonischemia driven TLR. An ABSORB BVSs 3.0 mm scaffold was implanted in the mid-LAD lesion (postprocedural angiography: **g**, white arrows indicate the scaffolded segment). Immediately after the procedure, OCT demonstrated a good expansion of the scaffold without any malapposition (**b** and **c**). Planned angiography at 1 year showed late lumen enlargement with, on OCT (**e** and **f**), malapposed and stacked struts (late discontinuity). The patient remained asymptomatic but the investigator, concerned by the malapposed struts observed at 1 year, performed a nonprotocol mandated angiography at 2 years. Two-year angiography demonstrated a patent scaffolded segment with further angiographic lumen enlargement (**g**). OCT (**h**, **i**, and **j**) and IVUS (**k** and **l**) showed malapposed struts in the scaffolded segment. Despite the absence of documented ischemia, an additional metallic stent in the previously scaffolded segment was implanted followed by postdilatation with a larger balloon. (Modified illustration reproduced from Onuma Y et al., *JACC Cardiovasc Interv.* 2014;7(12):1400–11. With permission.)

late discontinuities occur frequently as part of the programmed process of bioresorption [2]. The question remains whether the late discontinuities are bystander findings or a cause of the late event, and if so, what is the trigger to induce VLST.

As demonstrated in ABSORB Cohort B and ABSORB Japan, late discontinuity is generally a benign structural evolution during the bioresorption process and does not cause any clinical consequences if struts are well covered. However, in case struts are not covered by neointima and late discontinuity lets protrude part of the struts into the lumen and brings thrombogenic proteoglycan into contact with blood, late discontinuity could be a malignant potential cause of ScT. "Uncovered" late discontinuity could be critical, whereas late discontinuity itself would not be a culprit of ScT. Therefore, enhancement of neointimal coverage and firm tissue encapsulation of strut would be a key to prevent ScT associated with late discontinuity. Prevention of malapposition by either BVSs-specific implantation strategy (e.g., a mandatory postdilatation larger than nominal balloon) or OCT-guided implantation, and new generation BVSs with thinner struts could contribute to early neointimal coverage and consequent reduction of the incidence of late and very late ScT.

## CONCLUSION

The acute fracture is a rare iatrogenic phenomenon that has been anecdotally associated with anginal symptoms, which could be completely prevented by respecting the range of expansion. Late discontinuity is observed in 25–40% of patients in whom at the time of follow-up the struts are fully covered or embedded in tissue. In the majority of cases where the scaffold struts are well covered at an early time point, late discontinuities should be viewed as a serendipitous OCT finding of a normal bioresorption process. The discontinuities might have a pathological relationship in case of very late scaffold thrombosis. It should still be investigated whether the late discontinuities are bystander findings or a cause of the late event, and if so, what is the trigger to induce VLST.

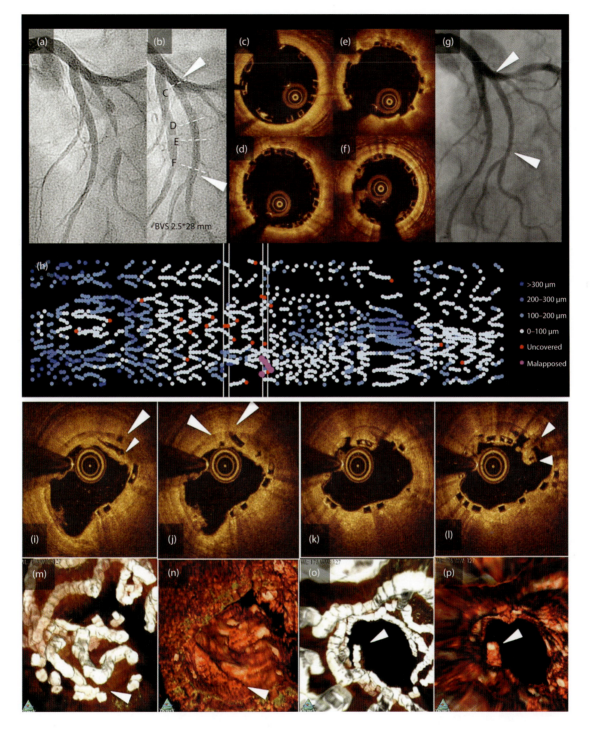

Figure 8.5.10 A case of late discontinuities without clinical consequences. A 2.5 × 28 mm ABSORB scaffold was implanted to treat a coronary stenosis in the diagonal branch **(a)**. After implantation **(b)**, optical coherence tomography showed the absence of strut disruption **(c–f)**, and a protrusion of plaque **(e** and **f)**. Final angiography showed excellent angiographic result **(g)**. OCT at 2 years (foldout view: **h**) demonstrated in the middle of BVSs covered and overhang struts (arrow heads in **i, j**, and **k**) and malapposed and overhang struts with back tissue bridge (arrow head in **l**), indicating late discontinuities. In the corresponding 3-D OCT reconstructions with **(n** and **p)** or without tissue enhancement **(m** and **o)**, two rings were overlapping with tissue coverage. One ring was protruding in the lumen from the vessel wall **(o)**, but this was integrated in the vessel wall by tissue extending behind struts **(p)**. (Modified illustration reproduced from Onuma Y et al., *EuroIntervention*. 2016;12(9):1090–1101. With permission.)

Table 8.5.3  Imaging findings of acute and subacute scaffold thrombosis

| Number | Indication for index PCI | Time (day) | ScT type | Imaging modality | Malapposition | Incomplete lesion coverage | Under-deployment | Acute disruption | Overlap | Acute Recoil | Other findings |
|---|---|---|---|---|---|---|---|---|---|---|---|
| 1 | SAP | 1 | Subacute ScT | OCT | – | | | YES | | | Calcified lesion, Asymmetrical apposition |
| 2 | SAP | 2 | Subacute ScT | OCT | – | | – | – | YES | – | |
| 3 | SAP | 7 | Subacute ScT | OCT | – | | – | – | – | – | Unknown mechanical cause |
| 4 | ACS | 0 | Acute ScT | OCT | YES | YES | – | – | – | – | |
| 5 | UAP | 0 | Acute ScT | OCT | – | | – | – | – | – | Calcified lesion |
| 6 | UAP | 0 | Acute ScT | OCT | YES | | – | – | – | – | |
| 7 | UAP | 7 | Subacute ScT | OCT | – | | – | – | – | YES | |
| 8 | UAP | 16 | Subacute ScT | OCT | | | | | | | Organized thrombus in distal scaffold |
| 9 | UAP | 18 | Subacute ScT | IVUS | – | | – | – | – | – | Recent DAPT cessation/No specific mechanical cause |
| 10 | NSTEMI | 8 | Subacute ScT | OCT | | | YES | – | – | – | Calcified lesion |
| 11 | STEMI | 0 | Acute ScT | OCT | – | | – | – | – | – | Unknown mechanical cause |
| 12 | STEMI | 0 | Acute ScT | IVUS | – | YES | – | – | – | – | Protrusion into lumen |
| 13 | STEMI | 0 | Acute ScT | OCT | YES | | – | – | – | – | |
| 14 | STEMI | 0 | Acute ScT | OCT | – | YES | YES | – | – | – | Calcified lesion |
| 15 | STEMI | 4 | Subacute ScT | OCT | | | | | | | Ticagrelor was stooped on day 3 after PCI/No specific mechanical cause |
| 16 | STEMI | 6 | Subacute ScT | OCT | YES | | – | – | – | – | |
| 17 | STEMI | 7 | Subacute ScT | OCT | – | | – | – | – | – | Unknown mechanical cause |
| Total number | | | | | 4 | 3 | 2 | 1 | 1 | 1 | |

Source: Reproduced from Sotomi Y et al., *EuroIntervention*. 2017;12(14):1747–1756. With permission.
Abbreviations: ACS = acute coronary syndrome; IVUS = intravascular ultrasound; "–" means "NO"; NSTEMI = non-ST segment elevation myocardial infarction; OCT = optical coherence tomography; SAP = stable angina pectoris; ScT = scaffold thrombosis; STEMI = ST segment elevation myocardial infarction; UAP = unstable angina pectoris.

Table 8.5.4  Imaging findings of late and very late scaffold thrombosis

| Number | Indication for index PCI | Time (day) | ScT type | Imaging | Malapposition | Late Discontinuity | Peri-strut low intensity area | Uncovered strut | Under-deployment | Incomplete lesion coverage | Recoil | Restenosis | Neoathero-sclerosis | Bifurcation | Other findings |
|---|---|---|---|---|---|---|---|---|---|---|---|---|---|---|---|
| 1 | SAP | 112 | Late ScT | OCT | – | | | | YES | – | | – | | | |
| 2 | SAP | 129 | Late ScT | OCT | – | | | YES | – | – | | – | | YES | |
| 3 | SAP | 161 | Late ScT | OCT | YES | YES | – | | YES | – | | – | | | |
| 4 | SAP | 263 | Late ScT | OCT | – | | YES | | YES | – | | – | | | Neovessel |
| 5 | SAP | 447 | Very Late ScT | IVUS | YES | | | | YES | – | | – | | | |
| 6 | SAP | 480 | Very Late ScT | IVUS | – | | | | | – | YES | – | | | |
| 7 | SAP | 540 | Very Late ScT | OCT | YES | | | | | – | | – | | | |
| 8 | SAP | 570 | Very Late ScT | OCT | YES | | – | | | – | | – | | | |
| 9 | SAP | 570 | Very Late ScT | OCT | YES | YES | | YES | | | | – | | | |
| 10 | SAP | 675 | Very Late ScT | OCT | YES | YES | | | | | | – | | | |
| 11 | SAP | 1320 | Very Late ScT | OCT | YES | | | | | | | – | | | |
| 12 | ACS | 47 | Late ScT | OCT | – | | | | | | | YES | – | | |
| 13 | ACS | 142 | Late ScT | OCT | – | | | | | YES | | – | – | | |
| 14 | ACS | 371 | Very Late ScT | OCT | YES | | | | | | | – | | | |
| 15 | UAP | 73 | Late ScT | OCT | | | | | | | | | | | Unknown mechanical cause |
| 16 | UAP | 602 | Very Late ScT | IVUS | | YES | | | YES | YES | | – | | | |
| 17 | UAP | 730 | Very Late ScT | OCT | | YES | | | | | | – | | | |
| 18 | NSTEMI | 243 | Late ScT | OCT | | | YES | | | | | | | | |
| 19 | NSTEMI | 420 | Very Late ScT | OCT | | | | | | YES | | | | | |
| 20 | NSTEMI | 584 | Very Late ScT | OCT | – | YES | YES | – | – | – | YES | | | | |
| 21 | NSTEMI | 630 | Very Late ScT | OCT | – | | – | YES | – | – | | | | | |
| 22 | STEMI | 104 | Late ScT | OCT | – | | | | | | | YES | YES | | Neovessels, ruptured restenosis |
| 23 | STEMI | 349 | Late ScT | OCT | – | – | YES | – | | | YES | | | | |
| 24 | STEMI | 540 | Very Late ScT | OCT | – | – | – | YES | | | | | | | |
| 25 | STEMI | 562 | Very Late ScT | OCT | YES | YES | YES | – | | | | | | | Asymmetrical apposition |
| 26 | STEMI | 570 | Very Late ScT | OCT | | YES | | | | | | | | | |
| Total number | | | | | 9 | 8 | 5 | 4 | 4 | 3 | 3 | 2 | 1 | 1 | |

*Source:* Reproduced from Sotomi Y et al., *EuroIntervention.* 2017;12(14):1747–1756. With permission.
*Abbreviations:* ACS = acute coronary syndrome; IVUS = intravascular ultrasound; "–" means "NO"; NSTEMI = non-ST segment elevation myocardial infarction; OCT = optical coherence tomography; SAP = stable angina pectoris; ScT = scaffold thrombosis; STEMI = ST segment elevation myocardial infarction; UAP = unstable angina pectoris.

(a) Acute and subacute scaffold thrombosis

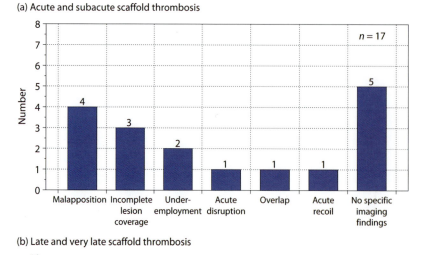

(b) Late and very late scaffold thrombosis

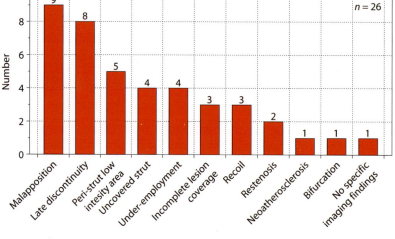

Figure 8.5.11 Imaging findings of scaffold thrombosis in acute/subacute **(a)** and late/very late phase **(b)** summarized in Tables 8.5.3 and 8.5.4 are presented as bar graphs. The vertical axis shows the number of each finding observed in the 43 case reports (acute and subacute: $n = 17$; late and very late: $n = 26$). (Reproduced from Sotomi Y et al., *EuroIntervention*. 2017;12(14):1747–1756. With permission.)

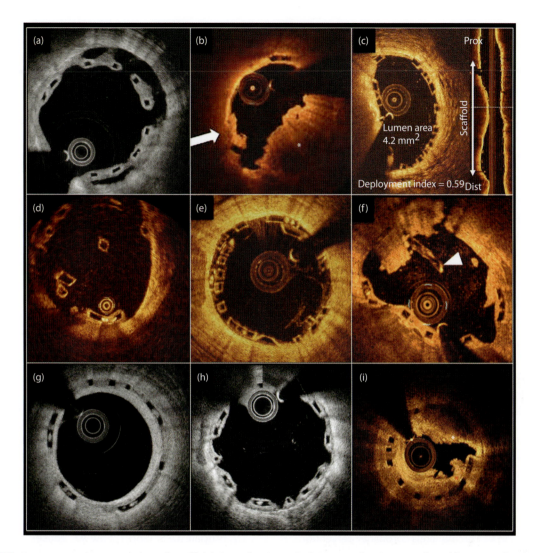

Figure 8.5.12 Representative examples of scaffold thrombosis underlying mechanisms explored by optical coherence tomography. In the acute and subacute ScT, strut malapposition (a), incomplete lesion coverage [(b), possible ruptured plaque (white arrow), uncovered thrombus (white asterisk)] under-deployment (c) were the leading mechanical causes, followed by acute disruption (d) and overlap (e). In the late and very late ScT, malapposition (a), late discontinuity (f, white arrowhead), and peri-strut low intensity area (g) were leading features, followed by uncovered struts (h) and neoatherosclerosis ((i), mural thrombus [red asterisk] with highly attenuating area [white asterisk]). (Modified illustration reproduced from Sotomi Y et al., *EuroIntervention*. 2017;12(14):1747–1756. With permission.)

# REFERENCES

1. Onuma Y, Serruys PW. Bioresorbable scaffold: The advent of a new era in percutaneous coronary and peripheral revascularization? *Circulation*. 2011;123(7):779–97.

2. Onuma Y, Serruys PW, Muramatsu T, Nakatani S, van Geuns RJ, de Bruyne B, Dudek D, Christiansen E, Smits PC, Chevalier B, McClean D, Koolen J, Windecker S, Whitbourn R, Meredith I, Garcia-Garcia HM, Veldhof S, Rapoza R, Ormiston JA. Incidence and imaging outcomes of acute scaffold disruption and late structural discontinuity after implantation of the absorb Everolimus-Eluting fully bioresorbable vascular scaffold: Optical coherence tomography assessment in the ABSORB cohort B Trial (A Clinical Evaluation of the Bioabsorbable Everolimus Eluting Coronary Stent System in the Treatment of Patients with De Novo Native Coronary Artery Lesions). *JACC Cardiovasc Interv*. 2014;7(12):1400–11.

3. Serruys PW, Onuma Y, Ormiston JA, de Bruyne B, Regar E, Dudek D, Thuesen L, Smits PC, Chevalier B, McClean D, Koolen J, Windecker S, Whitbourn R, Meredith I, Dorange C, Veldhof S, Miquel-Hebert K, Rapoza R, Garcia-Garcia HM. Evaluation of the second generation of a bioresorbable everolimus drug-eluting vascular scaffold for treatment of de novo coronary artery stenosis: Six-month clinical and imaging outcomes. *Circulation*. 2010;122(22):2301–12.

4. Serruys PW, Onuma Y, Dudek D, Smits PC, Koolen J, Chevalier B, de Bruyne B, Thuesen L, McClean D, van Geuns RJ, Windecker S, Whitbourn R, Meredith I, Dorange C, Veldhof S, Hebert KM, Sudhir K, Garcia-Garcia HM, Ormiston JA. Evaluation of the second generation of a bioresorbable everolimus-eluting vascular scaffold for the treatment of de novo coronary artery stenosis: 12-month clinical and imaging outcomes. *J Am Coll Cardiol.* 2011;58(15):1578–88.

5. Onuma Y, Serruys PW, Ormiston JA, Regar E, Webster M, Thuesen L, Dudek D, Veldhof S, Rapoza R. Three-year results of clinical follow-up after a bioresorbable everolimus-eluting scaffold in patients with de novo coronary artery disease: The ABSORB trial. *EuroIntervention.* 2010;6(4):447–53.

6. Ormiston JA, De Vroey F, Serruys PW, Webster MW. Bioresorbable polymeric vascular scaffolds: A cautionary tale. *Circ Cardiovasc Interv.* 2011;4(5):535–8.

7. Onuma Y, Sotomi Y, Shiomi H, Ozaki Y, Namiki A, Yasuda S, Ueno T, Ando K, Furuya J, Igarashi K, Kozuma K, Tanabe K, Kusano H, Rapoza R, Popma JJ, Stone GW, Simonton C, Serruys PW, Kimura T. Two-year clinical, angiographic, and serial optical coherence tomographic follow-up after implantation of an everolimus-eluting bioresorbable scaffold and an everolimus-eluting metallic stent: Insights from the randomised ABSORB Japan trial. *EuroIntervention.* 2016;12(9):1090–101.

8. Capodanno D, Gori T, Nef H, Latib A, Mehilli J, Lesiak M, Caramanno G, Naber C, Di Mario C, Colombo A, Capranzano P, Wiebe J, Araszkiewicz A, Geraci S, Pyxaras S, Mattesini A, Naganuma T, Munzel T, Tamburino C. Percutaneous coronary intervention with everolimus-eluting bioresorbable vascular scaffolds in routine clinical practice: Early and midterm outcomes from the European multicentre GHOST-EU registry. *EuroIntervention.* 2015;10(10):1144–53.

9. Gao R, Yang Y, Han Y, Huo Y, Chen J, Yu B, Su X, Li L, Kuo HC, Ying SW, Cheong WF, Zhang Y, Su X, Xu B, Popma JJ, Stone GW. Bioresorbable vascular scaffolds versus metallic stents in patients with coronary artery disease: ABSORB China Trial. *J Am Coll Cardiol.* 2015;66(21):2298–309.

10. Kimura T, Kozuma K, Tanabe K, Nakamura S, Yamane M, Muramatsu T, Saito S, Yajima J, Hagiwara N, Mitsudo K, Popma JJ, Serruys PW, Onuma Y, Ying S, Cao S, Staehr P, Cheong WF, Kusano H, Stone GW. A randomized trial evaluating everolimus-eluting Absorb bioresorbable scaffolds vs. everolimus-eluting metallic stents in patients with coronary artery disease: ABSORB Japan. *Eur Heart J.* 2015;36(47):3332–42.

11. Sabate M, Windecker S, Iniguez A, Okkels-Jensen L, Cequier A, Brugaletta S, Hofma SH, Raber L, Christiansen EH, Suttorp M, Pilgrim T, Anne van Es G, Sotomi Y, Garcia-Garcia HM, Onuma Y, Serruys PW. Everolimus-eluting bioresorbable stent vs. durable polymer everolimus-eluting metallic stent in patients with ST-segment elevation myocardial infarction: Results of the randomized ABSORB ST-segment elevation myocardial infarction-TROFI II trial. *Eur Heart J.* 2016;37(3):229–40.

12. Serruys PW, Chevalier B, Dudek D, Cequier A, Carrie D, Iniguez A, Dominici M, van der Schaaf RJ, Haude M, Wasungu L, Veldhof S, Peng L, Staehr P, Grundeken MJ, Ishibashi Y, Garcia-Garcia HM, Onuma Y. A bioresorbable everolimus-eluting scaffold versus a metallic everolimus-eluting stent for ischaemic heart disease caused by de-novo native coronary artery lesions (ABSORB II): An interim 1-year analysis of clinical and procedural secondary outcomes from a randomised controlled trial. *Lancet (London, England).* 2015;385(9962):43–54.

13. Abizaid A, Ribamar Costa J, Jr., Bartorelli AL, Whitbourn R, van Geuns RJ, Chevalier B, Patel T, Seth A, Stuteville M, Dorange C, Cheong WF, Sudhir K, Serruys PW, investigators AE. The ABSORB EXTEND study: Preliminary report of the twelve-month clinical outcomes in the first 512 patients enrolled. *EuroIntervention.* 2015;10(12):1396–401.

14. Kraak RP, Hassell ME, Grundeken MJ, Koch KT, Henriques JP, Piek JJ, Baan J, Jr., Vis MM, Arkenbout EK, Tijssen JG, de Winter RJ, Wykrzykowska JJ. Initial experience and clinical evaluation of the Absorb bioresorbable vascular scaffold (BVS) in real-world practice: The AMC Single Centre Real World PCI Registry. *EuroIntervention.* 2015;10(10):1160–8.

15. Brugaletta S, Gori T, Low AF, Tousek P, Pinar E, Gomez-Lara J, Scalone G, Schulz E, Chan MY, Kocka V, Hurtado J, Gomez-Hospital JA, Munzel T, Lee CH, Cequier A, Valdes M, Widimsky P, Serruys PW, Sabate M. Absorb bioresorbable vascular scaffold versus everolimus-eluting metallic stent in ST-segment elevation myocardial infarction: 1-year results of a propensity score matching comparison: The BVS-EXAMINATION Study (bioresorbable vascular scaffold-a clinical evaluation of everolimus eluting coronary stents in the treatment of patients with ST-segment elevation myocardial infarction). *JACC Cardiovasc Interv.* 2015;8(1 Pt B):189–97.

16. Cassese S, Byrne RA, Ndrepepa G, Kufner S, Wiebe J, Repp J, Schunkert H, Fusaro M, Kimura T, Kastrati A. Everolimus-eluting bioresorbable vascular scaffolds versus everolimus-eluting metallic stents: A meta-analysis of randomised controlled trials. *Lancet.* 2016;387(10018):537–44.

17. Lipinski MJ, Escarcega RO, Baker NC, Benn HA, Gaglia MA, Jr., Torguson R, Waksman R. Scaffold thrombosis after percutaneous coronary intervention with ABSORB bioresorbable vascular scaffold: A systematic review and meta-analysis. *JACC Cardiovasc Interv.* 2016;9(1):12–24.

18. Stone GW, Gao R, Kimura T, Kereiakes DJ, Ellis SG, Onuma Y, Cheong WF, Jones-McMeans J, Su X, Zhang Z, Serruys PW. 1-year outcomes with the Absorb bioresorbable scaffold in patients with coronary artery disease: A patient-level, pooled meta-analysis. *Lancet*. 2016;387(10025):1277–89.

19. Sotomi Y, Suwannasom P, Serruys PW, Onuma Y. Possible mechanical causes of scaffold thrombosis: Insights from case reports with intracoronary imaging. *EuroIntervention*. 2017;12(14):1747–56.

20. Fernandez-Rodriguez D, Brugaletta S, Otsuki S, Sabate M. Acute Absorb bioresorbable vascular scaffold thrombosis in ST-segment elevation myocardial infarction: To stent or not to stent? *EuroIntervention*. 2014;10(5):600; discussion 600.

21. Jaguszewski M, Wyss C, Alibegovic J, Luscher TF, Templin C. Acute thrombosis of bioabsorbable scaffold in a patient with acute coronary syndrome. *Eur Heart J*. 2013;34(27):2046.

22. Karanasos A, van Geuns RJ, Zijlstra F, Regar E. Very late bioresorbable scaffold thrombosis after discontinuation of dual antiplatelet therapy. *Eur Heart J*. 2014;35(27):1781.

23. Karanasos A, Van Mieghem N, van Ditzhuijzen N, Felix C, Daemen J, Autar A, Onuma Y, Kurata M, Diletti R, Valgimigli M, Kauer F, van Beusekom H, de Jaegere P, Zijlstra F, van Geuns RJ, Regar E. Angiographic and optical coherence tomography insights into bioresorbable scaffold thrombosis: Single-center experience. *Circ Cardiovasc Interv*. 2015;8(5).

24. Miyazaki T, Panoulas VF, Sato K, Naganuma T, Latib A, Colombo A. Acute stent thrombosis of a bioresorbable vascular scaffold implanted for ST-segment elevation myocardial infarction. *Int J Cardiol*. 2014;174(2):e72–4.

25. Abu Sharar H, Katus HA, Bekeredjian R. Pitfalls of bioresorbable vascular scaffold thrombosis—Be sure to cover it all. *Int J Cardiol*. 2014;177(3):1067–8.

26. Ishibashi Y, Onuma Y, Muramatsu T, Nakatani S, Iqbal J, Garcia-Garcia HM, Bartorelli AL, Whitbourn R, Abizaid A, Serruys PW, Investigators AE. Lessons learned from acute and late scaffold failures in the ABSORB EXTEND trial. *EuroIntervention*. 2014;10(4):449–57.

27. Raber L, Brugaletta S, Yamaji K, O'Sullivan CJ, Otsuki S, Koppara T, Taniwaki M, Onuma Y, Freixa X, Eberli FR, Serruys PW, Joner M, Sabate M, Windecker S. Very late scaffold thrombosis: Intracoronary imaging and histopathological and spectroscopic findings. *J Am Coll Cardiol*. 2015;66(17):1901–14.

28. Schiattarella GG, Magliulo F, D'Alise G, Mannacio V, Ilardi F, Trimarco B, Esposito G, Cirillo P. The pitfalls of managing thrombosis of an Absorb-treated bifurcation. *Int J Cardiol*. 2014;174(3):e93–5.

29. Hamm C. 30-days follow up of the German–Austrian–ABSORB Register: GABI-R. In Euro PCR. Paris, France; 2015.

30. Azzalini L, Al-Hawwas M, L'Allier PL. Very late bioresorbable vascular scaffold thrombosis: A new clinical entity. *EuroIntervention*. 2015;11(1):e1–2.

31. Azzalini L, L'Allier PL. Bioresorbable vascular scaffold thrombosis in an all-comer patient population: Single-center experience. *J Invasive Cardiol*. 2015;27(2):85–92.

32. Chevalier B, Serruys PW. The 2-year clinical outcomes of the ABSORB II trial: First randomized comparison between the Absorb everolimus eluting bioresorbable vascular scaffold and the XIENCE everolimus eluting stent. In *Transcatheter Cardiovascular Therapeutics*. San Francisco, CA, USA; 2015.

33. Cortese B, Piraino D, Ielasi A, Steffenino G, Orrego PS. Very late bioresorbable vascular scaffold thrombosis due to late device recoil. *Int J Cardiol*. 2015;189:132–3.

34. Cuculi F, Puricel S, Jamshidi P, Valentin J, Kallinikou Z, Toggweiler S, Weissner M, Munzel T, Cook S, Gori T. Optical coherence tomography findings in bioresorbable vascular scaffolds thrombosis. *Circ Cardiovasc Interv*. 2015;8(10):e002518.

35. Ho HH, Er Ching M, Ong PJ, Ooi YW. Subacute bioresorbable vascular scaffold thrombosis: A report of 2 cases. *Heart Vessels*. 2015;30(4):545–8.

36. Ielasi A, Cortese B, Steffenino G. Late structural discontinuity as a possible cause of very late everolimus-eluting bioresorbable scaffold thrombosis. *JACC Cardiovasc Interv*. 2015;8(10):e171–2.

37. Meincke F, Spangenberg T, Heeger CH, Bergmann MW, Kuck KH, Ghanem A. Very late scaffold thrombosis due to insufficient strut apposition. *JACC Cardiovasc Interv*. 2015;8(13):1768–9.

38. Timmers L, Stella PR, Agostoni P. Very late bioresorbable vascular scaffold thrombosis following discontinuation of antiplatelet therapy. *Eur Heart J*. 2015;36(6):393.

39. Yahagi K, Virmani R, Kesavamoorthy B. Very late scaffold thrombosis of everolimus-eluting bioresorbable scaffold following implantation in STEMI after discontinuation of dual antiplatelet therapy. *Cardiovasc Interv Ther*. 2017;32(1):53–5.

40. Radu MD. The clinical atlas of intravascular optical coherence tomography for iPad. *Eur Heart J*. 2012;33(10):1174–5.

41. Prabhu S, Hossainy S. Modeling of degradation and drug release from a biodegradable stent coating. *J Biomed Mater Res A*. 2007;80(3):732–41.

42. Oberhauser JP, Hossainy S, Rapoza RJ. Design principles and performance of bioresorbable polymeric vascular scaffolds. *EuroIntervention*. 2009;5(Supplement F):F15–22.

# The incidence and potential mechanism of side-branch occlusion after implantation of bioresorbable scaffolds: Insights from ABSORB II

YUKI ISHIBASHI, TAKASHI MURAMATSU, YOHEI SOTOMI, YOSHINOBU ONUMA, AND PATRICK W.J.C. SERRUYS

## INTRODUCTION

Despite advances in interventional technology, the incidence of postprocedural cardiac marker elevation has not substantially decreased since the first serial assessment 20 years ago. As of now, these postprocedural cardiac marker elevations are considered to represent periprocedural myocardial injury (PMI) with worse long-term outcome potential.

## SIDE-BRANCH OCCLUSION

Side-branch occlusion (SBO) has been implicated as a contributing factor to the development of periprocedural myocardial infarction (PMI) after percutaneous coronary intervention [1–3]. PMI has been associated with unfavorable late clinical outcomes, including an increased risk of cardiac mortality [4–6]. Mechanisms to explain the incidence of SBO after the metallic platform stent implantation have included mechanical vessel straightening and enlargement of the stented vessel, bifurcation carina shift, and/or coronary plaque shift into the orifice of the side branch [7–9]. In addition, the increased strut thicknesses of the first-generation drug-eluting stents (DESs) has been implicated in contributing to a higher incidence of SBO compared with the thinner strut second-generation DESs [10,11].

## SBO AFTER IMPLANTATION OF ABSORB SCAFFOLDS IN THE HISTORICAL DATA

The bioresorbable everolimus-eluting scaffold (ABSORB; Abbott Vascular, Santa Clara, CA) was developed to provide a novel approach to treat coronary artery stenosis with transient vessel support and drug delivery [12,13]. The performance of the second-generation ABSORB was investigated in the ABSORB Cohort B Trial which reported excellent clinical results [14,15]. However, the clinical relevance of this technology in comparison with metallic drug eluting stents still remains a matter of debate due to the absence of randomized comparative data between the ABSORB and conventional metallic drug-eluting stents. The ABSORB II randomized controlled trial (ClinicalTrials.gov NCT01425281) is the first randomized clinical trial assessing the clinical outcomes in 501 patients treated with either the ABSORB or the everolimus-eluting metallic stent (XIENCE; Abbott Vascular, Santa Clara, CA).

In a nonrandomized comparison using historical data, ABSORB scaffold was associated with a higher incidence of postprocedural side branch occlusion (SBO) compared with the EES [16]. Considering the greater vessel wall area covered by the strut of ABSORB scaffold (26%) compared with the EES (12%), there is a greater probability of covering the orifice of side branches with the ABSORB scaffold [16]. Given the increased strut thickness of the ABSORB, a potential concern exists that it might be associated with a higher incidence of periprocedural myocardial injury and myocardial infarction compared to newer-generations of DESs.

## INCIDENCE OF CARDIAC BIOMARKER RISE: INSIGHTS FROM ABSORB II

As recently described, we compared the peak value of the three cardiac biomarker (CB) values postprocedure according to six rise categories (CB: >1 × ULN, >2 × ULN, >3 × ULN, >5 × ULN, >10 × ULN, > 35 × ULN and >70 × ULN) after scaffold or stent implantation. In the present study, the rise of three CB subcategorized in seven different ranges was comparable between the two treatment arms (Table 8.6.1). Among the patients with postdilatation, the peak ratio of CKMB postprocedure was significantly higher in the ABSORB arm than in the EES arm ($1.43 \pm 2.41$ vs. $1.00 \pm 1.89$, $p = 0.02$). The current protocol did not recommend postdilatation of the ABSORB device with a balloon larger than 0.25 mm with respect to the nominal size of the device. The postprocedural CB rise with the patients who underwent postdilatation seems to justify retrospectively this conservative recommendation.

## QUALITATIVE AND QUANTITATIVE ANGIOGRAPHIC ASSESSMENT OF SBO: INSIGHTS FROM ABSORB II

In the present analysis, a total of 335 patients with 988 side branches in the ABSORB arm and 166 patients with 503 side branches in the EES arm were assessed. Incidence of

any "angiographic complications" (Figure 8.6.1) was similar between the two treatment arms (ABSORB; 16.4% vs. EES; 19.9%, $p = 0.39$) as well as the incidence of side branch occlusion (SBO) (5.3% vs. 7.6%, $p = 0.07$) (Table 8.6.2). The incidence of postprocedural SBO in the obstruction segment was significantly lower in the ABSORB arm compared with the EES arm (4.3% vs. 6.8%, $p = 0.046$) although there were no significant differences in the incidence of SBO according to the RVD size (RVD ≤ 0.5 mm, 0.5 < RVD ≤ 1.0, 1.0 < RVD) (Figure 8.6.2). At variance with a previous report [16], the ABSORB showed a trend toward lower incidence of postprocedural SBO compared with the EES. Of note, most of the side branch occlusions occurred in small side branches of RVD < 1.0 mm in both of treatment arms (Table 8.6.2). Although the nominal sizes of devices used ($3.01 \pm 0.31$ mm vs. $3.05 \pm 0.28$ mm, $p = 0.10$) and frequency of postdevice dilatation were comparable (60.7% vs. 58.8%, $p = 0.67$), the nominal balloon size and the pressure used during either implantation or postdilatation was larger and higher in the EES arm, so that the expected balloon diameter tended to be larger accordingly ($3.29 \pm 0.35$ mm vs. $3.35 \pm 0.37$ mm, $p = 0.15$) [17], the acute gain in minimal lumen diameter (QCA measurement by Core Lab) was significantly larger in the EES arm ($1.15 \pm 0.38$ mm vs. $1.46 \pm 0.38$ mm, $p < 0.001$) [17]. Whether the aggressive (post)dilatation may have resulted in a higher incidence of postprocedural SBO in the EES arm—due to the presence of the bifurcation carina shift and/or plaque shift into the orifice of the side branch [18]—remains speculative.

Table 8.6.1 Comparison of the peak value of cardiac biomarker rise postprocedure

| | CK 464/487 (95.3%) | | | CKMB 475/487 (97.5%) | | | cTn 473/487 (97.1%) | | |
|---|---|---|---|---|---|---|---|---|---|
| | ABSORB (n = 306) | XIENCE (n = 158) | p value | ABSORB (n = 315) | XIENCE (n = 160) | p value | ABSORB (n = 316) | XIENCE (n = 157) | p value |
| Mean ± SD | 0.71 ± 0.63 | 0.65 ± 0.64 | 0.380 | 1.33 ± 2.12 | 1.09 ± 1.65 | 0.180 | 12.09 ± 30.24 | 8.28 ± 20.20 | 0.138 |
| >1 × ULN | 16.7% (51/306) | 8.9% (14/158) | 0.024 | 32.1% (101/315) | 26.3% (42/160) | 0.205 | 62.3% (197/316) | 62.4% (98/157) | 1.000 |
| >2 × ULN | 5.2% (16/306) | 1.9% (3/158) | 0.135 | 13.7% (43/315) | 10.0% (16/160) | 0.304 | 48.1% (152/316) | 45.9% (72/157) | 0.696 |
| >3 × ULN | 1.3% (4/306) | 1.9% (3/158) | 0.694 | 7.3% (23/315) | 6.3% (10/160) | 0.849 | 38.3% (121/316) | 36.9% (58/157) | 0.841 |
| >5 × ULN | 0% (0/306) | 0.6% (1/158) | 0.341 | 5.1% (16/315) | 2.5% (4/160) | 0.232 | 29.7% (94/316) | 25.5% (40/157) | 0.386 |
| >10 × ULN | 0% (0/306) | 0% (0/158) | 1.000 | 0.6% (2/315) | 0.6% (1/160) | 1.000 | 19.0% (60/316) | 15.3% (24/157) | 0.372 |
| >35 × ULN | 0% (0/306) | 0% (0/158) | 1.000 | 0% (0/315) | 0% (0/160) | 1.000 | 6.0% (19/316) | 3.8% (6/157) | 0.387 |
| >70 × ULN | 0% (0/306) | 0% (0/158) | 1.000 | 0% (0/315) | 0% (0/160) | 1.000 | 3.5% (11/316) | 1.3% (2/157) | 0.236 |

Note: 14 patients presented with recent myocardial infarction at entry with normalized CKMB according to the protocol were excluded for post CB analysis.

Abbreviations: ABSORB = bioresorbablevascular scaffold(s); CK = creatine kinase; CKMB = creatine kinase-myoband; cTn = cardiac troponin; EES = everolimus-eluting metallic stent(s); ULN = upper limit of normal.

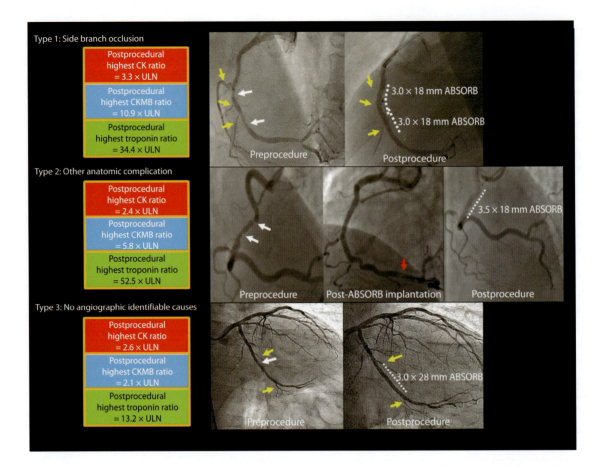

**Figure 8.6.1** According to the underlying angiographic mechanisms, the periprocedural MI after revascularization was classified into three types: Type 1 denotes cardiac biomarker rise due to side-branch occlusion, Type 2 denotes cardiac biomarker rise due to other anatomic complications, and Type 3 denotes cardiac biomarker rise without any identifiable anatomic causes in the coronary artery. Preprocedure angiography showed a focal stenosis (white arrows), side branches in the target lesion (yellow arrows), and distal embolization was observed after device implantation (red arrow).

## INCIDENCE AND PREDICTORS OF PERIPROCEDURAL MI: INSIGHTS FROM ABSORB II

In the protocol, MI without distinction of being spontaneous or periprocedural MI (PMI) is defined by elevation of total creatine kinase (CK) to >2 times normal along with elevated or "positive" creatine kinase myocardial band (CKMB). In addition, the SCAI definition requires elevation of cardiac biomarkers, preferably CKMB: (1) the SCAI definition (CKMB rise > 10 × ULN or troponin rise > 70 × ULN in the case of absence of CKMB); (2) the universal third definition {Troponin rise > 5 × ULN with either either (a) symptoms suggestive of myocardial ischemia (>20 min) or (b) new ischemic ECG changes [new or presumed new significant ST-segment-T wave (ST-T) changes or new left bundle branch block (LBBB) or development of pathological Q waves in the ECG], or (c) angiographic findings consistent with procedural complication (angiographic loss of patency of a major coronary artery or a side branch, or persistent slow- or no-flow or embolization), or (d) imaging

demonstration of new loss of viable} were also used and analyzed post hoc.

Per protocol PMI (WHO definition) occurred in 13/335 (3.9%) in the ABSORB arm and 2/166 (1.2%) in the EES arm ($p = 0.16$) (Table 8.6.3). We have reviewed as post hoc analysis that the PMI rates according to the third universal definition and the SCAI definition were 14.2% versus 10.6% and 0.6% vs. 0.6%, respectively (Table 8.6.3). Incidence of PMI per protocol according to "anatomic complications" assessed by angiography was similar between the two treatment arms. When the clinical adjudication was based on the combination of cardiac biomarker rise, ECG, and clinical symptoms, the impact of using different cut-points of cardiac biomarker rise on the PMI was not so emphasized. However, if the criteria solely based on cardiac biomarker (i.e., SCAI definition), the availability of cardiac biomarker influences the results. In the SCAI definition, CKMB is recommended at the first place and troponin is only used in the absence of CKMB. In the same population, the PMI rate of the SCAI definition could vary from 0.6% (100% CKMB available) to 2.7% (CKMB not available). This dataset is

Table 8.6.2 Anatomic complications assessed by angiography

| Per patient analysis | ABSORB (N = 335 pts) | EES (N = 166 pts) | p value |
|---|---|---|---|
| Any anatomic complications assessed by angiography | 16.4% (56/335) | 19.9% (33/166) | 0.39 |
| Type 1 anatomic complication assessed by angiography | – | – | – |
|   Side-branch occlusion, % (N) | 12.5% (43/335) | 15.7% (26/166) | 0.41 |
|   Side-branch occlusion after predilatation | 0% (0/335) | 0% (0/166) | 1.00 |
|   Side-branch occlusion after device implantation | 12.5% (43/335) | 15.7% (26/166) | 0.41 |
|   Side-branch occlusion improvement after NTG | 0.9% (3/335) | 0% (0/166) | 0.55 |
|   Side-branch occlusion after procedure | 11.6% (40/335) | 15.7% (26/166) | 0.26 |
| Type 2 anatomic complication assessed by angiography | – | – | – |
|   Abrupt closure, % (N) | 0% (0/335) | 1.8% (2/166) | 0.11 |
|   Distal embolization, % (N) | 0.3% (1/335) | 0% (0/166) | 1.00 |
|   Coronary perforation, % (N) | 0.6% (2/335) | 0% (0/166) | 1.00 |
|   Flow limiting dissection (NHLBI type F), % (N) | 0.3% (1/335) | 0% (0/166) | 1.00 |
|   Coronary dissection after predilatation (NHLBI D or E), % (N) | 1.8% (6/335) | 1.2% (2/166) | 1.00 |
|   Coronary dissection after device implantation, % (N) | 0.3% (1/335) | 0.6% (1/166) | 1.00 |
|   Thrombus during procedure, % (N) | 0.3% (1/335) | 0% (0/166) | 1.00 |
|   Disruption of collateral flow, % (N) | 0.3% (1/335) | 1.2% (2/166) | 0.26 |
| **Per side branch analysis** | **N = 998 side-branches** | **N = 503 side-branches** | |
| Incidence of side branch occlusion after procedure | 5.3% (52/988) | 7.6% (39/503) | 0.07 |
| Location of occluded side branch | – | – | – |
|   Outside scaffold segment | 0% (0/988) | 0% (0/503) | 1.00 |
|   To-be-scaffold segment outside obstruction | 0.9% (9/988) | 1.0% (5/503) | 1.00 |
|   Obstruction segment | 4.3% (42/988) | 6.8% (34/503) | 0.046 |
| Reference vessel diameter of occluded side branch | – | – | – |
|   Reference vessel diameter > 1.0 mm | 0.9% (9/988) | 1.2% (6/503) | 0.59 |
|   0.5 < reference vessel diameter ≤ 1.0 mm | 2.9% (29/988) | 4.2% (21/503) | 0.22 |
|   Reference vessel diameter ≤ 0.5 mm | 1.3% (13/988) | 2.4% (12/503) | 0.14 |

*Abbreviations:* ABSORB = bioresorbablevascular scaffold(s); EES = everolimus-eluting metallic stent(s).

unique in that almost all patients have two types of cardiac biomarkers, irrespective of the presence of suspected symptoms for PMI.

In the Spirit IV trial which randomized 3687 patients in a 2:1 fashion to receive either everolimus eluting stents or paclitaxel eluting stents, the total stent length was a strong predictor of PMI by criteria using CK or troponin [19]. In the present study, by multivariable analysis, treatment with overlapping devices was the independent determinant of per protocol PMI (OR: 5.07, 95% CI:1.78–14.41, $p = 0.002$), while there was overall no significant difference in PMI between the two device types (ABSORB vs. EES). In the ABSORB arm, the treatment with overlapping was associated with risk of PMI with a 3.59 OR ($p = 0.03$), while it was not significantly different with a 5.07 OR ($p = 0.28$) in the EES arm. However, $p$ for interaction was not significantly different ($p$ for interaction, $p = 0.65$). One MI (non-Q-wave) was attributed to definite scaffold thrombosis involving overlapping scaffolds. Of note, in a juvenile porcine model [20], overlapping ABSORB scaffolds showed delayed healing on histology and OCT and slower tissue coverage than in nonoverlapping scaffolds: the coverage of the overlapping

segment was 80.1% and 99.5% at 28 and 90 days after implantation, respectively, suggesting that complete coverage in humans may take up to 18 months. Similar findings [21]—delayed healing and promotion of inflammation at sites of overlap—have been reported in the atherosclerotic rabbit model implanted with EES, suggesting the general detrimental effect and potential biohazard of overlapping devices. Adjacent implantation of scaffolds instead of true overlapping may circumvent this problem.

## TARGET VESSEL MI WITH RESPECT TO D$_{MAX}$

A total of 1248 patients received ABSORB scaffolds in the ABSORB Cohort B (ABSORB Clinical Investigation, Cohort B) study (N = 101), ABSORB EXTEND (ABSORB EXTEND Clinical Investigation) study (N = 812), and ABSORB II (ABSORB II Randomized Controlled Trial) trial (N = 335). The incidence of major adverse cardiac events (MACE) (a composite of cardiac death, any myocardial infarction [MI], and ischemia-driven target lesion revascularization) was analyzed according to the D$_{max}$

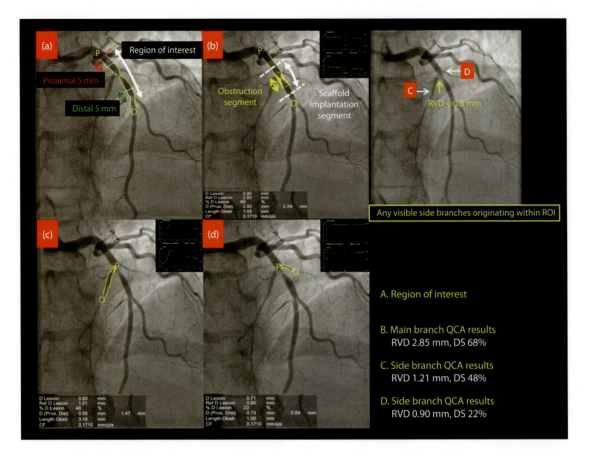

Figure 8.6.2 Preprocedural quantitative coronary angiography (QCA) analyses are shown. The QCA analysis delineates 5-mm proximal (**a**, red double arrow) and distal segment. (**a**, green double arrow) to the intended device implantation site (**b**, white double arrow). Any visible side branches originating from this region of interest were analyzed. The conventional QCA analysis automatically delineates an obstruction segment in the main branch (**b**, yellow double arrow). An example of side branch analysis is shown in (**c** and **d**). DS = diameter stenosis; RVD = reference vessel diameter.

Table 8.6.3 Incidence of periprocedural MI

|  | ABSORB arm | EES arm | *p* value |
|---|---|---|---|
| Per protocol PMI | 3.9% (13/335) | 1.2% (2/166) | 0.16 |
| SCAI definition PMI | 0.6% (2/315) | 0.6% (1/160) | 1.0 |
| TUD definition PMI | 14.6% (46/316) | 10.8% (17/157) | 0.31 |

*Abbreviations:* PMI = periprocedural myocardial infarction; SCAI = The Society for Cardiovascular Angiography and Interventions; TUD = The Universal Third.

($D_{max}$ is defined inside of the "landing zone") subclassification of scaffold oversize group versus scaffold nonoversize group. Of 1248 patients, preprocedural $D_{max}$ was assessed in 1232 patients (98.7%). In 649 (52.7%) patients, both proximal and distal $D_{max}$ values were smaller than the nominal size of the implanted scaffold (scaffold oversize group), whereas in 583 (47.3%) of the patients, the proximal and/or distal $D_{max}$ were larger than the implanted scaffold (scaffold nonoversize group). They clearly demonstrate that implanting ABSORB scaffolds in a vessel with both proximal and distal $D_{max}$ smaller than the device nominal size is associated with a higher risk of MACE (6.6% vs. 3.3%, $p < 0.01$). The difference in 1-year MACE was observed in the scaffold oversize group and was mainly driven by a higher MI rate (4.5% vs. 2.1%, $p < 0.01$). Scaffold expansion below nominal diameters can lead to a denser polymer surface pattern and a higher polymer-to-artery ratio. Furthermore, the expanding radial force may be suboptimal in these underdeployed configurations; presumably, these unfavorable final expansion diameters might cause microthrombus formation at the strut level and side-branch occlusion. However, no statistically significant difference in the incidence of overall angiographic complications could be documented at the end of the procedure for the patients who sustained MI within 1 month (scaffold oversize group: 3.1% vs. scaffold nonoversize group: 1.7%, $p = 0.14$) (Table 8.6.4).

**Table 8.6.4** Incidence of TVMI in scaffold oversize group versus scaffold nonoversize group

| | Scaffold oversize group (N = 649) | Scaffold nonoversize group (N = 583) | p value |
|---|---|---|---|
| TVMI at 12 months after index procedure, % (n) | 4.5 (29/649) | 2.1(12/583) | 0.025 |
| TVMI within 1 month after index procedure, % (n) | 3.5 (23/649) | 1.9 (11/583) | 0.08 |

*Abbreviation:* TVMI = target vessel myocardial infarction.

## CONCLUSIONS

1. There were no statistically significant differences in the incidence of CB rise and PMI between ABSORB and EES. Overlapping of scaffolds or stents might be a precipitating factor of myocardial injury. As demonstrated in the present study, which collected all three CB, binary definition of PMI is not only dependent on the selection of CB but also on the thresholds of the CB rise, which are arbitrarily chosen.

2. Implantation of an oversized ABSORB scaffold in a relatively small vessel appears to be associated with higher 1-year MACE rates driven by more frequent early MI.

## REFERENCES

1. Meier B, Gruentzig AR, King SB III et al. Risk of side branch occlusion during coronary angioplasty. *Am J Cardiol.* 1984;53:10–4.
2. Holmes DR Jr., Holubkov R, Vlietstra RE et al. Comparison of complications during percutaneous transluminal coronary angioplasty from 1977 to 1981 and from 1985 to 1986: The National Heart, Lung, and Blood Institute percutaneous transluminal coronary angioplasty registry. *J Am Coll Cardiol.* 1988;12:1149–55.
3. Porto I, Selvanayagam JB, Van Gaal WJ et al. Plaque volume and occurrence and location of periprocedural myocardial necrosis after percutaneous coronary intervention: Insights from delayed enhancement magnetic resonance imaging, thrombolysis in myocardial infarction myocardial perfusion grade analysis, and intravascular ultrasound. *Circulation.* 2006;114:662–9.
4. Califf RM, Abdelmeguid AE, Kuntz RE et al. Myonecrosis after revascularization procedures. *J Am Coll Cardiol.* 1998;31:241–51.
5. Prasad A, Singh M, Lerman A, Lennon RJ, Holmes DR Jr., Rihal CS. Isolated elevation in troponin T after percutaneous coronary intervention is associated with higher long-term mortality. *J Am Coll Cardiol.* 2006;48:1765–70.
6. Jensen LO, Maeng M, Kaltoft A et al. Stent thrombosis, myocardial infarction, and death after drug-eluting and bare-metal stent coronary interventions. *J Am Coll Cardiol.* 2007;50:463–70.
7. Fischman DL, Savage MP, Leon MB et al. Fate of lesion-related side branches after coronary artery stenting. *J Am Coll Cardiol.* 1993;22:1641–6.
8. Mazur W, Grinstead WC, Hakim AH et al. Fate of side branches after intracoronary implantation of the Gianturco-Roubin flex-stent for acute or threatened closure after percutaneous transluminal coronary angioplasty. *Am J Cardiol.* 1994;74:1207–10.
9. Farooq V, Serruys PW, Heo JH et al. New insights into the coronary artery bifurcation hypothesis-generating concepts utilizing 3-dimensional optical frequency domain imaging. *J Am Coll Cardiol Intv.* 2011;4:921–31.
10. Popma JJ, Mauri L, O'Shaughnessy C et al. Frequency and clinical consequences associated with sidebranch occlusion during stent implantation using zotarolimus-eluting and paclitaxel-eluting coronary stents. *Circ Cardiovasc Interv.* 2009;2:133–9.
11. Lansky AJ, Yaqub M, Hermiller JB et al. Side branch occlusion with everolimus-eluting and paclitaxel-eluting stents: Three-year results from the SPIRIT III randomised trial. *EuroIntervention.* 2010;6:J44–52.
12. Serruys PW, Ormiston JA, Onuma Y et al. A bioabsorbable everolimus-eluting coronary stent system (ABSORB): 2-year outcomes and results from multiple imaging methods. *Lancet.* 2009;373:897–910.
13. Ormiston JA, Serruys PW, Regar E et al. A bioabsorbable everolimus-eluting coronary stent system for patients with single de-novo coronary artery lesions (ABSORB): A prospective open-label trial. *Lancet.* 2008;371:899–907.
14. Serruys PW, Onuma Y, Dudek D et al. Evaluation of the second generation of a bioresorbable everolimus-eluting vascular scaffold for the treatment of de novo coronary artery stenosis: 12-month clinical and imaging outcomes. *J Am Coll Cardiol.* 2011;58:1578–88.
15. Serruys PW, Ormiston J, van Geuns RJ et al. A polylactide bioresorbable scaffold eluting everolimus for treatment of coronary stenosis: 5-year follow-up. *J Am Coll Cardiol.* 2016 23;67(7):766–76.
16. Muramatsu T, Onuma Y, Garcia-Garcia HM et al., for the ABSORB-EXTEND Investigators. Incidence and short-term clinical outcomes of small side branch occlusion after implantation of an everolimus-eluting bioresorbable vascular scaffold: An interim report of 435 patients in the ABSORB-EXTEND single-arm trial in comparison with an everolimus-eluting

metallic stent in the SPIRIT first and II trials. *J Am Coll Cardiol Intv*. 2013;6:247–57.

17. Serruys PW, Chevalier B, Dudek D et al. A bioresorbable everolimus-eluting scaffold versus a metallic everolimus-eluting stent for ischaemic heart disease caused by de-novo native coronary artery lesions (ABSORB II): An interim 1-year analysis of clinical and procedural secondary outcomes from a randomised controlled trial. *Lancet*. 2015;385:43–54.

18. Pervaiz MH, Sood P, Sudhir K et al. Periprocedural myocardial infarction in a randomized trial of everolimus-eluting and paclitaxel-eluting coronary stents: Frequency and impact on mortality according to historic versus universal definitions. *Circ Cardiovasc Interv*. 2012;5:150–6.

19. Park DW, Kim YH, Yun SC et al. Frequency, causes, predictors, and clinical significance of peri-procedural myocardial infarction following percutaneous coronary intervention. *Eur Heart J*. 2013;34:1662–9.

20. Farooq V, Serruys PW, Heo JH et al. Intracoronary optical coherence tomography and histology of overlapping everolimus-eluting bioresorbable vascular scaffolds in a porcine coronary artery model: The potential implications for clinical practice. *J Am Coll Cardiol Intv*. 2013;6:523–32.

21. Nakazawa G, Nakano M, Otsuka F et al. Evaluation of polymer-based comparator drug-eluting stents using a rabbit model of iliac artery atherosclerosis. *Circ Cardiovasc Interv*. 2011;4:38–46.

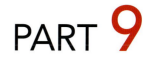# PART 9

# Tips and tricks to implant BRSs

# Tips and tricks for implanting BRSs: Sizing, pre- and postdilatation

AKIHITO TANAKA, RICHARD J. JABBOUR, AND ANTONIO COLOMBO

## INTRODUCTION

Bioresorbable scaffolds (BRSs) have numerous potential advantages over metallic stents due to the complete reabsorption process that occurs 3–4 years postimplantation [1].

Recent randomized trials have demonstrated noninferiority of BRSs to newer generation drug eluting stents (DESs) in relatively simple lesion subsets [2–6]. Furthermore, several real-world registries have reported acceptable outcomes even in complex lesions [7,8]. BRSs therefore are an attractive option for the interventional cardiology community and are increasingly being adopted into clinical practice.

Recent reports however have raised concerns about a higher incidence of scaffold thrombosis (ST) when compared to DESs [9,10]. The majority of events occurred within 30 days, and was most likely due to suboptimal implantation techniques leading to underexpansion and malapposition [11].

In contrast to BRSs, metallic stents have been used in clinical practice far longer, and progressive design iterations have resulted in easy to use devices, resulting in a less important role for procedural optimization strategies [12]. Current BRSs, however, have several limitations mainly due to the device's bulky struts, and are much less forgiving to poor implantation strategies. Therefore, the requirement of a dedicated implantation strategy is recommended to ensure the best possible clinical outcomes. In this chapter, we shall discuss the various tips and tricks to implant current generation BRSs.

## MECHANICAL AND PHYSICAL PROPERTIES OF BRSS

Several types of BRSs are in development [13] and currently the ABSORB BRSs (Abbott Vascular, Santa Clara, CA) is most commonly used in clinical practice. BRSs are distinctly different in design from DESs. For example, the ABSORB BRSs has thicker struts than the XIENCE Xpedition (Abbott Vascular, Santa Clara, CA) metallic stent (157 μm vs. 89 μm, respectively) [14]. Similarly, the strut width is greater with ABSORB: 191 μm/140 μm hoop and link parts with a 3.0 mm ABSORB, and only 89 μm with Xpedition [14]. Larger struts lead to a greater percentage vessel wall device coverage (27% for 3.0 mm ABSORB vs. 13%) and larger crossing profiles (1.43 mm for 3.0 mm ABSORB vs. 1.14 mm) [14]. In addition, the devices are mounted on different balloons. The delivery balloon of the ABSORB scaffold is highly compliant and should not be inflated above the recommended nominal pressure in order to avoid overdilating lesion segments. This specific feature demands a need for postdilatation. It is very important to appreciate these features when using current generation BRSs.

## PREDILATATION

Adequate lesion preparation is of paramount importance when implanting BRSs for both scaffold delivery and especially optimal scaffold expansion. BRSs have larger crossing profiles [14], and therefore reduced deliverability when compared to metallic DESs. Furthermore, current BRSs have reduced radial strength [14,15] and a tendency for greater acute recoil [16]. Although direct implantation is a possibility in soft lesions [17], since inadequate lesion preparation correlates with underexpansion [16,18,19], predilatation is recommended for almost all lesions. Either semi- or noncompliant balloons sized at 1:1 to vessel reference diameter can be used. Short noncompliant balloons inflated to high pressures are recommended if a balloon indentation remains. The operator must confirm complete expansion without indentation before BRSs deployment.

Furthermore, the use of adjunctive devices including cutting or scoring balloons is encouraged especially in heavily calcified lesions [20]. Importantly, clinicians should be aware of the compliance of these devices and they should be downsized in order to avoid excessive vessel injury. Although no clear evidence exists, operators should also have a low threshold to perform rotational atherectomy in lesions with a high calcific burden.

## BRSS SIZING

Due to the inherent limitations of BRSs, careful sizing before deployment is required [21]. First, large vessels (reference diameter >4.0 mm) are a contraindication to BRSs implantation because the largest ABSORB scaffold diameter is 3.5 mm with corresponding maximum post-implantation diameter of 4 mm. Expansion above this threshold can lead to breaks in scaffold struts. Second, it is important to note that an undersized BRSs can lead to malapposition, which is thought to be a major cause of both early and late scaffold thrombosis [11,22]. Malapposition is especially difficult to correct after deployment with BRSs due to the limited expansion capabilities of the device. Third, as described previously, an oversized scaffold increases the percentage of vessel coverage by BRSs, which may cause side branch occlusions (Figure 9.1.1) [23–25] and microthrombus formation [26]. In addition, edge dissections can occur postinflation. Hence, sizing of BRSs should be carefully done before implantation to avoid both over- and undersizing.

Although not mandatory, intravascular imaging for sizing is strongly recommended, especially in cases with diffuse disease, small vessel diameters, and large differences in diameter between proximal and distal landing sites. Quantitative coronary angiography can be used for objective estimation [26]; however, the operator should keep in mind it frequently underestimates the diameters particularly in diffuse disease.

BRSs should probably be avoided in target lesions with large differences in diameter (>0.5 mm) between proximal and distal ends. This is because malapposition could occur if undersized proximally, and if overexpanded the struts may fracture. Conversely, if oversized distally, vessel injury could occur on inflation and there will be an increased percentage of vessel wall device coverage.

## BRSS DELIVERY

The crossing profile of current BRSs is much larger than metallic stents, resulting in reduced deliverability. Therefore, sufficient lesion preparation is necessary to facilitate scaffold delivery. If difficulties arise in delivering BRSs across a lesion, the use of a more supportive wire or buddy wire technique may help. Additionally, the use of a child catheter may facilitate delivery [21,27]. All sizes of ABSORB BRSs can be delivered through a 7 Fr child catheter, for example, the Guideliner® 7F (Vascular Solutions, Inc., Minneapolis, MN). A 2.5 mm and 3.0 mm ABSORB BVSs can be delivered through a 6 Fr guide system with a child catheter. Examples include the 5 Fr

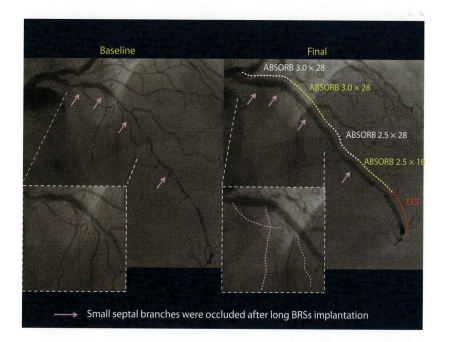

**Figure 9.1.1** A case of small side branch occlusions after BRSs implantation. Baseline angiogram demonstrated long diffuse disease in the left anterior descending artery involving multiple small branches. Four ABSORB BRSs and EESs were implanted over the entire length. Final angiogram revealed several septal branch occlusions. Pink dotted lines and arrows indicate occluded side branches. BRSs = bioresorbable scaffolds; EES = everolimus-eluting metallic stent.

Heratrail™ (Terumo, Tokyo, Japan) or Guideliner® 6 Fr; preloading into the extension tube outside the patient's body is recommended with the latter. Importantly, a 3.5 mm ABSORB BRSs cannot be delivered with a 6 Fr child catheter.

If resistance is felt when trying to deliver a BRSs, it is important to avoid continued attempts to advance the device due to the risk of dislodgement. There should be a low threshold in replacing the device when there is concern regarding scaffold distortion.

## IMPLANTATION TECHNIQUE

The ABSORB BRSs has two fluoroscopically visible platinum markers: the distal platinum marker is 0.3 mm proximal to the distal end and the proximal marker is at least 0.7 mm distal to the proximal end of the device. Both the proximal and distal ends of the scaffold are located on the balloon markers. When implanting BRSs in lesions that require multiple BRSs, it is important to know the relationship between the markers and scaffold body (Figure 9.1.2).

Although the clinical significance of overlapping scaffolds has not been clearly evaluated, it is of concern due to the increased strut thickness of current BRSs. The neointimal coverage of BRSs struts are delayed at the overlapping site [28], and also overlapping struts appear to be more thrombogenic [29]. A recent case report described

a case of coronary artery perforation occurring at the level of scaffold overlapping site, which was thought to be related to excessive vessel wall stretch [30]. Considering these concerns, strut overlap with current BRSs should be minimized [21]. Recently, we have adopted a "side by side" implantation technique to minimize overlap. We achieve this by placing the balloon marker of the proximal scaffold just before the scaffold marker of the distal scaffold (Figure 9.1.2).

Due to the bulky nature of the device, when implanting multiple BRSs in the same vessel, we recommend implanting distally to proximally in the majority of cases to avoid both the risk of not being able to pass a second BRSs through the proximal scaffold, and the possibility of strut fracture when crossing. When stenting ostially, which requires precise proximal positioning, we do implant from proximal to distal to control minimal overlapping. In such situations, high pressure postdilatation of the proximal BRSs should occur before implanting distally and care must also be taken when delivering the distal BRSs through the proximal scaffold.

During BRSs deployment, it is recommended to inflate gradually in 2 atm increments every 5 seconds [21]. Also long inflations (at least 30 seconds) may achieve better scaffold expansion [31]. The BRSs delivery balloon is more compliant than the metallic stent delivery balloon. Therefore, the operator should avoid using at high pressures, which can result in uneven balloon overexpansion

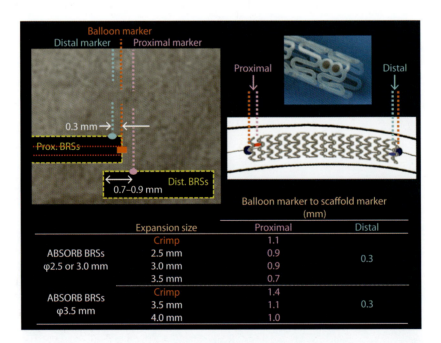

Figure 9.1.2 Relationship of balloon and scaffold markers to the proximal and distal edge of the scaffold. Fluoroscopic image (top left panel) demonstrates the relationship of the distal platinum scaffold marker, the balloon marker, and the scaffold. It can be seen (top right panel) that the BRSs edge is at the center of the balloon marker which is 0.3 mm distal to the distal scaffold platinum marker and between 0.7 and 1.4 mm proximal to the proximal scaffold platinum marker depending on scaffold and expansion size. BRSs = bioresorbable scaffolds.

and elongation, and the possibility of scaffold fractures and/or vessel injury [32].

## POSTDILATATION

Recent trials have demonstrated that the BRSs acute lumen gain was lower when compared to DESs when inflated to similar pressures even in simple lesion subsets [2–5]. An intravascular imaging study also indicated that BRSs expand more asymmetrically [33]. Caiazzo et al. reported that studies of BRSs, implantation with high postdilation rates (over 90%) and pressures (over 20 atm) were associated with lower rates of ST [34]. These data suggest the importance of high-pressure postdilation to achieve optimal expansion and better clinical outcomes [17,21,35,36]. It is important to stress that damage to the ABSORB scaffold occurs because of oversizing and not because of high pressure.

Overexpansion can cause strut disconnections and a focal loss of mechanical support [37]; therefore, judicious balloon sizing is important. Nonoversized noncompliant balloons (1:1 scaffold/postdilation balloon diameter) with high pressures (more than 20 atm) are an initial safe strategy [38]. When further postdilatation is required, higher pressures with the same balloon or a different balloon with diameter equal to scaffold size plus a maximum of 0.5 mm can be used.

## FINAL ASSESSMENT

As described above, BRSs. underexpansion is more common with current BRSs, (Figure 9.1.3). In addition, the need for more aggressive pre and postdilation to obtain optimal scaffold expansion may cause more frequent edge dissections (Figure 9.1.4). Prior reports have indicated malapposition and underexpansion to be the main causes of ST [4,11]. The latter also appears to be one of the predominant causes of restenosis [39]. It is frequently difficult to detect by angiographic assessment alone. A low threshold for intravascular imaging at the end of the procedure is recommended to confirm adequate expansion and evaluate the presence of edge injuries or malapposition, which may lead to better clinical outcomes [21]. In our experience, approximately 1 in 4 cases require further intervention based on intravascular imaging findings even after high pressure postdilatation.

## FLIP SIDE OF DEDICATED IMPLANTATION STRATEGY

On the flip side, higher procedural costs with longer procedure and fluoroscopy times and greater contrast use are inevitable [40]. However, this has to be balanced with the likely reduction in ST and in-scaffold restenosis when the previously mentioned strategies are utilized.

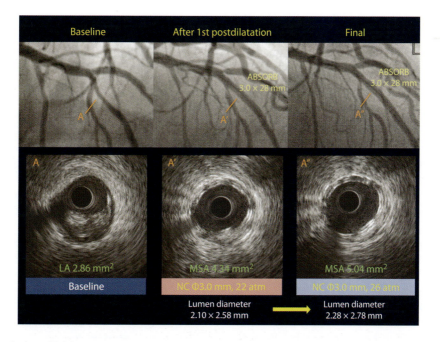

Figure 9.1.3 IVUS guided scaffold optimization. An ABSORB BRSs 3.0 × 28 mm was deployed after predilatation. After postdilatation with a 3.0 mm NC balloon (22 atm), the angiographic result seemed acceptable. MSA was 4.34 mm² by IVUS evaluation, and a further aggressive dilatation with the same NC balloon (26 atm) was then carried out. Final IVUS revealed an increase in MSA to 5.04 mm². This case illustrates the importance of intravascular imaging even after high-pressure postdilatation. IVUS = intravascular ultrasound; LA = lumen area; MSA = minimal scaffold area; NC = noncompliant; SA = scaffold area.

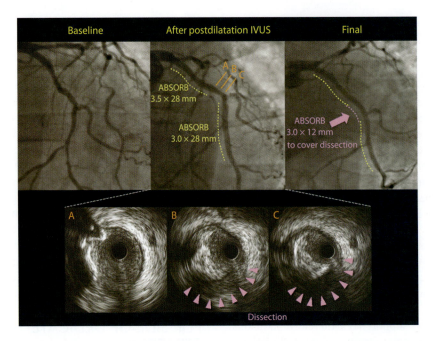

**Figure 9.1.4** Detection of edge dissections by IVUS. After predilation, a 3.0 × 28 mm and a 3.5 × 28 mm ABSORB BRSs were deployed to treat tandem lesions in the left circumflex artery, followed by postdilatation with a 3.0 mm NC balloon (20 atm) and a 3.5 mm NC balloon (20 atm), respectively. The angiographic result demonstrated a degree of stenosis at the gap between the two BRSs, but the angiographic result seemed acceptable. However, IVUS imaging detected a major edge dissection, and another ABSORB BRSs 3.0 × 12 mm was then deployed at the scaffold gap. IVUS = intravascular ultrasound.

## CONCLUSION

Current BRSs have several limitations, which make them less forgiving to suboptimal implantation techniques. As BRS use is becoming more frequent in daily clinical practice, we must keep it in mind that current generation BRSs require a dedicated implantation technique to maximize the chance of favorable clinical outcomes.

## REFERENCES

1. Onuma Y, Serruys PW. Bioresorbable scaffold: The advent of a new era in percutaneous coronary and peripheral revascularization? *Circulation.* 2011;123:779–97.
2. Ellis SG, Kereiakes DJ, Metzger DC, Caputo RP, Rizik DG, Teirstein PS, Litt MR et al. Everolimus-eluting bioresorbable scaffolds for coronary artery disease. *N Engl J Med.* 2015;373:1905–15.
3. Gao R, Yang Y, Han Y, Huo Y, Chen J, Yu B, Su X et al. Bioresorbable vascular scaffolds versus metallic stents in patients with coronary artery disease: ABSORB China trial. *J Am Coll Cardiol.* 2015;66:2298–309.
4. Kimura T, Kozuma K, Tanabe K, Nakamura S, Yamane M, Muramatsu T, Saito S et al. A randomized trial evaluating everolimus-eluting Absorb bioresorbable scaffolds vs. everolimus-eluting metallic stents in patients with coronary artery disease: ABSORB Japan. *Eur Heart J.* 2015;66:2298–309.
5. Serruys PW, Chevalier B, Dudek D, Cequier A, Carrie D, Iniguez A, Dominici M et al. A bioresorbable everolimus-eluting scaffold versus a metallic everolimus-eluting stent for ischaemic heart disease caused by de-novo native coronary artery lesions (ABSORB II): An interim 1-year analysis of clinical and procedural secondary outcomes from a randomised controlled trial. *Lancet.* 2015;385:43–54.
6. Puricel S, Arroyo D, Corpataux N, Baeriswyl G, Lehmann S, Kallinikou Z, Muller O et al. Comparison of everolimus- and biolimus-eluting coronary stents with everolimus-eluting bioresorbable vascular scaffolds. *J Am Coll Cardiol.* 2015;65:791–801.
7. Capodanno D, Gori T, Nef H, Latib A, Mehilli J, Lesiak M, Caramanno G et al. Percutaneous coronary intervention with everolimus-eluting bioresorbable vascular scaffolds in routine clinical practice: Early and midterm outcomes from the European multicentre GHOST-EU registry. *EuroIntervention.* 2014;10:1144–53.
8. Costopoulos C, Latib A, Naganuma T, Miyazaki T, Sato K, Figini F, Sticchi A et al. Comparison of early clinical outcomes between ABSORB bioresorbable vascular scaffold and everolimus-eluting stent implantation in a real-world population. *Cathet Cardiovasc Interv.* 2014;85:E10–5.
9. Lipinski MJ, Escarcega RO, Baker NC, Benn HA, Gaglia MA, Jr., Torguson R, Waksman R. Scaffold thrombosis after percutaneous coronary intervention

with ABSORB bioresorbable vascular scaffold: A systematic review and meta-analysis. *JACC Cardiovasc Interv.* 2016;9:12–24.

10. Cassese S, Byrne RA, Ndrepepa G, Kufner S, Wiebe J, Repp J, Schunkert H et al. Everolimus-eluting bioresorbable vascular scaffolds versus everolimus-eluting metallic stents: A meta-analysis of randomised controlled trials. *Lancet.* 2016;387:537–44.

11. Karanasos A, Van Mieghem N, van Ditzhuijzen N, Felix C, Daemen J, Autar A, Onuma Y et al. Angiographic and optical coherence tomography insights into bioresorbable scaffold thrombosis: Single-center experience. *Circ Cardiovasc Interv.* 2015 May;8(5).pii:e002369.

12. Colombo A, Ruparelia N. Who is thrombogenic: The scaffold or the doctor? Back to the future! *JACC Cardiovasc Interv.* 2016;9:25–7.

13. Wiebe J, Nef HM, Hamm CW. Current status of bioresorbable scaffolds in the treatment of coronary artery disease. *J Am Coll Cardiol.* 2014;64:2541–51.

14. Ormiston JA, Webber B, Ubod B, Darremont O, Webster MW. An independent bench comparison of two bioresorbable drug-eluting coronary scaffolds (Absorb and DESolve) with a durable metallic drug-eluting stent (ML8/Xpedition). *EuroIntervention.* 2015;11:60–7.

15. D'Ascenzo F, Frangieh AH, Templin C. Radial strength and expansion of scaffold struts remain a concern when considering a PCI with bioresorbable vascular scaffold. *Int J Cardiol.* 2015;191:254–5.

16. Danzi GB, Sesana M, Arieti M, Villa G, Rutigliano S, Aprile A, Nicolino A et al. Does optimal lesion preparation reduce the amount of acute recoil of the absorbe BVS? Insights from a real-world population. *Cathet Cardiovasc Interv.* 2015;86.984–991.

17. Suarez de Lezo J, Martin P, Mazuelos F, Novoa J, Ojeda S, Pan M, Segura J et al. Direct bioresorbable vascular scaffold implantation: Feasibility and midterm results. *Cathet Cardiovasc Interv.* 2015 Aug 13. doi:10.1002/ccd.26133.

18. Mattesini A, Secco GG, Dall'Ara G, Ghione M, Rama-Merchan JC, Lupi A, Vicenconte N et al. ABSORB biodegradable stents versus second-generation metal stents: A comparison study of 100 complex lesions treated under OCT guidance. *JACC Cardiovasc Interv.* 2014;7:741–50.

19. Brown AJ, McCormick LM, Braganza DM, Bennett MR, Hoole SP, West NE. Expansion and malapposition characteristics after bioresorbable vascular scaffold implantation. *Cathet Cardiovasc Interv.* 2014;84:37–45.

20. Miyazaki T, Panoulas VF, Sato K, Latib A, Colombo A. Bioresorbable vascular scaffolds for heavily calcified lesions: How to tackle the rugged passage? *J Invasive Cardiol.* 2015;27:E167–8.

21. Tamburino C, Latib A, van Geuns RJ, Sabate M, Mehilli J, Gori T, Achenbach S et al. Contemporary practice and technical aspects in coronary intervention with bioresorbable scaffolds: A European perspective. *EuroIntervention.* 2015;11:45–52.

22. Raber L, Brugaletta S, Yamaji K, O'Sullivan CJ, Otsuki S, Koppara T, Taniwaki M et al. Very late scaffold thrombosis: Intracoronary imaging and histopathological and spectroscopic findings. *J Am Coll Cardiol.* 2015;66:1901–14.

23. Kawamoto H, Jabbour RJ, Tanaka A, Latib A, Colombo A. The bioresorbable scaffold: Will oversizing affect outcomes? *JACC Cardiovasc Interv.* 2016;9:299–300.

24. Sato K, Panoulas VF, Kawamoto H, Naganuma T, Miyazaki T, Latib A, Colombo A. Side branch occlusion after bioresorbable vascular scaffold implantation: Lessons from optimal coherence tomography. *JACC Cardiovasc Interv.* 2015;8:116–8.

25. Muramatsu T, Onuma Y, Garcia-Garcia HM, Farooq V, Bourantas CV, Morel MA, Li X et al. Incidence and short-term clinical outcomes of small side branch occlusion after implantation of an everolimus-eluting bioresorbable vascular scaffold: An interim report of 435 patients in the ABSORB-EXTEND single-arm trial in comparison with an everolimus-eluting metallic stent in the SPIRIT first and II trials. *JACC Cardiovasc Interv.* 2012;6:247–57.

26. Ishibashi Y, Nakatani S, Sotomi Y, Suwannasom P, Grundeken MJ, Garcia-Garcia HM, Bartorelli AL et al. Relation between bioresorbable scaffold sizing using QCA-Dmax and clinical outcomes at 1 year in 1,232 patients from 3 study cohorts (ABSORB Cohort B, ABSORB EXTEND, and ABSORB II). *JACC Cardiovasc Interv.* 2015;8:1715–26.

27. Naganuma T, Ishiguro H, Panoulas VF, Fujino Y, Mitomo S, Kawamoto H, Nakamura S et al. Which child catheter should we choose to deliver a bulky bioresorbable vascular scaffold? *Int J Cardiol.* 2016;203:781–2.

28. Farooq V, Serruys PW, Heo JH, Gogas BD, Onuma Y, Perkins LE, Diletti R et al. Intracoronary optical coherence tomography and histology of overlapping everolimus-eluting bioresorbable vascular scaffolds in a porcine coronary artery model: The potential implications for clinical practice. *JACC Cardiovasc Interv.* 2013;6:523–32.

29. Kolandaivelu K, Swaminathan R, Gibson WJ, Kolachalama VB, Nguyen-Ehrenreich KL, Giddings VL, Coleman L et al. Stent thrombogenicity early in high-risk interventional settings is driven by stent design and deployment and protected by polymer-drug coatings. *Circulation.* 2011;123:1400–9.

30. Pichette M, Chevalier F, Genereux P. Coronary artery perforation at the level of two-overlapping bioresorbable vascular scaffolds: The importance of vessel sizing and scaffold thickness. *Cathet Cardiovasc Interv.* 2015;86:686–91.

31. Sorrentino S, De Rosa S, Ambrosio G, Mongiardo A, Spaccarotella C, Polimeni A, Sabatino J et al. The duration of balloon inflation affects the luminal diameter of coronary segments after bioresorbable vascular scaffolds deployment. *BMC Cardiovasc Disord.* 2015;15:169.

32. Kawamoto H, Jabbour RJ, Tanaka A, Latib A, Colombo A. Contained coronary rupture following bioresorbable scaffold implantation in a small vessel. *Int J Cardiol.* 2016;209:24–25.

33. Brugaletta S, Gomez-Lara J, Diletti R, Farooq V, van Geuns RJ, de Bruyne B, Dudek D et al. Comparison of in vivo eccentricity and symmetry indices between metallic stents and bioresorbable vascular scaffolds: Insights from the ABSORB and SPIRIT trials. *Cathet Cardiovasc Interv.* 2012;79:219–28.

34. Caiazzo G, Kilic ID, Fabris E, Serdoz R, Mattesini A, Foin N, De Rosa S et al. Absorb bioresorbable vascular scaffold: What have we learned after 5 years of clinical experience? *Int J Cardiol.* 2015;201:129–136.

35. Belardi JA, Albertal M. Bioresorbable drug-eluting scaffold restenosis: Larger is probably better. *Cathet Cardiovasc Interv.* 2015;85:1162–3.

36. Naganuma T, Latib A, Panoulas VF, Sato K, Miyazaki T, Colombo A. Why do we need post-dilation after implantation of a bioresorbable vascular scaffold even for a soft lesion? *JACC Cardiovasc Interv.* 2014;7:1070–2.

37. Foin N, Lee R, Mattesini A, Caiazzo G, Fabris E, Kilic D, Chan JN et al. Bioabsorbable vascular scaffold overexpansion: Insights from in vitro post-expansion experiments. *EuroIntervention.* 2015;11. pii:20141213–04.

38. Fabris E, Caiazzo G, Kilic ID, Serdoz R, Secco GG, Sinagra G, Lee R et al. Is high pressure postdilation safe in bioresorbable vascular scaffolds? Optical coherence tomography observations after noncompliant balloons inflated at more than 24 atmospheres. *Cathet Cardiovasc Interv.* 2015. doi: 10.1002/ccd.26222.

39. Longo G, Granata F, Capodanno D, Ohno Y, Tamburino CI, Capranzano P, La Manna A et al. Anatomical features and management of bioresorbable vascular scaffolds failure: A case series from the GHOST registry. *Cathet Cardiovasc Interv.* 2015;85:1150–61.

40. Sato K, Latib A, Panoulas VF, Kawamoto H, Naganuma T, Miyazaki T, Colombo A. Procedural feasibility and clinical outcomes in propensity-matched patients treated with bioresorbable scaffolds vs. new-generation drug-eluting stents. *Can J Cardiol.* 2015;31:328–34.

# Approach to bifurcation lesions

ASHOK SETH AND BABU EZHUMALAI

---

**Patient: D.K.S.**

- 53-year-old male
- Diabetic
- Presented with breathlessness on exertion (NYHA Class III)
- Echo: LVEF 55%
- CT coronary angiography showed LAD (90%) and diagonal (90%) bifurcation lesion

---

**Patient: M.G.D.**

- 63-year-old male
- Hypertensive
- Presented with chronic stable angina (CCS Class III)
- Echo: LVEF 60%
- Coronary angiography revealed mid-RCA 80% lesion → treated with ABSORB BVSs 3.5 × 18 mm; calcified LAD/D2 bifurcation lesion Medina 1,1,1

---

**Patient: G.D.S.**

- 62-year-old male
- Recent anterior wall STEMI (not thrombolyzed)
- Echo: LVEF 55%
- Coronary angiography revealed bifurcation lesion (Medina 1,1,1) involving proximal LAD and first large diagonal

---

**Patient: V.S.S.**

- 68-year-old male
- Diabetic for 14 years
- Hypertensive
- Quit smoking 3 years ago
- Presented with breathlessness on exertion (NYHA Class III)
- Echo: LVEF 55%
- Underwent coronary angiography which revealed CAD TVD
- Ostium of PDA showed 90% lesion and it was treated with XIENCE V 2.25 × 18 mm
- Distal LM bifurcation lesion Medina 0,1,1 involving osteum of LAD and circumflex arteries
- Calcified lesion extending from osteoproximal to mid-LAD

---

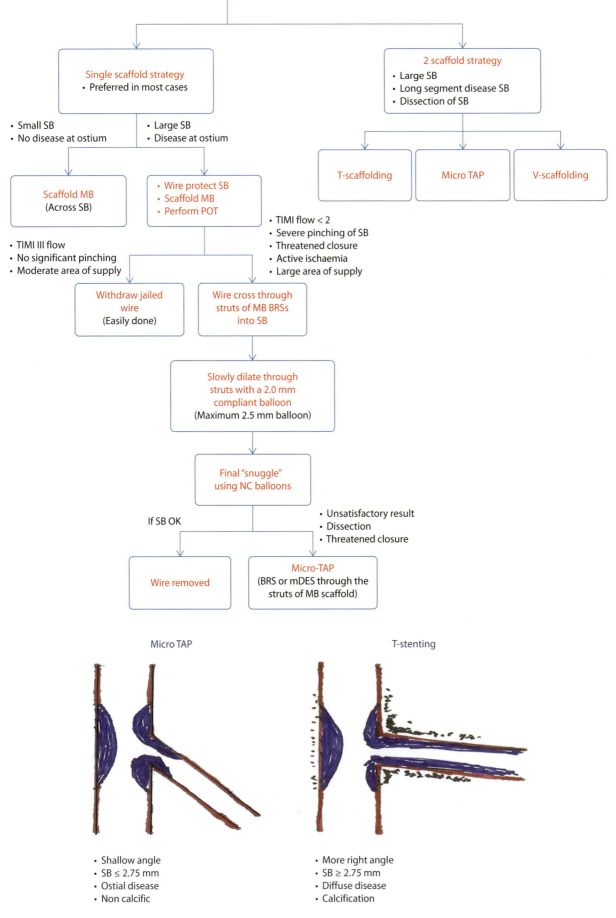

Single scaffold strategy
• Preferred in most cases

2 scaffold strategy
• Large SB
• Long segment disease SB
• Dissection of SB

• Small SB
• No disease at ostium

• Large SB
• Disease at ostium

T-scaffolding

Micro TAP

V-scaffolding

Scaffold MB
(Across SB)

• Wire protect SB
• Scaffold MB
• Perform POT

• TIMI flow < 2
• Severe pinching of SB
• Threatened closure
• Active ischaemia
• Large area of supply

• TIMI III flow
• No significant pinching
• Moderate area of supply

Withdraw jailed wire
(Easily done)

Wire cross through struts of MB BRSs into SB

Slowly dilate through struts with a 2.0 mm compliant balloon
(Maximum 2.5 mm balloon)

Final "snuggle" using NC balloons

If SB OK

• Unsatisfactory result
• Dissection
• Threatened closure

Wire removed

Micro-TAP
(BRS or mDES through the struts of MB scaffold)

Micro TAP

T-stenting

• Shallow angle
• SB ≤ 2.75 mm
• Ostial disease
• Non calcific

• More right angle
• SB ≥ 2.75 mm
• Diffuse disease
• Calcification

Tips for V-scaffolding

a.  Two 2.5 mm ABSORB™ go through a 7F large lumen guiding catheter. However not possible to insert two 3.0 mm/3.3 mm ABSORB.

b.  Thus, an ABSORB BRSs in branch A + balloon in branch B followed by an ABSORB BRSs in branch B and a balloon in branch A.

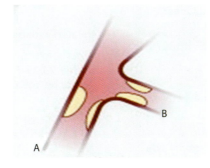

c.  ABSORB™ to go in first through guide followed by balloon, not vice versa, as even the shaft of a balloon provides resistance when large profile 3.0 mm or 3.5 mm ABSORB is passed through a 7F guiding catheter.

**Final "snuggle"**
Not a kissing balloon
(Low pressure simultaneous dilatation with very little protrusion of SB balloon into the MB)

**To lie or curl up together closely and comfortably**

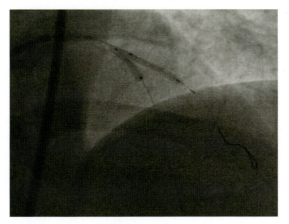

Final snuggle
3 × 12 NC balloon in LAD and 2.5 × 15 NC balloon in D1 at 7 atm

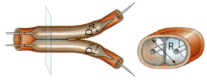  **Do not recommend** high pressure kissing balloon

# VIDEOS

## DKS

Video 9.2.1  Baseline coronary angiography demonstrating LAD and diagonal bifurcation lesion (Medina 0.1.1.): https://youtu.be/t70uLLA4dLk.

Video 9.2.2  Pre-dilatation of LAD and diagonal with non-compliant balloon: https://youtu.be/DJoWqjQnesY.

Video 9.2.3  Absorb BRS is deployed in LAD: https://youtu.be/-n94MwYV7OY.

Video 9.2.4  Proximal optimization technique: https://youtu.be/IouEH5FD4rc.

Video 9.2.5  Guidewire crossing into the diagonal side branch through the struts of main branch LAD: https://youtu.be/VjuBIXh-3Hc.

Video 9.2.6  Struts of the main branch crossed and dilated with 2mm compliant balloon: https://youtu.be/qCqXMvH227Y.

Video 9.2.7  Absorb BRS negotiated through the struts of main branch into diagonal side branch: https://youtu.be/psr32rpQ1R4.

Video 9.2.8  Micro-TAP technique: https://youtu.be/jVVB8GajDlc.

Video 9.2.9  Final snuggle balloon dilatation: https://youtu.be/hop7WXfxfMc.

Video 9.2.10  Final result: https://youtu.be/dsn7zEO2km0.

Video 9.2.11  OCT run: https://youtu.be/7ipz09uAEmU.

## GDS

Video 9.2.12  Coronary angiography demonstrating LAD and diagonal bifurcation lesion (medina 1.1.1.); plan: two scaffold strategy (T stenting): https://youtu.be/s_DKFwXvU1g.

Video 9.2.13  Pre-dilatation of side branch (diagonal) and main branch (LAD) with non-compliant balloons: https://youtu.be/pm4HBLUFoNY.

Video 9.2.14  Deployment of Absorb BRS in side branch: https://youtu.be/ptm6kN6zdR4.

Video 9.2.15  Post-dilatation of side branch with non-compliant balloon: https://youtu.be/X75E1rj_l-I.

Video 9.2.16  Deployment of Absorb BRS in LAD followed by post-dilatation: https://youtu.be/_8FNVT0nA9I.

Video 9.2.17  Guidewire crossing into the diagonal side branch through the struts of main branch LAD: https://youtu.be/eg3nU5HPQTo.

Video 9.2.18  Struts of the main branch crossed and dilated with balloon: https://youtu.be/Dg4qAxUf5jA.

Video 9.2.19  Final snuggle balloon dilatation: https://youtu.be/tgKx3NWxJMw.

Video 9.2.20  Coronary angiography depicting T stenting of LAD and diagonal: https://youtu.be/q4TxpDI4H4c.

Video 9.2.21  Dissection in proximal LAD: https://youtu.be/cT2fQ9KvaLA.

Video 9.2.22  Absorb BRS deployed in ostioproximal LAD: https://youtu.be/tqPq9bXv8uk.

Video 9.2.23  CT coronary angiography performed at 1 year of follow-up: https://youtu.be/3BomswOqicc.

## MGD

Video 9.2.24  Coronary angiography demonstrating calcified LAD and diagonal bifurcation lesion (medina 1.1.1.).

Video 9.2.25  Rotational atherectomy of LAD performed with 1.5mm burr: https://youtu.be/2IDMMqHZ2fg.

Video 9.2.26  Rotational atherectomy of diagonal also performed with 1.5mm burr: https://youtu.be/jBSlD366dqI.

Video 9.2.27  Pre-dilatation of LAD with non-compliant balloon: https://youtu.be/TYrWQTK1xpE.

Video 9.2.28  Absorb BRS deployed in distal LAD and then post-dilated: https://youtu.be/7mL42nx7PRM.

Video 9.2.29  Pre-dilatation of Diagonal with non-compliant balloon: https://youtu.be/OQn_nW1-pfE.

Video 9.2.30  Absorb BRS deployed in LAD at the bifurcation: https://youtu.be/EIpqJMTztXA.

Video 9.2.31  Absorb BRS being passed through the struts of main branch into side branch: https://youtu.be/-a9rISdt64Q.

Video 9.2.32 Deployment of Absorb BRS in diagonal; micro-TAP technique: https://youtu.be/EGgC8SHw5fc.

Video 9.2.33 Final simultaneous snuggle balloon dilatation: https://youtu.be/_s3DSAWGmR4.

Video 9.2.34 Angiography demonstrating good result at bifurcation but dissection in distal diagonal: https://youtu.be/QuOGspE2U5U.

Video 9.2.35 Deployment of Absorb BRS in distal diagonal: https://youtu.be/g3JNsJyJmjQ.

Video 9.2.36 Marker-to-marker overlap of scaffolds in diagonal followed by post-dilatation: https://youtu.be/0JqK-qROgH0.

Video 9.2.37 Final result: https://youtu.be/Jxw-pkxbGsM.

Video 9.2.38 OCT run: https://youtu.be/M8f_dB2INmo.

## VSS

Video 9.2.39 Coronary angiography demonstrating distal left main bifurcation lesion (Medina 0.1.1) involving ostioproximal LAD and ostial LCX: https://youtu.be/bOMv1MAN4sQ.

Video 9.2.40 Rotational atherectomy of calcified lesion in LAD: https://youtu.be/wCPDE_JH4SE.

Video 9.2.41 Pre-dilatation of the lesion with non-compliant balloon: https://youtu.be/iv6TVuNqECM.

Video 9.2.42 Deployment of Absorb BVS in mid LAD and post-dilatation with non-compliant balloon: https://youtu.be/XdYgsBRuful.

Video 9.2.43 Deployment of Absorb BVS in proximal LAD and post-dilatation with non-compliant balloon: https://youtu.be/lQkfHTX9SQA.

Video 9.2.44 Ostium of LAD and LCX were dilated with cutting balloon: https://youtu.be/LqVuf_sXuaQ.

Video 9.2.45 V-stenting of LAD and LCX: https://youtu.be/JAfZfHeLEl0.

Video 9.2.46 V-stenting performed using Absorb BVS in one branch and non-compliant balloon in another branch: https://youtu.be/i-TxJ3M_qJA.

Video 9.2.47 Final simultaneous v dilatation with balloons in LAD and LCX: https://youtu.be/z_0KSF7_auY.

Video 9.2.48 Final result: https://youtu.be/ZaHYprRMfwk.

# PART 10

# Emerging technologies (pre-CE mark, pre-FA, pre-PMDA, and pre-CFDA)

# Abbott: Current and next generation ABSORB scaffold

LAURA E. LEIGH PERKINS, BYRON J. LAMBERT, AND RICHARD J. RAPOZA

Permanent drug eluting stents (DESs) have revolutionized the interventional treatment of obstructive coronary artery disease (CAD); though accruing evidence indicates that, through a variety of mechanisms, the permanence of DESs detracts from their serving as the panacea for CAD [1,2]. Bioresorbable scaffolds serve as a novel approach to circumvent the shortcomings of permanent metallic implants by offering similar performance attributes to restore patency to occluded coronary arteries and prevent restenosis, but then superseding the basic mechanical and pharmacologic DESs functionality by benignly resorbing, thus allowing for the restoration of more normal arterial function. The ABSORB™ bioresorbable vascular scaffold (BVSs) (Abbott Vascular, Santa Clara, CA) has set the stage for the new bioresorbable era as the lead technology of its kind, demonstrating through novel endpoints that the potential advantages of this technology appear to be significant. In this chapter, the design and performance features of the ABSORB BVSs are detailed.

## SCAFFOLD COMPOSITION

The ABSORB BVSs is a balloon-expandable, drug-eluting device composed of the following components:

- A bioresorbable poly(L-lactide) (PLLA) scaffold backbone
- A coating comprised of the active pharmaceutical ingredient everolimus and bioresorbable poly(D,L-lactide) (PDLLA)
- Four platinum marker beads, two each embedded at the proximal and distal ends of the scaffold for radiopacity
- A delivery system that leverages technology advancements of the XIENCE family of products, incorporating design features from the XIENCE Xpedition® and XIENCE Alpine™ delivery systems

## PROCESS DEVELOPMENT

Development of a bioresorbable vascular scaffold and delivery system to meet the clinical and regulatory needs requires a broad cross-functional product development team. In brief, the manufacturing process for these systems includes manufacture of a balloon catheter; manufacture of the BVSs proper–extrusion, expansion, and lasing; coating of the scaffold with the drug/active agent; crimping the coated scaffold onto the balloon catheter; sealing the device into a sterile barrier package [3]; and terminal sterilization [4,5] of the finished product.

## MECHANICAL PROPERTIES

### Expansion capability

The ABSORB BVSs system allows for postdilatation of 0.5 mm above the nominal deployment diameter. Thus, for the 3.0 mm labeled product, the postdilatation diameter is 3.5 mm.

### Recoil

Minimizing acute scaffold recoil ensures that the final deployed diameter of a scaffold is representative of the labeled diameter of the scaffold and delivery system. Moreover, low recoil improves apposition to the vessel wall, providing the appropriate geometry for vessel support and limiting acute lumen area loss. Investigations have demonstrated that the *in vivo* acute stent recoil of the ABSORB BVSs is slightly higher though not significantly different from that of the XIENCE V™ (Abbott Vascular, Santa Clara, CA) [6,7].

### Radial strength

Radial strength is the attribute that describes a device's ability to support the vessel. A principal design objective of the

ABSORB BVSs is to maintain vessel support for a minimum of 3 months in order to forego acute recoil, minimize constrictive remodeling, and maintain lumen patency until the vessel has stabilized following revascularization; this design objective has been confirmed through radial strength testing [8]. However, unlike metallic stents, the supportive ability of ABSORB BVSs dissipates as the PLLA degrades (Figure 10.1.1). When the PLLA scaffold backbone number average molecular weight ($M_n$) has decreased sufficiently, radial strength also declines. Additionally, examination of samples following radial strength testing has revealed that scaffold discontinuities became increasingly prevalent following the 12-month time point, thus further contributing to the programmed decline of radial strength and the scaffold's assumed passivity.

## MECHANISM OF BIORESORPTION

Hydrolysis is the governing mechanism for the degradation of PLA *in vivo* and *in vitro* and results in the successive loss of molecular weight, strength, and mass (Figure 10.1.1). As the degradation of PLA occurs through bulk degradation, the molecular weight degradation and mass loss profiles are consistent between different scaffold sizes available in the ABSORB product matrix. The PLLA and PDLLA of ABSORB degrade to L- and D-lactic acid, which is readily converted to lactate. Lactate is in turn metabolized into carbon dioxide and water via the Krebs cycle and also serves as a source of energy in anaerobic metabolism.

## PERFORMANCE PROFILE

The performance profile of ABSORB BVSs is described by three phases that span its lifecycle: *revascularization*, *restoration*, and *resorption*. These phases parallel the generalized description of degradation for PLA, where molecular weight, strength, and mass successively begin to decline (Figure 10.1.1). The initial molecular weight and the rate of molecular weight degradation govern the time scales associated with loss of support and loss of mass; therefore, the time scales presented herein are unique for ABSORB BVSs based on its 100 kDa starting $M_n$.

During the initial phase of *revascularization* (implant to 6 months), the ABSORB BVSs maintains radial strength relative to only a minor decline in molecular weight (ca. 24%) [9]. During this initial performance phase, the artery stabilizes to its newly restored patency, and struts become sequestered in a benign, re-endothelialized neointima [10]. From 6 to 18 months, the phase of *restoration*, the ABSORB BVSs transitions from its DESs-like functionality to a passive device due to its progressive and collective decline in molecular weight (ca. 74% decrease) and acquisition of discontinuities. This phasic transition allows for a gradual transition of function from the scaffold to the artery, and sets the stage for the potential benefits detailed hereafter. After approximately 18 months, ABSORB is largely a passive device undergoing benign *resorption*, the third and final phase of its performance profile. The scaffold is completely degraded by approximately 36 months postimplant. Importantly, as

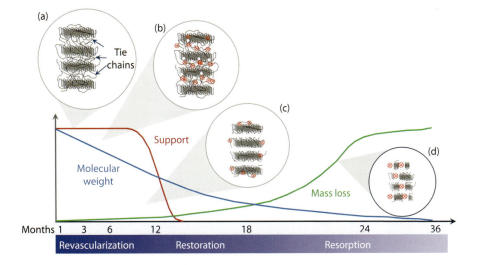

Figure 10.1.1 Conceptual representation of performance characteristics of ABSORB BVSs. **(a)** ABSORB BVSs is composed of PLLA, a semicrystalline polymer that includes crystallites (load-bearing elements) and amorphous tie chains (binders). **(b)** Initially, hydrolysis preferentially cleaves amorphous tie chains, leading to a decrease in molecular weight (blue) without altering radial strength. **(c)** When enough tie chains are broken, there is a decrease in the radial support offered by the scaffold (red). **(d)** Mass loss (green) begins when lactide monomers/oligomers are sufficiently small to escape the matrix and can be resorbed into the tissue to ultimately be metabolized into carbon dioxide and water via the Krebs cycle. (From Perkins L, Sheehy A, Lane J, Kamberi M, Benham J, Kossuth MB et al. Mechanistic insight into the transitional performance of a bioresorbable vascular scaffold: A correlation of in vitro and in vivo methods. Annual Meeting of the International Society of Applied Cardiovascular Biology, Cleveland, OH, 2014.)

PLA degradation is hydrolytically driven, this time scale is largely independent of species and the disease state [11,12]. Through the later stages of the resorption process, the preexisting struts of the ABSORB BVSs are progressively integrated into the arterial wall by connective tissue replacement to yield an artery with minimal evidence of the preexisting scaffold.

## DRUG ELUTION PROFILE

The ABSORB BVSs is coated with everolimus, a semisynthetic antiproliferative macrolide, in PDLLA in a 1:1 drug:polymer ratio. PDLLA, being more amorphous than PLLA, is used to contain and control the release of everolimus. The ABSORB BVSs has the same 100 μg/cm² everolimus dose density as the XIENCE family of drug-eluting stents (DESs). Preclinical pharmacokinetic studies have demonstrated that the ABSORB BVSs maintains a statistically bioequivalent drug release profile to that of the XIENCE V, with 78% everolimus elution at 28 days and 96% everolimus elution at 90 days [9]. Therapeutic concentrations of everolimus are maintained in target arteries for at least 28 days following implantation while maintaining a safe systemic profile.

## POTENTIAL ADVANTAGES OF THE TECHNOLOGY

DESs have revolutionized percutaneous coronary intervention (PCI), reducing the potential for target lesion revascularization (TLR) from near 30% with BMS to less than 10% [13]. However, with patients living longer after PCI, a "rebound effect" has been noted with DESs whereby the problem with TLR at 1 year with BMS has been shifted to 5 to 10 years with DESs [14–17]. Delayed vascular healing [1], chronic inflammation related to the durable polymeric material used in the controlled drug release formulations and/or the permanent metallic platform [18,19], late acquired malapposition [20], stent fracture [21], and neoatherosclerosis [22–24] are some of the means by which the adverse outcomes of in-stent restenosis and/or late and very late stent thrombosis have been attributed to DESs use [1,23,25–27]. Additional drawbacks attributed to the use of permanent implants include: distortion of vessel angulation and flow dynamics, restriction of vascular motion, hindrance both of future vascularization as well as of noninvasive imaging and impairment of access and flow to side branches [28–30]. Each of these handicaps of permanent implants may be circumvented through the use of a bioresorbable scaffold.

Preclinical and clinical evidence accrued to date on the ABSORB BVSs have provided valuable insight into the potential benefits of this next generation technology whereby the performance of ABSORB supersedes the basic mechanical and pharmacological functionality of DESs by benignly resorbing and allowing the treated

artery to adapt and remodel. Preclinical studies conducted in normal porcine coronary arteries have illustrated progressive lumen gain via expansive vascular remodeling [9,31], normalization of in-segment lumen area with the reference vessel, and both restoration of in-segment pulsatility [31] and vasomotility [32], with each of these potential benefits being coordinated with the projected loss of the scaffold's *in vivo* radial strength around 12 months postimplant (Figure 10.1.2) [8]. These benefits of ABSORB have been obtained while maintaining an *in vivo* safety profile comparable to that of XIENCE V [9].

These preclinical indicators, while obtained in non-diseased coronary arteries, have aptly foreshadowed both the clinical safety and efficacy of the ABSORB BVSs and the same technology-unique outcomes of lumen gain and a restoration of vasomotility reported in ABSORB clinical trials [10,12,33,34]. In addition, plaque reduction has been observed clinically as a late observation (2 to 3 years) as a result of the changing dynamics and expansive remodeling that the ABSORB BVSs arteries undergo once the scaffold assumes a more passive role (Figure 10.1.3) [12]. Sequestration of the plaque ("capping") and the prevention of neoatherosclerosis are other potential benefits still under investigation clinically and preclinically in diseased porcine coronary arteries [35–38]. Exactly how these outcomes unique to this bioresorbable technology result in tangible clinical benefits remains to be elucidated, though results regarding a reduction of angina and of repeat revascularizations with ABSORB BVSs as compared to permanent implants have sparked the interest and enthusiasm of the interventional community (Figure 10.1.3) [39–41].

## STATUS OF REGULATORY APPROVAL

The ABSORB BVSs currently has CE approval and regulatory approval in multiple geographies including the United States, Japan, Korea, Taiwan, India, Brazil, Canada, and Australia and is seeking approval in China. ABSORB BVSs is marketed globally in over 80 countries, including Europe, the Middle East, and parts of Asia Pacific and Latin America.

## CONCLUSION

Abbott Vascular's ABSORB BVSs initiated the next era of commercial bioresorbable interventional technologies whose objective is to perform as well as the preceding permanent technologies while circumventing its shortcomings. The extensive *in vivo* imaging interrogations conducted clinically in ABSORB patients and preclinical investigations provide evidence that ABSORB BVSs may be able to perform as well as DESs while mitigating DES-associated risks and providing more durable, long-term efficacy through its unique performance profile as compared to permanent implants.

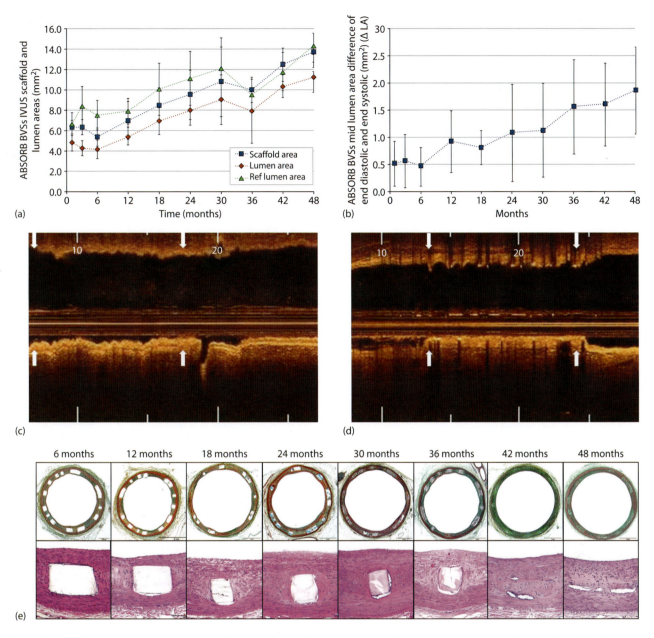

Figure 10.1.2 Graphical representation of benign expansive remodeling **(a)** and the restoration of pulsatility **(b)** observed in ABSORB BVSs implanted porcine coronary arteries based on intravascular ultrasound (IVUS); comparison in normalization of lumen area between ABSORB BVSs and XIENCE V implanted arteries assessed by optical coherence tomography (OCT) **(c, d)**; and vascular safety and benign integration of struts into the arterial wall illustrated histologically **(e)**. **(a)** IVUS reference vessel lumen area (green), scaffold area (blue), and lumen area (red) within the scaffolded region for ABSORB BVSs implanted arteries from 1 to 48 months. At 12 months and later time points, there is progressive and corresponding increase in each parameter, illustrating how ABSORB BVSs allows the artery to remodel in response to increased physiologic demand related to animal growth. **(b)** Absolute difference between end-diastolic and end-systolic mid-scaffold lumen area (ΔLA) in ABSORB BVSs implanted porcine coronary arteries from 1 to 48 months. Arteries demonstrate a continuous increase in ΔLA indicating a progressive return of pulsatility in the implanted region. **(c, d)** Longitudinal OCT pullbacks of ABSORB BVSs **(c)** and XIENCE V **(d)** implanted porcine coronary arteries at 42 to 48 months postimplant, illustrating the normalization in the lumen area of ABSORB BVSs implanted arteries. **(e)** Morphological changes in ABSORB BVSs implanted porcine coronary arteries which show progressive integration of connective tissue from 36 to 48 months, following complete degradation at 36 months. (Data adapted from Lane JP, Perkins LEL, Sheehy AJ, Pacheco EJ, Frie MP, Lambert BJ et al. *JACC Cardiovasc Interv.* 2014;7:688–95, and images on file with Abbott Vascular.)

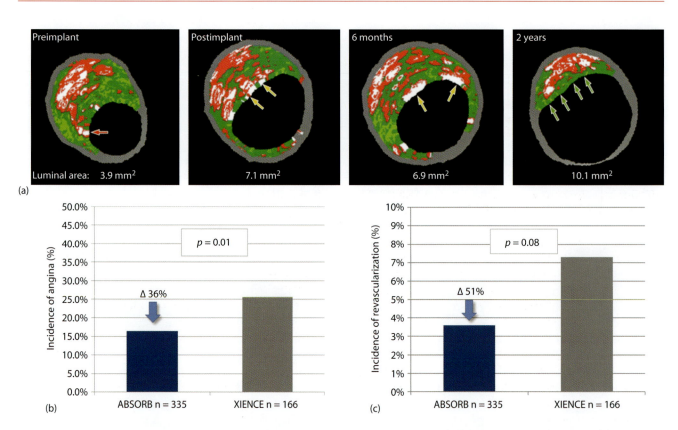

(a)

(b)

(c)

**Figure 10.1.3** Clinical results obtained from ABSORB Cohort A and ABSORB II clinical trials relating to lumen gain, capping of the plaque and plaque regression **(a)** and the reduction in the incidence of angina **(b)** and repeat revascularization **(c)**. **(a)** Serial assessment by (IVUS) radiofrequency backscattering. Prior to implantation, a large plaque with a necrotic core is evident, with the necrotic core being in contact with the lumen (red arrow). Immediately after ABSORB implantation, two struts are depicted as pseudo-dense calcium (yellow arrows). At 6 months, the two struts remain visible (yellow arrows). At 2 years, the struts evidenced as pseudo-dense calcium are no longer visible, and a fibrous cap (green arrows) sequesters the necrotic core. The lumen has enlarged from 7.1 mm² immediately postimplant to 10.1 mm² at 2 years. **(b)** Incidence in reported angina from ABSORB II trial. There was a 36% reduction ($p = 0.01$) in reported angina in patients receiving ABSORB BVSs versus XIENCE V. **(c)** Incidence in revascularizations from ABSORB II trial. A 51% reduction in repeat revascularizations was reported for patients receiving ABSORB BVSs versus XIENCE V. ([a] Reprinted with permission from Serruys PW, Ormiston JA, Onuma Y, Regar E, Gonzalo N, Garcia-Garcia HM et al. *Lancet.* 2009;373:897–910; [b] from Serruys PW, Chevalier B, Dudek D, Cequier A, Carrié D, Iniguez A et al. *Lancet.* 2014;385:43–54; [c] from Serruys PW, Chevalier B, Dudek D, Cequier A, Carrié D, Iniguez A et al. *Lancet.* 2014;385:43–54.)

# REFERENCES

1. Joner M, Finn AV, Farb A, Mont EK, Kolodgie FD, Ladich E et al. Pathology of drug-eluting stents in humans: Delayed healing and late thrombotic risk. *J Am Coll Cardiol.* 2006;48:193–202.
2. Iqbal J, Onuma Y, Ormiston J, Abizaid A, Waksman R, Serruys P. Bioresorbable scaffolds: Rationale, current status, challenges, and future. *Eur Heart J.* 2014;35:765–76.
3. International Standards Organization. Packaging for terminally sterilized medical devices Part 1: Requirements for materials, sterile barrier systems and packaging. ISO 11607–1:2006.
4. International Standards Organization. Sterilization of health care products—Radiation—Part 1: Requirements for the development validation and routine control of a sterilization process for medical devices. ISO 11137–1:2006.
5. Lambert B, Martin J. Sterilization of implants and devices. In: Ratner BD, Hoffman AS, Schoen FJ, editors. *Biomaterials Science*, Elsevier; 2013. p. 1339–53.
6. Tanimoto S, Serruys PW, Thuesen L, Dudek D, de Bruyne B, Chevalier B et al. Comparison of in vivo acute stent recoil between the bioabsorbable everolimus-eluting coronary stent and the everolimus-eluting cobalt chromium coronary stent: Insights from the ABSORB and SPIRIT trials. *Cathet Cardiovasc Interv.* 2007;70:515–23.
7. Onuma Y, Serruys PW, Gomez J, de Bruyne B, Dudek D, Thuesen L et al. Comparison of in vivo acute stent recoil between the bioresorbable everolimus-eluting coronary scaffolds (revision 1.0 and 1.1) and the

metallic everolimus-eluting stent. *Cathet Cardiovasc Interv.* 2011;78:3–12.

8. Kossuth MB, Perkins L, Rapoza R. Design Principles of Bioresorbable Polymeric Scaffolds. *Int Cardiol Clin.* 2016;5:349–355

9. Otsuka F, Pacheco E, Perkins LEL, Lane JP, Wang Q, Kamberi M et al. Long-term safety of an everolimus-eluting bioresorbable vascular scaffold and the cobalt-chromium XIENCE V stent in a porcine coronary artery model. *Circ Cardiovasc Interv.* 2014;7:330–42.

10. Ormiston JA, Serruys PW, Onuma Y, van Geuns R-J, de Bruyne B, Dudek D et al. First serial assessment at 6 months and 2 years of the second generation of absorb everolimus-eluting bioresorbable vascular scaffold. *Circ Cardiovasc Interv.* 2012;5:620–632.

11. Campos CM, Ishibashi Y, Eggermont J, Nakatani S, Cho YK, Dijkstra J et al. Echogenicity as a surrogate for bioresorbable everolimus-eluting scaffold degradation: Analysis at 1-, 3-, 6-, 12-, 18-, 24-, 30-, 36- and 42-month follow-up in a porcine model. *Int J Cardiovasc Imaging.* 2015;31:471–482.

12. Serruys PW, Onuma Y, García-García HM, Muramatsu T, van Geuns R-J, de Bruyne B et al. Dynamics of vessel wall changes following the implantation of the Absorb everolimus-eluting bioresorbable vascular scaffold: A multi-imaging modality study at 6, 12, 24 and 36 months. *EuroIntervention.* 2014;9:1271–84.

13. Garg S, Serruys PW. Coronary stents: Current status. *J Am Coll Cardiol.* 2010;56:S1–S42.

14. Natsuaki M, Morimoto T, Furukawa Y, Nakagawa Y, Kadota K, Yamaji K et al. Late adverse events after implantation of sirolimus-eluting stent and bare-metal stent: Long-term (5–7 years) follow-up of the coronary revascularization demonstrating outcome study—Kyoto Registry Cohort 2. *Circ Cardiovasc Interv.* 2014;7:168–179.

15. Brodie BR, Pokharel Y, Garg A, Kissling G, Hansen C, Milks S et al. Very late hazard with stenting versus balloon angioplasty for ST-elevation myocardial infarction: A 16-year single-center experience. *J Interv Cardiol.* 2014;27:21–8.

16. Spoon DB, Psaltis PJ, Singh M, Holmes DR, Gersh BJ, Rihal CS et al. Trends in cause of death after percutaneous coronary intervention. *Circulation.* 2014;129(12):1286–94.

17. Ko BS, Meredith IT. New DES: A new step forward? *Minerva Cardioangiol.* 2012;60:41–56.

18. Yamaji K, Kubo S, Inoue K, Kadota K, Kuramitsu S, Shirai S et al. Association of localized hypersensitivity and in-stent neoatherosclerosis with the very late drug-eluting stent thrombosis. *PLoS One.* 2014;9:e113870.

19. Nebeker JR, Virmani R, Bennett CL, Hoffman JM, Samore MH, Alvarez J et al. Hypersensitivity cases associated with drug-eluting coronary stents: A review of available cases from the Research on Adverse Drug Events and Reports (RADAR) project. *J Am Coll Cardiol.* 2006;47:175–81.

20. Hassan AK, Bergheanu SC, Stijnen T, van der Hoeven BL, Snoep JD, Plevier JW et al. Late stent malapposition risk is higher after drug-eluting stent compared with bare-metal stent implantation and associates with late stent thrombosis. *Eur Heart J.* 2009;31:1172–80.

21. Otsuka F, Vorpahl M, Nakano M, Foerst J, Newell JB, Sakakura K et al. Pathology of second-generation everolimus-eluting stents versus first-generation sirolimus- and paclitaxel-eluting stents in humans. *Circulation.* 2014;129:211–23.

22. Alfonso F, Fernandez-Vina F, Medina M, Hernandez R. Neoatherosclerosis: The missing link between very late stent thrombosis and very late in-stent restenosis. *J Am Coll Cardiol.* 2013;61(12):e155.

23. Nakazawa G. Stent thrombosis of drug eluting stent: Pathological perspective. *J Cardiol.* 2011;58:84–91.

24. Al Mamary A, Dariol G, Napodano M. Neo-atherosclerosis in very late stent thrombosis of drug eluting stent. *J Saudi Heart Assoc.* 2014;26:226–30.

25. Inoue T, Croce K, Morooka T, Sakuma M, Node K, Simon DI. Vascular inflammation and repair: Implications for re-endothelialization, restenosis, and stent thrombosis. *JACC Cardiovasc Interv.* 2011;4:1057–66.

26. Nakazawa G, Finn AV, Joner M, Ladich E, Kutys R, Mont EK et al. Delayed arterial healing and increased late stent thrombosis at culprit sites after drug-eluting stent placement for acute myocardial infarction patients: An autopsy study. *Circulation.* 2008;118:1138–45.

27. Virmani R, Farb A, Guagliumi G, Kolodgie FD. Drug-eluting stents: Caution and concerns for long-term outcome. *Coron Artery Dis.* 2004;15:313–8.

28. Onuma Y, Muramatsu T, Kharlamov A, Serruys PW. Freeing the vessel from metallic cage: What can we achieve with bioresorbable vascular scaffolds? *Cardiovasc Interv Ther.* 2012;27:141–54.

29. Serruys PW, Garcia-Garcia HM, Onuma Y. From metallic cages to transient bioresorbable scaffolds: Change in paradigm of coronary revascularization in the upcoming decade? *Eur Heart J.* 2012;33:16–25.

30. Felix C, Everaert B, Diletti R, Van Mieghem N, Daemen J, Valgimigli M et al. Current status of clinically available bioresorbable scaffolds in percutaneous coronary interventions. *Neth Heart J.* 2015;23:153–160.

31. Lane JP, Perkins LEL, Sheehy AJ, Pacheco EJ, Frie MP, Lambert BJ et al. Lumen gain and restoration of pulsatility after implantation of a bioresorbable vascular scaffold in porcine coronary arteries. *JACC Cardiovasc Interv.* 2014;7:688–95.

32. Gogas B, Benham J, Hsu S, Sheehy A, Lefer D, Goodchild T et al. Vasomotor function comparative assessment at 1 and 2 years following implantation of the ABSORB everolimus-eluting bioresorbable vascular scaffold and the XIENCE V

everolimus-eluting metallic stent in porcine coronary arteries: Insights from in vivo angiography, ex vivo assessment, and gene analysis and the stented/scaffolded segments and the proximal and distal edges. *JACC Cardiovasc Interv.* 2016;9:728–741.

33. Abizaid A, Costa JR, Jr., Bartorelli AL, Whitbourn R, van Geuns RJ, Chevalier B et al. The ABSORB EXTEND study: Preliminary report of the twelve-month clinical outcomes in the first 512 patients enrolled. *EuroIntervention.* 2014; 9-online publish-ahead-of-print April 2014.

34. Serruys PW, Onuma Y, Dudek D, Smits PC, Koolen J, Chevalier B et al. Evaluation of the second generation of a bioresorbable everolimus-eluting vascular scaffold for the treatment of de novo coronary artery stenosis 12-month clinical and imaging outcomes. *J Am Coll Cardiol.* 2011;58:1578–88.

35. Brugaletta S, Radu MD, Garcia-Garcia HM, Heo JH, Farooq V, Girasis C et al. Circumferential evaluation of the neointima by optical coherence tomography after ABSORB bioresorbable vascular scaffold implantation: Can the scaffold cap the plaque? *Atherosclerosis.* 2012;22:106–112.

36. Wang Q, Perkins LE, Sheehy A, McGregor J, Cheng Y, Gongora CA et al. TCT-629 effect of the absorb bioresorbable vascular scaffold (BVS) on coronary plaque regression in a familial hypercholesterolemic swine: 1-year follow-up. *J Am Coll Cardiol.* 2014;64:B183.

37. Karanasos A, Simsek C, Gnanadesigan M, van Ditzhuijzen NS, Freire R, Dijkstra J et al. OCT assessment of the long-term vascular healing response 5 years after everolimus-eluting bio-resorbable vascular scaffold. *J Am Coll Cardiol.* 2014;64:2343–56.

38. Bourantas CV, Farooq V, Zhang Y-J, Muramatsu T, Gogas BD, Thuesen L et al. Circumferential distribution of the neointima at six-month and two-year follow-up after a bioresorbable vascular scaffold implantation: A substudy of the ABSORB Cohort B Clinical Trial. *EuroIntervention.* 2015;10:1299–306.

39. Serruys PW, Chevalier B, Dudek D, Cequier A, Carrié D, Iniguez A et al. A bioresorbable everolimus-eluting scaffold versus a metallic everolimus-eluting stent for ischaemic heart disease caused by de-novo native coronary artery lesions (ABSORB II): An interim 1-year analysis of clinical and procedural secondary outcomes from a randomised controlled trial. *Lancet.* 2014;385:43–54.

40. Smits PC. ABSORB EXTEND: An interim report on the 36-month clinical outcomes from the first 250 patients enrolled. *J Am Coll Cardiol.* 2014; 64:B180.

41. Whitbourn RJ. TCT-31 ABSORB EXTEND: An interim report on the 24-month clinical outcomes from the first 250 patients enrolled. *J Am Coll Cardiol.* 2013;62:B11.

42. Serruys PW, Ormiston JA, Onuma Y, Regar E, Gonzalo N, Garcia-Garcia HM et al. A bioabsorbable everolimus-eluting coronary stent system (ABSORB): 2-year outcomes and results from multiple imaging methods. *Lancet.* 2009;373:897–910.

# 10.2

# Emerging technologies: Overview of the field

YOSHINOBU ONUMA, YOHEI SOTOMI, YUKI KATAGIRI, AND PATRICK W.J.C. SERRUYS

Bioresorbable scaffolds offer the possibility of transient scaffolding of the vessel to prevent acute vessel closure and recoil while also transiently eluting an antiproliferative drug to counteract the constrictive remodeling and excessive neointimal hyperplasia. The concept of a transient coronary device that disappears after doing its job fits the physiological demand to restore the vessel structure and seems attractive both to physicians and patients. Following the successful and intriguing findings observed in the first-in-human trials, the four products, ABSORB, Desolve, ART, and Magmaris scaffolds succeeded to acquire a CE mark.

As of September 2016, 28 companies have been developing the bioresorbable scaffolds (Table 10.2.1). The most commonly used biodegradable material is PLLA (26 products), followed by magnesium (6 products). The other materials used were tyrosine polycarbonate, salicylic acid polymer, and iron. Except for the four products that got the CE mark, 11 scaffolds were undergoing clinical trials for regulatory approval.

Since the first generation devices have a relatively thick strut, which is compromising the practical deliverability of the device, the reiteration of scaffolds is considered necessary and is ongoing. The newer generation devices are aiming at the thinner struts ≤120 micron with a smaller crossing profile compared to the currently available version of the bioresorbable devices.

Table 10.2.1 Overview of the current status of bioresorbable scaffolds

| Company | Product name | Biodegradable material used for backbone | Coating | Drug elution | Other features | Phase of development |
|---|---|---|---|---|---|---|
| Abbott | ABSORB | PLLA | PDLLA | Everolimus | Strut thickness 150 μm | CE mark, FDA approval |
| Abbott | ABSORB GT1 | PLLA | PDLLA | Everolimus | Strut thickness 150 μm | CE mark, FDA approval |
| ART | ART Pure | PDLLA | None | None | NA | CE mark |
| BIOTRONIK | Magmaris | WE43 alloy, 93% Mg, and 7% rare earth elements | PLLA | Sirolimus | Strut thickness 150 μm | CE mark |
| Elixir | DESolve 100 | PLLA | Bioresorbable polymer | Novolimus | Strut thickness 100 μm | CE mark |
| Elixir | DESolve 150 | PLLA | Bioresorbable polymer | Novolimus | Strut thickness 150 μm | CE mark |
| Elixir | DESolve XL | PLLA | Bioresorbable polymer | Novolimus | NA | CE mark |
| REVA | Fantom | Desaminotyrosine polycarbonate | Desaminotyrosine polycarbonate | Sirolimus | Strut thickness 125 μm | CE mark approval submitted |
| Amaranth Medical | APTITUDE | PLLA | NA | Sirolimus | Strut thickness 120 μm | Clinical studies underway |
| Amaranth Medical | FORTITUDE | PLLA | Bioresorbable polymer | Sirolimus | Strut thickness 150 μm | Clinical studies underway |
| Boston Scientific | FAST | PLLA | PLGA | Everolimus | Strut thickness 100 μm | Clinical studies underway |
| Huaan | XINSORB | PLA/PCL/PGA | PDLLA+PLLA | Sirolimus | Strut thickness 160 μm | Clinical studies underway |
| Kyoto Medical | IGAKI-TAMAI | PLLA | None | None | Strut thickness 170 μm | Clinical studies underway |
| Lepu | NeoVas | PLLA | PDLA | Sirolimus | Strut thickness 170 μm | Clinical studies underway |
| Manli Cardiology | Mirage | PLLA | PLLA | Sirolimus | Strut thickness 125 μm for <=3 mm and 150 μm for ≥3.5 mm | Clinical studies underway |
| Meril | MeRes100 | PLLA | PDLLA | Sirolimus | Strut thickness 100 μm | Clinical studies underway |
| MicroPort | Firesorb | PLLA | PDLLA | Sirolimus | 100 μm (2.5, 2.75 mm) and 125 μm (3.0, 4.0 mm) | Clinical studies underway |
| Xenogenics | Ideal BioStent | Polylactide anhydride mixed with a polymer of salicylic acid with a sebacic acid linker | Salicilate linked with adipic acid | Sirolimus | Strut thickness 175 μm | Clinical studies underway |
| Arterius | ArterioSorb | PLLA | Bioresorbable polymer | Sirolimus | 2 versions: 95 and 120 μm (3.5 mm device) | Preclinical study underway |
| Cardionovum | ReNATURAL (M) ReNATURAL (P) | (M) = metal, (P) = PLLA | NA | Sirolimus | NA | Preclinical study underway |

(Continued)

Table 10.2.1 (Continued) Overview of the current status of bioresorbable scaffolds

| Company | Product name | Biodegradable material used for backbone | Coating | Drug elution | Other features | Phase of development |
|---|---|---|---|---|---|---|
| Elixir | AMITY | PLLA | Bioresorbable polymer | Novolimus | Strut thickness 100 µm | Preclinical study underway |
| Elixir | DESolve Cx | PLLA | Bioresorbable polymer | Novolimus | Strut thickness 120 µm | Preclinical study underway |
| Envision Scientific | IMBIBE | Magnesium | Nanocarrier layer: Top-coat that carries sirolimus, Sandwich layer: Scaffold degradation-controlling jacket with PLA and sirolimus | Sirolimus | Strut thickness 120 µm | Preclinical study underway |
| LifeTech | LifeTech Iron-Based BRSs | Nitrided iron | "Special" polymer | Sirolimus | Strut thickness 70 to 80 µm | Preclinical study underway |
| Medtronic | Mg Spiral | Magnesium | "Family of degradable polymers" | Sirolimus | Strut thickness 120 µm | Preclinical study underway |
| OrbusNeich | On-AVS | PLLA, PLCL, PDLA | PLLA+PDLA | Sirolimus | Strut thickness 150 µm, coated with CD34 antibody | Preclinical study underway |
| QualiMed | Unity BRSs | Magnesium | PLGA | Sirolimus | Strut thickness 120 µm | Preclinical study underway |
| S3V | Avatar | Not available | Bioresorbable polymer | NA | NA | Preclinical study underway |
| Scitech | Scitech MBRS | Magnesium | NA | None | NA | Preclinical study underway |
| Terumo | Terumo/ART DCBS | PDLLA | Bioresorbable polymer | Sirolimus | Strut thickness 170 µm | Preclinical study underway |
| Zorion Medical Corporation | ZMED | Magnesium/PLGA | NA | NA | NA | Preclinical study underway |
| Abbott | Next-Gen ABSORB | PLLA | PDLLA | Everolimus | Strut thickness 100 µm | In development |
| Sahajanand | Sahajanand Bioabsorbable | PLLA | Bioresorbable polymer | Sirolimus | NA | In development |
| Amaranth Medical | MAGNITUDE | PLLA | Bioresorbable polymer | Sirolimus | Strut thickness 100 µm | No information |
| MicroPort | Firefalcon | PLLA | NA | NA | NA | No information |
| Shanghai Bio-Heart | Galaxy | PLA | Bioresorbable polymer | Sirolimus | NA | No information |

Abbreviations: ASA = salicylic acid; BRSs = bioresorbable scaffolds; NA = data not available; PCL = polycaprolactone; PDLA = poly-D-lactide; PDLLA = poly(L-lactide-co-D,L-lactide); PGA = polyglycolic acid; PLA = poly(lactic acid); PLGA = poly lactic-co-glycolic acid; PLLA = poly-L-lactide; TMC = trimethylene carbonate.

# MeRes100™—A sirolimus eluting bioresorbable vascular scaffold system

ASHOK SETH, BABU EZHUMALAI, SANJEEV BHATT, AND PRATIK VASANI

## BACKGROUND

The concept of a "temporary stent" to provide acute benefits in treatment of severe coronary stenosis and its eventual disappearance in order to free the vessel of metal caging is not just attractive but also represents an ultimate long-term goal of returning the arteries to their original physiological state [1]. The research on bioresorbable scaffolds (BRSs) has been challenging over the last 15 years. Increasing insight into biomaterial science of polymers and technological innovation among polymer scientists, device industry, and experienced interventionalists has led to the creation of the first generation of BRSs. The front-runner in this development process with pivotal randomized trials, large registry data, routine "real life" clinical use, and approval in more than 60 countries has been the ABSORB™ Bioresorbable Vascular Scaffold System (Abbott Vascular, Santa Clara, CA) [2]. The potential long-term benefits, which have been identified and outlined as the "final frontier," are only going to be proven over long-term studies though more and more supportive data keeps appearing every month [3].

However, there are limitations of the first-generation BRSs like ABSORB. It is a thick strut device with restrictive implantation characteristics (like gradual inflation deployment over 45–60 seconds, limited expansion characteristics of no more than 0.5 mm above its nominal size), limited sizes up to 3.5 mm in diameter (and hence meant only for vessels up to 4 mm in diameter) [4], limited lengths, and inadequate radiopacity. The device is difficult to track and cross especially in calcified and tortuous anatomy. In simple terms, it is not a stent but a new device and hence has its learning curve [5]. This limits its use in complex real life cases. Thus, newer device modifications are needed to expand the use of BRSs from a niche device to a workhorse stent. The increased applicability would also be determined by economics of the procedure in most parts of the world. Thus, the target is to progress to an economical BRSs with performance characteristics that bring it as close as possible to the metallic drug eluting stent (mDES) in most lesion subsets, thus overcoming some of the limitations of the first-generation BRSs.

The MeRes100–Sirolimus Eluting Bioresorbable Vascular Scaffold System is an investigational device (developed by Meril Life Sciences Pvt. Ltd., Vapi, Gujarat, India), which is undergoing first-in-human clinical trials in India. It has a novel scaffold architecture, low strut thickness, low profile delivery system, high radial strength, high flexibility and deliverability, improved radiopacity, convenient side branch access, multiple length and size matrix, and conventional storage methods (Table 10.3.1).

## DEVICE DESCRIPTION

The MeRes100–Sirolimus Eluting BRSs comprises the following components:

1. A balloon expandable BRSs made from polymer—poly-L-lactide (PLLA)
2. A topcoat comprising an antiproliferative agent—sirolimus ($1.25\ \mu gm/mm^2$) eluting from PDLLA polymer base
3. A rapid exchange PTCA balloon catheter that acts as the scaffold delivery system

Poly-L-lactide (PLLA) is one of the commonly available commercial aliphatic polyesters that possess excellent biocompatibility, biodegradability, a high mechanical strength, and good shaping and molding properties. PLLA used in MeRes100 construction is a semicrystalline polymer with the glass transition temperature of around 55°C–60°C and the melting temperature of around 180°C.

Table 10.3.1 Advantages of MeRes100 over first-generation BRSs

| | |
|---|---|
| Low strut thickness | 100 µm (±10%) |
| Low profile delivery system | Low crimping profile of 1.2 mm for a 3.00 mm diameter scaffold |
| Hybrid design | Closed cells at the edges and open cells along the length of the device |
| High radial strength | Strut-width variability in design maintains high radial strength starting above 22N without any loss in flexibility despite low strut thickness |
| High flexibility and deliverability | MeRes100 samples (3.00 × 19 mm scaffolds) produced low ultimate forces of 1.85N required to track the device and 8.77N of ultimate force required to push the device versus 2.09N and 8.81N required, respectively, to track and push the commercially available ABSORB control samples (3.00 × 18 mm scaffolds) |
| Improved radiopacity | Couplets of three tri-axial platinum radiopaque markers are fixed circumferentially 120° apart from each other at either end of the scaffold |
| Convenient side branch access | Open cells allow easy access of side branch |
| Large size matrix | Diameters of (mm) 2.25, 2.50, 2.75, 3.00, 3.25, 3.50, 4.00, 4.50 and lengths of (mm) 8, 13, 16, 19, 24, 29, 32, 37, 40 |
| Conventional storage methods | MeRes100 BRSs is sterilized using e-beam radiation and can be stored below 25°C |

PLLA is a recognized biocompatible and bioresorbable polymer that undergoes hydrolytic degradation in the body producing lactic acid, lactides, and oligomers which are decomposed in the body via well-known Kreb's cycle and eventually eliminated as carbon dioxide and water.

The MeRes100 scaffold strut thickness is maintained around 100 µm (±10%). The scaffold is laser cut to form an articulating mix of crowns and connectors. The resultant design (Figure 10.3.1) is an intelligent "hybrid" comprising closed cells at the edges and open cells along the length of the device. Additionally, the design incorporates strut-width variability; thus, the scaffold maintains high radial strength without any loss in flexibility despite low strut thickness. The open cells ensure sufficient side branch

access. The percentage of vessel wall area covered by the scaffold is 28.5% for the 3.0 mm device. In order to address the inadequate radiopacity with the current generation of BRSs, in the MeRes100, couplets of three tri-axial platinum radiopaque markers are fixed circumferentially 120° apart from each other at either end of the scaffold. These markers assist scaffold positioning when viewed in two orthogonal planes and ensure adequate visibility during post-deployment high-pressure dilatations.

The scaffold is mounted between the radiopaque markers of a rapid exchange balloon expandable delivery system. This thin strut BRSs has low crimping profile (1.2 mm for a 3.00 mm diameter scaffold) and higher trackability and pushability. In a series of MeRes100 samples tested on

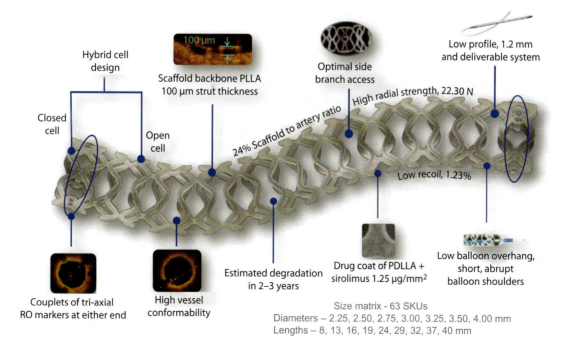

Figure 10.3.1 MeRes100–sirolimus eluting bioresorbable vascular scaffold.

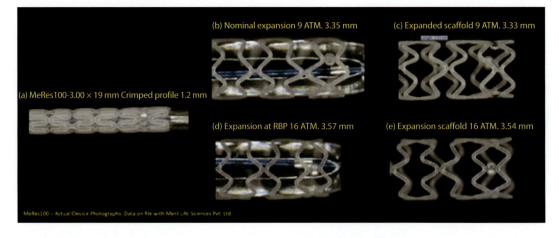

Figure 10.3.2 MeRes100–Crimped and expanded actual device images at NP 9 ATM and RBP 16 ATM.

ASTM standard test equipment for flexibility and deliverability, MeRes100 samples (3.00 × 19 mm scaffolds) produced low ultimate forces of 1.85N required to track the device and 8.77N of ultimate force required to push the device versus 2.09N and 8.81N required, respectively, to track and push the commercially available ABSORB control samples (3.00 × 18 mm scaffolds) [6].

The device demonstrates uniformity of expansion without any strut deformity, minor or major notching, no strut fractures at nominal pressures of 9 ATM and this is evenly observed beyond the balloon rated burst pressures (RBP) of 16 ATM (Figure 10.3.2).

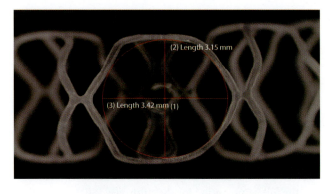

Figure 10.3.3 MeRes100 3.00 × 19. Open cell expansion using a 3.00 mm balloon at 16 ATM.

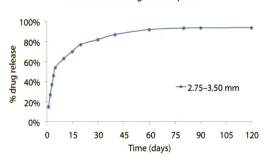

Cummulative drug release profile

Figure 10.3.4 MeRes100—*In vitro* drug release kinetics.

MeRes100 side branch accessibility tests demonstrate that the struts withstand the balloon expansion pressures without any link fractures or trauma to surrounding cells and the remaining structures. Figure 10.3.3 demonstrates the circular diameter available after expansion of a cell with 3.00 mm diameter balloon at 16 ATM.

The active drug coating is sirolimus in the dose of 1.25 µgm/mm$^2$. The drug is formulated in a 1:1 mixture with biocompatible bioabsorbable polymer, i.e., poly-DL-lactide (PDLLA), which acts as a drug reservoir and controls drug release rate. The coating is thin (<5 µm), uniform, and does not web, crack, or lump. The drug is timed to elute over a period of 120 days with 75% of drug elution happening during the first 30 days (Figure 10.3.4) [7].

MeRes100 is manufactured in a wide range of sizes—diameters (mm) of 2.25, 2.50, 2.75, 3.00, 3.25, 3.50, 4.00, 4.50 and lengths of (mm) 8, 13, 16, 19, 24, 29, 32, 37, 40 thus allowing the operators to choose from a wide matrix partially resolving the unmet clinical need to treat a variety of real life lesion morphologies. The device is sterilized using e-beam radiation and can be stored below 25°C, thus ensuring ease of transport and storage at various points along the distribution system.

## DEGRADATION, LOSS IN RADIAL STRENGTH, MOLECULAR WEIGHT AND CHANGE IN CRYSTALLINITY

Simulated in vitro degradation study performed as per ASTM standards demonstrates that MeRes100 BRSs retains its radial strength up to 6 months. Breakdown of PLLA on further hydration occurs leading to loss in molecular weight. Inversely, the crystallinity increases temporarily as the amorphous base degrades faster and then drops over a period of 6 months. The scientific hypothesis here is that during the 6 months post-deployment the scaffold endothelializes and the vessel no longer needs additional support allowing for its ultimate degradation estimate to be beyond 2 years, liberating the vessel of its primary implant [1]. Both animal model testing and in-house sophisticated degradation models developed by Meril have substantiated this correlation.

*In vitro* degradation testing demonstrates three critical parameters of the *in vitro* scaffold degradation analysis (Figures 10.3.5, 10.3.6, and 10.3.7). The scaffold is made of high molecular weight PLLA ranging 275–300 kDa. The design coupled with improved manufacturing process generates a scaffold with high radial strength starting above 22N. As the scaffold undergoes hydrolytic degradation, there is a gradual reduction in radial strength and beyond 3 months, the values drop to 14N, which is still sufficient to maintain the hoop strength while the vessel undergoes simultaneous healing and prevents recoil-led restenosis. An inversely proportional relationship is observed between molecular weight loss and temporary spike in crystallinity, which is temporary aggregation of large chain semicrystalline PLLA, which populates as the smaller chain PLLA cleaves preferentially. This can be correlated along with representative OCT images (Figure 10.3.8) from porcine coronary artery implantation at 90-day's time point demonstrating intact scaffold, no loss in vessel diameter, uniform and thin neointimal coverage, and absence of scaffold fractures [8].

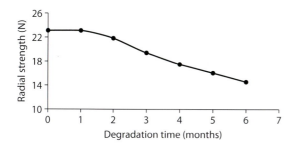

Figure 10.3.5 Loss in radial strength.

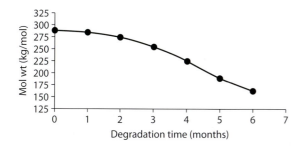

Figure 10.3.6 Loss in molecular weight.

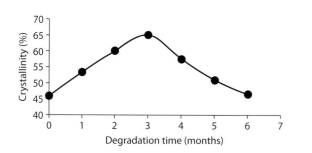

Figure 10.3.7 Change in crystallinity.

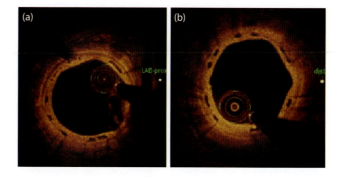

Figure 10.3.8 Ninety-day OCT image of MeRes100 3.00 × 19 implanted in (a) proximal LAD and (b) distal LAD porcine coronary artery.

## IN VIVO AND IN VITRO BENCH PERFORMANCE

Extensive *in vivo* biocompatibility tests and *in vitro* performance testing has been undertaken as per standard stent and BRSs testing guidelines prescribed as per ISO guidelines; US FDA guidance document; ASTM standard guidelines; D-618-stent practice document and WK-35909–standard guide to test absorbable stents [6]. Tests involved radial strength measurement, percentage recoil, fatigue resistance, 3-point bend test, pushability, trackability, radial force, percentage change in length, dislodgement force, uniformity of expansion, and ring strength test. All the samples passed both biocompatibility and engineering bench tests as per the guidelines.

## PRECLINICAL PROOF OF CONCEPT

The purpose of the preclinical studies of MeRes100 were to evaluate the acute operational performance, acute and intermediate biomechanics, intermediate durability and patency, biocompatibility, and pharmacokinetics (pK) of sirolimus elution, in a porcine model in comparison to ABSORB BRSs (Abbott Vascular, Santa Clara, CA), a mDES, i.e., XIENCE V everolimus eluting stent (Abbott Vascular, Santa Clara, CA), and BioMime Sirolimus Eluting Stent (Meril Life Sciences, India).

The follow-up period for the study was 180 days. A subset of these animals was used to get pK data on release profile of sirolimus into blood and local arterial tissue surrounding the scaffold.

Test devices MeRes100 and control devices (ABSORB EE BRS, XIENCE V EES, and BioMime SES) were implanted in Yucatan mini-swines in LCx, LAD, and RCA. All implanted arterial sites were imaged with angiography and OCT. There was no animal mortality or any serious adverse event (such as device thrombosis, MI, hypersensitivity, or acute/chronic mechanical device failure). No clinically relevant abnormalities were observed in the health status of animals nor in the clinical pathology (hematology and serum chemistry). Acute operational performance, acute and chronic biomechanics, and chronic patency were found satisfactory. MeRes100 BRSs demonstrated appropriate acute operational performance, adequate acute and chronic biomechanics, and favorable patency and neointimal growth when compared to benchmark ABSORB BRSs, mDES XIENCE V, and BioMime [8].

The purpose of the pK substudy was to evaluate release of sirolimus into the blood stream and in surrounding arterial tissue following implantation of MeRes100 BRSs in a porcine model up to 180 days. There was no animal mortality or any serious adverse event within the period of the study. MeRes100 BRSs demonstrated gradual release of sirolimus with a minor proportion released into the blood stream, and sustained presence with gradual decline in arterial tissue up to 180 days. The blood concentrations peaked between 1 and 4 hours. The levels were clinically acceptable as the peak was never higher than 9 ng/mL. The levels gradually declined below quantifiable limit (<0.100 ng/mL) in all animals at day 14 and beyond. The arterial tissue concentration gradually declined over time. At 90 days, the concentrations were about 50% lower than at 28 days. At 180 days, the concentrations were detectable, yet about 90% lower than at 28 days [9].

## MERES-1 FIM CLINICAL TRIAL

MeRes100 is currently an investigational device and is being studied in a phase-II safety and feasibility study in India. MeRes-1 is a prospective, multicenter, single arm, open label, pilot clinical Study of MeRes100 Sirolimus Eluting Bioresorbable Vascular Scaffold System in the treatment of *de novo* native coronary artery lesions [10].

The MeRes-1 study has been approved by the [DCG(I)] (Indian FDA) and has completed enrollment of 108 patients in 16 sites across India. Angiographic inclusion criteria involves a maximum of two treatable *de novo* lesions (maximum one per native epicardial vessel) located in a major artery or branch, with a reference vessel diameter between 2.75, 3.0, and 3.5 mm by online QCA and target lesion length ≤20 mm. The MeRes-1 study has completed enrollment and all subjects have cleared 6 months primary end-points.

The primary safety endpoint is ischemia-driven major adverse cardiac event (ID MACE) at 6 months. Clinical endpoints include ischemia-driven MACE, ischemia-driven TVF, TLR, TVR, scaffold thrombosis at 30 days, 6 months, and at 1, 2, and 3 years. Additionally acute device and procedural success have been determined.

A subset population has undergone angiographic ($n = 36$), IVUS ($n = 12$), OCT ($n = 12$) follow-up at 6 and 24 months and MSCT ($n = 12$) follow-up at 12 months with core lab analysis. A subset population has also undergone pK to measure time taken to reach maximum concentration ($T_{max}$) level in the blood after implantation of the scaffold, maximum concentration of the drug obtained in peripheral venous blood ($C_{max}$), mean initial ($T_{\frac{1}{2}i}$) and terminal ($T_{\frac{1}{2}T}$) half life period of the drug in venous blood, area under the curve (AUC) of the blood drug

concentration, and time taken for the drug to go below detectable levels by LCMS (Primary end points presented by Seth A. at TCT 2016).

## SUMMARY AND CONCLUSIONS

The MeRes100 Sirolimus Eluting BRSs represents a second generation BRS with a novel architecture, thinner struts, lower profile, and a variety of lengths and diameters, thus progressing closer to a user-friendly, workhorse device. Preclinical engineering and animal study data demonstrate extremely favorable characteristics and similar vascular tissue responses as seen with ABSORB (Abbott Vascular, Santa Clara, CA) BRSs up to 3 months. Longer animal data is awaited. The first-in-human study, MeRes-1 has demonstrated 0% MACE, 0% ST and low late loss of 0.15+0.23 mm at 6 months follow-up, primary safety and efficacy data have been presented at TCT 2016. Development of MeRes100 from India would also help to lower the cost of BRSs, which is a limitation for its widespread use not just in emerging countries but also in the developed world.

## REFERENCES

1. Serruys PW et al. Bioresorbable scaffolds. *The PCREAPCI Textbook*. 2012. Chapter 4/Part 3/Intervention 1/Volume 2.
2. Collet C, de Winter RJ, Onuma Y, Serruys PW. The Absorb bioresorbable vascular scaffold for the treatment of coronary artery disease. *Expert Opin Drug Deliv*. 2016; 13:1489–1499.
3. Onuma Y, Serruys PW. Bioresorbable scaffold: To advent of a new era in percutaneous coronary and peripheral revascularization? *Circulation* 2011; 123:779–97.
4. Serruys P et al. Coronary stents: Looking forward. *J Am Coll Cardio* 2010; 56:S43–S78.
5. Seth A, Kumar V. Bioresorbable scaffold: "Looking at the 'real world' through a plastic tube." *Catheter Cardiovasc Interv* 2014; 84:53–4.
6. Internal bench testing data. File with Meril Life Sciences Pvt. Ltd., Vapi, Gujarat, India.
7. Seth A, Onuma Y, Costa R, Chandra P, Bahl VK, Manjunath CN, Mahajan AU, Kumar V, Goel PK, Wander GS, Kalarickal MS, Kaul U, Kumar VKA, Rath PC, Trehan V, Sengottuvelu G, Mishra S, Abizaid A, Serruys PW. First-in-human evaluation of a novel poly-L-lactide based sirolimus-eluting bioresorbable vascular scaffold for the treatment of de novo native coronary artery lesions: MeRes-1 trial. *EuroIntervention*. 2017.
8. Kaluza G. Evaluation of MeRes sirolimus eluting bioresorbable scaffold system in porcine coronary arteries. 2014. Preclinical data on file with Meril Life Sciences Pvt. Ltd., Vapi, Gujarat, India.

9. Seth A, Chandra P, Mahajan AU, Nanjappa MC, Kumar V, Goel PK, Wander GS, Bahl VK, Kalarickal MS, Kumaran AV, Kaul U, Rath PC, Mishra A, Trehan VK, Ganeshwala G, Koshy AG. TCTAP A-058 favorable outcomes for systemic pharmacokinetic study of sirolimus-eluting bioresorbable vascular scaffold system in treating de novo native coronary artery lesion: A sub study of MeRes-1 Trial. *Journal of the American College of Cardiology.* 2017; 69:S31.

10. Seth A. MeRes-1—A prospective, multicenter, single arm, open label, pilot clinical study of MeRes 100 sirolimus eluting bioresorbable vascular scaffold system in the treatment of de novo native coronary artery lesions. Clinical Trials Registration—CTRI/2015/04/005706.

# XINSORB bioresorbable vascular scaffold

JUNBO GE AND LI SHEN

The XINSORB bioresorbable vascular scaffolds (BVSs) is a fully absorbable scaffold mounted on a balloon dilatation catheter. XINSORB BVSs was designed and fabricated by Shandong Huaan Biotechnology Co. Ltd. This scaffold was composed of bioabsorbable PLLA (poly-L-lactic acid) as its backbone. The molecular weight of PLLA used for XINSORB BVSs was 300 kDa. Bioabsorbable polymer, poly-D-L-lactic acid (PDLLA) carrying sirolimus was coated on the struts with a thin layer and controlled the release of antiproliferative drug. The scaffold was carefully mounted on a prewrapped balloon automatically by mounting equipment. This balloon-expandable scaffold could then be crimped down and constrained on the delivery system, able to return to that design shape when expanding the balloon in the coronary artery. The device was sterilized using an e-beam sterilization method.

Shandong Huaan started first-in-human with XINSORB on September 5, 2013. Thirty patients were included in the first short-term efficacy and safety clinical trial. Based on excellent clinical results after 6-months implantation, Shandong Huaan started to enroll a 1200 patient study in 2014 and concluded the enrollment in May 2016.

Figure 10.4.1 demonstrates the performance of XINSORB BVSs during the FIM trial. As shown in Figure 10.4.1, most struts were embedded and apposed at 6 months after implantation. During 24 months following up, we can see that all struts were embedded completely. The scaffolds were partially absorbed at 24 months follow-up based on visual assessment.

The design of the XINSORB BVSs used in the clinical trial is circumferential zig-zag hoops, strut thickness 160 μm, linked either directly or by straight bridges. The expanded scaffold covers 20–29% of the vessel wall depending on different sizes, and provides uniform vessel wall support and drug application. The radial strength of XINSORB is more than 40 kPa, tested by Instron using a two flat plate testing method. The scaffold has great security on the balloon during the scaffold delivery, which is comparable to the DESs on the market. Therefore, dislodgement will be unlikely. XINSORB BVSs contains four platinum marker beads, two embedded at each end. These are clearly visible on fluoroscopy and easily differentiated from calcium by their roundness and high radio-opacity. They facilitate precise postdilatation and additional scaffold placement because stent ends can be accurately located.

The XINSORB BVSs (Shandong Huaan) is made up of a backbone of PLLA coated with a thin layer of poly-D,L-lactide (PDLLA) and elutes sirolimus. PLLA is a fully biodegradable semicrystalline polymer, which forms a conglomeration of crystalline and amorphous phases when it solidifies. The structure and the state of this polymer change in relation to temperature and deformation history. PDLLA is a biodegradable polymer coating PLLA, which forms, similar to the PLLA, an amorphous phase when it solidifies at room and physiological temperatures. The PDLLA allows controlled release of the drug such that ~80% of sirolimus is eluted within 30 days. The absorption process of PLLA and PDLLA is by bulk erosion and occurs via hydrolysis, producing lactic acid, and subsequently degrades via the Krebs cycle, and small particles <2 μm in diameter are phagocytozed by macrophages. With regard to preclinical trials and *in vitro* degradation study, it seems that the XINSORB BVSs can hold radial strength over 3 months during the revascularization period, and then gradually loses its strength. The complete absorption of the scaffold could occur within 2–3 years after implantation.

The XINSORB BVSs is coated with a thin layer of poly-D,L-lactide (PDLLA) and elutes sirolimus. The dose of sirolimus on the XINSORB BVSs was 8–16 μg/mm. The drug release profile of the XINSORB BVSs was evaluated by immersing the stent in 20 mL of phosphate buffer solution (PBS) containing 4% FBS (Hyclone, pH7.4) at 37°C in a shaking incubator. At each time point (12 h, 24 h, 48 h, 3 days, 7 days, 14 days, and 28 days), the samples were quickly collected using a syringe and the concentration of sirolimus in PBS was measured with high-performance liquid chromatography (HPLC, Agilent 1100).

*In vitro* release profile of sirolimus from XINSORB BVSs and Excel stents was obtained and shown in Figure 10.4.2. Both of them have very similar release profiles. The release

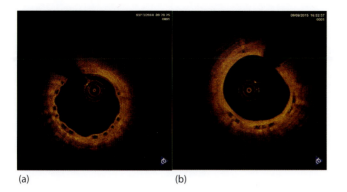

(a)　　　　　　　　(b)

**Figure 10.4.1** The strut apposition at 6 and 24 months after implantation. **(a)** 6 months. **(b)** 24 months follow-up.

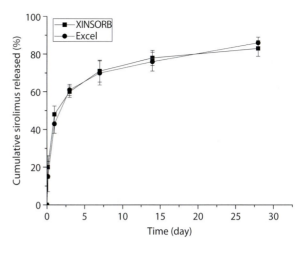

**Figure 10.4.2** Drug release profile of XINSORB BVSs.

of sirolimus from XINSORB BVSs and Excel stents was observed to go through two stages; with an initial sirolimus of approximately 75% (78% for XINSORB BVSs and 76% for Excel stents) within the first 2 weeks and subsequently a more slow release. All the loaded sirolimus reaches a release plateau of greater than 80% (83% for XINSORB BVSs and 86%

for Excel stents) within 4-weeks' incubation in PBS. The sirolimus release in the first stage was mainly dominated by diffusion, and then shifted to a degradation-controlled stage after 2 weeks. About 80% of sirolimus eluted from the polymer in 28 days *ex vivo*.

# NeoVas™ bioresorbable coronary scaffold system

YALING HAN AND YAO-JUN ZHANG

The bioresorbable scaffolds (BRSs), while providing a temporary vessel scaffold, gradually resorbed free of any caging, eventually restoring the vessel wall physiology and vasomotion, has been heralded as the fourth revolution in interventional cardiology. Currently, there are several BRSs available with different compositions (e.g., polymer or metallic alloy), strengths, and weaknesses in China. The NeoVas™ scaffold (Lepu Medical, Beijing, China) is a balloon expandable BRSs, and consists of four components: a poly-L-lactic acid platform, poly-D, L-lactide acid polymer, antiproliferative drug sirolimus (15.3 µg/mm scaffold lengths), and radiopaque markers at the ends (Figure 10.5.1). The mean strut thickness of the NeoVas scaffold is 170 µm, which consists of a backbone thickness of 160 µm and polymer thickness of 10 µm. The device crossing profile is 1.40 mm and 6-French

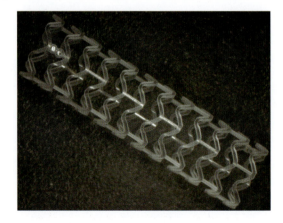

**Figure 10.5.1** The NeoVas bioresorbable coronary scaffold system.

catheter compatible. The kinetic release data indicated that approximately 75% of the drug releases within 1 month after scaffold implantation. The NeoVas scaffold has to be kept at a temperature between 0 and 10°C to ensure device stability and a shelf life of up to 1 year.

The performance of NeoVas scaffold was first tested in 31 patients with simple *de novo* lesions in the first-in-man (FIM) study. At 6-month follow-up, there was only one patient with target lesion revascularization (TLR). Angiographic follow-up demonstrated a mean late lumen loss of 0.26 mm. In this FIM study, multiple imaging modalities were performed with intravascular ultrasound (IVUS) and optical coherence tomography (OCT) at baseline, 6 months, and 2 years as well as multislice computed tomography at 1-, 3-, and 5-year follow-up. Serial IVUS examinations showed a slight reduction in the minimal scaffold cross-sectional area (from $7.11 \pm 1.56$ mm$^2$ poststenting, to $6.74 \pm 1.38$ mm$^2$ at 6 months, $p = 0.131$). Similar results were found at OCT-based cross-sectional level analysis with a nonsignificant decreased minimal scaffold area ($8.27 \pm 1.61$ mm$^2$ at baseline, to $8.02 \pm 1.35$ mm$^2$ at 6 months). Although these preliminary results are encouraging, further extensive studies are necessary to investigate the safety and efficacy of the scaffold. At present, the NeoVas pivotal trial has been designed to evaluate the effectiveness of the device in a broader number of patients to provide sufficient evidence for the Chinese Food and Drug Administration approval. It is a single-blind, multicenter, randomized trial in which no less than 600 patients with simple *de novo* lesions will be enrolled. The 1-year clinical follow-up is expected to be presented in the first quarter of 2017.

# ArterioSorb™ bioresorbable scaffold by Arterius Ltd.

RASHA AL-LAMEE

## INTRODUCTION

There remains a need to develop a fully bioresorbable scaffold (BRSs) that combines the most favorable properties of a BRSs with those of a permanent metallic stent. The ultimate BRSs that will lead to a practice-changing alternative to permanent metallic stenting will have the following properties:

1. Comparable radial strength to metallic stents, without compromising flexibility
2. Strut thickness and scaffold geometry of the best-in-class metallic stents
3. The integrity and strength of a polymer scaffold, during the remodeling phase of the arterial wall (normally 6 months postimplantation)
4. Flexibility and ease of implantation that is comparable to metallic stents
5. No polymer degradation until the stent is fully encapsulated in the intimal layer of the arterial wall, with full reabsorption taking place within 24 months, "leaving nothing behind"
6. No degradation of the polymer during the preuse storage phase, and properties that allow the BRSs to be stored at room temperature
7. Cost comparability to drug eluting stents (DESs)
8. A wide portfolio of diameters and lengths comparable to metallic stents

None of the BRSs products currently in market or in the clinical evaluation stage fulfill all of these criteria entirely. Advances in polymer processing technology will be the key to the development of a scaffold with the characteristics above. The ArterioSorb™ scaffold (Arterius Ltd., Bradford, United Kingdom) is manufactured using a patented die-drawing processing technique that results in improved radial strength. This unique scaffold is currently undergoing preclinical testing with extremely promising results.

## POLYMER PROCESSING TECHNOLOGY

Manufacturing of polymer scaffolds with mechanical properties closer to their metal counterparts introduces significant challenges. Polymers generally do not have the necessary material properties to facilitate the required crimping on a balloon catheter, expansion, and the provision of radial support to the target vessel. A number of different processing approaches has been developed to improve the material properties of polymers for BRSs including blow molding, dip coating, and annealing. However, all of these processes have failed to deliver the required mechanical performance and subsequently the current BRSs devices remain bulky with poor radial strength and deliverability. These processes are also expensive leading to the significantly higher prices of current BRSs devices. Unless the mechanical issues are tackled and the cost of the manufactured stent becomes comparable to DESs, BRSs will fail to realize its potential in the worldwide stent market.

ArterioSorb is produced from the FDA approved polymer poly-L-lactic acid (PLLA). The PLLA polymer is manufactured using a unique technology that enables the cost-effective manufacture of the bioresorbable polymeric scaffold with high strength and stiffness and greater flexibility. The manufacturing method is a combination of *melt processing* (extrusion) and *die-drawing* (solid phase orientation), as pictured in Figure 10.6.1. Die-drawing is a process whereby a polymeric material is heated to a temperature between its glass transition and melting temperature, and pulled through a die to change its cross-sectional area. This results in polymeric orientation that gives the material added strength and allows it to maximize its potential mechanical performance.

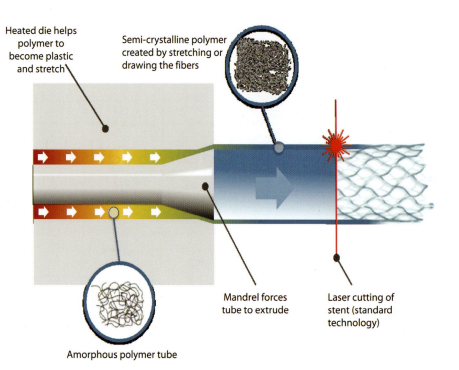

Figure 10.6.1 Arterius die-drawing manufacturing technique.

The tensile strength of ArterioSorb manufactured from the die-drawing technology is significantly higher than that of other devices (see Table 10.6.1). This is due to the highly oriented (molecularly aligned) materials made by this technology.

The die-drawing process produces material with high tensile strength that allows for plastic deformation at low strain. This reduces stent recoil, increases radial strength, and allows the manufacture of a stent with thinner struts (≤100 μm strut thickness), with enhanced physical performance similar to that of metal alloy stents. The strain required to break the polymer is increased from around 6% to more than 70%, allowing for a greater range of expansion for the scaffold (see Table 10.6.2).

The oriented polymer bioresorbable tubes are made either by batch or by continuous solid-phase die-drawing processes directly downstream from an extruder, and do not require further orientation steps, as in the case of the methods used to produce other scaffolds. This therefore streamlines the manufacturing procedure allowing it to be more cost-effective than other manufacturing processes. See Table 10.6.3 for a comparison of the manufacturing techniques used for BRSs. The proprietary die-drawing

Table 10.6.2 Comparison of die-drawn orientated tube to extruded tube

| Sample | Tensile modulus (MPa) | Yield strength (MPa) | UTS (MPa) | Strain to break (%) |
|---|---|---|---|---|
| Extruded tube | 2767 | 77.0 | 77.0 | 6 |
| Oriented tube | 4908 | 110.0 | 252.0 | 71 |

manufacturing technique for ArterioSorb has shown excellent results from bench-testing to date.

## SCAFFOLD DESIGN

ArterioSorb is a tubular scaffold composed of rows of cells parallel to the longitudinal axis with at least one cell in each row being a central cell. The design is based on closed-cell (with connectors) and open-cell (with less connectors) modules with increasing cell size as one moves away from the center. The smaller cells at the center provide increased structural support where the stenosis is most severe. Moreover, within the center of the stent the level of material

Table 10.6.1 Comparison of die-drawn orientated PLLA to other materials

| Material | PLLA | Oriented PLLA | Stainless steel | Cobalt chromium | Magnesium alloy |
|---|---|---|---|---|---|
| Ultimate tensile strength (MPa) | ~30–50 | 252 | 670 | 820–1200 | 280 |
| Tensile modulus (GPa) | 1.2–3.0 | 4.9 | 193 | 243 | 45 |
| Elongation (%) | 2–6 | 71 | 48 | 35–55 | 23 |

Table 10.6.3 Arterius die-drawing technology and the strength of PLLA tubing in comparison with the methods used by the main competitors

| Company | Processing method | Steps required | Material | Tensile modulus (MPa) | Ultimate strength (MPa) | Strain to break (%) |
|---|---|---|---|---|---|---|
| Arterius | Die-drawing of extruded tubing | 1-batch and continuous process | PLLA (FDA approved solid polymer) | 4908 | 252 | 71 |
| Zeus Inc (biodegradable tube manufacture) | Extrusion tubing | 1 | PLLA (FDA approved solid polymer) | 2767 | 77 | 6 |
| Abbott vascular | Blow-molding of extruded tubing | 1-batch process | PLLA (FDA approved solid polymer) | Not reported | 140 | 48 |
| Elixir | PLLDA dissolved in a solvent onto a mandrel to form a tube followed by annealing of the tube for up 72 hours and final heat annealing | 4–5 batch processes | PLLA (dissolved in an organic solvent) | Not reported | Not reported | 20 |
| ART | Annealing of the stent made from a tube | 5 batch processes | PLLA (specifically synthesized) | Not reported | Not reported | Not reported |
| Amaranth medical | Dip coating on mandrel to form a tube from PLLA solution | 2–20 batch processes | PLLA (in-house polymer synthesis and dissolved in an organic solvent) | 2708 | 73 | 97 |

is at its highest; therefore, a larger dose of drug will be delivered in the central region of the lesion where the severity is likely to be higher. The design provides high radial strength and yet appropriate flexibility for ease of implantation. The design also delivers a thinner strut thickness leading to lower coverage of the artery wall and the potential for reduced restenosis. An example of the computer-aided design is illustrated in Figure 10.6.2.

Many prototypes of the open-cell design, for greater flexibility, have been manufactured and extensively bench tested. The two most successful designs were selected for the Arterius preclinical trials. The first iteration of ArterioSorb had a strut thickness of 140 microns. A comparison of the ArterioSorb design with a number of other scaffolds is seen in Figure 10.6.3.

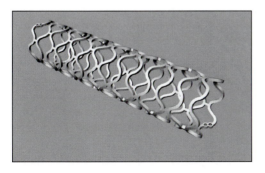

Figure 10.6.2 ArterioSorb computer-aided design.

## BIORESORPTION

For a BRSs to be as effective as the currently available DESs, it should have excellent radial strength that is maintained for at least 3–6 months postdevice implantation. The scaffold then needs to resorb after vessel integrity has been restored as a permanent scaffold is no longer necessary.

The five stages of the bioresorption mechanism of PLLA scaffold result in degradation of the polymer to carbon dioxide and water. The first stage involves hydration of the polymer, due to water absorption from the surrounding tissue. In the second stage, the water hydrolyzes the ester bond of PLLA, resulting in the degradation of the polymer. During the third stage, the polymer loses its cohesive strength leading to formation of many short segments with low molecular weights. In the fourth stage, these short segments are hydrolyzed further to form hydrophilic monomers that can be phagocytized by macrophages. After phagocytosis, in the fifth stage the soluble monomer (l-lactate) is catabolized to pyruvate and ultimately to carbon dioxide and water through the Kerbs cycle leading to full resorption [1].

ArterioSorb will need to fully bio-resorb within a 12–24 month time frame with gradual resorption process commencing after the scaffold has allowed arterial remodeling and become completely encapsulated within the vessel wall [2]. The unique die-drawing process allows the crystallinity of the PLLA molecules to be adjusted

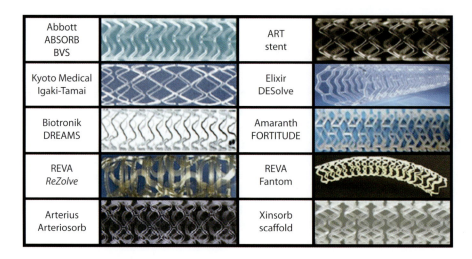

Figure 10.6.3 Comparison of the ArterioSorb scaffold design to other devices.

allowing the scaffold resorption time to be controlled in relation to clinical need.

The construction of ArterioSorb ensures sufficient radial and longitudinal strength to enable the vessel to recover its natural shape while avoiding recoil and malapposition. It also ensures that the shape and integrity of the scaffold is not affected by changes in the environment such as heat, cold, and humidity.

## RADIO-OPACITY OF MARKERS

Poor visibility of BRSs can lead to difficulty in implantation resulting in lengthening of procedural times and procedural complications. The first iteration of ArterioSorb 3.25 mm had Tantalum radiopaque markers placed at the proximal and distal ends of the device to make it visible during the implantation and postdilation procedures. Animal testing showed that the ArterioSorb markers were easily visible at each end of the scaffold leading to ease of implantation (see Figure 10.6.4).

## DRUG COATING AND ELUTION PROFILE

The ideal BRSs will need to be coated with the optimum drug in terms of its antiproliferative action and its drug elution profile in order to reduce restenosis rates and the need

for revascularization [3,4]. The drug must be eluted gradually over time to ensure the lowest restenosis rates but this elution profile must be balanced with the need for endothelialization of the scaffold, which is necessary to prevent late stent thrombosis [5–7].

ArterioSorb is coated with a bioabsorbable (PDLLA) polymer containing the active drug to reduce restenosis rates. The ArterioSorb formulation has been investigated utilizing a 1:1 ratio of the active drug rapamycin and low molecular weight bioresorbable PDLLA as a carrier. Scaffolds from two sizes of ArterioSorb were coated and the drug content was measured. The initial drug loading was measured to be $117.2 \pm 1.3$ µg, equivalent to 1.02 µg/mm$^2$, with the target drug loading being 1 µg/mm$^2$. After 11 weeks of *in vitro* drug release measurements, $76.0 \pm 1.3\%$ of the original drug content was eluted.

The elution curves for the two initial scaffold sizes are shown in Figure 10.6.5 as compared to the values for competitor products. It can be seen that drug release from the ArterioSorb coating is slower than those of the competitor products. After 28 days, Abbott's ABSORB and XIENCE V stents have released 75 and 78% of their drug coating, respectively, whereas the ArterioSorb scaffold has released

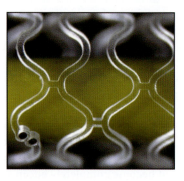

Figure 10.6.4 Image of ArterioSorb drug-coated scaffolds with twin-radiopaque markers.

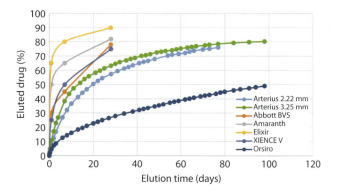

Figure 10.6.5 Rapamycin release profile of ArterioSorb in comparison to other BRSs devices and metallic DESs (XIENCE and Orsiro).

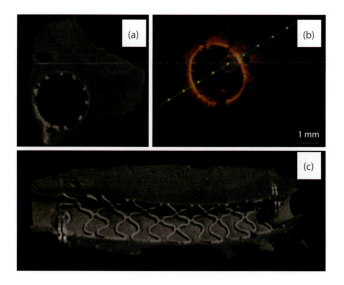

Figure 10.6.6 3D micro-CT and OCT images of ArterioSorb implanted in pig arteries during the pilot study. **(a)** Cross-sectional micro-CT image of ArterioSorb. **(b)** OCT image of ArterioSorb. **(c)** Longitudinal micro-CT image of ArterioSorb.

only 57%. However, by 14 weeks, 75–80% of sirolimus from ArterioSorb was released.

## PRECLINICAL EVALUATION: ANIMAL PILOT STUDY

The first preclinical trial was a pilot animal study performed in conjunction with AccelLAB in Canada to evaluate ArterioSorb for acute performance.

Key parameters of the pilot study that were tested at that time included:

- Introduction and deliverability
- Visibility by angiography
- Deployment and expansion performance
- Device sizing

This pilot study was conducted in a total of two pigs, with a protocol aligned with FDA Guidance for Industry. The Regulatory Compliance and Quality Consulting were subcontracted to provide regulatory expertise to the project. A total of 6 scaffolds were implanted in each pig. The technicians rated the performance at implantation as generally excellent. All devices were easy to position and deploy, with no complications encountered during delivery, deployment, or withdrawal. Furthermore, the scaffolds were clearly visible by angiographic evaluation due to the radiopaque markers, and showed no abnormality following implantation, with complete perfusion of the blood flow.

Optical coherence tomography (OCT) showed good apposition of the struts to the vessel wall as illustrated in Figure 10.6.6.

The conclusion of the pilot study in September 2014 was that ArterioSorb showed excellent overall implantation behavior in the pigs' coronary arteries (see Figure 10.6.7).

## PRECLINICAL EVALUATIONS: 30-DAY AND 90-DAY ANIMAL TRIAL

The 30-day and 90-day animal studies were designed to assess the safety and efficacy of the first generation of Rapamycin-coated ArterioSorb in a pig coronary artery model. A total of 12 hybrid farm pigs were enrolled in the study (6 animals per cohort). The control used for comparison was the metallic Orsiro DESs (Biotronik Ltd., Berlin, Germany). The operator was blinded to the identity of each device implanted. Deployment was controlled by quantitative coronary angiography with a target stent/artery ratio of between 1.1 and 1.2:1 to avoid oversizing but ensure vessel contact.

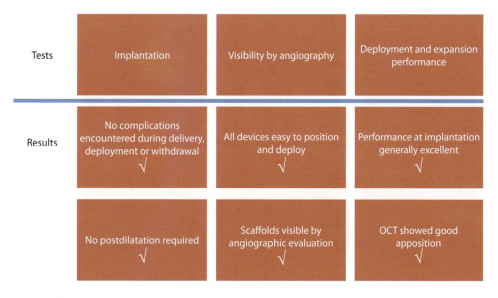

Figure 10.6.7 Acute preclinical trial summary.

A standard antiplatelet regimen of aspirin and clopidogrel was used.

Postdeployment QCA and OCT were used to document device apposition for comparison with the endpoint. At 30 days and 90 days, the animals were given a terminal anesthetic. QCA and OCT were repeated at this stage. The safety criteria (vessel patency, strut coverage, BRSs integrity) were assessed. The arteries were then excised and 7 of each were sectioned for cross-sectional histology and the strut areas, endothelial coverage, and neointimal areas quantified. Selected sections were examined for inflammatory responses using appropriate antibodies and standardized scoring systems. The remaining 7 pairs of BRSs were sectioned longitudinally for similar analysis.

The results of the 30- and 90-day animal trials showed good acute performance of the scaffold when compared to Osiro with good biocompatibility.

## FUTURE PLANS

Initial bench and preclinical testing of ArterioSorb has shown promising results. Further iterations of the scaffold are now being developed with continued bench testing to ensure that the strength of the scaffold continues to improve and with lower levels of strut thickness. The strut thickness of ArterioSorb is now 97 microns and is currently undergoing a thorough program of bench testing with plans for further animal trials later this year prior to first-in-human trials in the near future.

## SUMMARY

The use of the novel die-drawing technique in the manufacture of ArterioSorb has resulted in the production of a scaffold with extremely promising results in terms of thinner strut thickness with greater radial strength. The scaffold design and geometry continues to be improved with ongoing bench testing and further animal trials planned prior to a first-in-human trials.

## ACKNOWLEDGMENTS

Arterius Ltd. is based in Bradford University's Bioincubator Centre in the United Kingdom. Arterius Ltd. works in partnership with a consortium consisting of the Computational Design Group at Southampton University, United Kingdom; the Industrial Research Centre in Polymer Engineering, Bradford University, United Kingdom; and the Department of Surface Characterisation and Drug Distribution at Nottingham University, United Kingdom to design, manufacture, and put into preclinical evaluation the ArterioSorb scaffold. The author would like to thank Dr. Kadem Al-Lamee and the team at Arterius Ltd. for providing preclinical data for the publication of this manuscript.

## REFERENCES

1. Ormiston JA, Serruys PW, Regar E, Dudek D, Thuesen L, Webster MW, Onuma Y et al. A bioabsorbable everolimus-eluting coronary stent system for patients with single de-novo coronary artery lesions (ABSORB): A prospective open-label trial. *Lancet.* 2008;371:899–907.

2. Onuma Y, Serruys PW, Perkins LE, Okamura T, Gonzalo N, Garcia-Garcia HM, Regar E et al. Intracoronary optical coherence tomography and histology at 1 month and 2, 3, and 4 years after implantation of everolimus-eluting bioresorbable vascular scaffolds in a porcine coronary artery model: An attempt to decipher the human optical coherence tomography images in the ABSORB trial. *Circulation.* 2010;122:2288–300.

3. Sousa JE, Costa MA, Abizaid AC, Rensing BJ, Abizaid AS, Tanajura LF, Kozuma K et al. Sustained suppression of neointimal proliferation by sirolimus-eluting stents: One-year angiographic and intravascular ultrasound follow-up. *Circulation.* 2001;104:2007–11.

4. Stone GW, Ellis SG, Cox DA, Hermiller J, O'Shaughnessy C, Mann JT, Turco M et al. One-year clinical results with the slow-release, polymer-based, paclitaxel-eluting TAXUS stent: The TAXUS-IV trial. *Circulation.* 2004;109:1942–7.

5. Daemen J, Wenaweser P, Tsuchida K, Abrecht L, Vaina S, Morger C, Kukreja N et al. Early and late coronary stent thrombosis of sirolimus-eluting and paclitaxel-eluting stents in routine clinical practice: Data from a large two-institutional cohort study. *Lancet.* 2007;369:667–78.

6. Virmani R, Guagliumi G, Farb A, Musumeci G, Grieco N, Motta T, Mihalcsik L et al. Localized hypersensitivity and late coronary thrombosis secondary to a sirolimus-eluting stent: Should we be cautious? *Circulation.* 2004;109:701–5.

7. Wenaweser P, Daemen J, Zwahlen M, van Domburg R, Juni P, Vaina S, Hellige G et al. Incidence and correlates of drug-eluting stent thrombosis in routine clinical practice. 4-year results from a large 2-institutional cohort study. *J Am Coll Cardiol.* 2008;52:1134–40.

# IBS™ bioresorbable scaffold by Lifetech

DEYUAN ZHANG, WENJIAO LIN, AND HAIPING QI

## DEVICE DESCRIPTION

The iron-based bioresorbable coronary scaffold (IBS™) of Lifetech Scientific is shown in Figure 10.7.1. The sinusoid rings of the scaffold, composed of 6–10 crowns, are connected together by 3–5 omega-shaped connectors circumferentially to cover a diameter range of 2.0–4.0 mm and a length range of 8–38 mm, which is exactly the same as mainstream permanent coronary stents. The scaffold, only 50–55 μm thick, weighs 2.6–23 mg for the entire range of available specifications, which is much less than the daily iron dosage transferred by hemoglobin in an adult blood system. A set of integrated gold marks, weighing 0.2 mg, is placed at each end of the scaffold to ensure enough radiopacity.

The platform of the IBS is made of a nitrided iron material composed of approximately 99.5 wt.% iron and less than 0.1 wt.% nitrogen, which, however, could lead to significant elevation of the mechanical properties and faster *in vivo* corrosion rate without compromise of plasticity and biocompatibility by dispersive precipitation of iron nitride with diameter from tens of nanometers to 2 microns in iron substrate [1]. Moreover, there is a nanoscaled surface coating on iron platform to delay the onset of iron corrosion about 2–3 months, avoiding early nonuniform corrosion or premature fracture. The outermost layer on the struts is the proprietary polymer film with sirolimus inside to control drug release and create a predesigned local environment in which iron can corrode fast into soluble corrosion products.

The manufacturing process of the IBS is described as follows. First, pure iron scaffolds are laser-cut from the as-drawn pure iron tubings (OD1.6 mm, wall 0.09 mm) manufactured by Lifetech Scientific (Shenzhen, China). Second, vacuum glow discharge nitriding technique is applied to obtain the nitrided iron scaffolds using an in-house designed vacuum nitriding furnace. All the nitrided iron scaffolds are chemically polished to the designated size. Gold radiopaque marks are then loaded to both ends of the as-polished scaffold in an integrated form. Further, the scaffold will be coated with a polymeric layer carrying therapeutic drugs and then be crimped onto an unfolded balloon of a delivery catheter to form a scaffold system. The sterilization is subsequently conducted to the packaged scaffold system to obtain a finished product. The nitrogen filled aluminum foil pouch ensures IBS 1 year shelf life when stored at room temperature.

## MECHANICAL PERFORMANCE AND SUPPORT DURATION

The IBS (3.0 × 18 mm) with 53 μm thick strut weighs 8 mg and has an original radial strength comparable to the current workhorse stents, e.g., XIENCE Prime (Abbott Vascular, Santa Clara, CA) and Resolute Integrity™ (Medtronic, Minneapolis, MN) as shown in Table 10.7.1. The mechanical performances of IBSs are noninferior to the current workhorse stents, which ensures capacities of overdilation and side branch dilation the same as that of cobalt-based alloy stent. The percentage surface area of the IBS was ~13% while the reported data for XIENCE Prime™ is ~13.3% for the specification of 3.0 × 18 mm. Further, due to the ultra-thin strut, the crossing profile of IBS decreases accordingly, leading to the improvement of its crossability in terms of flexibility, pushing force, and withdrawing force. The IBSs is designed to keep original radial force unchanged in the first 2 or 3 months and then corrode fast with quick reduction of radial force, and totally lose its integrity in about 8 months after implantation. As discussed above, scaffolding force of the IBS (123 kPa comparable to XIENCE Prime) is unchanged during the first 3 months, and then drops down to near zero in about 8 to 10 months. Adequate scaffold radial force at 4 months is ensured as a design target.

## DRUG ELUTING PROFILE

The sirolimus release profile of IBS is shown in Figure 10.7.2. It has been found that polymer degradation and iron corrosion have a strong influence on the drug release profile.

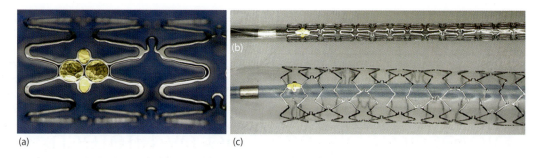

**Figure 10.7.1** Iron-based bioresorbable drug-eluting coronary scaffold (IBS) with gold radiopaque marks. Iron-based bioresorbable drug-eluting coronary scaffold (IBS) with gold radiopaque marks. **(a)** Bare iron-based scaffold after polishing, **(b)** IBS crimped on a balloon catheter, and **(c)** IBS expanded to nominal diameter.

**Table 10.7.1** Comparison of mechanical performance

| 3.0 × 18 mm | Metallic strut thickness (µm) | Crossing profile (mm) | Radial strength (kPa) | Recoil at nominal pressure (%) | Foreshortening at nominal pressure (%) | Maximal expansion diameter (mm) |
|---|---|---|---|---|---|---|
| IBS | 53 | 1.04 ± 0.02 | 123 ± 3 | 3.4 ± 0.2 | 0.4 ± 0.1 | 4.4 |
| XIENCE Prime | 81 | 1.13 ± 0.02 | 116 ± 6 | 3.6 ± 0.6 | −2.4 ± 1.0 | 4.4 |
| Resolute Integrity | 89 | 1.19 ± 0.05 | 147 ± 10 | 3.6 ± 0.9 | −2.4 ± 0.1 | 5.4 |

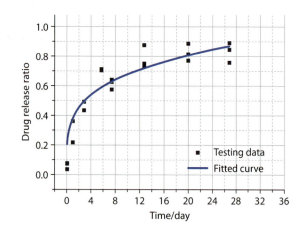

**Figure 10.7.2** *In vivo* drug release profile of IBS.

## CORROSION MECHANISM AND BIORESORPTION DURATION

The Pourbaix diagrams of iron corrosion under the physiological conditions were calculated and drawn in Figure 10.7.3. From the diagrams, it can be seen that the corrosion products of iron are $Fe_3(PO_4)_2 \cdot 8H_2O$ and $Fe(OH)_3$ at pH = 7.4 when phosphates ($PO_4^{3-}$ and/or $HPO_4^{2-}$ and/or $H_2PO_4^-$) exist in solution (Figure 10.7.3a). The corrosion products of iron are $Fe(OH)_2$, $Fe(OH)_3$, $Fe_3O_4$, and $Fe_2O_3$ at pH = 7.4 when phosphates are exhausted (Figure 10.7.3a and b). Based on the results above, the Gibbs free energies of different reactions in iron corrosion process at pH = 7.4 are calculated under the assumed physiological conditions. Based on the calculation results, the standard molar Gibbs free energy change

of different reactions was defined as the gaps of free energy between product and reactant, which represented the driving force of transformation between the different components. Therefore, the calculated reaction routes of iron with oxygen and phosphor consumption were as shown in Figure 10.7.3c. Considering the stability of substance, the different kinds of arrows represent different reaction speeds roughly in the reaction route diagram. On the initial corrosion stage, Fe transforms to $Fe_3(PO_4)_2$ at physiological environment and [P] ($PO_4^{3-}$ and/or $HPO_4^{2-}$ and/or $H_2PO_4^-$) is consumed, and it is difficult that $Fe_3(PO_4)_2$ change to $Fe(OH)_3$. Fe transforms to $Fe(OH)_2$ when [P] is exhausted, and then $Fe(OH)_2$ changes to $Fe(OH)_3$ immediately when $O_2$ presents and $Fe(OH)_3$ can change to FeOOH easily by a dehydration reaction. $Fe_3O_4$ is obtained under local anoxic conditions and lack of [P] due to corrosion products covering on iron scaffold strut and low diffusion velocity of $O_2$ and [P] ions. $Fe_2O_3$ can be obtained from $Fe(OH)_3$ or $Fe_3O_4$. When polymer monomer exists due to the degradation of polymer coating, iron and its solid corrosion products may react with monomer into soluble complex.

Accordingly, the possible corrosion products of iron scaffold *in vivo* are $Fe_3O_4$ and $Fe_2O_3$ (in original strut position), $Fe_3(PO_4)_2$, and FeOOH (both precipitated in tissue round struts). The theoretical analysis above has been verified by tests of the explanted *in vivo* specimen of IBS using energy dispersive spectrometer (EDS), X-ray photoelectron-spectroscopy (XPS), X-ray diffraction (XRD), transmission electron microscopy (TEM), infrared spectrometer (IR spectrometer), and Raman photography.

During the ongoing corrosion, only a very small portion of iron becomes iron ions or soluble complex and could be carried away by blood or tissue fluid. The rest becomes two kinds of solid corrosion products. One is mainly $Fe_3O_4$ in

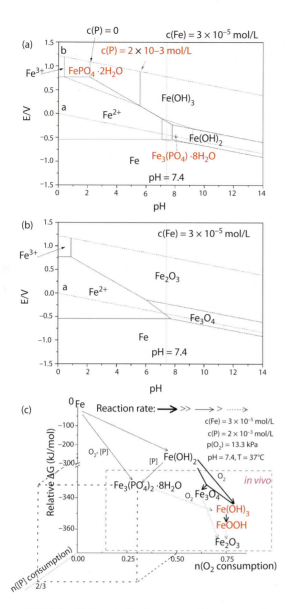

the original position with or without polymer around them as indicated in Figure 10.7.4a, which continuously reduces by reaction with polymer monomer to soluble products, another is a combination of FeOOH and $Fe_3(PO_4)_2$, which precipitated in tissue as dispersive small particulates when soluble iron ion or complex become oversaturated due to the elevation of pH value where it is far away from the original strut position as indicated in Figure 10.7.4a. The real 3D profile of the scaffold reconstructed by the microcomputed tomography (Micro-CT, Skyscan1172, Bruker, Germany) is shown in Figure 10.7.4b. It could be found that the struts turn thinner, become fractured, and some nearly disappear, leaving nebulous corrosion products (a combination of FeOOH and $Fe_3(PO_4)_2$) dispersed in tissue far away from the original struts, after 6 months *in vivo* corrosion.

The iron matrix of IBS is kept intact for the first 2–3 months to achieve long enough scaffolding for blood vessels, and then corrodes fast and loses integrity at about 6–8 months after implantation, and totally becomes corrosion products at around 1 year, which means intact iron disappears.

The bioresorption of iron-based scaffold includes the bioresorption of iron ions or soluble complex and the solid corrosion products. It is easily understood that the iron ions or soluble complex combines with albumens related with iron metabolism, and then transfers to other organs and can be either absorbed or excreted by the body finally. As regards to the solid corrosion products, large particulates can be phagocytized by phagocytes (Figure 10.7.5a) and/or other somatic cells, e.g., smooth muscle cells and lymphocytes (Figure 10.7.5b), while the small particulates can move in body fluid in an intercellular path (Figure 10.7.5c), and settle down in a lymph gland finally or congregate in adventitia (Figure 10.7.5d).

From the discussion above, it is known that the metabolism of solid corrosion products is a long-term process, perhaps taking 4 years or longer after implantation. Therefore, our further work will focus on reducing or eliminating solid corrosion products during iron corrosion by more accurate control of iron corrosion.

Figure 10.7.3 **(a, b)** Pourbaix diagrams of iron corrosion under the physiological conditions; **(c)** the possible reaction routes *in vivo* based on thermodynamics with $O_2$ and [P] consumption.

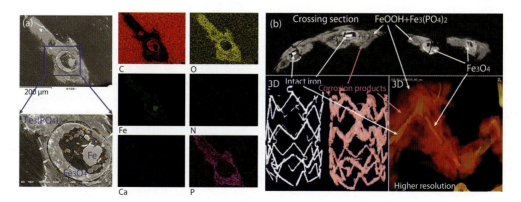

Figure 10.7.4 **(a)** Scanning electron microscope (SEM)/energy dispersive spectrometer (EDS) and **(b)** microcomputed tomography (micro-CT) images of IBS after 6 months implantation in rabbit abdominal aorta. (From Lin WJ, Zhang DY, Zhang G, Sun HT, Qi HP, Chen LP, Liu ZQ et al. *Mater Des* 2016; 91:72–79.)

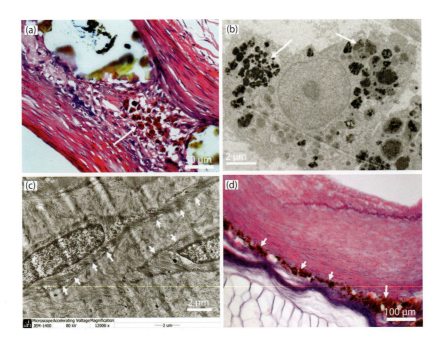

Figure 10.7.5 Corrosion particulates in (a) macrophages, (b) somatic cell, (c) cytoplasm matrix between smooth muscle cells, and (d) adventitia, as indicated by the white arrows.

## POTENTIAL ADVANTAGES AND DISADVANTAGES

The advantages of IBS are listed below:

1. Pure iron shows inferior mechanical performance to permanent stent materials, but a lot of methods can be used to enhance its mechanical performance. Nitriding technology makes it possible that the IBS made of nitrided iron-based alloy with very thin struts could still show high mechanical performance, comparable to those of the best permanent stents. Moreover, similar stent design to current permanent stents allows IBS the same overdilation and side-branch dilation capability, specifications coverage, and procedural manipulation without any compromise. These merits entitle IBS the only potential bioresorbable scaffold to cover all specifications of the current permanent stents, when compared with the bioresorbable polymer-based and magnesium-based scaffolds.
2. In comparison with the polymer scaffold, corrosion speed of iron scaffold can be adjusted easily by many ways, so we can set a best corrosion timeframe, for example, effective scaffolding for 4 months, uncaging at 6 months, and total loss of structural integrity at 1 year or so.

3. IBS made of pure iron with trace nitrogen is safe in terms of biocompatibility in comparison to other stent material design with many toxic metallic elements alloyed, such as rare earth elements, nickel, and chromium.

The disadvantages of IBS are listed below according to their severity:

1. Despite the fact that the solid corrosion products of IBS scattered in tissue could remain there biosafely, a long time is needed for them to be cleared away.
2. IBS is just MRI safe with strong image artefacts before most of the iron is cleared away.
3. Production of IBS is much more complicated and needs strict control.

## REFERENCES

1. Lin WJ, Zhang G, Cao P, Zhang DY, Zheng YF, Wu RX et al. Cytotoxicity and its test methodology for a bioabsorbable nitrided iron stent. *J Biomed Mater Res Part B Appl Biomater*. 2015;103:764–776.
2. Lin WJ, Zhang DY, Zhang G, Sun HT, Qi HP, Chen LP, Liu ZQ et al. Design and characterization of a novel biocorrodible iron-based drug-eluting coronary scaffold. *Mater Des*. 2016;91:72–79.

# INDEX